AMERICAN COLLEGE OF CLINICAL PHARMACY

Updates In Therapeutics:
The Pharmacotherapy Preparatory Course

2010 Edition

VOLUME 2

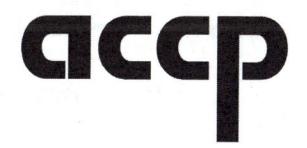

accp

Director of Professional Development: Nancy M. Perrin, M.A., CAE
Project Manager, Education: Emma F. Webb, M.A.
Medical Editor: Kimma J. Sheldon, Ph.D.
Desktop Publisher: Jen DeYoe, B.F.A., ACE
Project Manager, Publications: Janel Mosley

For order information or questions, contact:
American College of Clinical Pharmacy
13000 W. 87th St. Parkway
Lenexa, KS 66215-4530
Phone: (913) 492-3311
Fax: (913) 492-0088
accp@accp.com
http://www.accp.com

Copyright© 2010 by the American College of Clinical Pharmacy. All rights reserved. This book is protected by copyright. No part of this publication may be reproduced, stored in a retrieval system, or transmitted, in any form or by any means, electronic or mechanical, including photocopy, without prior written permission of the American College of Clinical Pharmacy.

Printed in the United States of America.

To properly cite this book:
Author(s). Chapter name. In: Bressler L, DeYoung, G.R., El-Ibiary, S., et al. Updates in Therapeutics: The Pharmacotherapy Preparatory Course, 2010 ed. Lenexa, KS: American College of Clinical Pharmacy, **year:pages**.

Note: The authors and publisher of the Pharmacotherapy Preparatory Course recognize that the development of this material offers many opportunities for error. Despite our very best efforts, some errors may persist into print. Drug dosage schedules are, we believe, accurate and in accordance with current standards. Readers are advised, however, to check other published sources to be certain that recommended dosages and contraindications are in agreement with those listed in this book. This is especially important in the cases of new, infrequently used, or highly toxic drugs.

ISBN-13: 978-1-932658-71-2
ISBN-10: 1-932658-71-8

Continuing Pharmacy Education:
The American College of Clinical Pharmacy is accredited by the Accreditation Council for Pharmacy Education as a provider of continuing pharmacy education. The Universal Activity Numbers are: Pharmacotherapy Preparatory Course for home study, 2010 Edition: Pediatrics; Geriatrics; Fluids, Electrolytes, and Nutrition; and Endocrine and Metabolic Disorders, Activity No. 0217-0000-10-013-H01-P; 4.50 contact hours; Biostatistics: A Refresher and Clinical Trials, Activity No. 0217-0000-10-014-H01-P; 3.00 contact hours; Critical Care and Ambulatory Care, Activity No. 0217-0000-10-015-H01-P; 3.00 contact hours; Neurology and General Psychiatry, Activity No. 0217-0000-10-016-H01-P; 2.50 contact hours; Infectious Diseases, HIV/Infectious Diseases, Nephrology, and Gastrointestinal Disorders, Activity No. 0217-0000-10-017-H01-P; 4.00 contact hours; Oncology Supportive Care; Men's and Women's Health; and Pharmacokinetics: A Refresher, Activity No. 0217-0000-10-018-H01-P; 3.50 contact hours; Acute Care Cardiology and Outpatient Care Cardiology, Activity No. 0217-0000-10-019-H01-P; 3.00 contact hours.

To earn continuing pharmacy education credit for the home study version of the 2010 Pharmacotherapy Preparatory Course, you must successfully complete and submit the Web-based post test associated with each program within the course by not later than October 31, 2011. Statements of continuing pharmacy education credit will be available at www.accp.com within 4 weeks of submission of the Web-based post test.

The American College of Clinical Pharmacy (ACCP) has compiled the materials in this course book for pharmacists to use in preparing for the Board of Pharmaceutical Specialties (BPS) Pharmacotherapy Specialty Certification Examination. There is no intent or assurance that all of the knowledge on the examination will be covered in the ACCP process. Although ACCP does use the BPS Content Outline in creating the material for this course, ACCP does not know the specific content of any particular BPS examination. BPS guidelines prohibit any overlap of individuals writing the examination and developing preparatory materials.

Program Goals and Target Audience

Updates in Therapeutics: The Pharmacotherapy Preparatory Course is designed to help pharmacists who are preparing for the Board of Pharmacy Specialties certification examination in Pharmacotherapy as well as those seeking a general review and refresher on disease states and therapeutics. The program goals are:

1. To present a high-quality, up-to-date overview of disease states and therapeutics;
2. To provide a framework to help attendees prepare for the specialty certification examination in pharmacotherapy; and
3. To offer participants an effective learning experience using a case-based approach with a strong focus on the thought processes needed to solve patient care problems in each therapeutic area.

Faculty

Linda R. Bressler, Pharm.D., BCOP
Clinical Associate Professor
Director of Regulatory Affairs
(Cancer and Leukemia Group B)
University of Illinois
Chicago, Illinois

G. Robert DeYoung, Pharm.D., BCPS
Clinical Pharmacist, Ambulatory Care
Advantage Health Physicians and
St. Mary's Health Care
Grand Rapids, Michigan

Shareen El-Ibiary, Pharm.D., BCPS
Associate Professor of Pharmacy Practice
Department of Pharmacy Practice
Midwestern University College of Pharmacy-Glendale
Glendale, Arizona

Edward F. Foote, Pharm.D., FCCP, BCPS
Associate Professor
Wilkes University
Wilkes Barre, Pennsylvania

Ila M. Harris, Pharm.D., FCCP, BCPS
Associate Professor
Medical School
Department of Family Medicine and Community
Health, University of Minnesota
Bethesda Family Medicine
St. Paul, Minnesota

Brian Hemstreet, Pharm.D., BCPS
Associate Professor
University of Colorado at Denver and
Health Sciences Center
Aurora, Colorado

Brian K. Irons, Pharm.D., BCPS, BC-ADM
Division Head - Primary Care
Associate Professor - Department of
Pharmacy Practice
School of Pharmacy
Texas Tech University Health Sciences Center
Lubbock, Texas

William A. Kehoe, Pharm.D., FCCP, BCPS
Professor of Clinical Pharmacy and Psychology
Chairman, Department of Pharmacy Practice
University of the Pacific
Stockton, California

Judith Kristeller, Pharm.D., BCPS
Associate Professor
Wilkes University
Wilkes Barre, Pennsylvania

Kirsten H. Ohler, Pharm.D., BCPS
Clinical Assistant Professor
University of Illinois Medical Center at Chicago
Chicago, Illinois

Norma J. Owens, Pharm.D., FCCP, BCPS
Professor and Chair
Pharmacy Department
University of Rhode Island
Providence, Rhode Island

Robert L Page II, Pharm.D., MSPH, FCCP, FASHP, FAHA, FASCP, BCPS, CGP
Associate Professor of Clinical Pharmacy and
Physical Medicine
Schools of Pharmacy and Medicine
University of Colorado
Aurora, Colorado

Jo E. Rodgers Pharm.D., BCPS
Clinical Associate Professor
Division of Pharmacotherapy and
Experimental Therapeutics
School of Pharmacy
University of North Carolina, Chapel Hill,
North Carolina

Melody Ryan, Pharm.D., BCPS
Associate Professor
University of Kentucky
Lexington, Kentucky

Curtis L. Smith, Pharm.D., BCPS
Professor
Ferris State University
Grand Ledge, Michigan

Faculty Disclosures

Consultancies: Brian Hemstreet (Conexus Health); Robert Page (Astra Zeneca); Jo Rodgers (Arca Discovery, Astellas, Canyon Pharmaceuticals, Inc.).

Speaker's Bureau: Edward Foote (American Regent); Brian Hemstreet (AstraZeneca)

Other: Norma Owens (Steere House Nursing Home and Rehabilitation Center).

Nothing to Disclose: Linda Bressler; G. Robert DeYoung; Shareen El-Ibiary; Ila Harris; Brian Irons; William Kehoe; Judith Kristeller; Kirsten Ohler; Melody Ryan; Curtis Smith.

Acknowledgments

Teresa M. Bailey, Pharm.D., BCPS
Associate Professor
College of Pharmacy
Ferris State University
Kalamazoo, Michigan

Debra J. Barnette, Pharm.D., BCPS
Ambulatory Care Coordinator
University of North Carolina
Chapel Hill, North Carolina

Lisa Anne Boothby, Pharm.D., BCPS
Clinical Research Pharmacist
Drug Information Coordinator
Pharmacy Administration
Columbus Regional Healthcare System
Columbus, Georgia

Linda R. Bressler, Pharm.D., BCOP
Clinical Associate Professor
Department of Pharmacy Practice, College of Pharmacy
Director of Regulatory Affairs
Cancer and Leukemia Group B
University of Illinois
Chicago, Illinois

G. Robert DeYoung, Pharm.D., BCPS
Clinical Pharmacist, Ambulatory Care
Advantage Health Physicians
St. Mary's Health Care
Grand Rapids, Michigan

Shareen El-Ibiary, Pharm.D., BCPS
Associate Professor of Pharmacy Practice
Department of Pharmacy Practice
Midwestern University College of Pharmacy-Glendale
Glendale, Arizona

Edward F. Foote, Pharm.D., FCCP, BCPS
Associate Professor
Wilkes University
Wilkes Barre, Pennsylvania

Ila M. Harris, Pharm.D., FCCP, BCPS
Associate Professor
Medical School
Department of Family Medicine and Community Health
University of Minnesota
Bethesda Family Medicine
St. Paul, Minnesota

Brian A. Hemstreet, Pharm.D., BCPS
Associate Professor
Department of Clinical Pharmacy, School of Pharmacy
University of Colorado at Denver and Health Sciences Center
Denver, Colorado

Trudy M.R. Hodgman, Pharm.D., BCPS
Critical Care Pharmacist
Northwest Community Healthcare
Arlington Heights, Illinois

Brian K. Irons, Pharm.D., BCPS, BC-ADM
Division Head - Primary Care
Associate Professor - Department of Pharmacy Practice
School of Pharmacy
Texas Tech University Health Sciences Center
Lubbock, Texas

William A. Kehoe, Pharm.D., M.A., FCCP, BCPS
Professor of Clinical Pharmacy and Psychology
Chairman, Department of Pharmacy Practice
T.J. Long School of Pharmacy and Health Sciences
University of the Pacific
Stockton, California

Judith Kristeller, Pharm.D., BCPS
Associate Professor
Wilkes University
Wilkes Barre, Pennsylvania

Kirsten H. Ohler, Pharm.D., BCPS
Clinical Assistant Professor
University of Illinois Medical Center at Chicago
Chicago, Illinois

Norma J. Owens, Pharm.D., FCCP, BCPS
Professor and Chair
Pharmacy Department
University of Rhode Island
Providence, Rhode Island

Robert Lee Page, II, Pharm.D., FCCP, FAHA, BCPS
Associate Professor of Clinical Pharmacy and Physical Medicine
Schools of Pharmacy and Medicine
University of Colorado
Aurora, Colorado

Jo E. Rodgers Pharm.D., BCPS
Clinical Associate Professor
Division of Pharmacotherapy and Experimental Therapeutics
School of Pharmacy
University of North Carolina, Chapel Hill, North Carolina

Melody Ryan, Pharm.D., BCPS
Associate Professor
Department of Pharmacy Practice and Science
College of Pharmacy
University of Kentucky
Lexington, Kentucky

Gordan S. Sacks, Pharm.D., BCNSP, FCCP
Clinical Professor and Chair
Pharmacy Practice Division, School of Pharmacy
University of Wisconsin – Madison, Madison, Wisconsin

Lisa A. Sanchez, Pharm.D.
President
PE Applications
Highlands Ranch, Colorado

Curtis L. Smith, Pharm.D., BCPS
Professor
Ferris State University
Lansing, Michigan

Anne P. Spencer, Pharm.D., BCPS
Associate Professor of Pharmacy and Clinical Sciences
College of Pharmacy
Medical University of South Carolina
Charleston, South Carolina

Ceressa T. Ward, Pharm.D., BCPS
Clinical Coordinator
Emory Crawford Long Hospital
Atlanta, Georgia

Eric T. Wittbrodt, Pharm.D., FCCP, BCPS
Medical Education and Research Liaison
Medical Affairs
Tap Pharmaceutical Products Inc.
Voorhees, New Jersey

Reviewers

The American College of Clinical Pharmacy and the authors would like to thank the following individuals for their review of the Updates of Therapeutics: The Pharmacotherapy Preparatory Course.

Rita R. Alloway, Pharm.D., BCPS, FCCP
Research Professor of Medicine
Director, Transplant Clinical Research
University of Cincinnati College of Medicine
Cincinnati, Ohio

Kathleen M. Bungay-Massaro, Pharm.D., M.S., FCCP
Associate Professor
Northeastern University
School of Pharmacy
Boston, Massachusetts

Juliana Chan, Pharm.D.
Research Associate Professor
University of Illinois – Chicago
College of Pharmacy
Chicago, Illinois

Paul G. Cuddy, Pharm.D., M.B.A.
Associate Professor and Senior Associate Dean
University of Missouri Kansas City
School of Medicine
Kansas City, Missouri

Chris Destache, Pharm.D., FCCP
Professor of Pharmacy Practice
Internal Medicine, Medical Microbiology and Immunology
Creighton University Schools of Pharmacy &
Health Professions and Medicine
Omaha, Nebraska

Mike Dorsch, Pharm.D., M.S., BCPS
Clinical Pharmacist, Cardiology
Adjunct Clinical Assistant Professor
University of Michigan Health System and
College of Pharmacy
Ann Arbor, Michigan

David P. Elliott, Pharm.D., FCCP
Professor
West Virginia University
Department of Clinical Pharmacy
Charleston, West Virginia

Susan C. Fagan, Pharm.D., BCPS
Jowdy Professor and Associate Head
Department of Clinical and Administrative Pharmacy
Assistant Dean
College of Pharmacy
University of Georgia Medical College of Georgia
Augusta, Georgia

Elizabeth A. Farrington, Pharm.D., FCCP, BCPS
Clinical Assistant Professor
UNC Hospitals
Chapel Hill, North Carolina

Marcus Ferrone, Pharm.D., BCNSP
Assistant Professor of Clinical Pharmacy
Director, Drug Products Services Laboratory
University of California, San Francisco
San Francisco, California

Douglas N. Fish, Pharm.D., BCPS, FCCP
Professor and Interim Chair,
Department of Clinical Pharmacy
Clinical Associate Professor of Medicine
Division of Pulmonary Sciences and Critical Care Medicine
Department of Medicine, School of Medicine
University of Colorado Denver
Aurora, Colorado

Andrea S. Franks, Pharm.D., BCPS
Associate Professor
Director of Education
College of Pharmacy, Knoxville Campus
University of Tennessee
Knoxville, Tennessee

Barry E. Gidal, Pharm.D.
Division Chair
Professor of Pharmacy and Neurology
University of Wisconsin
School of Pharmacy
Madison, Wisconsin

Thomas G. Hall, Pharm.D., BCPS
Director, Department of Pharmacy
Missouri Baptist Medical Center
Pharmacy Department
Saint Louis, Missouri

Y.W. Francis Lam, Pharm.D., FCCP
Associate Professor of Pharmacology and Medicine
Clinical Associate Professor
James O. Burke Endowed Centennial Fellow in Pharmacy
University of Texas Health Sciences Center at San Antonio
Department of Pharmacology
San Antonio, Texas

Thomas P. Lombardi, Pharm.D., FASHP
Supervisor
Clinical Pharmacy Services
St. Peter's Hospital,
Albany, New York

Jim Koeller, RPh., M.S.
Professor
University of Texas at Austin
College of Pharmacy
Pharmacotherapy Division
Clinical Professor
University of Texas Health Science Center at San Antonio School of Medicine Pharmacotherapy Education & Research Center
San Antonio, Texas

Nancy Mason, Pharm.D.
Director, Experiential Training Program
Clinical Associate Professor of Pharmacy
Department of Clinical Sciences, College of Pharmacy
Clinical Pharmacist, Nephrology
University of Michigan Health Systems
Ann Arbor, Michigan

Joseph E. Mazur, Pharm.D., BCPS, BCNSP
Clinical Pharmacy Manager
Critical Care Clinical Specialist, MICU
Clinical Associate Professor
South Carolina College of Pharmacy
Mount Pleasant, South Carolina

Ian R. McNicholl, Pharm.D., BCPS (AQ-Infectious Diseases), AAHIVE
Associate Clinical Professor
Clinical Pharmacy Specialist
Positive Health Program
University of California – San Francisco
San Francisco, California

Varsha Mehta, M.S.,(CRDSA), Pharm.D., FCCP
Clinical Associate Professor
Pharmacy, Pediatrics and Communicable Diseases
Clinical Pharmacist Neonatal Critical Care
University of Michigan
Ann Arbor, Michigan

David I. Min, Pharm.D., FCCP
Associate Professor
College of Pharmacy
Western University of Health Sciences
Pomona, California

Mark A. Newnham, Pharm.D., BCPS, BCNSP
Clinical Coordinator
Pharmacy Service
Lawnwood Regional Medical Center and Heart Institute
Ft Pierce, Florida

Keith M. Olsen, Pharm.D., FCCP, FCCM
Professor and Chair
Department of Pharmacy Practice
University of Nebraska Medical Center
Omaha, Nebraska

Christine K. O'Neil, Pharm.D., FCCP, BCPS, CGP
Professor
Duquesne University
Wexford, Pennsylvania

Theresa Prosser, Pharm.D., FCCP, BCPS
Professor of Pharmacy Practice
Saint Louis College of Pharmacy
Saint Louis, Missouri

Ralph H. Raasch, Pharm.D., FCCP, BCPS
Associate Professor
UNC School of Pharmacy
Chapel Hill, North Carolina

Toni L. Ripley, Pharm.D., BCPS, (AQ Cardiology)
Associate Professor
University of Oklahoma College of Pharmacy
Oklahoma City, Oklahoma

Mario L. Rocci, Jr., Ph.D.
Executive Vice-President
Prevalere Life Sciences, Inc.
Whitesboro, New York

Cynthia A. Sanoski, Pharm.D., FCCP, BCPS
Associate Professor and Chair of the Department
of Pharmacy Practice
Jefferson School of Pharmacy
Philadelphia, Pennsylvania

Larry W. Segars, Pharm.D., DrPH, FCCP, BCPS
Chair, Department of Pharmacology & Microbiology
Associate Professor of Pharmacology & Preventive Medicine
Kansas City University of Medicine & Biosciences
Kansas City, Missouri

Sarah A. Spinler, Pharm.D., FAHA, FCCP, BCPS (AQ Cardiology)
Professor of Clinical Pharmacy
Residency and Fellowship Program Coordinator
Philadelphia College of Pharmacy
University of the Sciences in Philadelphia
Philadelphia, Pennsylvania

Kevin M. Sowinski, Pharm.D., FCCP
Professor
Purdue University
School of Pharmacy and Pharmaceutical Sciences
Indianapolis, Indiana

Danielle M. Stitt, Pharm.D. (reviewed in conjunction with David P. Elliott, Pharm.D., FCCP)
PGY-2 Geriatric Resident
Charleston Area Medical Center
Charleston, West Virginia

Kimberly B. Tallian, Pharm.D., FASHP, FCCP, BCPP
Psychiatry Pharmacy Specialist
University of California, San Diego
San Diego, California

Barbara S. Wiggins, Pharm.D., FCCP, BCPS (AQ Cardiology)
Pharmacy Clinical Specialist
Clinical Assistant Professor
University of Virginia Health System
Richmond, Virginia

Patricia R. Wigle, Pharm.D.,BCPS
Associate Professor
James L. Winkle College of Pharmacy
University of Cincinnati Medical Center
Cincinnati, Ohio

Michael Z. Wincor, Pharm.D.
Associate Dean
Globalization and Continuing Professional Development
Associate Professor of Clinical Pharmacy,
Psychiatry and the Behavioral Sciences
University of Southern California
Schools of Pharmacy and Medicine
Los Angeles, California

Table of Contents

Infectious Diseases..2-1
Pneumonia; Urinary Tract Infections; Skin and Soft Tissue Infections; Diabetic Foot Infections; Osteomyelitis; Central Nervous System Infections; Endocarditis; Peritonitis/Intra-abdominal Infections; Medical/Surgical Prophylaxis

HIV/Infectious Diseases..2-43
Human Immunodeficiency Virus; Opportunistic Infections in Patients with HIV; Tuberculosis

Nephrology...2-83
Acute Renal Failure; Drug-Induced Renal Damage; Renal Replacement Therapy; Chronic Kidney Disease; Renal Replacement Therapy; Complications of Chronic Kidney Disease; Dosage Adjustments in Renal Insufficiency

Gastrointestinal Disorders...2-115
Gastroesophageal Reflux Disease; Peptic Ulcer Disease; Upper Gastrointestinal Bleeding; Inflammatory Bowel Disease; Complications of Alcoholic Liver Disease; Viral Hepatitis

Oncology Supportive Care..2-177
Antiemetics; Pain Management; Febrile Neutropenia; Colony-Stimulating Factors; Thrombocytopenia; Anemia/Fatigue; Chemoprotectants; Oncology Emergencies

Men's and Women's Health...2-205
Osteoporosis; Hormone Replacement Therapy; Drugs in Pregnancy and Lactation; Complications in Pregnancy; Contraception; Sexually Transmitted Diseases; Prostatic Infections; Male Sexual Dysfunction

Pharmacokinetics: A Refresher..2-259
Basic Relationships; Absorption; Distribution; Clearance; Non-Linear Pharmacokinetics; Noncompartmental Pharmacokinetics; Data Collection and Analysis; Pharmacokinetics in Renal Disease

Acute Care Cardiology...2-287
Decompensated Heart Failure; Dysrhythmias; Acute Coronary Syndromes; Pulmonary Arterial Hypertension; Hypertensive Urgency and Emergency

Outpatient Cardiology..2-327
Heart Failure; Atrial Fibrillation; Hypertension; Coronary Artery Disease; Chronic Stable Angina

ADDITIONAL RESOURCES

Types of Economic and Humanistic Outcomes Assessments..................................2-363
From the ACCP publication, "Pharmacoeconomics and Outcomes"

Policy, Practice, and Regulatory Issues..2-411
HIPAA, IRB, and Informed Consent; Prescription Drug Approval Process; Investigational Drug Service; JCAHO, ORYX, NCQA, and HEDIS

The Board of Pharmaceutical Specialties "2010 Candidate's Guide"........................2-435
Printed courtesy of the Board of Pharmaceutical Specialties

INFECTIOUS DISEASES

CURTIS L. SMITH, PHARM.D., BCPS
FERRIS STATE UNIVERSITY
LANSING, MICHIGAN

INFECTIOUS DISEASES

CURTIS L. SMITH, PHARM.D., BCPS
FERRIS STATE UNIVERSITY
LANSING, MICHIGAN

Learning Objectives:

1. Describe appropriate treatment of patients with pneumonia, urinary tract infections, central nervous system infections, skin and soft tissue infections, osteomyelitis, intra-abdominal infections, and endocarditis.

2. Identify appropriate preventive therapy for pneumonia, central nervous system infections, endocarditis, and surgical wound infections.

Self-Assessment Questions:

Answers to these questions may be found at the end of this chapter.

1. P.E. is a 56-year-old man who comes to the clinic with a 3-day history of fever, chills, pleuritic chest pain, malaise, and cough productive of sputum. In the clinic, his temperature is 102.1°F (38.9°C) (all other vital signs are normal). His chest radiograph shows consolidation in the right lower lobe. His white blood cell count (WBC) is 14.4/mm³, but all other laboratory values are normal. He is given a diagnosis of community-acquired pneumonia. He has not received any antibiotics in 5 years and has no chronic disease states. Which of the following is the best empiric therapy for P.E.?

    A. Doxycycline 100 mg orally 2 times/day.
    B. Cefuroxime axetil 250 mg orally 2 times/day.
    C. Levofloxacin 750 mg/day orally.
    D. Trimethoprim-sulfamethoxazole double strength orally 2 times/day.

2. H.W. is a 38-year-old woman who presents with high temperature, malaise, dry cough, nasal congestion, and severe headaches. Her symptoms began suddenly 3 days ago, and she has been in bed since then. She reports no other illness in her family, but several people have recently called in sick at work. Which one of the following is best for H.W.?

    A. Azithromycin 500 mg, followed by 250 mg/day orally, for 4 more days.
    B. Amoxicillin-clavulanic acid 875 mg orally 2 times/day.
    C. Oseltamivir 75 mg 2 times/day orally for 5 days.
    D. Symptomatic treatment only.

3. A study is designed to assess the risk of pneumococcal pneumonia in elderly patients 10 years or more after their pneumococcal vaccination, compared with elderly patients who have never received the vaccination. Which one of the following study designs is best?

    A. Case series.
    B. Case-control study.
    C. Prospective cohort study.
    D. Randomized clinical trial.

4. N.R. is a 28-year-old woman who presents to the clinic with a 2-day history of dysuria, frequency, and urgency. She has no significant medical history, and the only drug she takes is oral contraceptives. Which one of the following is the best empiric therapy for N.R.?

    A. Oral amoxicillin 3 g in a single dose.
    B. Oral ciprofloxacin 500 mg 2 times/day for 7 days.
    C. Oral trimethoprim-sulfamethoxazole (TMP/SMZ) double strength 2 times/day for 3 days.
    D. Oral cephalexin 500 mg 4 times/day for 3 days.

5. B.Y. is an 85-year-old woman who is bedridden and lives in a nursing home. She is chronically catheterized, and her urinary catheter was last changed 3 weeks ago. Today, her urine is cloudy, and a urinalysis shows many bacteria. B.Y. is not complaining of any symptoms. A urine culture is obtained. Which one of the following therapies should B.Y. receive?

    A. No therapy because she is chronically catheterized and has no symptoms.
    B. No antibiotic therapy, but the catheter should be changed.
    C. Oral ciprofloxacin 500 mg 2 times/day for 7 days and a new catheter.
    D. Oral ciprofloxacin 500 mg 2 times/day for 14-21 days without a change in catheter.

6. A patient with poor renal function is given a diagnosis of methicillin-resistant *Staphylococcus aureus* (MRSA) endocarditis. An initial 1-g dose of vancomycin is given. The patient has the following characteristics: height 5'10"; weight 72 kg (158 lb); and creatinine 4.2 mg/dL. The vancomycin half-life in this patient is 35 hours, and its volume of distribution is 0.7 L/kg. Which one of the following is correct in determining when the patient will reach a concentration of 10 mcg/L and require another dose?

    A. About 18 hours from the time of the first dose.
    B. About 35 hours from the time of the first dose.

C. About 70 hours from the time of the first dose.
D. Initial dose inadequate to achieve a concentration of 10 mcg/mL.

7. V.E. is a 44-year-old man who presents to the emergency department with a warm, erythematous, and painful right lower extremity. There is no raised border at the edge of the infection. Three days ago, he had scratched his leg on a barbed wire fence on his property. He has had a temperature as high as 101.8°F (38°C) with chills. Doppler studies of his lower extremity are negative. Blood cultures were drawn, and they are negative to date. Which one of the following is the best empiric therapy for V.E.?
   A. Nafcillin 2 g intravenously every 6 hours. The infection may worsen, and necrotizing fasciitis needs to be ruled out.
   B. Penicillin G, 2 million units intravenously every 4 hours. This is probably erysipelas.
   C. Piperacillin-tazobactam 3.375 g intravenously every 6 hours. Surgical debridement is vitally important.
   D. Enoxaparin 80 mg subcutaneously 2 times/day and warfarin 5 mg/day orally.

8. R.K. is a 36-year-old woman who presents to the emergency department with a severe headache and neck stiffness. Her temperature is 99.5°F (37.5°C). After a negative computed tomographic scan of the head, a lumbar puncture is performed, showing the following: glucose 54 mg/dL (peripheral, 104), protein 88 mg/dL, and WBC 220/mm^3 (100% lymphocytes). The Gram stain shows no organisms. Which one of the following options describes the best therapy for R.K.?
   A. This is obviously an aseptic (probably viral) meningitis, and no antibiotics are necessary.
   B. Administer ceftriaxone 2 g intravenously every 12 hours until the cerebrospinal fluid (CSF) cultures are negative for bacteria.
   C. Administer ceftriaxone 2 g intravenously every 12 hours and vancomycin 1000 mg intravenously every 12 hours until the CSF cultures are negative for bacteria.
   D. Administer acyclovir 500 mg intravenously every 8 hours until the CSF culture results are complete.

9. L.G. is a 49-year-old woman with a history of mitral valve prolapse. She presents to her physician's office complaining of malaise and a low-grade fever. Her physician notes that her murmur is louder than normal and orders blood cultures and an echocardiogram. Large vegetation is observed on L.G.'s mitral valve, and her blood cultures are growing *Enterococcus faecalis* (susceptible to all antibiotics). Which one of the following is the best therapy for L.G.?
   A. Penicillin G plus gentamicin for 2 weeks.
   B. Vancomycin plus gentamicin for 2 weeks.
   C. Ampicillin plus gentamicin for 4-6 weeks.
   D. Cefazolin plus gentamicin for 4-6 weeks.

10. N.L. is a 28-year-old woman with no significant medical history. She reports to the emergency department with fever and severe right lower quadrant pain. She has had a dull pain for the past few days, but it suddenly became severe during the past 8 hours. Her temperature is 103.5°F (39.7°C), and she has rebound tenderness on abdominal examination. She is taken to surgery immediately, and a perforated appendix is diagnosed and repaired. Which one of the following is an appropriate follow-up antibiotic regimen?
    A. Vancomycin 1000 mg intravenously every 12 hours plus metronidazole 500 mg intravenously every 8 hours.
    B. Ceftriaxone 1 g/day intravenously plus ciprofloxacin 400 mg intravenously every 12 hours.
    C. Ertapenem 1 g/day intravenously.
    D. No antibiotics needed after surgical repair of a perforated appendix.

Infectious Diseases

I. **PNEUMONIA**

   A. Introduction
   1. Pneumonia is the most common cause of death attributable to infectious diseases (very high rates in the elderly) and the seventh most common cause of death in the United States.
   2. Hospital-acquired pneumonia is the second most common nosocomial infection (0.6%–1.1% of all hospitalized patients)—there is an increased incidence in patients in the intensive care unit recovering from thoracic or upper abdominal surgery and the elderly.
   3. Mortality rates
      a. Community-acquired pneumonia without hospitalization: less than 1%
      b. Community-acquired pneumonia with hospitalization: about 14%
      c. Nosocomial: about 33%–50%

   B. Community-Acquired Pneumonia
   1. Definition: Acute infection of the pulmonary parenchyma, accompanied by the presence of an acute infiltrate consistent with pneumonia on chest radiograph or auscultatory findings. In patients not hospitalized or patients in a long-term care facility for 14 days or more before symptoms appear
   2. Symptoms of community-acquired pneumonia are listed below (must have any two). Elderly patients often have fewer and less severe findings (mental status changes are common).
      a. Fever or hypothermia
      b. Rigors
      c. Sweats
      d. New cough with or without sputum (90%)
      e. Chest discomfort (50%)
      f. Onset of dyspnea (66%)
      g. Fatigue, myalgias, abdominal pain, anorexia, and headache
   3. Predictors of a complicated course in community-acquired pneumonia are listed below. Hospitalization should be based on the severity of illness scores (e.g., CURB-65, PSI [pneumonia severity index]).
      a. Age older than 65 years
      b. Comorbid illness (diabetes mellitus, congestive heart failure, lung disease, renal failure, liver disease)
      c. High temperature: more than 101°F (38°C)
      d. Bacteremia
      e. Altered mental status
      f. Immunosuppression (e.g., steroid use, cancer)
      g. High-risk etiology (*S. aureus*, *Legionella*, gram-negative bacilli, anaerobic aspiration)
      h. Multilobe involvement or pleural effusions

   C. Hospital-Acquired Pneumonia
   1. Hospital-acquired pneumonia—pneumonia that occurs 48 hours or more after admission and was not incubating at the time of admission
   2. Ventilator-associated pneumonia—pneumonia that arises more than 48–72 hours after endotracheal intubation
   3. Health care–associated pneumonia—pneumonia developing in a patient who was hospitalized in an acute care hospital for 2 or more days within 90 days of the infection; resides in a nursing home or long-term care facility; received recent intravenous antibiotic therapy,

chemotherapy, or wound care within the past 30 days of the current infection; or attended a hospital or hemodialysis clinic

Risk factors for hospital-acquired pneumonia:
    a. Intubation and mechanical ventilation
    b. Supine patient position
    c. Enteral feeding
    d. Oropharyngeal colonization
    e. Stress bleeding prophylaxis
    f. Blood transfusion
    g. Hyperglycemia
    h. Immunosuppression/corticosteroids
    i. Surgical procedures: thoracoabdominal, upper abdominal, thoracic
    j. Immobilization
    k. Nasogastric tubes
    l. Prior antibiotic therapy
    m. Admission to the intensive care unit
    n. Elderly
    o. Underlying chronic lung disease

D. Table 1. Microbiology

Table 1. Incidence of Pneumonia by Organism

Community Acquired (%)		Hospital Acquired (%)	
Unidentifiable	40–60	Unidentifiable	50
M. pneumoniae	13–37	*S. aureus*	10
S. pneumoniae	9–20	*Pseudomonas aeruginosa*	8
H. influenzae	3–10	*Enterobacter* sp.	5
C. pneumoniae	1–17	*Klebsiella pneumoniae*	4
Legionella pneumophila	0.7–13	*Candida*	3
Viruses	Common	*Acinetobacter* sp.	2
Others:	Uncommon	*Serratia marcescens*	2
S. aureus		*Escherichia coli*	2
Moraxella catarrhalis		*S. pneumoniae*	1
PCP			
Anaerobes			
Gram-negative bacilli (e.g., *K. pneumoniae*)			
Specific populations in community-acquired pneumonia: Alcoholics: *S. pneumoniae*, oral anaerobes, gram-negative bacilli (i.e., *Klebsiella*) Nursing home: *S. pneumoniae*, *H. influenzae*, gram-negative bacilli, *S. aureus* COPD: *S. pneumoniae*, *H. influenzae*, *M. catarrhalis* Postinfluenza: *H. influenzae*, *S. aureus*, *S. pneumoniae* Exposure to water: *Legionella* Poor oral hygiene: oral anaerobes HIV infection: PCP, *S. pneumoniae*, *M. pneumoniae*, *Mycobacterium*		Issues in hospital-acquired pneumonia: - *P. aeruginosa* is transmitted by health care workers' hands or respiratory equipment - *S. aureus* is transmitted by health care workers' hands - Enterobacteriaceae endogenously colonize hospitalized patients' airways (healthy people seldom have gram-negative upper airway colonization) - Stress changes respiratory epithelial cells so that gram-negative organisms can adhere - Up to 70% of patients in the intensive care unit have gram-negative upper airway colonization, and 25% of them will become infected through aspiration	

COPD = chronic obstructive pulmonary disease; HIV = human immunodeficiency virus; PCP *Pneumocystis* pneumonia.

Patient Case

1. R.L. is a 68-year-old man who presents to the emergency department complaining of coughing and shortness of breath. His symptoms, which began 4 days ago, have worsened during the past 24 hours. He is coughing up yellow-green sputum, and he complains of chills with a temperature of 102.4°F (39°C). His medical history includes coronary artery disease with a myocardial infarction 5 years ago, congestive heart failure, hypertension, and osteoarthritis. He rarely drinks alcohol and has not smoked since his myocardial infarction. His medications on admission include lisinopril 10 mg/day, hydrochlorothiazide 25 mg/day, and acetaminophen 650 mg 4 times/day. On physical examination, he is alert and oriented, with the following vital signs: temperature 101.8°F (38°C); heart rate 100 beats/minute; respiratory rate 24 breaths/minute; and blood pressure 142/94 mm Hg. His laboratory results were normal except for blood urea nitrogen (BUN) 32 mg/dL (serum creatinine 1.23 mg/dL). Blood gases were pH 7.44; pCO$_2$ 35; pO$_2$ 82; and O$_2$ sat 90%. A sputum specimen is not available. If R.L. were hospitalized, which one of the following would be the best empiric therapy for him?
   A. Ampicillin-sulbactam 1.5 g intravenously every 6 hours.
   B. Piperacillin-tazobactam 4.5 g intravenously every 6 hours plus gentamicin 180 mg intravenously every 12 hours.
   C. Ceftriaxone 1 g intravenously every 24 hours plus azithromycin 500 mg/day intravenously.
   D. Doxycycline 100 mg intravenously every 12 hours.

E. Therapy
   1. Community-acquired pneumonia (duration, at least 5 days)
      a. Empiric treatment of nonhospitalized patients
         i. Previously healthy and no antibiotic therapy in the past 3 months
            (a) Macrolide (macrolide: clarithromycin or azithromycin if *H. influenzae* is suspected)
            (b) Doxycycline
         ii. Comorbidities (chronic obstructive pulmonary disease, diabetes mellitus, chronic renal or liver failure, congestive heart failure, malignancy, asplenia, or immunosuppression) OR recent antibiotic therapy (within the past 3 months)
            (a) Respiratory fluoroquinolone (moxifloxacin, gemifloxacin, or levofloxacin [750 mg])
            (b) Macrolide (or doxycycline) with high-dose amoxicillin (1 g 3 times/day) or amoxicillin-clavulanate (2 g 2 times/day) or a cephalosporin (ceftriaxone, cefuroxime, or cefpodoxime)
      b. Empiric treatment of hospitalized patients with moderately severe pneumonia
         i. Respiratory fluoroquinolone (moxifloxacin, gemifloxacin, or levofloxacin [750 mg])
         ii. Ampicillin, ceftriaxone, or cefotaxime (ertapenem in select patients) plus a macrolide (or doxycycline)
      c. Empiric treatment of hospitalized patients with severe pneumonia requiring intensive care unit treatment
         i. Ampicillin-sulbactam, ceftriaxone, or cefotaxime plus either a respiratory fluoroquinolone or azithromycin (may need to add other antibiotics if *P. aeruginosa* or MRSA is suspected)
      d. Treatment duration—at least 5 days, with 48–72 hours afebrile and no more than one sign of clinical instability (elevated temperature, heart rate, or respiratory rate; decreased systolic blood pressure; or arterial oxygen saturation) before discontinuation of therapy

Infectious Diseases

> **Patient Case**
> 2. B.P. is a 66-year-old woman who underwent a two-vessel coronary artery bypass graft 8 days ago and has been on a ventilator in the surgical intensive care unit since then. Her temperature is now rising, and a tracheal aspirate shows many WBC and gram-negative rods. Her medical history includes coronary artery disease with a myocardial infarction 2 years ago, chronic obstructive pulmonary disease, and hypertension. Which one of the following is the best empiric therapy for B.P.?
> A. Ceftriaxone 1 g/day intravenously plus gentamicin 140 mg intravenously every 12 hours plus linezolid 600 mg intravenously every 12 hours.
> B. Piperacillin-tazobactam 4.5 g intravenously every 6 hours.
> C. Levofloxacin 750 mg/day intravenously plus linezolid 600 mg intravenously every 12 hours.
> D. Cefepime 2 g intravenously every 12 hours plus tobramycin 140 mg intravenously every 12 hours plus vancomycin 15 mg/kg intravenously every 12 hours.

2. Hospital-acquired pneumonia
   a. Early onset (less than 5 days) and no risk factors for multidrug-resistant (MDR)* organisms
      i. Organisms: *S. pneumoniae, Haemophilus influenzae*, methicillin-sensitive *S. aureus* (MSSA), *Escherichia coli, Klebsiella pneumoniae, Enterobacter* species, *Proteus* species
         (a) Third-generation cephalosporin (cefotaxime or ceftriaxone)
         (b) Fluoroquinolone (levofloxacin, moxifloxacin, ciprofloxacin)
         (c) Ampicillin-sulbactam
         (d) Ertapenem

   b. Late onset (5 days or longer) or risk factors for MDR organisms
      i. Organisms: Those listed above for early onset plus *Pseudomonas aeruginosa, K. pneumoniae* (extended-spectrum b-lactamase positive), *Acinetobacter* species, MRSA, and *Legionella pneumophila*
         (a) Ceftazidime or cefepime plus aminoglycoside or fluoroquinolone (cipro-, levo)
         (b) Imipenem, meropenem, or doripenem plus aminoglycoside or fluoroquinolone (ciprofloxacin, levofloxacin)
         (c) Piperacillin-tazobactam plus aminoglycoside or fluoroquinolone (ciprofloxacin, levofloxacin)
         (d) Vancomycin or linezolid should be used only if MRSA risk factors (e.g., history of MRSA infection/colonization, recent hospitalization or antibiotic use, presence of invasive health care devices) are present or there is a high incidence locally (greater than 10%–15%).

   c. Treatment duration—Efforts should be made to decrease duration of therapy to as short as 7 or 8 days (14 days for pneumonia secondary to *P. aeruginosa*).

   *Risk factors for MDR organisms
      i. Antibiotic therapy within the past 90 days
      ii. Hospitalization of 5 days or more
      iii. High resistance in community or hospital unit
      iv. Risk factors for health care–associated pneumonia
      v. Immunosuppressive disease and/or therapy

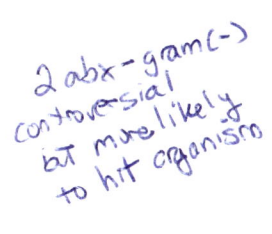

Patient Case

3. B.P., who eventually improves, is transferred to a regular floor. She cannot remember receiving any recent vaccinations. Which one of the following vaccinations do you recommend for this patient?
   A. B.P. does not need any vaccinations.
   B. B.P. should receive pneumococcal vaccine now and the influenza vaccine in the fall.
   C. B.P. should receive the influenza vaccine in the fall, but because of her current infection, the pneumococcal vaccine is unnecessary.
   D. B.P. should receive the pneumococcal vaccine now, but she is not in a group in which influenza vaccine is recommended.

F. Influenza
   1. Characteristics of influenza infection
      a. Epidemic with significant mortality
      b. Epidemics begin abruptly → peak in 2–3 weeks → resolve in 5–6 weeks
      c. Occurs almost exclusively in the winter months (December–April)
      d. Average overall attack rates of 10%–20%
      e. Mortality greatest in those older than 65 years (especially with heart and lung disease): more than 80% of deaths caused by influenza are from this age group (20,000 deaths/year in the United States)
   2. Is it a cold or the flu? (Table 2)

Table 2. Differentiating the Symptoms of Cold and Influenza

Signs and Symptoms	Influenza	Cold
Onset	Sudden	Gradual
Temperature	Characteristic, high (> 101°F [38°C]) of 3 or 4 days' duration	Rare
Cough	Dry; can become severe	Hacking
Headache	Prominent	Rare
Myalgia (muscle aches/pains)	Usual; often severe	Slight
Tiredness and weakness	Can last up to 2–3 weeks	Very mild
Extreme exhaustion	Early and prominent	Never
Chest discomfort	Common	Mild to moderate
Stuffy nose	Sometimes	Common
Sneezing	Sometimes	Usual
Sore throat	Sometimes	Common

   3. Pathophysiology
      a. Type A
         i. Influenza further grouped by variations in hemagglutinin and neuraminidase (e.g., H1N1, H1N2)
         ii. Changes through antigenic drift or shift; a pandemic can occur with one "shift"
         iii. Causes epidemics every 1–3 years
      b. Type B
         i. Type B influenza carries one form of hemagglutinin and one form of neuraminidase.
         ii. Changes through antigenic drift (minor mutations from year to year); when enough "drifts" occur, an epidemic is likely
         iii. Causes epidemics every 5 years

Infectious Diseases

4. Prevention
   a. Amantadine, rimantadine
      i. Prevents about 50% of infections and 70%–90% of illnesses (similar to the influenza vaccine)
      ii. Dose/recommendations: short term (5–7 weeks or the duration of the epidemic); prophylaxis during a presumed outbreak of influenza A in patients who cannot receive vaccine (or 2 weeks only if the vaccine is given at the same time)
      iii. Not recommended unless testing shows increased susceptibility
   b. Neuraminidase inhibitors
      i. Oseltamivir (Tamiflu)
         (a) Oseltamivir 75–150 mg/day orally for 6 weeks during peak influenza season showed 74% protective efficacy.
         (b) Begin oseltamivir 75 mg/day orally for at least 7 days within 2 days of close contact with an infected individual.
      ii. Zanamivir (Relenza)
         (a) Zanamivir 10 mg/day through inhalation for 4 weeks during peak influenza season showed 67% protective efficacy.
5. Therapy
   a. Treat only if patient has severe symptoms (clinical deterioration or lower respiratory tract infection) or is at higher risk of complications – use only the neuraminidase inhibitors
   b. Amantadine (Symmetrel); rimantadine (Flumadine)
      i. Inhibits viral uncoating and release of viral nucleic acid by inhibiting M2 protein
         (a) Only effective against influenza A virus
         (b) Decreases the duration of signs and symptoms by 1 day
      ii. Adverse effects
         (a) Central nervous system
         (b) Peripheral edema
         (c) Orthostatic hypotension
      iii. Dose
         (a) 100 mg orally 2 times/day
         (b) Elderly patients should not receive more than 100 mg/day.
         (c) Adjust for renal disease (amantadine > rimantadine).
         (d) Therapy duration is 3–7 days.
         (e) Initiate treatment within 1–2 days of symptoms.
         (f) Not recommended unless testing shows increased susceptibility
   c. Oseltamivir (Tamiflu)
      i. Inhibits neuraminidase; symptoms disappear 1–1.5 days sooner.
      ii. Adverse effects: gastrointestinal (nausea and vomiting)
      iii. Dose
         (a) A total of 75 mg orally 2 times/day for 5 days; decrease dose to 75 mg/day orally in patients with creatinine clearance less than 30 mL/minute
         (b) Initiate within 48 hours of symptom onset.
   d. Zanamivir (Relenza)
      i. Inhibits neuraminidase; symptoms disappear 1–1.5 days sooner
      ii. Adverse effects: bronchospasm, cough
      iii. Dose
         (a) Two inhalations (5 mg/inhalation) 2 times/day for 5 days
         (b) Initiate within 48 hours of symptom onset.

G. Pneumonia Immunizations
1. Pneumococcal vaccine
    a. Characteristics
        i. Pneumococcal vaccine contains 23 purified capsular polysaccharide antigens of *S. pneumoniae*.
        ii. The 23 capsular types account for 85%–90% of invasive *S. pneumoniae* infection.
        iii. All six serotypes that commonly cause drug-resistant *S. pneumoniae* (DRSP) infection are in the vaccine.
        iv. Antibody levels remain elevated for at least 5 years.
    b. Recommendations (Table 3)

Table 3. Pneumococcal Vaccine Recommendations

Vaccination-Recommended Group	Revaccination
Immunocompetent People	
- People ≥ 65 years	- Second dose of vaccine if patient received vaccine ≥ 5 years previously and was < 65 years at the time of vaccination
- People 2–64 years old with chronic cardiovascular disease, chronic pulmonary disease, diabetes mellitus, alcoholism, chronic liver disease, or CSF leaks; adult asthmatics or adult smokers	- Not recommended
- People 2–64 years old with functional or anatomic asplenia	- Single revaccination recommended after 5 years (for anyone ≥ 2 years)
- People 2–64 years old living in special environments or social settings	- Not recommended
Immunocompromised People	
- Immunocompromised people ≥ 2 years old, including those with HIV infection, leukemia, lymphoma, Hodgkin disease, multiple myeloma, generalized malignancy, chronic renal failure, or nephrotic syndrome; those receiving immunosuppressive chemotherapy (including corticosteroids); and those who have received an organ or bone marrow transplant	- Single revaccination recommended after 5 years (for anyone ≥ 2 years)

CSF = cerebrospinal fluid; HIV = human immunodeficiency virus.

2. Influenza vaccine
    a. Characteristics
        i. Each year's vaccine contains two strains of type A and one strain of type B—selected by worldwide surveillance and antigenic characterization.
        ii. Prevents illness in 70%–90% of healthy people younger than 65 years
        iii. Prevents illness in 53%, hospitalization in 50%, and death in 68% of the elderly
        iv. Administer yearly in September or October.
    b. Recommendations (Table 4)

Table 4. Influenza Vaccine Recommendations

Groups for Which Vaccination Is Recommended (Use Inactivated Vaccine Only)	
People at high risk of influenza-related complications	- Healthy individuals ≥ 50 years - Residents of nursing homes and other chronic care facilities - Adults and children with chronic cardiac or pulmonary conditions, including asthma (not hypertension) - People who required regular medical follow-up or were hospitalized during the past year because of chronic underlying diseases such as diabetes mellitus, renal dysfunction, anemia, immunosuppression, HIV, or asthma - People with any condition (e.g., cognitive dysfunction, spinal cord injuries, seizure disorders, other neuromuscular disorders) that can compromise respiratory function or the handling of respiratory secretions or that can increase the risk of aspiration - Children and teenagers receiving chronic aspirin therapy - Women who will be pregnant during the influenza season - Healthy children from 6 months to 18 years old
People who can transmit influenza to those at high risk	- All health care workers - Home care providers for people in high-risk groups - Household members of people in high-risk groups
Patients with HIV: - No risk to the patient and should be given to anyone receiving antiretrovirals - Studies show a decreased antibody response (< 60% have adequate response)	
Intranasal live-attenuated vaccine (FluMist): - Indicated for people 2–49 years old without underlying illnesses (including health care workers) - Use of inactivated vaccine is preferred for vaccinating household members, health care workers, and others who have close contact with immunosuppressed people	

HIV = human immunodeficiency virus.

II. URINARY TRACT INFECTIONS

A. Introduction
 1. Most common bacterial infection in humans: 7 million office visits per year; 1 million hospitalizations
 2. Many women (15%–20%) will have a urinary tract infection (UTI) during their lifetime.
 3. From ages 1–50, UTIs predominantly occur in women; after 50, men are affected because of prostate problems.

B. Microbiology (Table 5)

Table 5. Incidence of Urinary Tract Infections by Organism

Community Acquired (%)		Nosocomial (%)	
E. coli	73	E. coli	31
S. saprophyticus	13	P. aeruginosa	10
P. mirabilis	5	Other gram-negative bacilli	10
K. pneumoniae	4	K. pneumoniae	9
Enterococcus	2	S. aureus	6
		P. mirabilis	5
		Enterococcus	2
		Fungal	14

C. Predisposing Factors
   1. Age
   2. Female sex
   3. Diabetes mellitus
   4. Pregnancy
   5. Immunosuppression
   6. Urinary tract instrumentation
   7. Urinary tract obstruction
   8. Renal disease; renal transplantation
   9. Neurologic dysfunction

Patient Case
4. G.N. is a 62-year-old woman who presents to the clinic with a 3-day history of urinary frequency and dysuria. During the past 24 hours, she has had nausea, vomiting, and flank pain. One month before this visit, the patient received 3 days of cefpodoxime for an *E. coli* UTI. Six weeks before the *E. coli* UTI, the patient received a single 3-g dose of amoxicillin for UTI-like symptoms. This is her third UTI in 3 months. G.N. has a history of type 2 diabetes mellitus, which is poorly controlled with some diabetic-related complications. G.N. also has hypertension and a history of several episodes of deep venous thrombosis. Her medications include glyburide 5 mg/day orally, enalapril 10 mg orally 2 times/day, warfarin 3 mg/day orally, and metoclopramide 10 mg 4 times/day. On physical examination, she is alert and oriented, with the following vital signs: temperature 102.8°F (39°C); heart rate 120 beats/minute; respiratory rate 16 breaths/minute; blood pressure (supine): 140/75 mm Hg; and blood pressure (standing) 110/60 mm Hg. Her laboratory values were within normal limits except for increased international normalized ratio 2.7; BUN 26 mg/dL; serum creatinine 1.88 mg/dL; and WBC 12,000 (78 polymorphonuclear leukocytes, 7 band neutrophils, 10 lymphocytes, and 5 monocytes). Her urinalysis shows turbidity, 2+ glucose; pH 7.0; protein 100 mg/dL; 50–100 WBC; + nitrites; 3–5 red blood cells; and many bacteria and +casts. Which one of the following is the best empiric therapy for G.N.?
   A. TMP/SMZ double strength orally 2 times/day—duration of antibiotics: 7 days.
   B. Ciprofloxacin 400 mg intravenously 2 times/day and then 500 mg orally 2 times/day—duration of antibiotics: 10 days.
   C. Gentamicin 140 mg intravenously every 24 hours—duration of antibiotics: 3 days.
   D. Ampicillin-sulbactam 3 g intravenously every 6 hours and then amoxicillin-clavulanate 875 mg orally 2 times/day—duration of antibiotics: 10 days.

D. Clinical Presentation
   1. Lower UTI—cystitis (elderly patients may have only nonspecific symptoms, such as mental status changes, abdominal pain, and decreased eating or drinking)
      a. Dysuria
      b. Frequent urination
      c. Urgency
      d. Occasionally gross hematuria
      e. Occasionally foul-smelling urine
   2. Upper UTI—pyelonephritis (elderly patients may have only nonspecific symptoms, such as mental status changes, abdominal pain, and decreased eating or drinking)
      a. Frequency, dysuria, hematuria
      b. Suprapubic pain
      c. Costovertebral angle tenderness—flank pain
      d. Fever, chills
      e. Increased WBC
      f. Nausea, vomiting

3. Factors associated with complicated UTI
   a. Male sex
   b. Hospital-acquired
   c. Pregnancy
   d. Anatomic abnormality of the urinary tract
   e. Childhood UTIs
   f. Recent antimicrobial use
   g. Diabetes mellitus
   h. Indwelling urinary catheter
   i. Recent urinary tract instrumentation
   j. Immunosuppression
4. Recurrent cystitis
   a. Relapse: infection with the same organism within 14 days of discontinuing antibiotics for the preceding UTI
   b. Reinfection: infection with a completely different organism—most common cause of recurrent cystitis

E. Diagnosis
   1. Urinalysis (blood cultures will be positive in 20% of patients with upper UTIs)
      a. Polyuria (greater than 5-10 WBC)
      b. Bacteriuria (greater than 10^2 CFU [colony-forming units]/mL is diagnostic)
      c. Red blood cells
      d. Cloudiness
      e. Nitrite positive
      f. Leukocyte esterase positive
      g. Casts (if pyelonephritis)

F. Therapy
   1. Uncomplicated cystitis
      a. Three-day treatment regimen (vs. 5-10 days: equal in symptomatic but not bacteriologic cure)
         i. TMP/SMZ
         ii. Trimethoprim
         iii. Fluoroquinolone
      b. Alternatives
         i. Nitrofurantoin (7-day course)
         ii. Fosfomycin (single dose)
      c. Single-dose therapy
         i. Improved adherence; fewer adverse effects; cheaper
         ii. Reduced cure rates compared with a 3- or 7-day regimen
         iii. Inappropriate for patients with occult upper tract involvement
         iv. First-line antibiotics as listed above
   2. Pregnancy (pregnant women should be screened for bacteriuria and treated, even if asymptomatic)
      a. Antibiotics to avoid
         i. Fluoroquinolones
         ii. Tetracyclines
         iii. Aminoglycosides
         iv. TMP/SMZ (used frequently but avoidance recommended especially during the late third trimester)

b. Seven-day treatment regimen
   i. Amoxicillin
   ii. Nitrofurantoin
   iii. Cephalexin
   iv. TMP/SMZ
3. Recurrent cystitis
   a. Relapse
      i. Assess for pharmacologic reason for treatment failure.
      ii. Treat longer (for 2–6 weeks, depending on length of initial course).
   b. Reinfection (reassess need for continuous prophylactic antibiotics every 6–12 months)
      i. If patient has two or fewer UTIs in 1 year, use patient-initiated therapy for symptomatic episodes (3-day treatment regimens).
      ii. If patient has three or more UTIs in 1 year and they are temporally related to sexual activity, use post-intercourse prophylaxis with TMP/SMZ SS, cephalexin 250 mg, or nitrofurantoin 50-100 mg.
      iii. If patient has three or more UTIs in 1 year that are not related to sexual activity, use daily or 3 times/week prophylaxis with trimethoprim 100 mg, TMP/SMZ SS, cephalexin 250 mg, norfloxacin 200 mg, or nitrofurantoin 50–100 mg.
4. Uncomplicated pyelonephritis
   a. Outpatient therapy (if patient is not immunocompromised or does not have nausea and vomiting)
      i. TMP/SMZ
      ii. Fluoroquinolone
   b. Therapy duration
      i. Five to 14 days (5 days with levofloxacin, 14 days with TMP/SMZ)
5. Complicated UTIs
   a. Therapy
      i. Fluoroquinolone
      ii. Aminoglycoside
      iii. Extended-spectrum b-lactamase
   b. Therapy duration
      i. Five to 14 days (5 days with levofloxacin)
6. Catheter-related UTIs
   a. Short-term indwelling catheters
      i. About 5% of patients will develop one UTI per day; by 30 days, 75%–95% of patients with an indwelling catheter will have bacteriuria.
      ii. Preventive antimicrobial therapy is not recommended—it only increases the chance of selecting out resistant organisms.
      iii. Asymptomatic patients with bacteriuria should not be treated.
      iv. Symptomatic patients with bacteriuria should be treated with 7–10 days of antibiotics and catheter removal; a shorter course of therapy (5–7 days) should be used if the catheter cannot be removed.
      v. The most common organisms are *E. coli* (21.4%), *Candida* species (21.0%), *Enterococcus* species (14.9%), *P. aeruginosa* (10.0%), *K. pneumoniae* (7.7%), and *Enterobacter* species (4.1%).

b. Long-term indwelling catheters
    i. Virtually all patients will be bacteriuric with two to five organisms.
    ii. Asymptomatic patients should not be treated.
    iii. Symptomatic patients should be treated for a short period (7 days) to prevent resistance, and catheter replacement may be indicated.
7. Prostatitis and epididymitis
    a. Acute bacterial prostatitis
        i. Primarily gram-negative organisms
        ii. Therapy duration, 4 weeks
            (a) TMP/SMZ
            (b) Cephalosporins
            (c) Fluoroquinolones
    b. Chronic bacterial prostatitis
        i. Difficult to treat
        ii. Therapy duration, 1–4 months
            (a) TMP/SMZ
            (b) Fluoroquinolones
8. Epididymitis
    a. Older than 35 years; most likely caused by enteric organisms
    b. Therapy duration, 10 days to 4 weeks
        i. TMP/SMZ
        ii. Fluoroquinolones
    c. Younger than 35 years; most likely gonococcal or chlamydial infection
    d. Therapy duration, 10 days
        i. Ceftriaxone 250 mg intramuscularly once plus doxycycline 100 mg 2 times/day

III. SKIN AND SOFT TISSUE INFECTIONS

A. Cellulitis
   1. Description
      a. Acute spreading skin infection that primarily involves the deep dermis and subcutaneous fat
      b. Nonelevated and poorly defined margins
      c. Warmth, pain, erythema and edema, and tender lymphadenopathy
      d. Malaise, fever, and chills
      e. Usually, patient has had previous minor trauma, abrasions, ulcers, or surgery (could be as little as tinea infections, psoriasis, or eczema).
      f. Often, patients have impaired lymphatic drainage.
   2. Microorganism—usually *S. pyogenes* and occasionally *S. aureus* (rarely other organisms)
   3. Treatment: 5–10 days (infection may worsen when treatment begins—must differentiate from necrotizing fasciitis)
      a. Anti-staphylococcal penicillin (nafcillin, oxacillin, or dicloxacillin)
      b. Penicillin G if definitively streptococcal
      c. Alternatives
         i. Clindamycin
         ii. β-Lactamase inhibitor combinations
         iii. First-generation cephalosporin
         iv. Vancomycin or linezolid for MRSA cellulitis

B. Erysipelas
   1. Description
      a. Acute spreading skin infection that primarily involves the superficial dermis
      b. Spreads rapidly through the lymphatic system in the skin (patients may have impaired lymphatic drainage)
      c. Usually occurs in infants and the elderly
      d. Most commonly occurs on the legs and feet (Facial erysipelas can occur, but they are less common.)
      e. Warmth, erythema, and pain
      f. Edge of infection is elevated and sharply demarcated from the surrounding tissue.
      g. Systemic signs of infection are common, but blood cultures are positive only 5% of the time.
   2. Microorganism: group A streptococcus (*S. pyogenes*) but occasionally groups G, C, and B are seen
   3. Treatment: 7–10 days (infections may worsen when treatment begins)
      i. Penicillin G
      ii. Clindamycin

C. Necrotizing Fasciitis
   1. Description
      a. Acute, necrotizing cellulites that involve the subcutaneous fat and superficial fascia
      b. Infection extensively alters surrounding tissue, leading to cutaneous anesthesia or gangrene.
      c. Very painful
      d. Streptococcal infection: either spontaneous or attributable to varicella, minor trauma (cuts, burns, and splinters), surgical procedures, or muscle strain; mixed infection generally secondary to abdominal surgery or trauma
      e. Significant systemic symptoms, including shock and organ failure
   2. Microorganisms
      a. *S. pyogenes*
      b. Mixed infection with facultative and anaerobic bacteria
   3. Treatment
      a. Surgical debridement: most important therapy and often requires repeated debridement
      b. Antibiotics are not curative; given in addition to surgery (if used early, may be effective alone)
      c. Empiric therapy: b-lactamase inhibitor combinations plus clindamycin plus ciprofloxacin, carbapenems, cefotaxime plus clindamycin or metronidazole
      d. Streptococcal necrotizing fasciitis: high-dose intravenous penicillin plus clindamycin

D. Varicella-Zoster Virus Immunization
   1. Shingles vaccine (Zostavax)
      a. Characteristics
         i. Zoster vaccine is a live, attenuated vaccine, identical to the chicken pox vaccine (Varivax) but with significantly more plaque-forming units of virus per vaccination.
         ii. Significantly decreases the number of cases and the burden of illness in vaccinated patients (50% effective, but decreases with age). In addition, significantly decreases the incidence and persistence of post-herpetic neuralgia (40% effective)

b. Recommendations
   i. One dose – all adults 60 years and older (regardless of chicken pox or zoster history)
   ii. Not indicated for treatment of active herpes zoster infections or post-herpetic neuralgia

IV. DIABETIC FOOT INFECTIONS

A. A diabetes complication that most often leads to hospitalization
B. Twenty-five percent of people with diabetes develop foot infections; 1 in 15 requires amputation.

Patient Case

5. G.N. returns to the clinic in 6 months with no urinary symptoms, but her chief complaint is now an ulcer on her right foot. She has recently returned from vacation in Florida and thinks she might have stepped on something while walking barefoot on the beach. Her foot is not sore but is red and swollen around the ulcer. The ulcer is deep, and the infection may involve the underlying bone. Her medications are the same as before, except that now, she also takes trimethoprim 100 mg 3 times/week for UTI. Vital signs are stable, and there is nothing significant on physical examination except the right foot ulcer. Laboratory values are within normal limits (serum creatinine 0.86 mg/dL). Which one of the following best describes the organism(s) likely responsible for G.N.'s foot ulcer?
   A. Multiple anaerobic organisms.
   B. *P. aeruginosa.*
   C. *S. aureus.*
   D. Polymicrobial with gram-positive, gram-negative, and anaerobic organisms.

C. Etiology
   1. Neuropathy: motor and autonomic
      a. Mechanical or thermal injuries lead to ulcerations without patient knowledge.
      b. Gait disturbances and foot deformities; maldistribution of weight on the foot
      c. Diminished sweating, causing dry, cracked skin
   2. Vasculopathy: decreased lower limb perfusion
   3. Immunologic defects (cellular and humoral)

D. Causative Organisms
   1. In general, polymicrobial (average, 2.1–5.8 microorganisms)
      a. *S. aureus*
      b. *Streptococcus*
      c. *Enterococcus*
      d. *Proteus*
      e. *E. coli*
      f. *Klebsiella*
      g. *Enterobacter*
      h. *P. aeruginosa*
      i. *Bacteroides fragilis*
      j. *Peptococcus*

E. Therapy
1. Preventive therapy
   a. Examine feet daily for calluses, blisters, trauma, etc.
   b. Wear properly fitting shoes.
   c. No barefoot walking
   d. Keep feet clean and dry.
   e. Have toenails cut properly.

Patient Case

6. Which one of the following is the best empiric therapy for G.N.?
   A. Nafcillin 2 g intravenously every 6 hours—duration of antibiotics: 6–12 weeks.
   B. Tobramycin 120 mg intravenously every 12 hours plus levofloxacin 750 mg/day intravenously—duration of antibiotics: 1–2 weeks.
   C. Piperacillin-tazobactam 4.5 g intravenously every 8 hours—duration of antibiotics: 1–2 weeks.
   D. Below-the-knee amputation followed by ceftriaxone 1 g intravenously every 24 hours—duration of antibiotics: 1 week.

---

2. Antimicrobial therapy
   a. Shallow, non–limb-threatening infections can be treated like cellulitis (penicillinase-resistant penicillin, first-generation cephalosporin, etc.).
   b. Deep, limb-threatening infections require more broad-spectrum agents.
      i. Ampicillin-sulbactam
      ii. Ticarcillin-clavulanate or piperacillin-tazobactam
      iii. Ertapenem
      iv. Fluoroquinolone plus clindamycin-metronidazole
      v. Cefoxitin
      vi. Third-generation cephalosporin plus clindamycin or metronidazole
   c. Treatment duration: 1–2 weeks if it is only a skin/soft tissue infection or 6–12 weeks if osteomyelitis

F. Topical Therapy
1. Becaplermin (Regranex)
   a. 0.01% gel of recombinant human platelet–derived growth factor
   b. Increases production of cells that repair wounds and form granulation tissue
   c. Improves complete healing from 35% to 50%
   d. May increase cancer mortality (but not cancer incidence)

G. Surgical Therapy
1. Drainage and debridement are very important.
2. Amputation: often required; if caught early, can maintain structural integrity of the foot

V. OSTEOMYELITIS

Patient Case

7. W.A. is a 55-year-old man who presents with weight loss, malaise, and severe back pain and spasms that have progressed during the past 2 months. He has also experienced loss of sensation in his lower extremities. Four months before this admission, he had surgery for a fractured tibia, followed by an infection treated with unknown antibiotics. W.A. has hypertension and diverticulitis. On physical examination, he is alert and oriented, with the following vital signs: temperature 99.4°F (37.4°C); heart rate 88 beats/minute; respiratory rate 14 breaths/minute; and blood pressure 130/85 mm Hg. His laboratory values are within normal limits, except for WBC 14,300, erythrocyte sedimentation rate 89 mm/hour, and C-reactive protein 12 mg/dL. Magnetic resonance imaging shows bony destruction of lumbar vertebrae 1 and 2, which is confirmed by a bone scan. A computed tomography–guided bone biopsy shows gram-positive cocci in clusters. Which one of the following is the best initial therapy for W.A.?

A. Vancomycin 15 mg/kg intravenously every 12 hours—duration of antibiotics: 6 weeks.
B. Nafcillin 2 g intravenously every 6 hours—duration of antibiotics: 2 weeks.
C. Levofloxacin 750 mg/day orally—duration of antibiotics: 6 weeks.
D. Ampicillin-sulbactam 3 g intravenously every 6 hours—duration of antibiotics: 2 weeks.

A. Introduction
  1. Infection of the bone with subsequent bone destruction
  2. Around 20 cases per 100,000

B. Characteristics (Table 6)

Table 6. Characteristics of Osteomyelitis

	Hematogenous Spread	**Contiguous Spread**	**Vascular Insufficiency**
Definition	Spread of bacteria through the bloodstream from a distant site	Spread of bacteria from an adjacent tissue infection or by direct inoculation	Infection results from insufficient blood supply to fight the bacteria
Patient population	Children (< 16 years) - Femur, tibia, humerus, vertebrae	Adults (25–50 years) - Femur, tibia, skull	Adults (> 50 years)
Predisposing factors	1. Bacteremia (IV catheters, IVDA, skin infections, URI, etc.) 2. Sickle cell anemia	1. Open reduction of fractures 2. Gunshot wound 3. Dental/sinus infections 4. Soft tissue infections	1. Diabetes 2. PVD 3. Post-CABG (sternum)

Common pathogens	Usually monomicrobial
	
	1. Children
	  S. aureus (60%–90%) *S. epidermidis, S. pyogenes, S. pneumoniae, H. influenzae, P. aeruginosa, Enterobacter, E. coli* (all < 5%)
	2. Adult
	  S. aureus and gram-negative bacilli
	3. Sickle cell anemia
	  Salmonella (67%)
	  S. pneumoniae
	4. IV drug abusers
	  P. aeruginosa
		Usually mixed infection
		
		S. aureus (60%)
		S. epidermidis
		Streptococcus
		Gram-negative bacilli
		  P. aeruginosa (foot punctures), *Proteus, Klebsiella, E. coli*
		Anaerobic (human bites, decubitus ulcers)
			Usually polymicrobial
			
			S. aureus
			S. epidermidis
			Streptococcus
			Gram-negative bacilli
			Anaerobic (*Bacteroides fragilis* group)
			
			Infected prosthesis:
			S. aureus
			S. epidermidis

CABG = coronary artery bypass graft; IV = intravenous; IVDA = intravenous drug abuse; PVD = pulmonary vascular disease; URI = upper respiratory infection.

C. Clinical Presentation
   1. Signs and symptoms
      a. Fever and chills
      b. Localized pain, tenderness, and swelling
      c. Neurologic symptoms if spinal cord compression
   2. Laboratory tests
      a. Elevated WBC
      b. Elevated erythrocyte sedimentation rate
      c. Elevated C-reactive protein
   3. Diagnostic tests
      a. Radiographic tests: Positive results lag behind infectious process.
      b. Computed tomography and magnetic resonance imaging scans
      c. Radionuclide imaging: positive as soon as 24–48 hours after infectious process begins

D. Empiric Therapy
   1. Neonates younger than 1 month
      a. Nafcillin plus cefotaxime OR
      b. Nafcillin plus an aminoglycoside
   2. Infants (1–36 months)
      a. Cefuroxime
      b. Ceftriaxone
      c. Nafcillin plus cefotaxime
   3. Pediatrics (older than 3 years)
      a. Nafcillin or cefazolin or clindamycin
   4. Adults
      a. Nafcillin or cefazolin or vancomycin
      b. Choose additional antibiotics on the basis of patient-specific characteristics.
   5. Patients with sickle cell anemia
      a. Nafcillin plus ampicillin
   6. Prosthetic joint infections
      a. Vancomycin plus rifampin or nafcillin plus rifampin

E. Therapy Length
   1. Acute osteomyelitis: 4–6 weeks
   2. Chronic osteomyelitis: 6–8 weeks of parenteral therapy and 3–12 months of oral therapy

F. Criteria for Effective Oral Therapy for Osteomyelitis
   1. Adherence
   2. Identified organism that is highly susceptible to the oral antibiotic used
   3. C-reactive protein less than 2.0 mg/dL
   4. Adequate surgical debridement
   5. Resolving clinical course

VI. CENTRAL NERVOUS SYSTEM INFECTIONS

A. Meningitis: Introduction
1. Incidence: about 8.6 cases per 100,000 population
2. More males than females
3. More common in children

B. Microbiology (Table 7)
1. Bacterial (septic meningitis)

Table 7. Bacterial Etiology of Meningitis, Based on Age

Age	Most Likely Organisms	Less Common Organisms
< 1 month (newborns)	S. agalactiae E. coli Klebsiella sp. Enterobacter sp.	Listeria monocytogenes Herpes simplex, type 2
1 month to 2 years	S. pneumoniae N. meningitidis S. agalactiae H. influenzae	Viruses E. coli
2–50 years	N. meningitidis S. pneumoniae	Viruses
> 50 years	S. pneumoniae N. meningitidis	L. monocytogenes; aerobic gram-negative bacilli; viruses

2. Other causes (aseptic meningitis)
   a. Viral
   b. Fungal
   c. Parasitic
   d. Tubercular
   e. Syphilis
   f. Drugs (e.g., TMZ/SMZ, ibuprofen)

C. Predisposing Factors
1. Head trauma
2. Immunosuppression
3. Central nervous system shunts
4. Cerebrospinal fluid fistula/leak
5. Neurosurgical patients
6. Alcoholism
7. Local infections
   a. Sinusitis
   b. Otitis media
   c. Pharyngitis
   d. Bacterial pneumonia
8. Splenectomized patients
9. Sickle cell disease
10. Congenital defects

D. Clinical Presentation
   1. Symptoms
      a. Fever, chills
      b. Headache, backache, nuchal rigidity, mental status changes, photophobia
      c. Nausea, vomiting, anorexia, poor feeding habits (infants)
      d. Petechiae/purpura (*N. meningitidis* meningitis)
   2. Physical signs
      a. Brudzinski sign
      b. Kernig sign
      c. Bulging fontanel

E. Diagnosis
   1. History and physical examination
   2. Lumbar puncture
      a. Increased opening pressure
      b. Composition in bacterial meningitis (Table 8)

Table 8. CSF Changes in Bacterial Meningitis

Component	Normal CSF	Bacterial Meningitis
Glucose	30–70 mg/dL (2/3 peripheral)	< 50 mg/dL (≤ 0.4 CSF:blood)
Protein	< 50 mg/dL	> 150 mg/dL
WBC	< 5/mm^3	> 1200/mm^3
pH	7.3	7.1
Lactic acid	< 14 mg/dL	> 35 mg/dL

CSF = cerebrospinal fluid; WBC = white blood cell count.

   c. Cerebrospinal fluid stains/studies
      i. Gram stain (microorganisms): helps identify organism in 60%–90% of cases
      ii. Latex agglutination: high sensitivity, 50%–100%, for common organisms
         (a) Not recommended routinely
         (b) Most useful in patients pretreated with antibiotics with subsequent negative CSF Gram stains and cultures
      iii. Acid-fast staining (tubercular meningitis)
      iv. India ink test (*Cryptococcus*)
      v. Cryptococcal antigen
      vi. Herpes simplex virus-polymerase chain reaction
   3. Laboratory findings
      a. Increased WBC with a left shift
      b. Cerebrospinal fluid Gram stain
      c. Cerebrospinal fluid cultures (positive in 75%–80% of bacterial meningitis cases)
      d. Blood cultures (±)
      e. C-reactive protein concentrations: high negative predictive value

Patient Case

8. D.M. is a 21-year-old university student who presents to the emergency department with the worst headache of his life. During the past few days, he has felt slightly ill but has been able to go to class regularly and eat and drink adequately. This morning, he awoke with a terrible headache and pain whenever he moved his neck. He has no significant medical history and takes no medications. He cannot remember the last time he received a vaccination. On physical examination, he is in extreme pain (10/10) with the following vital signs: temperature 102.4°F (39.1°C); heart rate 110 beats/minute; respiratory rate 18 breaths/minute; and blood pressure 130/75 mm Hg. His laboratory values are within normal limits, except for WBC 22,500 (82 polymorphonuclear leukocytes, 11 band neutrophils, 5 lymphocytes, and 2 monocytes). A computed tomography scan of the head was normal, so a lumbar puncture was performed with the following results: glucose 44 mg/dL (peripheral, 110); protein 220 mg/dL; and WBC 800/mm^3 (85% neutrophils, 15% lymphocytes). Gram staining shows abundant gram-negative cocci. Which one of the following is the best empiric therapy for D.M.?

   A. Penicillin G 4 million units intravenously every 4 hours plus dexamethasone 4 mg intravenously every 6 hours.
   B. Ceftriaxone 2 g intravenously every 12 hours.
   C. Ceftriaxone 2 g intravenously every 12 hours plus dexamethasone 4 mg intravenously every 6 hours.
   D. Ceftriaxone 2 g intravenously every 12 hours plus vancomycin 1000 mg intravenously every 12 hours.

F. Empiric Therapy
   1. Neonates younger than 1 month
      a. Ampicillin plus aminoglycoside OR
      b. Ampicillin plus cefotaxime
   2. Infants (1-23 months)
      a. Third-generation cephalosporin (cefotaxime or ceftriaxone) plus vancomycin
   3. Pediatrics and adults (2–50 years)
      a. Third-generation cephalosporin (cefotaxime or ceftriaxone) plus vancomycin
   4. The elderly (50 years and older)
      a. Third-generation cephalosporin (cefotaxime or ceftriaxone) plus ampicillin plus vancomycin
   5. Penetrating head trauma, post-neurosurgery, or CSF shunt
      a. Vancomycin plus cefepime, ceftazidime, or meropenem

G. Therapy for Common Pathogens
   1. *S. pneumoniae*
      a. A minimum inhibitory concentration (MIC) equal to 0.1 mcg/mL or less
         i. Penicillin G 4 million units intravenously every 4 hours
         ii. Ampicillin 2 g intravenously every 4 hours
         iii. Alternative: third-generation cephalosporin or chloramphenicol
      b. An MIC 0.1–1.0 mcg/mL
         i. Third-generation cephalosporin
         ii. Alternative: cefepime or meropenem
      c. An MIC 2.0 mcg/mL or greater
         i. Vancomycin plus a third-generation cephalosporin
         ii. Alternative: moxifloxacin

2. *Neisseria meningitidis*
    a. An MIC less than 0.1 mcg/mL
        i. Penicillin G 4 million units intravenously every 4 hours
        ii. Ampicillin 2 g intravenously every 4 hours
        iii. Alternative: third-generation cephalosporin or chloramphenicol
    b. An MIC 0.1–1.0 mcg/mL
        i. Third-generation cephalosporin
        ii. Alternative: chloramphenicol, fluoroquinolone, or meropenem
3. *H. influenzae*
    a. β-Lactamase negative
        i. Ampicillin 2 g intravenously every 4 hours
        ii. Alternative: third-generation cephalosporin, cefepime, chloramphenicol, or fluoroquinolone
    b. β-Lactamase positive
        i. Third-generation cephalosporin
        ii. Alternative: cefepime, chloramphenicol, or fluoroquinolone
4. *S. agalactiae*
    a. Penicillin G 4 million units intravenously every 4 hours
    b. Ampicillin 2 g intravenously every 4 hours
    c. Alternative: third-generation cephalosporin
5. *Listeria monocytogenes*
    a. Penicillin G 4 million units intravenously every 4 hours
    b. Ampicillin 2 g intravenously every 4 hours
    c. Alternative: TMZ/SMZ or meropenem

H. Therapy Length: Based on Clinical Experience, Not on Clinical Data
   1. *N. meningitidis:* 7 days
   2. *H. influenzae:* 7 days
   3. *S. pneumoniae:* 10–14 days
I. Adjunctive Corticosteroid Therapy
   1. Risks versus benefits
       a. Significantly less hearing loss and other neurologic sequelae in children receiving dexamethasone for *H. influenzae* meningitis
       b. Significantly improved outcomes, including decreased mortality, in adults receiving dexamethasone for *S. pneumoniae* meningitis
       c. May decrease antibiotic penetration
       d. Decreased penetration of vancomycin in animals after dexamethasone
   2. Dose and administration
       a. Give corticosteroids 10–20 minutes before or at same time as antibiotics.
       b. Dexamethasone 0.15 mg/kg every 6 hours for 2–4 days
       c. Use in children with *H. influenzae* meningitis or in adults with pneumococcal meningitis; however, may need to initiate before knowing specific causative bacteria

Patient Case

9. After D.M.'s diagnosis, there is concern about prophylaxis. Which one of the following is the best recommendation for meningitis prophylaxis?
   A. The health care providers in close contact with D.M. should receive rifampin 600 mg every 12 hours for four doses.
   B. Everyone in D.M.'s dormitory and in all his classes should receive rifampin 600 mg/day for 4 days.
   C. Everyone in the emergency department at the time of D.M.'s presentation should receive the meningococcal polysaccharide vaccine.
   D. Everyone in the emergency department at the time of D.M.'s presentation should receive rifampin 600 mg every 12 hours for four doses.

J. Prophylaxis
   1. *S. pneumoniae*
      a. Pneumococcal conjugate vaccine: 7 valent
         i. All children younger than 23 months
         ii. Children 24–59 months with high-risk status
            (a) Certain chronic diseases
            (b) Alaska Native or American Indian
            (c) African American
            (d) Day care attendees
      b. Pneumococcal polysaccharide vaccine: 23 valent
         i. Give to those at risk (see patient groups in pneumonia section above).
   2. *N. meningitidis*
      a. Chemoprophylaxis: for close contacts (household or day care) and exposure to oral secretions of index case
         i. Rifampin:
            (a) Adults: 600 mg every 12 hours × 4 doses
            (b) Children: 10 mg/kg every 12 hours × 4 doses
            (c) Infants (younger than 1 month): 5 mg/kg every 12 hours × 4 doses
         ii. Ciprofloxacin 500 mg orally × 1 (adults only)
         iii. Ceftriaxone 125-250 mg intramuscularly × 1
      b. Meningococcal polysaccharide vaccine (Menomune) and meningococcal conjugate vaccine (Menactra) (both lack serogroup B)
         i. Indications (use Menactra unless patient is older than 55 years)
            (a) Young adolescents (11-12 years)
            (b) College freshmen living in dormitories (4 cases per 100,000 per year, especially freshmen living in dormitories)
            (c) Military recruits
            (d) Travel to "meningitis belt" of Africa and Asia, Saudi Arabia for Islamic Hajj pilgrimage
            (e) People with asplenia (anatomic or functional)
            (f) People with terminal complement component deficiencies
            (g) Outbreaks of meningococcal disease

3. *H. influenzae*
   a. Chemoprophylaxis: for everyone in households with unvaccinated children
      i. Adults: rifampin 600 mg/day for 4 days
      ii. Children (1 month to 12 years): rifampin 20 mg/kg/day for 4 days
      iii. Infants younger than 1 month: rifampin 10 mg/kg/day for 4 days
   b. *H. influenzae* type B polysaccharide vaccine
      i. All children
      ii. Indications regardless of age
         (a) Asplenia (anatomic or functional)
         (b) Sickle cell disease
         (c) Hodgkin disease
         (d) Hematologic neoplasms
         (e) Solid-organ transplantation
         (f) Severely immunocompromised (non-HIV related)
      iii. Consider for people with HIV infection

K. Brain Abscess
   1. Pathophysiology
      a. Direct extension or retrograde septic phlebitis from otitis media, mastoiditis, sinusitis, and facial cellulitis
      b. Hematogenous: particularly lung abscess or infective endocarditis: 3%–20% have no detectable focus
   2. Signs and symptoms
      a. Expanding intracranial mass lesion: focal neurologic deficits
      b. Headache
      c. Fever
      d. Seizures
      e. Mortality is about 50%.
   3. Microbiology
      a. Usually polymicrobial
      b. *Streptococcus* in 50%–60%
      c. Anaerobes in about 40%
   4. Therapy
      a. Incision and drainage: by craniotomy or stereotaxic needle aspiration
      b. Suggested empiric regimens based on source of infection
         i. Otitis media or mastoiditis: metronidazole plus third-generation cephalosporin
         ii. Sinusitis: metronidazole plus third-generation cephalosporin
         iii. Dental sepsis: penicillin plus metronidazole
         iv. Trauma or post-neurosurgery: vancomycin plus third-generation cephalosporin
         v. Lung abscess, empyema: penicillin plus metronidazole plus sulfonamide
         vi. Unknown: vancomycin plus metronidazole plus third-generation cephalosporin
      c. Corticosteroids if increased intracranial pressure

VII. ENDOCARDITIS

Patient Case

10. T.S. is a 48-year-old man who presents to the emergency department complaining of fever, chills, nausea/vomiting, anorexia, lymphangitis in his right hand, and lower back pain. He has no significant medical history except for kidney stones 4 years ago. He has no known drug allergies. He is homeless and was an intravenous drug abuser (heroin) for the past year but quit 2 weeks ago. On physical examination, he is alert and oriented, with the following vital signs: temperature 100.8°F (38°C); heart rate 114 beats/minute; respiratory rate 12 breaths/minute; and blood pressure 127/78 mm Hg. He has a faint systolic ejection murmur, and his right hand is erythematous and swollen. His laboratory values were all within normal limits. He had an HIV test 1 year ago, which was negative. One blood culture was obtained that later grew MSSA. Two more cultures were obtained that are now growing gram-positive cocci in clusters. A transesophageal echocardiogram shows vegetation on the mitral valve. Which one of the following therapeutic regimens is appropriate for T.S.?
    A. Nafcillin intravenous therapy—antibiotic duration: 2 weeks.
    B. Nafcillin intravenously plus rifampin therapy—antibiotic duration: 6 weeks or longer.
    C. Nafcillin intravenously plus gentamicin intravenous therapy—antibiotic duration: 2 weeks of both antibiotics.
    D. Nafcillin intravenously plus gentamicin—antibiotic duration: 6 weeks (nafcillin) with first 3–5 days of gentamicin.

A. Introduction
   1. Infection of the heart valves or other endocardial tissue
   2. Platelet-fibrin complex becomes infected with microorganisms—vegetation
   3. Main risk factors include mitral valve prolapse, prosthetic valves, and intravenous drug abuse.
   4. Three or four cases per 100,000 population per year

B. Presentation/Clinical Findings
   1. Signs and symptoms
      a. Fever: low grade and remittent
      b. Cutaneous manifestations (50% of patients): petechiae (including conjunctival), Janeway lesions, splinter hemorrhage
      c. Cardiac murmur (90% of patients)
      d. Arthralgias, myalgias, low back pain, arthritis
      e. Fatigue, anorexia, weight loss, night sweats
   2. Laboratory findings
      a. Anemia: normochromic, normocytic
      b. Leukocytosis
      c. Elevated erythrocyte sedimentation rate and C-reactive protein
      d. Positive blood culture in 78%–95% of patients
   3. Complications
      a. Congestive heart failure: 38%–60% of patients
      b. Emboli: 22%–43% of patients
      c. Mycotic aneurysm: 5%–10% of patients

C. Microbiology (Table 9)
  1. Three to five blood cultures of at least 10 mL each should be drawn during the first 24–48 hours.
  2. Empiric therapy should be initiated only in acutely ill patients. In these patients, three blood samples should be drawn during a 15- to 20-minute period before initiating antibiotics.

Table 9. Incidence of Microorganisms in Endocarditis

Organism	Incidence (%)
Streptococcus	50
S. aureus	25
Enterococcus	8
Coagulase-negative *Staphylococcus*	7
Gram-negative bacilli	6
Candida albicans	2

D. Treatment (Table 10)

Table 10. Treatment Recommendation for Endocarditis

Organism	Recommended Therapy	Length of Therapy (weeks) Native Valve	Prosthetic Valve
Streptococcus viridans (with penicillin MIC ≤ 0.12 mcg/mL)	Penicillin G	4	—
	Penicillin G + gentamicin	2	6[a]
	Ceftriaxone	4	—
	Ceftriaxone + gentamicin	2	6[a]
	Vancomycin	4	6
Streptococcus viridans (with penicillin MIC > 0.12 mcg/mL)	Penicillin G + gentamicin	4[b]	6
	Ceftriaxone + gentamicin	4[b]	6
	Vancomycin	4	6
Staphylococcus—methicillin sensitive	Oxacillin or nafcillin - ± Gentamicin for 3–5 days - Plus rifampin in prosthetic valves	6	≥ 6[b]
	Cefazolin - ± Gentamicin for 3–5 days - Plus rifampin in prosthetic valves	6	≥ 6[b]
	Vancomycin (only if severe PCN allergy) - Plus rifampin in prosthetic valves	6	≥ 6[b]
Staphylococcus—methicillin resistant	Vancomycin - Plus rifampin in prosthetic valves	6	≥ 6[b]
Enterococcus	Penicillin G or ampicillin + gentamicin or streptomycin	4–6	6
	Vancomycin + gentamicin or streptomycin	6	6
Enterococcus—penicillin resistant	Ampicillin-sulbactam or vancomycin + gentamicin	6	6
E. faecium—penicillin, aminoglycoside, and vancomycin resistant	Linezolid	≥ 8	≥ 8
	Quinupristin-dalfopristin	≥ 8	≥ 8
E. faecalis—penicillin, aminoglycoside, and vancomycin resistant	Imipenem-cilastatin + ampicillin	≥ 8	≥ 8
	Ceftriaxone + ampicillin	≥ 8	≥ 8
HACEK group	Ceftriaxone	4	6
	Ampicillin-sulbactam	4	6
	Fluoroquinolone (cipro-, levo-, gati-, moxi)	4	6

[a]Gentamicin can be added for 2 weeks if creatinine clearance is greater than 30 mL/minute.
[b]Gentamicin for 2 weeks.
HACEK = [*Haemophilus, Actinobacillus Cardiobacterium, Eikenella, Kingella*] group; MIC = minimum inhibitory concentration; PCN = penicillin.

E. Prophylaxis (Table 11)
   1. Risk categories

Table 11. Endocarditis Prophylaxis

Conditions in Which Prophylaxis Is Necessary	Dental Procedures That Require Prophylaxis

- Prosthetic cardiac valves including bioprosthetic and homograft valves
- Previous bacterial endocarditis
- Congenital heart disease
   - Unrepaired cyanotic congenital heart disease
   - Completely repaired congenital heart defect with prosthetic material or device, during the first 6 months after the procedure
   - Repaired congenital heart disease with residual defects adjacent to or at the site of a prosthetic patch or device
- Cardiac transplant recipients who develop cardiac valvulopathy
	- Any dental procedure that involves the gingival tissues or periapical region of a tooth and for procedures that perforate the oral mucosa

	Other Procedures That Require Prophylaxis
	Respiratory tract - Tonsillectomy and/or adenoidectomy - Surgical operations that involve an incision or biopsy of the respiratory mucosa

F. Recommended Prophylaxis for Dental or Respiratory Tract Procedures (Table 12)

Table 12. Prophylaxis for Dental or Respiratory Tract Procedures

Situation	Agent	Regimen
Standard general prophylaxis	Amoxicillin	Adults: 2 g; children: 50 mg/kg 1 hour before procedure
Unable to take oral medications	Ampicillin	Adults: 2 g IM/IV; children: 50 mg/kg IM/IV within 30 minutes before procedure
	Cefazolin or ceftriaxone	Adults: 1 g IM/IV; children: 50 mg/kg IM/IV within 30 minutes before procedure
Allergic to penicillin	Clindamycin	Adults: 600 mg; children: 20 mg/kg 1 hour before procedure
	Cephalexin	Adults: 2 g; children: 50 mg/kg 1 hour before procedure
	Azithromycin or clarithromycin	Adults: 500 mg; children: 15 mg/kg 1 hour before procedure
Allergic to penicillin and unable to take oral medications	Clindamycin	Adults: 600 mg; children: 20 mg/kg IV within 30 minutes before procedure
	Cefazolin or ceftriaxone	Adults: 1 g IM/IV; children: 50 mg/kg IM/IV within 30 minutes before procedure

IM = intramuscularly; IV = intravenously.

Patient Case

11. Six months after treatment of his endocarditis, T.S. is visiting his dentist for a tooth extraction. Which of the following antibiotics is best for prophylaxis?
    A. Tooth extractions do not require endocarditis prophylaxis.
    B. Administer amoxicillin 2 g 1 hour before the extraction.
    C. Administer amoxicillin 3 g 1 hour before the extraction and 1.5 g 6 hours after the extraction.
    D. T.S. is not at increased risk of endocarditis and does not need prophylactic antibiotics.

Infectious Diseases

VIII. PERITONITIS/INTRA-ABDOMINAL INFECTIONS

A. Introduction
   1. Definition: inflammation of the peritoneum (serous membrane lining the abdominal cavity)
   2. Types
      a. Primary: spontaneous/idiopathic—no primary focus of infection
      b. Secondary: occurs secondary to an abdominal process

B. Primary Peritonitis
   1. Etiology
      a. Alcoholic cirrhosis and ascites (peritonitis occurs in 10% of these patients)
      b. Other: postnecrotic cirrhosis, chronic active hepatitis, acute viral hepatitis, congestive heart failure, systemic lupus erythematous, metastatic malignancy (common underlying problem is ascites)
   2. Microbiology
      a. *E. coli*
      b. *K. pneumoniae*
      c. *S. pneumoniae*
      d. Group A Streptococcus
   3. Pathogenesis
      a. Hematogenous: Portosystemic shunting increases bacteria in the blood, infecting ascitic collection.
      b. Lymphogenous
      c. Transmural through the intact gut wall from the lumen
      d. Vaginally through the fallopian tubes
   4. Clinical manifestations/diagnosis
      a. Fever
      b. Abdominal pain
      c. Nausea, vomiting, diarrhea
      d. Diffuse abdominal tenderness, rebound tenderness, hypoactive or no bowel sounds
      e. Ascitic fluid
         i. Protein: low because of hypoalbuminemia or dilution with transudate fluid from the portal system
         ii. White blood cell count: more than 300/mm^3 (85% have more than 1000/mm^3)—primarily granulocytes
         iii. pH: less than 7.35
         iv. Lactic acid: more than 25 mg/dL
         v. Gram stain: 60%–80% are negative, but diagnostic if it is positive

C. Secondary Peritonitis
   1. Etiology
      a. Injuries to the gastrointestinal tract including
         i. Peptic ulcer perforation
         ii. Perforation of a gastrointestinal organ
         iii. Appendicitis
         iv. Endometritis secondary to intrauterine device

v. Bile peritonitis
vi. Pancreatitis
vii. Operative contamination
viii. Diverticulitis
ix. Intestinal neoplasms
x. Secondary to peritoneal dialysis
2. Microbiology of intra-abdominal infections
   a. Stomach/proximal small intestine: aerobic and facultative gram-positive and gram-negative organisms
   b. Ileum: *E. coli, Enterococcus*, anaerobes
   c. Large intestine: obligate anaerobes (i.e., *Bacteroides, Clostridium perfringens*), aerobic and facultative gram-positive and gram-negative organisms (i.e., *E. coli, Streptococcus, Enterococcus, Klebsiella, Proteus, Enterobacter*)
3. Clinical manifestations/diagnosis
   a. Fever, tachycardia
   b. Increased WBC
   c. Abdominal pain aggravated by motion, rebound tenderness
   d. Bowel paralysis
   e. Pain with breathing
   f. Decreased renal perfusion
   g. Ascitic fluid
      i. Protein: high (more than 3 g/dL)—exudate fluid
      ii. White blood cell count: many, primarily granulocytes

D. Therapy
   1. Therapy is not necessary for
      a. Bowel injuries caused by trauma that are repaired within 12 hours (treat for less than 24 hours)
      b. Intraoperative contamination by enteric contents (treat for less than 24 hours)
      c. Perforations of the stomach, duodenum, and proximal jejunum (unless patient is on antacid therapy or has malignancy) (treat < 24 hours)
      d. Acute appendicitis without evidence of perforation, abscess, or peritonitis (treat < 24 hours)
   2. Mild to moderate community-acquired infection
      a. Cefoxitin
      b. Cefazolin, cefuroxime, ceftriaxone or cefotaxime plus metronidazole
      c. Ticarcillin/clavulanate
      d. Ertapenem
      e. Moxifloxacin
      f. Ciprofloxacin or levofloxacin plus metronidazole
      g. Tigecycline
   3. High risk or severity community-acquired or health care–acquired infection
      a. Piperacillin/tazobactam
      b. Ceftazidime or cefepime plus metronidazole
      c. Imipenem/cilastatin or meropenem or doripenem
      d. Ciprofloxacin or levofloxacin plus metronidazole (not for health care-acquired infections)
   4. Duration of therapy: 4–7 days (unless source control is difficult)

Infectious Diseases

IX. CLOSTRIDIUM DIFFICILE INFECTION

A. Introduction
1. *Clostridium difficile* is transmitted by the fecal-oral route.
2. Overgrowth in the gastrointestinal tract occurs after antibiotic therapy.
3. Risk factors: hospital stays, medical comorbidities, extremes of age, immunodeficiency states, advancing age, use of broad-spectrum antibiotics for extended periods
4. Production of endotoxins A and B causes pathogenesis.
5. Symptoms: watery diarrhea, abdominal pain, leukocytosis, gastrointestinal complications
6. New strain (BI/NAP-1) produces more enterotoxin, produces binary toxin, has increased sporulation capacity, and is resistant to fluoroquinolones. Increased risk of metronidazole failure, morbidity, and mortality

B. Therapy
1. Initial episode and first recurrence
   a. Metronidazole 500 mg orally or intravenously 3 or 4 times/day for 10–14 days
   b. Vancomycin 125 mg orally 4 times/day for 10–14 days
2. Second and third recurrences
   a. Can consider higher doses of vancomycin (500 mg orally 4 times/day)
   b. Taper therapy: vancomycin 125 mg orally 4 times/day for 14 days, 2 times/day for 7 days, and daily for 7 days
   c. Pulse therapy: recommended vancomycin course of therapy for initial episode (for 10–14 days), followed by vancomycin every other day for 8 days, and then every 3 days for 15 days
   d. Consider rifaximin 400 mg 2 times/day for 14 days.

X. MEDICAL/SURGICAL PROPHYLAXIS

A. Introduction
1. Prophylaxis: administration of the putative agent before bacterial contamination occurs
2. Early therapy: immediate or prompt institution of therapy as soon as the patient presents; usually contamination or infection will have preceded the initiation of therapy (e.g., dirty wounds)

Patient Case

12. You are a pharmacist who works closely with the surgery department to optimize therapy for patients undergoing surgical procedures at your institution. The surgeons provide you with principles of surgical prophylaxis that they believe are appropriate. Which one of the following provided principles is acceptable?
    A. Antibiotics should be redosed for extended surgical procedures; redose if the surgery lasts longer than 4 hours or involves considerable blood loss.
    B. All patients should be given antibiotics for 24 hours after the procedure; this will optimize prophylaxis.
    C. Preoperative antibiotics can be given up to 4 hours before the incision; this will make giving the antibiotics logistically easier.
    D. Vancomycin should be the antibiotic of choice for surgical wound prophylaxis because of its long half-life and activity against MRSA.

B. Classification of Surgical Procedures (Table 13)

Table 13. Classification of Surgical Procedures

Surgical Procedure	Infection Rate (%)
Clean: No entry is made in the respiratory, gastrointestinal, or genitourinary tracts or in the oropharyngeal cavity. In general, it is elective with no break in technique and no inflammation encountered	1–4
Clean contaminated: Entry in the respiratory, gastrointestinal, genitourinary, or biliary tracts or oropharyngeal cavity without unusual contamination. Includes clean procedures with a minor break in technique	5–15
Contaminated: Includes fresh traumatic wounds, gross spillage from the gastrointestinal tract (without a mechanical bowel preparation), a major break in technique, or incisions encountering acute, nonpurulent inflammation	16–25
Dirty: Includes procedures involving old traumatic wounds, perforated viscera, or clinically evident infection	30–45

C. Risk Factors for Postoperative Wound Infections
   1. Bacterial contamination
      a. Exogenous sources
         i. Flaw in aseptic technique
      b. Endogenous sources
         i. Most important except in clean procedures
         ii. Patient flora causes infection
   2. Host resistance
      a. Extremes of age
      b. Nutrition (i.e., malnourished patients)
      c. Obesity
      d. Diabetes mellitus
         i. Decreased wound healing and increased risk of infection
      e. Immunocompromised
      f. Hypoxemia
      g. Remote infection
      h. Presence of foreign body
         i. Healthy person tolerates inoculum of 10^5
         ii. In presence of foreign body, need only 10^2

D. Indications for Surgical Prophylaxis
   1. Common postoperative infection with low morbidity
   2. Uncommon postoperative infection with significant morbidity and mortality

E. Principles of Prophylaxis (Figure 1; Tables 14 and 15)
   1. Timing: Antibiotics must be present in the tissues at the time of bacterial contamination (incision) and throughout the operative period; "on-call" dosing is not acceptable.
      a. Conclusions
         i. Administering antibiotics any sooner than immediately preoperatively (within 60 minutes before incision) is unnecessary.
         ii. Initiating antibiotics postoperatively is no more effective than administering no prophylaxis.

b. Conclusions
   i. Antibiotics should be redosed for extended surgical procedures.
   ii. Redose if the surgery lasts longer than 4 hours (or more than 2 half-lives of the antibiotic) or involves considerable blood loss.

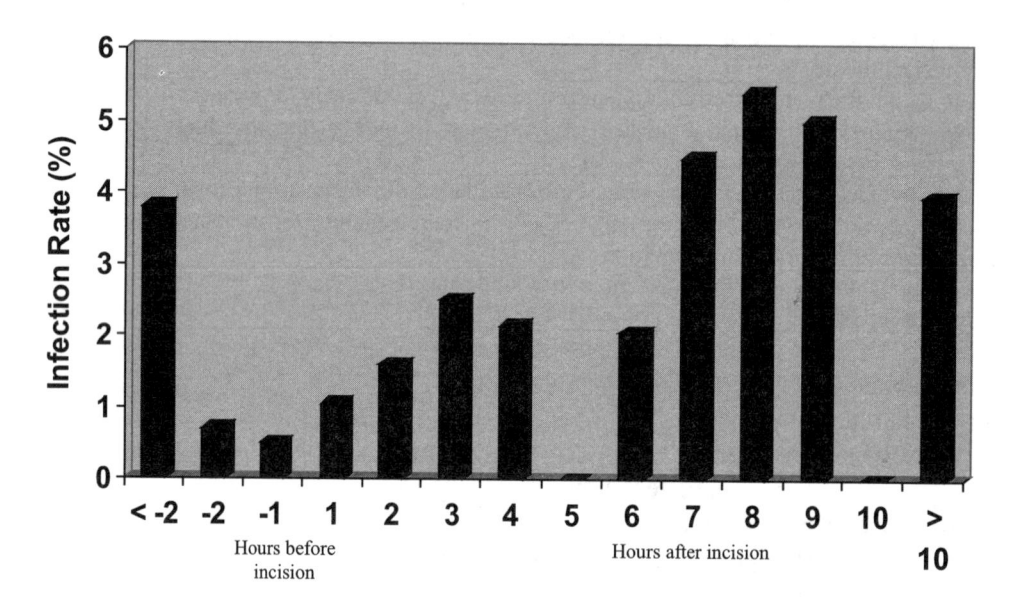

Figure 1. Principles of prophylaxis.

Information from Classen DC, Evans RS, Pestotnik SL, Horn SD, Menlove RL, Burke JP. The timing of prophylactic administration of antibiotics and the risk of surgical-wound infection. *N Engl J Med* 1992;326:281–6.

Table 14. Temporal Relation Between the Administration of Prophylactic Antibiotics and Rates of Surgical Wound Infection

Time of Administration[a]	No. of Patients	No. (%) of Infections	Relative Risk (95% CI)	Odds Ratio (95% CI)
Early	369	14 (3.8)	6.7 (2.9–14.7)	4.3 (1.8–10.4)
Preoperative	1708	10 (0.59)	1.0	
Perioperative	282	4 (1.4)	2.4 (0.9–7.9)	2.1 (0.6–7.4)
Postoperative	488	16 (3.3)	5.8 (2.6–12.3)	5.8 (2.4–13.8)
All	2847	44 (1.5)	—	—

[a]For the administration of antibiotics; "early" denotes 2–24 hours before the incision; "preoperative" 0–2 hours before the incision; "perioperative" within 3 hours after the incision; and "postoperative" more than 3 hours after the incision.
CI = confidence interval.

Table 15. Duration of Surgical Procedure and Risk of Infection

Duration of Surgical Procedures	Infections/Total Patients (%)	Infections/Standard Regimen Patients (%)	Infections/Cefoxitin Regimen Patients (%)
< 3 hours	0/46	0/29	0/17
≥ hours to ≤ 4 hours	4/46 (8.7)	2/21 (9.5)	2/25 (8.0)
> 4 hours	5/27 (18.5)	0/13	5/14 (35.7)

Information from Kaiser AB, Herrington JL Jr., Jacobs JK, Mulherin JL Jr., Roach AC, Sawyers JL. Cefoxitin versus erythromycin, neomycin, and cefazolin in colorectal operations. Importance of the duration of the surgical procedure. *Ann Surg* 1983;98:525–30.

2. Duration
    a. Most procedures, including gastrointestinal, orthopedic, and gynecologic procedures, require only antibiotics while the patient is in the operating room.
    b. Cardiac procedures may require 24 hours of antibiotics postsurgery.
3. Spectrum
    a. Need only activity against skin flora unless the operation violates a hollow viscus mucosa
    b. Gastrointestinal, genitourinary, hepatobiliary, and some pulmonary operations require additional antibiotics.
    c. Colorectal surgery is one procedure in which broad-spectrum aerobic and anaerobic coverage has been shown to be most effective.
    d. Attempt to avoid a drug that may be needed for therapy.
4. Adverse reactions/bacterial resistance
    a. Antibiotic prophylaxis should not cause greater morbidity than the infection it prevents.
    b. Overuse may lead to resistance, which could prevent further use of the antibiotic for surgical prophylaxis or other infections (duration of administration is an important factor).
5. Cost
    a. Prophylaxis can account for a significant portion of the antibiotic budget.
    b. Must be weighed against the cost of treating one person with a postoperative infection

F. Antibiotic Prophylaxis in Specific Surgical Procedures
   1. Gastrointestinal
      a. Gastric/duodenal
         i. Because of acidity, relatively little normal flora
         ii. Intragastric organisms and postoperative infections are increased with an increasing pH.
         iii. Indicated for morbid obesity, esophageal obstruction, decreased gastric acidity, or decreased gastrointestinal motility
         iv. Recommendation: cefazolin 1–2 g preinduction
      b. Biliary
         i. Biliary tract normally has no organisms.
         ii. Indicated for high-risk patients. (Often, intraoperative cholangiography shows unexpected common duct stones, so some studies recommend using antibiotics in all biliary surgery. In addition, studies have shown an increase in rates of infection without risk factors.)
         iii. Acute cholecystitis
         iv. Obstructive jaundice
         v. Common duct stones
         vi. Age older than 70 years
         vii. Recommendation: cefazolin (or cefoxitin) 1–2 g preinduction
      c. Appendectomy
         i. Acutely inflamed or normal appendix: less than 10% risk
         ii. Evidence of perforation: more than 50% risk (treatment required)
         iii. If perforated appendix, treat for 3–7 days
         iv. Recommendation: cefoxitin 1–2 g (or cefazolin plus metronidazole or ampicillin-sulbactam) preinduction

d. Colorectal
   i. A 30%–77% infection rate without antibiotics
   ii. One of the few surgical procedures in which coverage for aerobes and anaerobes has proved most effective
   iii. Preoperative antibiotics
      (a) Combined oral and parenteral regimens may be better than parenteral regimens alone.
      (b) Oral regimens are inexpensive; however, some data suggest they are less effective when used alone (without parenteral agents), have greater toxicity, and may increase the risk of *C. difficile* infections.
      (c) Recommendation: cefoxitin 1–2 g (or cefazolin plus metronidazole or ampicillin-sulbactam or ertapenem) preinduction OR gentamicin-tobramycin 1.5 mg/kg and clindamycin 600 mg–metronidazole 0.5–1 g preinduction with or without neomycin 1 g and erythromycin 1 g at 19, 18, and 9 hours before surgery or neomycin 2 g and metronidazole 2 g at 13 and 9 hours before surgery
      (d) Note: Mechanical bowel preparation is not recommended and may be harmful.
2. Obstetrics/gynecology
   a. Vaginal/abdominal hysterectomy
      i. Antibiotics have been found to be most effective in vaginal hysterectomies but generally are given for both procedures.
      ii. Recommendation: cefazolin or cefoxitin 1–2 g (or ampicillin-sulbactam) preinduction
   b. Cesarean section
      i. Recommendation: cefazolin 1–2 g after the cord is clamped

3. Cardiothoracic
   a. Cardiac surgery
      i. Antibiotics decrease risk of mediastinitis.
      ii. Recommendation: cefazolin or cefuroxime 1–2 g preinduction (plus intraoperative doses), if MRSA is probable or patient has been hospitalized, and then vancomycin
   b. Pulmonary resection (i.e., lobectomy and pneumonectomy)
      i. Recommendation: cefazolin or cefuroxime 1–2 g preinduction (or vancomycin)
   c. Vascular surgery
      i. High mortality with infected grafts
      ii. Recommendation: cefazolin 1 g preinduction and every 8 hours for three doses; if MRSA is probable, then use vancomycin
4. Orthopedic
   a. Prophylaxis is indicated when surgery involves prosthetic materials (i.e., total hip/knee, nail, or plate).
   b. Recommendation: cefazolin 1–2 g preinduction (or cefuroxime or vancomycin)
5. Head and neck
   a. Indicated for major surgical procedures when an incision is made through the oral or pharyngeal mucosa
   b. Recommendation: cefazolin 1–2 g or ampicillin-sulbactam 1.5–3 g preinduction or gentamicin 1.5 mg/kg and clindamycin 600–900 mg preinduction
6. Urologic
   a. In general, not recommended
   b. Indicated if patient has a positive urine culture before surgery (should treat and then operate)
   c. If therapy is unsuccessful, cover for the infecting organism and operate.

REFERENCES

Pneumonia
1. Mandell LA, Wunderink RG, Anzueto A, et al. Infectious Diseases Society of America/American Thoracic Society consensus guidelines on the management of community-acquired pneumonia in adults. Clin Infect Dis 2007;44(Suppl 2):S27–S72.
2. American Thoracic Society; Infectious Diseases Society of America. Guidelines for the management of adults with hospital-acquired, ventilator-associated, and healthcare-associated pneumonia. Am J Respir Crit Care Med 2005;171:388–416.
3. Chastre J, Fagon JY. Ventilator-associated pneumonia. Am J Respir Crit Care Med 2002;165:867–903.
4. Moscona A. Neuraminidase inhibitors for influenza. N Engl J Med 2005;353:1363–73.
5. Harper SA, Fukuda K, Uyeki TM, Cox NJ, Bridges CB; Advisory Committee on Immunization Practices (ACIP), Centers for Disease Control and Prevention (CDC). Prevention and control of influenza. Recommendations of the Advisory Committee on Immunization Practices (ACIP). MMWR Recomm Rep 2005;54:1–40.
6. Appelbaum PC. Resistance among *Streptococcus pneumoniae:* implications for drug selection. Clin Infect Dis 2002;34:1613–20.

Urinary Tract Infections
1. Warren JW, Abrutyn E, Hebel JR, Johnson JR, Schaeffer AJ, Stamm WE. Guidelines for antimicrobial treatment of uncomplicated acute bacterial cystitis and acute pyelonephritis in women. Clin Infect Dis 1999;29:745–58.
2. Treatment of urinary tract infections in nonpregnant women. ACOG Practice Bulletin No. 91. American College of Obstetricians and Gynecologists. Obstet Gynecol 2008;111:785–94.

Skin and Soft Tissue Infections
1. Swartz MN. Cellulitis. N Engl J Med 2004;350:904–12.
2. Stevens DL, Bisno AL, Chambers HF, et al. Practice guidelines for the diagnosis and management of skin and soft-tissue infections. Clin Infect Dis 2005;41:1373–406.
3. Lipsky BA, Berendt AR, Deery HG, et al. Diagnosis and treatment of diabetic foot infections. Clin Infect Dis 2004;39:885–910.

Osteomyelitis
1. Lew DP, Waldvogel FA. Osteomyelitis. Lancet 2004;364:369–79.

Central Nervous System Infections
1. Tunkel AR, Hartman BJ, Kaplan SL, et al. Practice guidelines for the management of bacterial meningitis. Clin Infect Dis 2004;39:1267–84.

Endocarditis
1. Wilson W, Taubert KA, Gewitz M, et al. Prevention of infective endocarditis. Guidelines from the American Heart Association. Circulation 2007;115:1656–8.
2. Baddour LM, Wilson WR, Bayer AS, et al. Infective endocarditis: diagnosis, antimicrobial therapy, and management of complications. Circulation 2005;111:3167–84.

Intra-abdominal Infections
1. Solomkin JS, Mazuski JE, Bradley JS, et al.; Infectious Diseases Society of America. Diagnosis and management of complicated intra-abdominal infection in adults and children: Guidelines by the Surgical Infection Society and the Infectious Diseases Society of America. Clin Infect Dis 2010;50:133-164.

Medical/Surgical Prophylaxis
1. American Society of Health-System Pharmacists. Therapeutic guidelines on antimicrobial prophylaxis in surgery. Am J Hosp Pharm 1999;56:1839–88.
2. American Society of Health-System Pharmacists. Therapeutic guidelines for nonsurgical antimicrobial prophylaxis. Am J Hosp Pharm 1999;56:1201–50.
3. Bratzler DW, Houck PM; Surgical Infection Prevention Guidelines Writers Workgroup. Antimicrobial prophylaxis for surgery: an advisory statement from the National Surgical Infection Prevention Project. Clin Infect Dis 2004;38:1706–15.

Infectious Diseases

ANSWERS AND EXPLANATIONS TO PATIENT CASES

1. Answer C
Although ampicillin-sulbactam has good activity against *H. influenza, Moraxella catarrhalis*, and *S. pneumoniae* (but not drug-resistant *S. pneumoniae* [DRSP]), it has no activity against atypical organisms (*L. pneumophila, M. pneumoniae, C. pneumoniae*). Current recommendations are to include a macrolide with a β-lactam antibiotic for hospitalized patients with community-acquired pneumonia. Piperacillin-tazobactam has good activity against *H. influenza, M. catarrhalis,* and *S. pneumoniae* (but not DRSP) and, with gentamicin, is excellent for pneumonia caused by most gram-negative organisms. However, this increased activity is not necessary for community-acquired pneumonia, and the combination has no activity against atypical organisms. Ceftriaxone plus azithromycin is the best initial choice. It has excellent activity against atypical organisms (because of azithromycin), *H. influenzae, M. catarrhalis,* and *S. pneumoniae* (even intermediate DRSP). Although doxycycline has activity against atypical organisms and most of the typical organisms that cause community-acquired pneumonia, it is not recommended as monotherapy in hospitalized patients. In addition, its activity against *S. pneumoniae* may be limited (if R.L. lives in an area with extensive DRSP). Doxycycline would not be the best initial choice.

2. Answer D
Ceftriaxone plus gentamicin plus linezolid is not good empiric therapy because ceftriaxone has limited activity against *P. aeruginosa*, and gentamicin has variable activity against *P. aeruginosa,* depending on the institution. Because B.P. has been on a ventilator and in an intensive care unit for 8 days, she is at increased risk of nosocomial pneumonia, specifically caused by *P. aeruginosa* (and possibly MRSA, depending on the institution). Although piperacillin-tazobactam has good activity against most of the common causes of nosocomial pneumonia (including *P. aeruginosa*), the most recent guidelines recommend two antibiotics with activity against *P. aeruginosa* for patients with severe nosocomial pneumonia, and she may require an antibiotic with MRSA activity. Levofloxacin has only moderate activity against *P. aeruginosa*, and two drugs should be used. Cefepime plus tobramycin plus vancomycin is the best empiric therapy because it includes two antibiotics with excellent activity against *P. aeruginosa* and another agent for MRSA.

3. Answer B
B.P. should receive vaccinations now. There are no contraindications to receiving either pneumococcal or influenza vaccine immediately after an episode of pneumonia. It is best to vaccinate whenever patients are available. B.P.'s age and medical history put her at risk of both pneumococcal disease and influenza. Therefore, administration of pneumococcal and influenza vaccines is indicated (if it is during the middle of influenza season and she was not vaccinated in the fall, she can receive the influenza vaccine now). B.P.'s age places her in a group needing both pneumococcal and influenza vaccines, regardless of the causative agent for her current infection.

4. Answer B
Although the treatment duration is correct for G.N.'s diagnosis (7 days), oral TMP/SMZ is inappropriate for complicated pyelonephritis. It will also interact with warfarin, increasing the risk of bleeding. Ciprofloxacin 400 mg intravenously 2 times/day and then 500 mg orally 2 times/day for 10 days is an appropriate choice and duration (7–14 days) for this complicated pyelonephritis (it may also interact with warfarin, but to a lesser extent than TMP/SMZ). It would be expected to have activity against the common organisms causing complicated pyelonephritis. Gentamicin for 3 days is too short a treatment duration, and ampicillin-sulbactam, followed by amoxicillin-clavulanate, is not recommended for complicated pyelonephritis.

5. Answer D
Diabetic foot infections are generally polymicrobial (average organisms, 2.5–5.8).

6. Answer C
Nafcillin has excellent activity against gram-positive organisms, but it would miss the gram-negative organisms and anaerobes often involved in moderate to severe diabetic foot infections. Tobramycin and levofloxacin would be good against aerobic organisms, but levofloxacin has only limited activity against anaerobes. Tobramycin may also not be a good choice for a patient with diabetes mellitus with long-term complications (because of the increased risk of nephrotoxicity). β-Lactamase inhibitor combinations are good agents because they have activity against the organisms that are often involved. Treatment duration may need to be extended if the bone is involved. Aggressive antibiotic treatment often prevents the need for an amputation.

7. Answer A
Because sensitivities of the gram-positive organism are still unknown, vancomycin is the best choice. In addition, the duration of therapy for osteomyelitis is 4–6 weeks. Therefore, the 2-week duration with nafcillin is too short. Although levofloxacin is advantageous because it can be given orally, it will probably not achieve adequate bone concentrations to eradicate *S. aureus* (the most likely organism). Ampicillin-sulbactam is effective against *S. aureus* (except for MRSA); its broad spectrum of activity is not necessary in this situation, and the duration is too short.

8. Answer D
Based on his presentation and laboratory values, D.M. has bacterial meningitis. The gram-negative cocci on Gram stain are most likely *N. meningitidis*. Penicillin is effective against *N. meningitides;* however, some strains are resistant, and until culture results are back, it is unwise to use this agent alone. Ceftriaxone alone is effective for meningococcal meningitis, but until the cultures actually grow *N. meningitides*, it is wise to maintain broader antibiotic activity. Dexamethasone is beneficial only in adults with pneumococcal meningitis (not meningococcal meningitis). Ceftriaxone is the appropriate empiric antibiotic therapy in this situation. Vancomycin is generally used empirically because of its activity against highly penicillin-resistant *S. pneumoniae*. After pneumococcal meningitis is ruled out on the basis of culture results, vancomycin can be discontinued.

9. Answer A
Only people in close contact to a patient with meningococcal meningitis require prophylaxis (primarily those who live closely with the patient and those who are exposed to oral secretions). The correct regimen is rifampin 600 mg every 12 hours for four doses. Although the vaccine is a good idea for those at future risk of acquiring this infection (e.g., college students living in dormitories), its use during an outbreak is very limited.

10. Answer D
The treatment duration is too short (nafcillin intravenously × 2 weeks) for *S. aureus* endocarditis. Only streptococcal endocarditis can be treated for 2 weeks. Although nafcillin intravenously plus rifampin therapy for 6 weeks or longer is an appropriate duration for MSSA, the rifampin does not need to be added in patients with native valve endocarditis. Nafcillin intravenously plus gentamicin intravenously × 2 weeks is too short for *S. aureus* endocarditis. Nafcillin intravenously × 6 weeks with gentamicin for the first 3–5 days is the recommended treatment for MSSA endocarditis. Gentamicin needs to be added for only 3–5 days to decrease the duration of bacteremia.

11. Answer B
T.S. is at increased risk of endocarditis because of his history of the disease. Tooth extractions require prophylaxis for those at risk. Amoxicillin 2 g, 1 hour before the tooth extraction, is the current recommended dose. The 2-g dose is adequate for protection, and a follow-up dose is not needed. Amoxicillin 3 g, 1 hour before the extraction, and 1.5 g, 6 hours after the extraction, is the older recommended dose. A follow-up dose is not needed.

12. Answer A
Redosing antibiotics for surgical prophylaxis is very important—especially for antibiotics with short half-lives, for extended surgical procedures, or for when there is extensive blood loss. Antibiotics given beyond the surgical procedure are generally unnecessary and only increase the potential for adverse drug reactions and resistant bacteria. Although preoperative antibiotics given up to 4 hours before the incision may improve the logistics of administering surgical prophylaxis, study results show that antibiotics need to be given as close to the time of the incision as possible (definitely within 2 hours). Vancomycin should not be used routinely for surgical prophylaxis. The Centers for Disease Control and Prevention does not recommend the use of vancomycin for "routine surgical prophylaxis other than in a patient with life-threatening allergy to b-lactam antibiotics."

ANSWERS AND EXPLANATIONS TO SELF-ASSESSMENT QUESTIONS

1. Answer A
The patient has community-acquired pneumonia that does not require hospitalization (CURB-65 score is 1 at most [no mention of mental status]). Because he has not received any antibiotics in the past 3 months and has no comorbidities, he is at low risk of DRSP. Therefore, the drug of choice is either a macrolide or doxycycline. Cefuroxime is not recommended for treatment of community-acquired pneumonia. Fluoroquinolones are only recommended if the patient has had recent antibiotics or has comorbidities. Trimethoprim-sulfamethoxazole is not used for community-acquired pneumonia.

2. Answer D
The symptoms in this patient (high temperature, malaise, dry cough, nasal congestion, and severe headaches) are most consistent with influenza; therefore, an antibacterial agent would not affect recovery. Oseltamivir should be initiated within 48 hours of symptom onset, and because this patient is more than 3 days out from symptom onset, oseltamivir will not affect recovery. Because of the viral etiology and time since symptom onset, symptomatic treatment is all that is indicated.

3. Answer B
A case-control study would be the most appropriate study design because it is the most ethical, cost-effective, timely methodology. A stronger study design—for instance, a prospective cohort study or a randomized, controlled trial—has many disadvantages if used to answer this question. In a prospective cohort study, too many patients would need to be observed because of the relatively low incidence of confirmed pneumococcal pneumonia. This study would therefore be too costly and take too long to complete. Randomized, controlled trials also have many disadvantages in this situation. First, patients would need to be vaccinated and then observed for at least 10 years. Second, too many patients would need to be observed because of the relatively low incidence of confirmed pneumococcal pneumonia. Third, it would be unethical to randomize half of the patients to no vaccination. This study would therefore be too costly, unethical, and time-consuming. A case series would evaluate only a small number of patients given a diagnosis of pneumococcal pneumonia 10 or more years after vaccination. It would not provide comparative data, nor would it provide a strong study design.

4. Answer C
Single-dose therapy is not recommended because of decreased cure rates and inadequate treatment of potential upper UTIs. Ciprofloxacin is an appropriate choice, but 7 days of therapy is not necessary. The best choice for this patient is TMP/SMZ double strength 2 times/day orally for 3 days. The patient should be counseled about the potential interaction between antibiotics and oral contraceptives. β-Lactams are not as effective as TMP/SMZ or fluoroquinolones, and data are limited on their use for 3 days.

5. Answer A
For the asymptomatic patient who is bedridden and chronically catheterized, with cloudy urine and bacteria shown by urinalysis, no therapy is indicated. All patients with chronic urinary catheters will be bacteriuric. Because this patient is asymptomatic, the catheter does not need to be replaced. If she were symptomatic, catheter replacement might be indicated. Antibiotics are not indicated; however, a 7-day course would be appropriate if treatment were instituted. A long course of treatment only increases the risk of acquiring resistant organisms.

6. Answer B
Using the equation $Cp = dose/V_d$, where V_d = volume of distribution, the concentration after the first dose can be calculated. The concentration is 19.8 mcg/mL. Therefore, it will take about 1 half-life to decrease to a concentration of 10 mcg/mL (i.e., 35 hours).

7. Answer A
Because cellulitis (which the patient appears to have) is most commonly caused by *Streptococcus* or *Staphylococcus*, nafcillin is the drug of choice (vancomycin could be initiated empirically if MRSA were a concern in this patient). Necrotizing fasciitis needs to be ruled out because other organisms may be involved, and surgery is crucial. Although penicillin is the treatment of choice for erysipelas, the patient probably has acute cellulitis (there is no raised border at the edge of the infection, which is indicative of erysipelas). Although piperacillin-tazobactam has activity against both *Streptococcus* and *Staphylococcus*, this treatment is too broad spectrum for an acute cellulitis. Because Doppler studies are negative, there is a low likelihood of a deep venous thrombosis.

8. Answer C

Even if a patient is believed to have aseptic meningitis after analysis of the CSF, antibiotics need to be given until CSF cultures are negative. In empiric therapy for bacterial meningitis in adults (i.e., when the CSF Gram stain is negative), ceftriaxone should be used in combination with vancomycin. The vancomycin is required for activity against resistant *S. pneumoniae*. Although the symptoms and CSF results are similar to what is expected for herpes simplex encephalitis, the use of acyclovir alone in this patient is inappropriate. Antibacterials must be used as well. Viral meningitis is generally caused by coxsackie virus, echovirus, and enterovirus, which are not treated with acyclovir.

9. Answer C

Enterococcal endocarditis should be treated for 4–6 weeks. The 2-week treatment regimen is indicated only for *S. endocarditis*. There is also no indication that the patient is penicillin allergic; thus, vancomycin should not be used as first-line treatment. Ampicillin plus gentamicin for 4-6 weeks is the regimen of choice for penicillin-susceptible, enterococcal endocarditis. Cephalosporins have no activity against *Enterococcus*; therefore, the regimen with cefazolin is inappropriate.

10. Answer C

A perforated appendix requires antibiotics after surgery for an intra-abdominal infection. The combination of vancomycin and metronidazole does not have adequate activity against aerobic, gram-negative organisms (e.g., *E. coli*). The combination of ceftriaxone and ciprofloxacin does not have adequate activity against anaerobic organisms (e.g., *B. fragilis* group). Ertapenem is a good choice for intra-abdominal infections, although it has limited activity against *Enterococcus*.

HIV/INFECTIOUS DISEASES

CURTIS L. SMITH, PHARM.D., BCPS

FERRIS STATE UNIVERSITY
LANSING, MICHIGAN

HIV/INFECTIOUS DISEASES

CURTIS L. SMITH, PHARM.D., BCPS

FERRIS STATE UNIVERSITY
LANSING, MICHIGAN

HIV/Infectious Diseases

Learning Objectives:

1. Describe appropriate treatment of patients with human immunodeficiency virus, including initiation and monitoring therapy.

2. Discuss appropriate treatment of the various acquired immunodeficiency syndrome opportunistic infections, including primary and secondary prophylaxis.

3. Describe appropriate treatment and preventive therapy for tuberculosis, including infections with drug-resistant organisms.

Self-Assessment Questions:

Answers to these questions may be found at the end of this chapter.

1. K.E. is a 29-year-old asymptomatic patient who is human immunodeficiency virus (HIV) positive. She recently found out she is pregnant and is estimated to be early in her first trimester. Her most recent CD_4 count was 170/mm^3, and her viral load was 100,000 copies/mL by reverse transcriptase–polymerase chain reaction. Which one of the following is the best treatment therapy for K.E. to prevent HIV transmission to her child?
   A. No drug therapy is needed—the risks to the fetus outweigh any benefits.
   B. Administer zidovudine 300 mg 2 times/day orally throughout the pregnancy, followed by zidovudine during labor and consequently to the baby for 6 weeks.
   C. No drug therapy is required now, but administer a single dose of nevirapine at the onset of labor.
   D. Administer a potent combination antiretroviral therapy regimen that includes zidovudine throughout the pregnancy.

2. R.E. is a 33-year-old man who has been HIV positive since 2005. Recently, his CD_4 counts started to decrease significantly, and his viral load started to increase. He is started on tenofovir, emtricitabine, and atazanavir-ritonavir. Which one of the following statements represents what R.E. should be told about his therapy?
   A. Watch for jaundice because atazanavir can cause hyperbilirubinemia.
   B. If you think you are having a drug-related adverse effect, simply cut the dose of all your drugs in half.
   C. Talk to your pharmacist about drug interactions because both atazanavir and tenofovir inhibit cytochrome P450 (CYP) 3A4.
   D. Tenofovir and emtricitabine cause additive peripheral neuropathy, so let your pharmacist know if you experience tingling in your extremities.

3. One year later, R.E. is concerned that his antiretroviral therapy is not working and asks if he should make some changes. Which one of the following statements best represents what to tell him?
   A. His therapy should be changed only if he is deteriorating clinically (e.g., having more opportunistic infections).
   B. His therapy should be changed if his viral load is detectable after an initial suppression to undetectable concentrations.
   C. If he is concerned about his regimen not being effective, then his atazanavir-ritonavir should be changed to fosamprenavir-ritonavir.
   D. Resistance most commonly occurs with emtricitabine, so this should be changed to lamivudine.

4. F.V. is a 42-year-old man who has been HIV positive for 10 years. He has been receiving potent combination antiretroviral therapy for the past 3 years, including zidovudine, lamivudine, and lopinavir-ritonavir. He is now experiencing hyperglycemia, fat redistribution, and lipid abnormalities. Which one of the following represents how F.V.'s drug-related symptoms should be managed?
   A. Add simvastatin for the lipid abnormalities and treat according to the recommendations from the National Cholesterol Education Program.
   B. Add pioglitazone for the glucose abnormalities.
   C. Change zidovudine to tenofovir.
   D. Change lopinavir-ritonavir to nevirapine.

5. P.P., a 43-year-old man who is HIV positive, presents to the clinic with a headache that has gradually worsened during the past 2 weeks. He does not feel very sick and has not experienced any focal seizures. His most recent CD_4 count was 35/mm^3. He has a laboratory profile performed with the following results: Gram's stain = negative; white blood cell count = 2 mg; protein = 35 mg/dL; glucose = 75 mg/dL (peripheral = 110 mg/dL); India ink = positive; and cryptococcal antigen = 1:1024. Which one of the following therapies should be used to treat P.P.?

A. Fluconazole 200 mg/day orally.
B. Amphotericin B 0.3 mg/kg/day alone.
C. Amphotericin B 0.3 mg/kg/day plus flucytosine 37.5 mg/kg every 6 hours.
D. Amphotericin B 0.7 mg/kg/day plus flucytosine 25 mg/kg every 6 hours for 2 weeks, followed by fluconazole 400 mg/day.

6. A study is performed to compare the incidence of active tuberculosis (TB) infection in patients receiving isoniazid (INH) versus rifampin (RIF) for latent TB infection. After completion of therapy (6 months for INH and 4 months for RIF), 0.3% in the INH group and 0.8% in the RIF group progress to active disease. Which one of the following represents how many patients would need to be treated with INH over RIF to prevent one progression to active disease?

A. 5.
B. 50.
C. 200.
D. Insufficient information to calculate this number.

7. G.T. is a 34-year-old woman positive for HIV who is brought to the emergency department by her boyfriend after experiencing headaches, a change in mental status, and loss of feeling on her right side. A computed tomographic scan shows two large ring-enhancing lesions in her brain. Her most recent CD_4 count was 85/mm^3, but that was 4 months ago. She currently takes no antiretroviral agents but takes dapsone for *Pneumocystis pneumonia* (PCP) prophylaxis. Which one of the following therapies should be used to treat G.T.?

A. Atovaquone for 4–6 weeks.
B. High-dose trimethoprim-sulfamethoxazole (TMP/SMX) plus clindamycin for 6 weeks.
C. Pyrimethamine plus sulfadiazine for 6 weeks.
D. Pyrimethamine plus clindamycin and leucovorin for 6 weeks.

8. A patient who is HIV positive receives a diagnosis of cryptococcal meningitis and begins taking amphotericin B and flucytosine. You want to keep flucytosine peak concentrations between 50 and 100 mcg/mL. Assuming a trough concentration of 25 mcg/mL, every-6-hour dosing, and 100% bioavailability, which one of the following doses would achieve a peak concentration within the desired range (flucytosine volume of distribution = 0.7 L/kg and half-life = 3 hours)?

A. 12.5 mg/kg.
B. 37.5 mg/kg.
C. 75 mg/kg.
D. 150 mg/kg.

9. P.I. is a 35-year-old woman who presents to the clinic with a 2-week history of night sweats, fatigue, weight loss, and a persistent cough. A purified protein derivative (PPD) is placed, and a sputum sample is taken; then, P.I. is sent home with a prescription for levofloxacin 750 mg/day orally. Two days later, her PPD is measured at 20-mm induration, and her sputum sample is positive for acid-fast bacilli. P.I., who has no pertinent medical history, has never been outside the United States. He lives in an area with an extremely low incidence of multidrug-resistant TB. Which of the following is the best therapy for P.I.?

A. INH 300 mg/day orally for 6 months.
B. INH, RIF, pyrazinamide (PZA), and ethambutol (EMB) for 2 months, followed by INH and RIF for 4 more months.
C. INH and RIF for 6 months.
D. Levofloxacin 750 mg/day orally for both TB and other bacterial causes of pneumonia.

10. A prospective, double-blind study compared the effects of two therapies—a potent combination antiretroviral therapy with a ritonavir-boosted protease inhibitor and a potent combination antiretroviral therapy with efavirenz—in 350 patients with HIV. Which one of the following statistical tests should be used to compare end points such as the mean change in viral load or mean change in CD_4 counts?

A. Analysis of variance.
B. Chi-square test.
C. Student's t-test.
D. Wilcoxon rank sum test.

I. **HUMAN IMMUNODEFICIENCY VIRUS (HIV)**

   A. Transmission of HIV
   1. Sexual transmission
      a. Homosexual or heterosexual
      b. Increases with increased number of sexual partners
      c. Prevention: condom
   2. Parenteral exposure to blood or blood products
      a. Intravenous drug abuser: increased with increased needle sharing
      b. Hemophiliacs/blood transfusions: decreased since 1985
   3. Universal precautions (Table 1)
      a. Purpose is prevention of parenteral, mucous membrane, and nonintact skin exposures to bloodborne pathogens
      b. Body fluids

   Table 1. Universal Precautions

Universal Precautions Apply to:	Universal Precautions Do Not Apply to:
Blood	Feces
Body fluids containing visible blood	Nasal secretions
Semen and vaginal secretions	Sputum
Tissue	Sweat
Cerebrospinal fluid	Tears
Synovial fluid	Urine
Pleural fluid	Vomitus
Peritoneal fluid	Breast milk
Pericardial fluid	Saliva (precautions recommended for dentistry)
Amniotic fluid	

   c. General guidelines
      i. Take care when using needles, scalpels, and other sharp instruments and when disposing of needles.
      ii. Use protective barriers (i.e., gloves, masks, and protective eyewear).
      iii. Wash hands and skin immediately if they are contaminated with body fluids to which universal precautions apply.
   4. Perinatal transmission
      a. Antepartum—through maternal circulation
      b. During delivery
      c. Postpartum—breastfeeding
      d. Zidovudine therapy decreases risk of transmission from 23% to 3%–4% (even lower with combination therapy).

   B. Diagnosis
   1. Enzyme-linked immunosorbent assay (ELISA)
      a. For ELISA: Expose patient sera to HIV antigen and check for antibodies to HIV.
      b. Positive: 1–6 months after the infection
      c. Sensitivity and specificity: 97%–100%

2. Western blot
   a. Confirms ELISA
   b. False-positive: 1 in 20,000
   c. False-negative: 1 in 250,000
3. Rapid HIV tests
   a. OraQuick Advance: finger-stick, whole blood, or oral fluid
   b. Uni-Gold Recombigen: finger-stick or whole blood
   c. Reveal G2, Multispot HIV-1/HIV-2: serum or plasma
4. Test for HIV RNA
   a. Detects HIV RNA in serum (tests for the virus, not for antibodies)
   b. Branched-chain DNA, VERSANT, and Quantiplex (Bayer)
      i. Signal amplification
      ii. Sensitive to 75 copies/mL of HIV RNA
   c. Reverse transcriptase–polymerase chain reaction, Amplicor HIV-1 Monitor (Roche)
      i. Sensitive to 50 copies/mL of HIV RNA
   d. Nucleic acid sequence–based amplification (NASBA), NucliSens (Organon Teknika)
      i. Sensitive to 40 copies/mL of HIV RNA
   e. Values expressed as copies of HIV RNA per milliliter or the log of copies of HIV RNA per milliliter
   f. Changes greater than 3-fold (about 0.5 log) are clinically significant.
5. Use of HIV RNA testing
   a. Acute HIV infection (diagnosis is received sooner than with older tests)
   b. Newly diagnosed HIV infection (for baseline value to follow)
   c. Every 3–4 months without therapy
   d. From 2 to 4 (no more than 8) weeks after starting or changing therapy (should detect a significant decrease)
   e. From 3 to 4 months after starting therapy (change therapy if decrease is limited)
   f. Every 3–4 months while on therapy (checking for increase—therapy failure)
   g. Whenever there is a clinical event or decrease in CD_4 count
6. Who should be screened for HIV?
   a. All patients aged 13–64 years (in all health care settings)
   b. Adults and adolescents at increased risk of HIV infection should be checked annually (intravenous drug users, those who have unprotected sex with several partners, men who have sex with men, men or women who have sex for money or drugs, people being treated for sexually transmitted diseases, recipients of several blood transfusions 1975–1985)
   c. Pregnant women
7. Case definition for HIV – 2008 (Table 2)

Table 2. Case Definition for HIV – 2008

Stage	Laboratory Evidence[a]	Clinical Evidence
Stage 1	Laboratory confirmation of HIV infection AND CD_4 count of $\geq 500/\mu L$ OR CD_4 percentage of ≥ 29	None required (but no AIDS-defining condition)
Stage 2	Laboratory confirmation of HIV infection AND CD_4 count of 200–499/μL OR CD_4 percentage of ≥ 14–28	None required (but no AIDS-defining condition)
Stage 3 (AIDS)	Laboratory confirmation of HIV infection AND CD_4 count of $< 200/\mu L$ OR CD_4 percentage of < 14	OR documentation of an AIDS-defining condition (with laboratory confirmation of HIV infection)
Stage unknown	Laboratory confirmation of HIV infection AND No information on CD_4 count or percentage	AND no information on presence of AIDS-defining conditions

[a]Laboratory confirmation: Positive result from an HIV antibody screening test (e.g., reactive enzyme immunoassay) confirmed by a positive result from a supplemental HIV antibody test (e.g., Western blot or indirect immunofluorescence assay test) OR positive result or report of a detectable quantity (i.e., within the established limits of the laboratory test) from any of the following HIV virologic (i.e., non-antibody) tests.
AIDS = acquired immunodeficiency syndrome; HIV = human immunodeficiency virus.

    8. Acquired immunodeficiency syndrome (AIDS)-defining conditions (Table 3)

Table 3. AIDS-Defining Conditions

• Candidiasis: bronchi, trachea, or lungs • Candidiasis: esophageal • Cervical cancer: invasive • Coccidioidomycosis: disseminated, or extrapulmonary • Cryptococcosis: extrapulmonary • Cryptosporidiosis: chronic intestinal (> 1 month in duration) • Cytomegalovirus disease (other than liver, spleen, or nodes) • Cytomegalovirus retinitis (with loss of vision) • Encephalopathy: HIV related • Herpes simplex: chronic ulcer(s) (> 1 month in duration); bronchitis, pneumonitis, or esophagitis • Histoplasmosis: disseminated or extrapulmonary • Isosporiasis: chronic intestinal (> 1 month in duration) • Kaposi sarcoma	• Lymphoma: Burkitt (or equivalent term) • Lymphoma: immunoblastic (or equivalent term) • Lymphoma: primary or brain • *Mycobacterium avium* complex or *M. kansasii*: disseminated or extrapulmonary • *M. tuberculosis*: any site (pulmonary or extrapulmonary) • *Mycobacterium*: other species or unidentified species; disseminated or extrapulmonary • *Pneumocystis* pneumonia • Pneumonia: recurrent • Progressive multifocal leukoencephalopathy • *Salmonella* septicemia (recurrent) • Toxoplasmosis of brain • Wasting syndrome caused by HIV

AIDS = acquired immunodeficiency syndrome; HIV = human immunodeficiency virus.

  C. Primary HIV Infection
    1. Characteristics of the primary HIV infection
      a. About 40%–60% develop symptoms from the primary infection.
      b. Abrupt onset: duration = 3–14 days
      c. Occurs 5 days to 3 months after HIV exposure (generally within 2–4 weeks)
      d. Fevers, sweats, lethargy, malaise, myalgias, arthralgias, headache, photophobia, diarrhea, sore throat, lymphadenopathy
      e. Treatment of an acute HIV infection is generally not recommended.

2. Progression of HIV
   a. Human immunodeficiency virus replicates actively at all stages of the infection.
   b. From 10^9 to 10^{10} virions are produced <u>every</u> day.
   c. Half-life of virions is about 6 hours.
3. Immunization of patients with HIV (no live virus vaccines if CD_4 count is less than $200/mm^3$)
   a. Influenza virus vaccine: annually (before the influenza season)
   b. Pneumococcal vaccine: once (ideally, before CD_4 count is less than $200/mm^3$)
   c. Hepatitis B vaccine: for all susceptible patients
   d. Hepatitis A vaccine: for all at-risk patients

D. Treatment of HIV
   1. Reverse transcriptase inhibitors (RTIs) (nucleoside [NRTI], nucleotide, and nonnucleoside [NNRTI])
      a. Reverse transcriptase: enzyme required to copy viral RNA to DNA
      b. Dideoxynucleoside analogs: inserted in growing DNA chain, terminating elongation
      c. See Tables 4 and 5 for RTI characteristics.
      d. Nonnucleoside NRTIs and nucleotide RTIs do not require phosphorylation.
   2. Protease inhibitors
      a. See Table 6 for protease inhibitor characteristics.

   3. Entry inhibitors
      a. Fusion inhibitors: enfuvirtide (Fuzeon); a.k.a.: T-20 and pentafuside
         i. Mechanism of action: HIV envelope protein gp120 binds to the cell's CD_4 receptor, resulting in exposure of chemokine coreceptors on the cell; attachment of gp120 to CD_4 receptor and coreceptors CCR5 or CXCR4 results in exposure of specific peptide sequence of gp 41; enfuvirtide binds to this gp 41 peptide sequence, preventing fusion.
         ii. Indications – treatment-experienced patients with HIV infection
         iii. Adverse effects – hypersensitivity reactions; local injection-site reactions (98%); pneumonia
         iv. Drug interactions – none
         v. Dosing – 90 mg (1 mL) 2 times/day subcutaneously (reconstitution required)
      b. CCR5 antagonist: maraviroc (Selzentry)
         i. Mechanism of action: binds to the CCR5 receptor of the CD_4 T cell
         ii. Indications – treatment-experienced patients with HIV infected solely with R5 strains
         iii. Adverse effects – abdominal pain, cough, dizziness, musculoskeletal symptoms, pyrexia, rash, upper respiratory tract infections, hepatotoxicity, orthostatic hypotension
         iv. Drug interactions – CYP3A substrate (watch CYP3A inducers and inhibitors)
         v. Dosing – 150–600 mg 2 times/day oral (depending on concomitant drug interactions)
   4. Integrase inhibitors: raltegravir (Isentress)
      a. Mechanism of action: inhibits strand transfer of viral DNA to host cell DNA
      b. Indications – treatment-experienced patients with HIV infection
      c. Adverse effects – nausea, headache, diarrhea, pyrexia, creatine kinase elevation
      d. Drug interactions – metabolized by uridine 5'-diphospho (UDP)-glucuronosyltransferases (UGTs); inducers of UGT1A1: RIF, efavirenz, tipranavir-ritonavir, and rifabutin
      e. Dosing – 400 mg 2 times/day orally

HIV/Infectious Diseases

Table 4. Nucleoside Reverse Transcriptase Inhibitors

	Zidovudine (AZT, ZDV, Retrovir, Combivir, Trizivir)	Didanosine (ddI, Videx)	Stavudine (d4T, Zerit)	Lamivudine (3TC, Epivir, Combivir, Epzicom, Trizivir)	Emtricitabine (FTC, Emtriva)	Abacavir (ABC, Ziagen, Epzicom, Trizivir)
Form	100-mg capsules, 300-mg tablets; 50 mg/5 mL liquid; 10 mg/mL injection	125-, 200-, 250-, 400-mg enteric-coated capsules	15-, 20-, 30-, 40-mg capsules 1 mg/mL solution 75, 100 mg extended release	150-, 300-mg tablets 10 mg/mL liquid Combivir: 150 mg of 3TC/300 mg of ZDV Epzicom: 300 mg of 3TC/600 mg of ABC	200-mg capsules 10 mg/mL liquid Truvada: 200 mg of FTC/300 mg of TDF	300-mg tablets 20 mg/mL liquid Trizivir: 300 mg of ABC/150 mg of 3TC/300 mg of ZDV
Dosing	200 mg TID or 300 mg BID	> 60 kg: 200 mg BID or 400 mg/day ≤ 60 kg: 125 mg BID or 250 mg/day	> 60 kg: 40 mg BID ≤ 60 kg: 30 mg BID	150 mg BID or 300 mg/day < 50 kg: 2 mg/kg BID	200 mg/day or 240 mg liquid/day	300 mg BID or 600 mg/day
Oral bioavailability	60%	40% Empty stomach	86%	86%	93%	83%
Serum half-life	1.1 hours	1.6 hours	1 hour	3–6 hours	10 hours	1.5 hours
Intracellular half-life	7 hours	> 20 hours	7.5 hours	18–22 hours	39 hours	12–26 hours
Elimination	Metabolized to ZDV glucuronide (GZDV) Renal excretion of GZDV	Renal excretion 50%	Renal excretion 50%	Renally excreted unchanged (70%)	Renal excretion	Metabolized by alcohol dehydrogenase and glucuronyl transferase Metabolites—renal
Major toxicity *All may cause lactic acidosis with hepatic steatosis	Bone marrow suppression, GI intolerance, headache, insomnia, asthenia, nail pigmentation, and myalgia	Pancreatitis (5%) Peripheral neuropathy (35%) Nausea, diarrhea	Peripheral neuropathy (20%–30%) Elevated liver enzymes	Diarrhea, nausea, abdominal pain, insomnia, and headaches (minimal toxicity)	Diarrhea, nausea, headache, rash, and hyperpigmentation	Hypersensitivity, fever, rash, GI symptoms, malaise, fatigue, anorexia, and myocardial infarction
Drug interactions	Myelosuppressive agents Rifampin	Fluoroquinolones, tetracycline; ketoconazole, dapsone; tenofovir		TMP/SMX may increase 3TC concentrations		Ethanol may increase ABC concentrations
Miscellaneous information	Activity in activated lymphocytes		Activity in activated lymphocytes	Resistance develops quickly with monotherapy Activity in resting macrophages	Activity in resting macrophages	Hypersensitivity reaction may be fatal—discontinue drug immediately Screen for HLA-B*5701 before initiation; cross-resistance with ddI and 3TC

BID = 2 times/day; GI = gastrointestinal; TID = 3 times/day; TMP/SMX = trimethoprim-sulfamethoxazole.

Table 5. Nonnucleoside and Nucleotide Reverse Transcriptase Inhibitors

	Nevirapine (Viramune)	Delavirdine (Rescriptor)	Efavirenz (Sustiva, Atripla)	Etravirine (Intelence)	Tenofovir DF (TDF, Viread, Truvada)
RTI type	Nonnucleoside	Nonnucleoside	Nonnucleoside	Nonnucleoside	Nucleotide
Form	200-mg tablets	100-, 200-mg tablets	50-, 100-, 200-mg capsules 600-mg tablets Atripla: 200 mg of FTC/300 mg of TDF/efavirenz 600 mg	100 mg tablets	300-mg tablets Truvada: 200 mg of FTC/300 mg of TDF
Dosing	200 mg/day for 14 days; then 200 mg PO BID	400 mg PO TID	600 mg PO qHS	200mg PO BID	300 mg/day PO
Oral bioavailability	> 90%	85%	42%	Take with food	40%
		Avoid antacids	Avoid with high-fat meal		Take with food
Serum half-life	25–30 hours	5.8 hours	40–55 hours	20–60 hours	10–14 hours
Elimination	Metabolized by CYP3A4; 80% excreted in urine (< 5% unchanged), 10% in feces	Metabolized by CYP3A4, 51% excreted in urine (< 5% unchanged), 44% in feces	Metabolized by CYP3A4, 14%–34% excreted in urine, 16%–61% in feces	Metabolized by CYP 3A4, 2C9, 2C19	Eliminated by renal filtration and active secretion
Major toxicity	Rash GI toxicity Increased LFTs—hepatotoxicity	Rash (less than nevirapine) Headache	Rash (less than delavirdine) CNS symptoms (insomnia, impaired concentration, nightmares, mania) Increased LFTs	Rash Nausea	GI toxicity Headache May cause lactic acidosis with hepatic steatosis (mitochondrial toxicity may be less)
Drug interactions	Induces CYP3A4 Watch rifampin, rifabutin, OCs, protease inhibitors, triazolam, midazolam	Inhibits CYP3A4 Separate administration with antacids and ddI	Induces CYP3A4	Induces CYP3A4 Inhibits CYP 2C9 and 2C19	Increases didanosine concentration—separate administration
Miscellaneous information	Extensive cross-resistance in class Do not initiate in women with CD_4^+ counts > 250 cells/mm^3 or in men with CD_4^+ counts > 400 cells/mm^3 (liver toxicity)	Extensive cross-resistance in class	Extensive cross-resistance in class Avoid in first trimester of pregnancy; do not use Atripla if CrCl < 50 mL/minute	Can dissolve in water for patients who cannot swallow May be effective against HIV strains resistant to efavirenz or nevirapine	May be effective against HIV strains resistant to other RTIs

BID = 2 times/day; CNS = central nervous system; CrCl = creatinine clearance; CYP = cytochrome P450; DM = diabetes mellitus; GI = gastrointestinal; HIV = human immunodeficiency virus; LFT = liver function test; OC = oral contraceptive; PO = orally; qHS = every night; RTI = reverse transcriptase inhibitor; TID = 3 times/day.

HIV/Infectious Diseases

Table 6. Protease Inhibitors

	Indinavir [IDV] (Crixivan)	Nelfinavir (Viracept)	Ritonavir [RTV] (Norvir)	Saquinavir [SQV] (Invirase)	Fosamprenavir [f-APV] (Lexiva)	Lopinavir-Ritonavir (Kaletra)	Atazanavir [ATV] (Reyataz)	Tipranavir [TPV] (Aptivus)	Darunavir [TMC 114] (Prezista)
Form	200-, 333-, 400-mg capsules; refrigerate capsules	250-, 625-mg tablets; 50 mg/g oral powder	100-mg capsules; 80 mg/mL liquid; refrigerate capsules	200-mg capsules, 500-mg tablets	700 mg tablets; 50 mg/mL liquid; prodrug of amprenavir	100/25, 200/50 mg tablets; 80/20 mg/mL solution	100-, 150-, 200-, 300-mg capsules	250-mg capsules	75-, 150-, 400-, 600-mg tablets
Dosing	800 mg q8h 800 mg + RTV 100 mg or 200 mg q12h	750 mg TID or 1250 mg BID	600 mg every 12 hours (300 mg q12h for 2 days, 400 mg q12h for 3 days, 500 mg q12h for 8 days) "Boosting dose" = 100–400 mg divided 1 or 2 times/day	1000 mg BID with ritonavir 100 mg; take within 2 hours of a meal	1400 mg BID (or 1400 mg + RTV 100–200 mg/day; or 700 mg + RTV 100 mg BID). With efavirenz: 700 mg + RTV 100 mg BID	400/100 mg BID or 800/200 mg/day with food. If taking efavirenz or nevirapine: 500 mg/125 mg BID	400 mg/day If taken with efavirenz: RTV 100 mg + ATV 400 mg/day If taken with efavirenz: RTV 100 mg + ATV 300 mg/day	500 mg BID with RTV 200 mg BID	800 mg/day with RTV 100 mg/day or 600 mg BID with RTV 100 mg BID
Oral bioavailability	65%; 1 hour before or 2 hours after meals (may take with low-fat meal)	20%–80%; take with meal or snack	65%–75%; take with food	Invirase: 4%	Fosamprenavir: T$_{max}$ of amprenavir occurs in 1.5–4 hours; take without respect to food	Solution take with food; take tablets without respect to food	Food increases absorption and bioavailability; take with food	Food increases absorption and bioavailability Take with food	Food increases absorption and bioavailability Take with food
Serum half-life	1.5–2 hours	3.5–5 hours	3–5 hours	1–2 hours	7–11 hours	5–6 hours	7 hours	6 hours	15 hours
Elimination	CYP3A4; renal—20%	CYP3A4	CYP 3A4 > 2D6 > 2C9/10	CYP3A4	CYP3A4	CYP3A4	CYP3A4	CYP3A4	CYP3A4
Major toxicity	Nephrolithiasis GI intolerance; alopecia, dry skin and lips; endocrine disturbances[a]	Diarrhea (mild); endocrine disturbances[a]	GI intolerance; paresthesias (circumoral and extremities); taste disturbances; asthenia; endocrine disturbances[a]	GI intolerance (mild); endocrine disturbances[a]	GI intolerance; rash; oral paresthesias; increased LFTs; endocrine disturbances[a]	GI intolerance; fatigue; asthenia; pancreatitis; endocrine disturbances[a]	Indirect hyperbilirubinemia, prolonged QT interval/heart block, endocrine disturbances[a]	Hepatotoxicity; rash (sulfa); endocrine disturbances[a]	Rash (sulfa); endocrine disturbances[a]
Drug interactions	Inhibits CYP3A4 (< RTV); ddI decreases absorption	Inhibits CYP3A4 (< RTV)	Inhibits CYP3A4, 2D6 (potent) ddI decreases absorption Induces glucuronyl transferases	Inhibits CYP3A4 (< RTV)	Inhibits CYP3A4 (< RTV)	Inhibits CYP 3A4, 2D6	Inhibits CYP3A4, PPIs, H$_2$ blockers, antacids	Inhibits CYP 3A4, 2D6	Inhibits CYP3A4
Miscellaneous information			Cross-resistance with IDV	Do not use with IDV			Less lipid effects	Good for PI-resistant virus	Good for PI-resistant virus (in 70%).

[a]Endocrine disturbances include insulin resistance (type 2 diabetes mellitus in 8%–10%), peripheral fat loss/central fat accumulation (in 50%), and lipid abnormalities (in 70%). BID = 2 times/day; CYP = cytochrome P450; GI = gastrointestinal; PI = protease inhibitor; q8h = every 8 hours; q12h = every 12 hours; TID = 3 times/day.

4. Prevention of maternal-fetal transmission
   a. Pregnant women with HIV receiving no antiretroviral therapy
      i. Women who meet criteria for beginning HIV therapy in adults should receive potent combination antiretroviral therapy (to prevent resistance); initiate therapy as soon as possible, even in the first trimester.
      ii. Women who do not meet criteria for beginning HIV therapy should still receive potent combination antiretroviral therapy (to prevent transmission); consider delaying therapy until after first trimester.
      iii. Use zidovudine as a component of therapy if possible.
      iv. Avoid efavirenz in the first trimester and avoid nevirapine if CD_4 is greater than $250/mm^3$.
      v. Women who have received antiretroviral therapy in the past but are currently on no therapy should have HIV antiretroviral resistance testing completed before initiating therapy.
      vi. Continue combination regimen through intrapartum period (with zidovudine infusion added), and treat baby for 6 weeks.
   b. Pregnant women with HIV receiving potent combination antiretroviral therapy
      i. Continue current combination regimens (preferably with zidovudine) if already receiving therapy. Avoid efavirenz in the first trimester.
      ii. Continue combination regimen through intrapartum period (with zidovudine infusion added), and treat baby for 6 weeks.
   c. Pregnant women with HIV in labor (with or without therapy during pregnancy)
      i. At labor, zidovudine 2 mg/kg intravenously for 1 hour followed by a 1-mg/kg/hour infusion until cord is clamped. Discontinue oral zidovudine but continue any other oral antiretrovirals (except stavudine).
      ii. Continue antiretroviral therapy as much as possible during labor.
      iii. For women who have not received antiretrovirals during pregnancy, consider single-dose nevirapine to mother at labor onset and to baby at 48 hours (consider also adding ZDV/3TC to mother for 7 days any time single-dose nevirapine is used, to prevent resistance).
   d. Infants born to mothers who are HIV positive
      i. Zidovudine 2 mg/kg every 6 hours for 6 weeks. Can consider additional antiretroviral agents in certain situations
5. Prevention of postexposure infection
   a. Use universal precautions.
   b. Occupational exposures: needle sticks or cuts (1 in 300 risk) and mucous membrane exposure (1 in 1000 risk)
   c. Nonoccupational exposures: treat if exposure of vagina, rectum, eye, mouth, mucous membrane, or nonintact skin with blood, semen, vaginal secretions, or breast milk of an individual with known HIV infection
   d. Recommended therapy for occupational exposure is outlined in Table 7.
   e. Recommended therapy for nonoccupational exposure is potent combination antiretroviral therapy.
   f. Postexposure prophylaxis can reduce HIV infection by about 80%.
   g. Occupational exposures: begin treatment within 1-2 hours; most effective if begun within 24-36 hours
   h. Nonoccupational exposures: Begin within 72 hours.
   i. Treatment should be administered for 4 weeks.

Table 7. Recommended Therapy for Postexposure Infection

Exposure Type	Severity	HIV-positive Class[a]	Recommended Prophylaxis[b]
Percutaneous exposure	Less severe	Class 1	Basic 2-drug regimen
		Class 2	Expanded ≥ 3-drug regimen
	More severe	Class 1 or 2	Expanded ≥ 3-drug regimen
Mucous membrane and nonintact skin exposure	Small volume	Class 1 or 2	Basic 2-drug regimen
	Large volume	Class 1	Basic 2-drug regimen
		Class 2	Expanded ≥ 3-drug regimen[c]

[a] Class 1: asymptomatic HIV infection or low viral load (< 1500 copies/mL); class 2: symptomatic HIV infection or high viral load.
[b] Basic 2-drug regimen: ZDV/3TC or FTC; d4T/3TC or FTC; TDF/3TC or FTC.
[c] Expanded 3-drug regimen: add LPV/RTV, ATV, f-APV, IDV/RTV, SQV/RTV, NFV, or EFV.

Patient Case

1. F.G. is a 27-year-old man who is HIV positive but asymptomatic. One year ago, his CD_4 count was 815/mm³, and his viral load was 1500 copies/mL (by reverse transcriptase–polymerase chain reaction). F.G. continues to be monitored; his CD_4 count has decreased (most recent was 240/mm³), and his viral load has increased (most recent was 60,000 copies/mL by reverse transcriptase–polymerase chain reaction). Which one of the following treatments should F.G. receive?

    A. Antiretroviral therapy should not be given because F.G.'s CD_4 count is still above 200/mm³.
    B. Initiate F.G. on zidovudine alone because his CD_4 count is still above 200/mm³.
    C. Initiate F.G. on combination therapy of zidovudine, lamivudine, and nevirapine.
    D. Initiate F.G. on combination therapy of tenofovir, emtricitabine, and atazanavir-ritonavir.

---

6. Treatment of the patient who is HIV positive
    a. Initiating potent combination antiretroviral therapy in an antiretroviral-naïve patient
        i. Any symptomatic patient who is HIV positive (regardless of CD_4 count)
        ii. CD_4 less than 350/mm³
        iii. Initiate therapy regardless of CD_4 T-cell count in pregnant women, patients with HIV-associated nephropathy, and patients coinfected with hepatitis B virus (HBV) when treatment for HBV infection is indicated.
        iv. Recommended in patients with CD_4 350–500/mm³ (lower strength of recommendation)
        v. Consider in patients with CD_4 greater than 500/mm³.
    b. Preferred therapy
        i. Efavirenz OR atazanavir-ritonavir OR darunavir-ritonavir OR raltegravir **PLUS** tenofovir-emtricitabine
    c. Alternative therapy
        i. One protease inhibitor (atazanavir-ritonavir, fosamprenavir-ritonavir [once or twice daily], lopinavir-ritonavir [once or twice daily], saquinavir-ritonavir) OR one NNRTI (efavirenz, nevirapine) **PLUS** two NRTIs (abacavir or zidovudine or tenofovir-emtricitabine or lamivudine)
    d. Acceptable therapy
        i. Efavirenz **PLUS** two NRTIs (didanosine-lamivudine or emtricitabine)
        ii. Atazanavir **PLUS** two NRTIs (abacavir or zidovudine-lamivudine)
    e. Regimens that need more data
        i. Maraviroc **PLUS** zidovudine-lamivudine
        ii. Raltegravir **PLUS** two NRTIs (abacavir or zidovudine-lamivudine)

iii. Darunavir-ritonavir or saquinavir-ritonavir **PLUS** two NRTIs (abacavir or zidovudine-lamivudine)
f. Regimens to be used with caution
   i. Nevirapine **PLUS** abacavir-lamivudine
   ii. Nevirapine **PLUS** tenofovir-emtricitabine
   iii. Fosamprenavir **PLUS** two NRTIs (abacavir or zidovudine or tenofovir-emtricitabine or lamivudine)
g. Not recommended regimens
   i. All monotherapies, dual NRTI regimens alone; triple NRTI regimens other than abacavir-lamivudine-zidovudine

---

Patient Cases

2. Six months after starting appropriate therapy, F.G.'s CD_4 count is 620/mm³, and his viral load is undetectable. Two years later, his CD_4 count decreases to 310/mm³, and his viral load is 15,000 copies/mL. Which one of the following changes is best to make to F.G.'s therapy?
   A. No changes should be made; wait until his viral load is again more than 50,000 copies/mL.
   B. Change tenofovir to abacavir because abacavir is a more potent antiretroviral.
   C. Change tenofovir and emtricitabine to abacavir and lamivudine.
   D. Change the entire regimen to abacavir, lamivudine, and fosamprenavir-ritonavir.

3. Which one of the following should be monitored now that F.G. is receiving fosamprenavir-ritonavir?
   A. Peripheral neuropathy.
   B. Drug interactions with drugs metabolized by CYP1A2.
   C. Endocrine disturbances such as hyperglycemia, fat redistribution, and lipid abnormalities.
   D. Nephrolithiasis.

---

h. Change therapy for the following reasons:
   i. Virologic failure
      (a) Not achieving HIV RNA less than 400 copies/mL by 24 weeks or less than 50 copies/mL by 48 weeks of therapy (continue therapy, but assess adherence and consider intensification)
      (b) Repeated detection of virus (more than 400 copies/mL) after initial suppression to undetectable levels
   ii. Immunologic failure
      (a) Failure to increase 50–100 cells/mm³ above the baseline CD_4 cell count during the first year of therapy
      (b) Failure to increase the CD_4 count above 350 cells/mm³
i. Options for treatment failure
   i. Perform resistance testing (while patient is on failing regimen or within 4 weeks of discontinuing).
   ii. Prior therapy with no resistance
      (a) Check adherence and address underlying causes. Consider reinitiating the same regimen.
      (b) Initiate a new regimen.
      (c) Intensify one therapy or pharmacokinetically boost one therapy.
   iii. Prior therapy with resistance – Start a new regimen with at least two and preferably three fully active agents.

iv. Extensive therapy with resistance – Resuppress viral load maximally or at least adequately to prevent clinical progression.
v. New regimen with at least two fully active agents not possible – Continue current regimen.
j. Resistance testing
  i. Types of testing
   (a) Genotypic
    (1) Testing for the presence of mutations known to cause drug resistance
    (2) Comparing the HIV-1 pol gene with a wild-type gene
    (3) Recommend to guide therapy in patients with virologic failure while on their first or second regimen.
   (b) Phenotypic
    (1) Test for inhibitory concentration needed to decrease HIV replication by 50% (IC_{50}).
    (2) Values are reported as fold changes in sensitivity.
    (3) An increase of more than 4-fold in IC_{50} = "sensitive."
    (4) A 4- to 10-fold increase in IC_{50} = "intermediate."
    (5) An increase of more than 10-fold in IC_{50} = "resistant."
    (6) Added to genotypic testing in patients with complex drug resistance mutation patterns
  ii. Indications
   (a) Recommended: virologic failure during potent combination antiretroviral therapy
   (b) Recommended: suboptimal suppression of viral load after initiation of potent combination antiretroviral therapy
   (c) Recommended: acute HIV infection before initiating therapy to determine whether a drug-resistant virus was transmitted
  iii. Benefits
   (a) Resistance testing is an independent indicator of virologic outcome (better short-term viral load response in those who had testing completed).
   (b) May also benefit patients by limiting drug exposures, toxicities, and expense
  iv. Limitations
   (a) The effect of resistance testing is limited in heavily treated patients.
   (b) The HIV RNA value must be 500-1000 copies/mL or more.
   (c) Current need for expert interpretation
   (d) Difficult-to-detect small mutant populations (less than 20%)
   (e) Cost: about $400-$500 per test

II. OPPORTUNISTIC INFECTIONS: PATIENTS WITH HIV

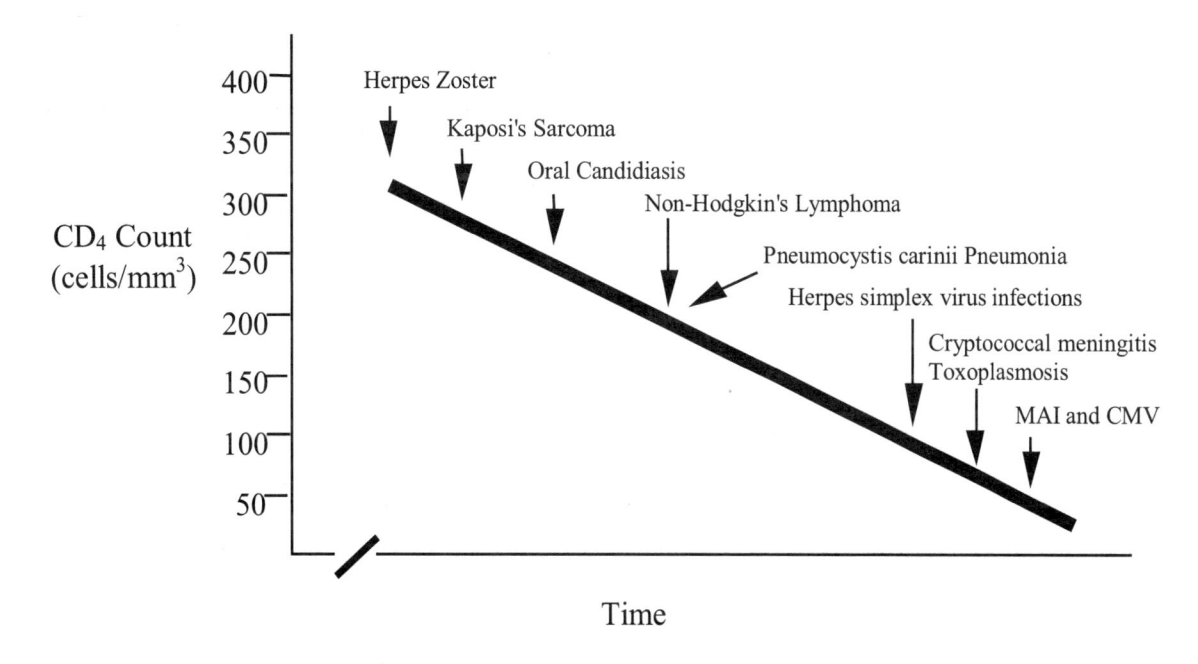

Figure 1. Relationship between CD_4 count and risk of HIV-related opportunistic infections.

A. Overview of HIV-Associated Infections
   1. Principle No. 1: The fungal, parasitic, and viral infections acquired by people who are infected with HIV are <u>rarely curable</u>. At best, the infection is controllable during an acute episode but usually <u>requires long-term suppressive therapy</u>.
   2. Principle No. 2: Most HIV-associated infections represent <u>endogenous reactivation</u> of previously acquired organisms and <u>do not represent a threat to others</u>.
   3. Principle No. 3: <u>Concurrent or consecutive infections</u> with different organisms are a common clinical occurrence in severely immunosuppressed people with HIV infection.
   4. Principle No. 4: The observed frequency in certain parasitic and fungal infections depends on the prevalence of asymptomatic infection with these pathogens in the local population.
   5. Principle No. 5: Infections associated with HIV are severe, often disseminated and atypical, and characterized by a high density of organisms.
   6. Principle No. 6: Certain B-cell–associated infections are seen with increased frequency in people with HIV infections (i.e., pneumococcal infection).

B. Categories of Acute Opportunistic Infections in the Setting of Potent Combination Antiretroviral Therapy
   1. Subclinical infections unmasked by immune reconstitution soon after beginning therapy (within 12 weeks) – continue antiretroviral therapy
   2. Infections beginning more than 12 weeks after onset of therapy; caused by either immune reconstitution or incomplete immunity – continue antiretroviral therapy
   3. Infections occurring because of failure of potent combination antiretroviral therapy – complete resistance testing and modify antiretroviral therapy

C. Initiating Potent Combination Antiretroviral Therapy in the Setting of Acute Opportunistic Infections
   1. Opportunistic infections with no effective therapy require prompt initiation of antiretroviral therapy: cryptosporidiosis, microsporidiosis, promyelocytic leukemia, and Kaposi sarcoma
   2. Antiretroviral therapy should begin within 2 weeks of acute opportunistic infections, except for TB, in which the infection should be treated first.

Patient Cases

4. Three years later, F.G. (from patient case questions 1–3) has not responded to any of his antiretroviral treatment regimens because of resistance or intolerance. His CD_4 count has decreased to 135/mm³. Against which one of the following infections should he receive primary prophylaxis?

   A. PCP.
   B. Cryptococcal meningitis.
   C. Cytomegalovirus (CMV).
   D. *Mycobacterium avium* complex (MAC).

5. B.L. is a 44-year-old man positive for HIV who arrives at the emergency department severely short of breath. He is an extremely nonadherent patient and has not seen a health care provider in more than 3 years. A chest radiograph shows pulmonary infiltrates in both lung fields. The following laboratory profile and tests are performed: sodium = 147 mEq/L; potassium = 4.2 mEq/L; chloride = 104 mEq/L; bicarbonate = 25.2 mEq/L; glucose = 107 mg/dL; blood urea nitrogen = 38 mg/dL; serum creatinine = 1.1 mg/dL; aspartate aminotransferase = 28 IU/L; alanine aminotransferase = 32 IU/L; lactate dehydrogenase = 386 IU/L; alkaline phosphate = 75 IU/L; pH = 7.45; partial pressure of oxygen = 63 mm Hg; partial pressure of carbon dioxide = 32 mm Hg; and oxygen saturation = 85%. Sputum Gram's stain is negative; silver stain is also negative. Which one of the following treatments should B.L. receive?

   A. Pentamidine intravenously with adjuvant prednisone therapy.
   B. TMP/SMZ for 21 days.
   C. TMP/SMZ intravenously with adjuvant prednisone therapy for 21 days.
   D. Atovaquone for 21 days.

D. *Pneumocystis pneumonia* (PCP)
   1. Clinical presentation
      a. Fever, shortness of breath, and nonproductive cough
      b. Increased lactate dehydrogenase
      c. Diffuse pulmonary infiltrates
      d. In general, with CD_4 counts less than 200/mm³
      e. Increased alveolar-arterial (A-a) gradient and decreased PaO_2—A-a gradient = 150—PaO_2—$PaCO_2$
   2. Diagnosis
      a. Induced sputum or bronchoalveolar lavage or transbronchial biopsy
      b. Methenamine silver stain of sputum sample
   3. Therapy
      a. Trimethoprim-sulfamethoxazole
         i. Dose = 5 mg/kg of TMP every 8 hours for 21 days (orally or intravenously)
         ii. Adverse effects (80% of patients, with 20%-60% requiring discontinuation)
            (a) Nausea and vomiting
            (b) Rash
            (c) Anemia, thrombocytopenia, leukopenia
         iii. Prophylaxis dose = TMP/SMZ double strength or single strength 1/day or 3 times/week (pediatric dose = 150 mg/m²/dose of TMP and 750 mg/m²/dose of SMZ)

b. Pentamidine
   i. Dose = 4 mg/kg/day for 21 days (intravenously)
   ii. Adverse effects
      (a) Hypotension
      (b) Rash
      (c) Electrolyte disturbances
      (d) Hypo- or hyperglycemia
      (e) Pancreatitis
   iii. Prophylaxis dose = 300 mg by nebulization (Respirgard) once monthly (can predose with β-agonist to diminish respiratory irritation)
c. Trimethoprim and dapsone
   i. Dose = 5 mg/kg of TMP every 8 hours and dapsone 100 mg/day for 21 days (orally only for mild to moderate PCP)
   ii. Adverse effects
      (a) Nausea and vomiting
      (b) Anemia
   iii. Prophylactic dose = dapsone 100 mg/day (pediatric dose = 1 mg/kg/day) or 50 mg/week with 50–75 mg of pyrimethamine and 25 mg of leucovorin
d. Clindamycin and primaquine
   i. Dose = 300–450 mg of clindamycin every 6 hours and primaquine 15–30 mg/day for 21 days (intravenous clindamycin may be used)
   ii. Adverse effects
      (a) Rash
      (b) Anemia, methemoglobinemia
e. Atovaquone (Mepron)
   i. Dose = 750 mg 2 times/day for 21 days (orally only for mild to moderate PCP)
   ii. Pediatric dose (less than 40 kg [88 lb]) = 40 mg/kg/day divided 2 times/day
   iii. Equal to TMP/SMX for PCP but not an antibacterial
   iv. Potential for decreased efficacy in patients with diarrhea (because of poor absorption)
   v. Adverse effects
      (a) Nausea and vomiting
      (b) Rash
      (c) Transient increase in liver function tests
      (d) Insomnia, headache, fever
   vi. Prophylactic dose = 1500 mg/day (alternative to TMP/SMX)
f. Adjuvant therapy
   i. Corticosteroids
      (a) Used in patients with severe PCP (A-a gradient of 35 or more or PaO_2 of 70 or less) – Start within 72 hours.
      (b) Decreases mortality
      (c) Dose = 40 mg 2 times/day of prednisone for 5 days, followed by 40 mg/day for 5 days, and then 20 mg/day for remainder of PCP therapy (use cautiously in patients with TB)
4. Prophylaxis
   a. Secondary prophylaxis in patients after PCP (may be discontinued if CD_4 count is more than 200/mm³ for 3 months or longer because of potent combination antiretroviral therapy)

b. Primary prophylaxis in patients with CD_4 count less than 200/mm³ (may be discontinued if CD_4 count is more than 200/mm³ for 3 months or longer because of potent combination antiretroviral therapy)

E. *Candida* Infections
  1. Oral *Candida* infections (thrush)
     a. More than 90% of patients with AIDS sometime during their illness
     b. Signs and symptoms
        i. Creamy white, curdlike patches on the tongue and other oral mucosal surfaces
        ii. Pain; decreased food and fluid intake
  2. *Candida* esophagitis
     a. Not always an extension of oral thrush (30% do not have oral thrush)
     b. Signs and symptoms
        i. Painful swallowing, obstructed swallowing, substernal pain
  3. Diagnosis
     a. Signs and symptoms of infection
     b. Fungal cultures/potassium hydroxide smear
  4. Therapy (oral candidiasis is easy to treat [3–14 days' duration], but it relapses within 30 days)
     a. Nystatin
        i. Indicated for mucous membrane and cutaneous *Candida* infections
        ii. Use for initial episodes in patients with CD_4 count more than 50/mm³.
        iii. Five milliliters (100,000 units/mL); swish and swallow 4 times/day
        iv. Poor adherence
     b. Clotrimazole—alternative to nystatin
        i. Use for initial episodes in patients with CD_4 count more than 50/mm³.
        ii. Mycelex troches 10 mg 5 times/day
        iii. Poor adherence (generally better tolerated than nystatin)
     c. Fluconazole
        i. Indicated for oropharyngeal and esophageal candidiasis
        ii. Two percent relapse on fluconazole versus 28% on placebo
        iii. Ten percent of patients develop fluconazole-resistant infections.
        iv. A total of 100-200 mg/day
     d. Itraconazole
        i. Indicated for oropharyngeal and esophageal candidiasis
        ii. Oral solution: 200 mg/day

Patient Case

6. G.H. is a 33-year-old man positive for HIV who presents to the clinic with a severe headache that has gradually worsened during the past 3 weeks. He also has memory problems and is always tired. He has refused antiretroviral therapy in the past, and his most recent CD_4 count was 75/mm³. He is given a diagnosis of *Cryptococcal meningitis* and is successfully treated. Which one of the following is the best follow-up therapy for G.H.?

   A. No maintenance treatment is required.
   B. Administer fluconazole 200 mg/day orally.
   C. Administer amphotericin B 1 mg/kg/week intravenously.
   D. G.H. is protected as long as he is also receiving PCP prophylaxis.

F. Cryptococcosis
   1. *C. neoformans*
   2. Occurs in 6%–10% of patients with AIDS
   3. In general, occurs in patients with CD_4 counts less than $100/mm^3$
   4. Acute mortality is 10%–25%, and 12-month mortality is 30%–60%.
   5. Worldwide distribution
      a. Found in aged pigeon droppings and nesting places (e.g., barns, window ledges)
      b. Organism must be aerosolized and inhaled; it then disseminates hematogenously.
   6. Signs and symptoms
      a. Almost always meningitis (66%–84%)
      b. Usually present for weeks or months (1 day to 4 months; average = 31 days)
      c. Insidious onset
         i. Low-grade fever (80%–90%)
         ii. Headaches (80%–90%)
         iii. Altered sensorium (20%): irritability, somnolence, clumsiness, impaired memory and judgment, behavioral changes
         iv. Seizures may occur late in the course (less than 10%).
         v. Minimal nuchal rigidity, meningismus, photophobia
   7. Diagnosis
      a. Cerebral spinal fluid (CSF) changes
         i. Patients with AIDS often have no CSF abnormalities except:
            (a) Positive CSF cultures
            (b) Cerebral spinal fluid India ink
            (c) Cerbral spinal fluid cryptococcal antigen titer (91%)
      b. Serum cryptococcal antigen more than 1:8
   8. Therapy
      a. Amphotericin B: 0.7–1 mg/kg/day (or liposomal amphotericin 4-6 mg/kg/day) PLUS flucytosine 25 mg/kg every 6 hours for at least 2 weeks, followed by fluconazole 400 mg/day for at least 8 weeks—commonly used in patients with AIDS
      b. Amphotericin B: 0.7–1 mg/kg/day (or liposomal amphotericin 4-6 mg/kg/day) for 4-6 weeks (or 1 month after negative cultures); alternative in patients with AIDS
      c. Amphotericin B: 0.7–1 mg/kg/day PLUS fluconazole 800 mg/day for 2 weeks, followed by fluconazole 800 mg/day for at least 8 weeks
      d. Fluconazole 1200mg/day PLUS flucytosine 25 mg/kg every 6 hours for 6 weeks
      e. Fluconazole 800-2000 mg/day for 10-12 weeks
   9. Outcome
      a. Therapeutic response: 42%–75%
      b. Length of therapy is controversial, but antifungals should probably be continued as long as CSF and other body fluid cultures are positive and for 1 month after negative cultures.
      c. Relapse: 50%–90% (with about 100% mortality)
   10. Prophylaxis
      a. Relapses usually occur within first year after therapy (less often with HAART therapy).
      b. Secondary prophylaxis: fluconazole 200 mg/day (may consider stopping if CD_4 count is more than $100/mm^3$ for 3 months or longer after potent combination anti-retroviral therapy; restart if CD_4 count decreases to less than $100/mm^3$)
      c. Primary prophylaxis: not indicated (decreases the incidence of cryptococcosis but does not decrease mortality and may lead to resistance)

Patient Cases

7. After treatment of his cryptococcal meningitis, G.H. is initiated on potent combination antiretroviral therapy. Two, 6, and 8 months after starting the therapy, his CD_4 counts are 212, 344, and 484/mm³, respectively. Which one of the following is the best follow-up therapy for G.H. now?
    A. Continue the fluconazole maintenance.
    B. Maintenance therapy with fluconazole should be given for at least 1 year; then, it can be discontinued because the CD_4 counts have increased.
    C. Maintenance therapy with fluconazole should be continued until CD_4 counts are greater than 500/mm³.
    D. Maintenance therapy with fluconazole can be discontinued.

8. J.C., a 36-year-old woman positive for HIV, has severe anemia. She has been tested for iron deficiency and has been taken off zidovudine and TMP/SMZ. She has also started to lose weight and to have severe diarrhea. A blood culture is positive for MAC. Which one of the following treatments is best for J.C.?
    A. Clarithromycin plus EMB for 2 weeks, followed by maintenance with clarithromycin alone.
    B. Azithromycin plus EMB for at least 12 months.
    C. Clarithromycin plus INH for 2 weeks, followed by maintenance with clarithromycin alone.
    D. EMB plus rifabutin indefinitely.

G. *M. avium* Complex (MAC)
　1. Organism characteristics
　　a. Complex is similar (main species are *M. avium* and *M. intracellulare*, which are not differentiated microbiologically).
　　b. Ubiquitous in soil and water
　　　i. Organisms gain access through the gastrointestinal tract.
　　　ii. After access, the organism spreads hematogenously.
　　c. Usually occurs in patients with HIV having a CD_4 count less than 50/mm³
　2. Signs and symptoms
　　a. Nonspecific
　　　i. Weight loss, intermittent fevers, chills, night sweats, abdominal pain, diarrhea, chronic malabsorption, and progressive weakness
　　　ii. Anemia
　3. Diagnosis
　　a. Blood culture
　　b. Bone marrow biopsy
　　c. Stool cultures (do not treat if cultured only in the stool)
　4. Therapy
　　a. The MAC is independently associated with risk of death, and treatment prolongs survival.
　　b. Suggested therapeutic regimen – macrolide plus ethambutol: clarithromycin 500 mg (7.5–15 mg/kg) 2 times/day (alternative: azithromycin 500–600 mg/day 10–20 mg/kg) **PLUS** ethambutol 15 mg/kg/day
　　　i. Other agents:
　　　　(a) Rifabutin (Mycobutin) 150-600 mg/day (added to regimen if patient has CD_4 less than 50/mm³, has a high mycobacterial load, or is not currently taking antiretrovirals; rifabutin dose chosen on the basis of other antiretrovirals because of drug-drug interactions)
　　　　(b) Ciprofloxacin 750 mg (10-15 mg/kg) 2 times/day
　　　　(c) Amikacin 10-15 mg/kg/day intravenously
　　c. Chronic maintenance therapy/secondary prophylaxis may be discontinued after 12 months of therapy if CD_4 count is more than 100/mm³ for 6 months or longer because of potent combination antiretroviral therapy <u>and</u> if patient is asymptomatic.

5. Prophylaxis
   a. Primary prophylaxis in patients with CD_4 counts less than 50/mm³ (may be discontinued if CD_4 count is more than 100/mm³ for 3 months or longer because of potent combination antiretroviral therapy)
      i. Clarithromycin 500 mg orally 2 times/day
         (a) Three times lower incidence of MAC bacteremia (vs. placebo)
      ii. Azithromycin 1200 mg orally once weekly
      iii. Rifabutin 300 mg/day (150 mg orally 2 times/day with food if there are gastrointestinal adverse effects)
         (a) Two times longer until a positive MAC culture (vs. placebo)
         (b) Decreased incidence of symptoms related to MAC
         (c) Adverse effects: rash, gastrointestinal disturbances, neutropenia, body fluid discoloration
         (d) **DO NOT** give alone to patients with active TB.

Patient Case

9. P.L. is a 44-year-old man positive for HIV who receives a diagnosis of CMV retinitis. He currently receives zidovudine, lamivudine, and efavirenz as antiretroviral agents; pyrimethamine-sulfadiazine for toxoplasmosis and PCP prophylaxis; and fluconazole for esophageal candidiasis. Which one of the following agents is the best empiric therapy?
   A. Ganciclovir intravenously or valganciclovir orally.
   B. Foscarnet intravenously.
   C. Cidofovir intravenously.
   D. Acyclovir intravenously.

H. Cytomegalovirus (CMV)
   1. Characteristics of CMV infection
      a. Fifty-three percent of Americans between 18 and 25 years old are CMV+.
      b. Eighty-one percent of Americans older than 35 years are CMV+.
      c. More than 95% of homosexual men are CMV+.
      d. About 90% of CMV infections are asymptomatic (if illness occurs, it resembles mononucleosis).
      e. Virus remains latent in the host after initial infection but may reactivate if patient becomes immunocompromised (especially cell-mediated immunity).
      f. Ninety percent of patients with AIDS develop CMV infections, and 25% experience life- or sight-threatening disease (pre-HAART [highly active antiretroviral therapy] data: pre-1996).
   2. Diagnosis of CMV infection
      a. Serology
         i. Detects exposure to CMV
      b. Virus isolation
         i. Tissue culture—requires up to 6 weeks
         ii. Shell vial technique—requires only 16 hours
            (a) Organism is incubated overnight and then detected by immunofluorescence microscopy with monoclonal antibodies.
      c. Cytology/histology
         i. Large (cytomegalic) cell with a large, central, basophilic, intranuclear inclusion ("owl's eye")
         ii. Low yield

3. Manifestations of CMV
   a. Gastrointestinal
      i. Colitis: 5%–10% of patients with AIDS
         (a) Diarrhea, abdominal pain, weight loss, anorexia, fever
      ii. Esophagitis/gastritis uncommon
      iii. Hepatitis: 33%–50% with histologic evidence but minimal clinical importance
      iv. Maintenance drugs not needed
   b. Pneumonia
      i. Cytomegalovirus is commonly in bronchial secretions; of questionable importance
      ii. Chest radiography results are similar to those seen with PCP.
      iii. Symptoms: shortness of breath; dyspnea on exertion; dry, nonproductive cough
      iv. Treat if:
         (a) Documented tissue infection
         (b) Cytomegalovirus is only pathogen
         (c) Deteriorating illness
      v. About 50%-60% of patients will respond; no need for maintenance
   c. Retinitis
      i. Occurs in 10%–15% of patients with AIDS; is clinically most important CMV infection
      ii. In general, patients have CD_4 counts less than $100/mm^3$.
      iii. Begins unilaterally and spreads bilaterally
      iv. Early complaints: "floaters," pain behind the eye
      v. In general, progressive; no spontaneous resolution (blindness in weeks to months)
      vi. Twenty-six percent progression, even with treatment; retinal detachment very common
4. Therapy for CMV infections
   a. Ganciclovir (Cytovene-IV, Cytovene), valganciclovir (Valcyte)
      i. Competes with deoxynucleosides, inhibiting viral DNA synthesis
      ii. Must be triphosphorylated; the rate-limiting step in this process is the first phosphorylation. Cytomegalovirus induces the production of the enzymes required to monophosphorylate ganciclovir but not acyclovir.
      iii. Valganciclovir is rapidly converted to ganciclovir in intestinal wall and liver (F of about 60%).
      iv. Adverse effects
         (a) A total of 65% have adverse effects, and 76% have moderate to severe neutropenia (25% less than $1000/mm^3$, 16% less than $500/mm^3$).
            (1) In general, after 10 days
            (2) Ganciclovir plus zidovudine: 82% will have severe hematologic toxicity
            (3) Patients receiving ganciclovir can tolerate only up to 300 mg/day of zidovudine.
         (b) Thrombocytopenia (9% less than $20,000/mm^3$)
         (c) Confusion; convulsions; dizziness; headache; thinking disorders
         (d) Nausea; vomiting; diarrhea; abnormal liver function tests
         (e) Possible reproductive toxicity
      vi. Dose
         (a) Induction: valganciclovir 900 mg orally 2 times/day for 14–21 days (alternative: ganciclovir 5 mg/kg intravenously every 12 hours for 14–21 days)
         (b) Maintenance: valganciclovir 900 mg/day orally (alternative: ganciclovir 5 mg/kg/day intravenously)
         (c) All (100%) patients will relapse in 1–8 weeks without maintenance.
         (d) Intravenous maintenance therapy requires establishment of central venous access.

vii. Local therapy
   (a) Intraocular implant (Vitrasert): designed to release 1 mcg/hour (replace after 6–8 months) plus valganciclovir 900 mg/day orally
   (b) Local therapy alone is associated with an increased incidence of ocular adverse effects, contralateral CMV retinitis, and extraocular CMV disease.
b. Foscarnet
   i. Inhibits viral-induced DNA polymerase; no effect on human DNA polymerase
   ii. Effective against all herpes viruses (especially CMV), HBV (±), and HIV
   iii. Foscarnet and ganciclovir are equally effective against CMV, but foscarnet decreases (by about 4 months) mortality because of its anti-HIV effects.
   iv. Adverse effects
      (a) Renal impairment
         (1) Especially occurs if the patient is dehydrated or taking other renal toxic drugs
         (2) A 2–3 times increase in serum creatinine (more than 50% had to discontinue)
         (3) Usually reversible
         (4) Prevented by administering 2.5 L/day of normal saline
      (b) Decrease in hemoglobin and hematocrit
      (c) Altered serum electrolytes (calcium, phosphorus, magnesium)
      (d) Penile ulcerations
   v. Preparation and dose
      (a) Commercial preparation is available in 500-mL glass bottles at 24 mg/mL; 24 mg/mL should be administered centrally. For peripheral administration, use 12 mg/mL.
      (b) One gram of foscarnet contains about 600 mg of sodium chloride.
      (c) Induction: 60 mg/kg every 8 hours or 90 mg/kg every 12 hours for 14–21 days (administer for 1 hour)
      (d) Maintenance: 90–120 mg/kg/day (administer for 2 hours)
      (e) Decrease dose by 3.5 mg/kg for each 0.1 mL/minute/kg of creatinine clearance below 1.6 mL/minute/kg.
      (f) Maintenance therapy requires establishment of central venous access.
c. Cidofovir (Vistide)
   i. Acts as a nucleoside monophosphate, inhibiting viral DNA polymerase
   ii. Intracellular activation required
   iii. Adverse effects
      (a) Renal impairment
      (b) Manifested as proteinuria and increased creatinine concentrations
      (c) Decreased with concurrent probenecid (2 g, 3 hours before infusion and 1 g, 2 and 8 hours after infusion—to decrease renal secretion) and saline hydration
      (d) Probenecid may cause nausea, vomiting, headache, fever, and flushing.
   iv. Neutropenia (15% of patients)
   v. Dose
      (a) Induction: 5 mg/kg/week for 2 weeks
      (b) Maintenance: 5 mg/kg every other week
      (c) Maintenance therapy does not require the establishment of central venous access.
5. Prophylaxis
   a. Secondary prophylaxis is required for all patients (see individual drugs for specific doses); it may be discontinued if the CD_4 count is more than 100/mm^3 for 3–6 months or longer because of potent combination antiretroviral therapy; restart secondary prophylaxis if the CD_4 count decreases to less than 100/mm^3.
   b. Primary prophylaxis not recommended. In patients with CD_4 counts less than 50/mm^3, regular funduscopic examinations are recommended.

I. Toxoplasmosis
   1. Description
      a. *Toxoplasma gondii* (protozoan)
      b. Felines are the hosts for sporozoite production (change litter box daily, wash hands after changing litter box or have someone else change the litter box, and, ideally, keep the cat indoors).
      c. A total of 15%–68% of adults in the United States are seropositive for *T. gondii*.
      d. Secondary to undercooked beef, lamb, or pork (stress avoidance in patients with HIV)
      e. Case-defining illness in 2.1% of patients with AIDS
   2. Signs and symptoms
      a. Fever, headache, altered mental status
      b. Focal neurologic deficits (60%): hemiparesis; aphasia; ataxia; visual field loss; nerve palsies
      c. Seizures (33%)
      d. Cerebral spinal fluid: mild pleocytosis, increased protein, normal glucose
   3. Diagnosis
      a. Brain biopsy: only definitive diagnosis but generally not done
      b. Antibodies or *T. gondii* isolation in serum or CSF
      c. Magnetic resonance imaging scan or computerized tomographic scan: multiple, bilateral, hypodense, ring-enhancing mass lesions (magnetic resonance imaging scan more sensitive than computerized tomographic scan)
   4. Therapy
      a. Standard therapy
         i. Pyrimethamine 50–75 mg/day (loading dose = 200 mg in two doses) **PLUS**
         ii. Sulfadiazine 1000–1500 mg every 6 hours (watch crystalluria)
            (a) Bone marrow suppression: thrombocytopenia, granulocytopenia, anemia
            (b) Folinic acid (leucovorin) 10–20 mg/day to reduce bone marrow effects of pyrimethamine
            (c) Duration: 6 weeks or after signs and symptoms resolve
      b. Alternative therapy
         i. Clindamycin
            (a) Dosage: 600–1200 mg intravenously every 6 hours for 6 weeks; after 3 weeks, can change to oral 600 mg every 8 hours
            (b) Used in combination with pyrimethamine-leucovorin for sulfa intolerance or by itself when bone marrow suppression occurs
         ii. Atovaquone
            (a) Dosage: 1500 mg orally 2 times/day
            (b) Used in combination with pyrimethamine-leucovorin or in combination with sulfadiazine or alone (monitor plasma concentrations if using alone)
         iii. Azithromycin
            (a) Dosage: 900–1200 mg/day orally
            (b) Used in combination with pyrimethamine (do not use alone for acute therapy)
         iv. Other alternatives: clarithromycin plus pyrimethamine, 5-FU (fluorouracil) plus clindamycin, dapsone plus pyrimethamine plus leucovorin, and minocycline or doxycycline combined with pyrimethamine plus leucovorin, sulfadiazine, or clarithromycin

5. Prophylaxis
   a. Relapse rates approach 80% without maintenance therapy.
   b. Toxoplasma-seropositive patients with a CD_4 count of 100/mm³ or less should receive primary prophylaxis.
   c. For primary prophylaxis, use TMP/SMZ or dapsone-pyrimethamine-leucovorin or atovaquone with or without pyrimethamine at doses used for PCP prophylaxis (may be discontinued if the CD_4 count is more than 200/mm³ for 3 months or longer because of potent combination antiretroviral therapy).
   d. For secondary prophylaxis, use the following (may be discontinued if the CD_4 count is more than 200/mm³ for 6 months or longer because of potent combination antiretroviral therapy):
      i. Pyrimethamine 25–50 mg/day plus leucovorin 10–25 mg/day with sulfadiazine 2–4 g/day
      ii. Clindamycin 600 mg every 8 hours can be substituted if sulfa intolerance occurs.
      iii. Atovaquone 750 mg orally every 6–12 hours with or without pyrimethamine-leucovorin

III. TUBERCULOSIS (TB)

A. Introduction
   1. *Mycobacterium tuberculosis*
      a. Factors associated with acquiring TB
         i. Exposure to individuals with active pulmonary TB
         ii. Geographic location
         iii. Low socioeconomic status
         iv. Nonwhite race
         v. Male sex
         vi. Acquired immunodeficiency syndrome
   2. Epidemiology (Figure 2)

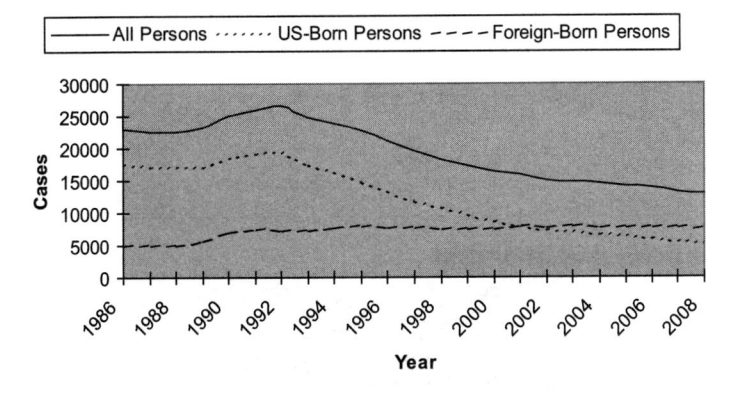

Figure 2. Epidemiology of tuberculosis.

B. Pathophysiology (Figure 3)
  1. Person-to-person transmission—Airborne droplets carrying *M. tuberculosis* are inhaled.
  2. Infection primarily pulmonary, although can occur in other organ systems

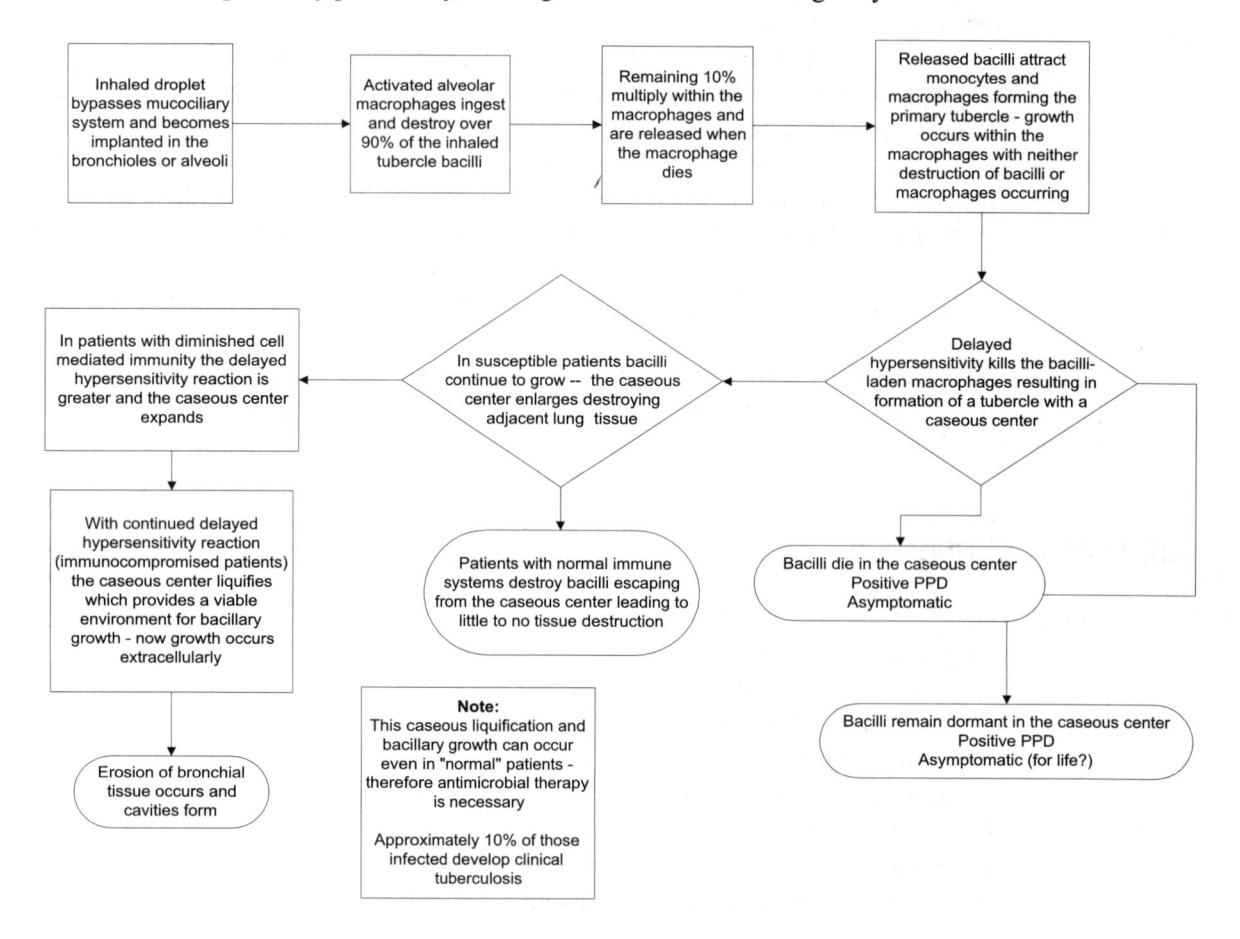

```
[Inhaled droplet bypasses mucociliary system and becomes implanted in the bronchioles or alveoli]
  → [Activated alveolar macrophages ingest and destroy over 90% of the inhaled tubercle bacilli]
  → [Remaining 10% multiply within the macrophages and are released when the macrophage dies]
  → [Released bacilli attract monocytes and macrophages forming the primary tubercle - growth occurs within the macrophages with neither destruction of bacilli or macrophages occurring]
  → ⬥ Delayed hypersensitivity kills the bacilli-laden macrophages resulting in formation of a tubercle with a caseous center ⬥
      → (Bacilli die in the caseous center / Positive PPD / Asymptomatic)
      → (Bacilli remain dormant in the caseous center / Positive PPD / Asymptomatic (for life?))
      → ⬥ In susceptible patients bacilli continue to grow -- the caseous center enlarges destroying adjacent lung tissue ⬥
          → (Patients with normal immune systems destroy bacilli escaping from the caseous center leading to little to no tissue destruction)
          → [In patients with diminished cell mediated immunity the delayed hypersensitivity reaction is greater and the caseous center expands]
              → [With continued delayed hypersensitivity reaction (immunocompromised patients) the caseous center liquifies which provides a viable environment for bacillary growth - now growth occurs extracellularly]
              → (Erosion of bronchial tissue occurs and cavities form)
```

Note:
This caseous liquification and bacillary growth can occur even in "normal" patients - therefore antimicrobial therapy is necessary

Approximately 10% of those infected develop clinical tuberculosis

Figure 3. Pathophysiology of tuberculosis.

C. Diagnosis (Table 8)

Table 8. Diagnosis of Tuberculosis

Nonspecific Signs and Symptoms	Radiology	Microbiology
Cough Malaise Weight loss Fever, chills Night sweats Pleuritic pain	Chest radiograph patchy or nodular infiltrates in upper lobes; cavitary lesions	Sputum smear for AFB Sputum culture for *Mycobacterium tuberculosis*

AFB = acid-fast bacillus.

1. Skin test for PPD (Table 9)
    a. Recommended dose is 5 tuberculin units/0.1 mL.
    b. Mantoux method
        i. Intradermal injection of tuberculin into forearm
        ii. Measure diameter of induration after 48–72 hours.
    c. False-negative tests occur in 15%–20% of people infected with *M. tuberculosis*, primarily in those recently infected or anergic.
    d. Two hundred fifty tuberculin units per 0.1 mL of solution can be used, but this is not recommended by the Centers for Disease Control and Prevention.
    e. Only 8% of people vaccinated with Bacille Calmette-Guérin at birth will react 15 years later.

Table 9. Recommendation for Purified Protein Derivative (PPD) Skin Test

Criterion for Positive Skin Test (mm)	Applicable Group
5	• Patients with chest radiograph consistent with TB • Close contacts of individuals with newly diagnosed infectious TB • Patients with HIV infection • Patients with documented defects in cellular immunity • Patients receiving prednisone ≥ 15 mg/day for ≥ 1 month
10	• Recent immigrants (within the past 5 years) from countries with a high prevalence of TB (even if they had BCG) • Intravenous drug abusers • Residents and employees of: prisons/jails, nursing homes, hospitals, and homeless shelters • Patients with diseases known to be associated with a higher risk of TB (diabetes mellitus, silicosis, leukemias and lymphomas, chronic renal failure), gastrectomy, and jejunoileal bypass • Children < 4 years
15	Patients with no identifiable risk factors

BCG = Bacille Calmette-Guérin; HIV = human immunodeficiency virus; TB = tuberculosis.

2. Interferon-gamma release assays/targeted blood tests
    a. QuantiFERON-TB Gold and T-SPOT.TB
    b. Blood test that detects the release of interferon-gamma in response to *M. tuberculosis* infection
    c. Greater sensitivity and specificity than the PPD test
    d. Most beneficial to verify a positive PPD in patients with a history of Bacille Calmette-Guérin vaccine
3. Booster effect
    a. The TB test can restimulate hypersensitivity in those exposed in the past.
    b. Occurs within 1 week of the test and persists for longer than 1 year
    c. Those with small TB test reactions can be retested in 1 week—if positive, it should be attributed to boosting of a subclinical hypersensitivity; chemoprophylaxis is not necessary.

HIV/Infectious Diseases

Patient Case

10. J.M. is a 42-year-old man who has a yearly PPD skin test because he works at a long-term care facility. Forty-eight hours after the PPD was placed, he had an 18-mm induration. This is the first time he has reacted to this test. His chest radiograph is negative. Which one of the following is best in view of J.M.'s positive PPD?
    A. No treatment is necessary, and J.M. should have another PPD skin test in 1 year.
    B. Another PPD skin test should be performed in 1 week to see whether this is a booster effect.
    C. J.M. should be monitored closely, but no treatment is necessary because he is older than 35 years.
    D. J.M. should be initiated on INH 300 mg/day orally for 6 months.

D. Therapy
   1. Treatment of latent TB infection
      a. The goal is to prevent latent (asymptomatic) infection from progressing to clinical disease.
      b. The treatment of latent TB infection should be instituted in the following groups with a positive PPD skin test:
         i. Close contacts of individuals with newly diagnosed infectious TB
         ii. Health care workers at facilities treating patients with TB
         iii. Foreign-born people from high-prevalence countries (immigration within 5 years)
         iv. Homeless people
         v. People working at or living in long-term care facilities
         vi. Patients with HIV infection
         vii. Recent converters (within a 2-year period)
         viii. People with abnormal chest radiographs that show fibrotic lesions—likely to represent old, healed TB
         ix. People with medical conditions that have been reported to increase the risk of TB: intravenous drug use, diabetes mellitus, silicosis, Hodgkin disease, leukemia, immunosuppressive therapy, corticosteroids, end-stage renal disease
      c. Dosing regimens
         i. Patients who are not infected with HIV:
            (a) Administer INH 300 mg/day or 900 mg 2 times/week for 6-9 months (or RIF alone for 4 months).
         ii. Patients who are infected with HIV:
            (a) Administer INH 300 mg/day for 9 months (or RIF alone for 4 months).
         iii. Areas with multidrug-resistant isolates:
            (a) Two drugs with activity against the isolate for 6-12 months

Patient Case

11. R.J. is a 32-year-old man positive for HIV infection who presents to the clinic with increased weight loss and night sweats, as well as a cough productive of sputum. He is currently receiving fosamprenavir-ritonavir 700 mg/100 mg 2 times/day, zidovudine 300 mg 2 times/day, lamivudine 150 mg 2 times/day, fluconazole 200 mg/day orally, and TMP/SMZ double strength daily. A sputum sample is obtained that is positive for acid-fast bacillus. R.J. lives in an area with a low incidence of multidrug-resistant TB. Which one of the following is the initial treatment of choice?
    A. Initiate INH, RIF, and PZA with no change in his HIV medications.
    B. Initiate INH, RIF, and PZA; increase the dosage of fosamprenavir-ritonavir; and use a higher dosage of RIF.
    C. Initiate INH, rifabutin, PZA, and EMB, with a lower dosage of rifabutin.
    D. Initiate INH, rifabutin, PZA, and EMB and decrease the dosage of fosamprenavir-ritonavir.

2. Treatment of active TB infection (Table 10)
   a. Principles of treatment
      i. Regimens must contain many drugs to which the organisms are susceptible.
      ii. Drug therapy must continue for a sufficient period.

Table 10. Pharmacotherapeutic Agents in the Treatment of Tuberculosis

First-line Agents	Second-line Agents
Isoniazid (INH)	Para-aminosalicylic acid
Rifampin (RIF)	Ethionamide
Pyrazinamide (PZA)	Cycloserine
Ethambutol (EMB)	Kanamycin-amikacin
Streptomycin (SM)	Capreomycin
	Fluoroquinolones
	Rifabutin
	Rifapentine

   b. Therapeutic options for patients without HIV infection (*Note*: Any regimen administered 2, 3, or 5 times/week should be done by directly observed therapy.)
      i. Option 1: INH, RIF, PZA, and EMB for 2 months (daily, 5 times/week, 3 times/week, or 2 times/week), followed by INH and RIF for 4 months (daily, 5 times/week, 3 times/week, or 2 times/week)
      ii. Option 2: INH, RIF, and EMB for 2 months (daily or 5 times/week), followed by INH and RIF for 7 months (daily, 5 times/week, or 2 times/week)
   c. Therapeutic options for patients with HIV
      i. Option 1: INH, RIF, PZA, and EMB for 2 months (daily, 5 times/week, or 3 times/week), followed by INH and RIF for 4 months (daily, 5 times/week, or 3 times/week)
      ii. Option 2: INH, RIF, and EMB for 2 months (daily or 5 times/week), followed by INH and RIF for 7 months (daily or 5 times/week)
   d. Concurrent therapy in patients with HIV
      i. Protease inhibitors and NNRTIs (except for efavirenz or nevirapine) should not be administered concurrently with RIF; NRTIs can be administered with RIF.
      ii. A washout period of 1–2 weeks may be necessary once RIF is discontinued before protease inhibitors or NNRTIs are initiated.
      iii. Rifabutin can be substituted for RIF; patients may take NNRTIs with rifabutin, but doses may need to be increased to 450–600 mg/day (see HIV guidelines).
      iv. Patients may take protease inhibitors with RIF but the rifabutin dose should be decreased to 150 mg every day or every other day (300 mg 3 times/week may be an option).
      v. Patients taking rifabutin and protease inhibitors or NNRTIs should have HIV RNA concentrations performed periodically.
   e. Known drug resistance to INH
      i. Administer RIF, PZA, and EMB for 6 months; rifabutin may be substituted for RIF in patients with HIV.
   f. Known drug resistance to RIF
      i. Administer INH, PZA, and EMB for 9–12 months; streptomycin may be added for the first 2 months to shorten the total treatment time to 9 months.

Patient Case

12. Which one of the following represents the best follow-up for R.J.?
    A. Treatment with the initial drugs should continue for 6 months.
    B. Treatment can be decreased to just INH and a rifamycin after 2 months for a total treatment of 18–24 months.
    C. Treatment can be decreased to just INH and a rifamycin after 2 months for a total treatment of 6 months; HIV RNA concentrations should be observed closely during therapy.
    D. Treatment can be decreased to INH, a rifamycin, and either PZA or EMB after 2 months for a total treatment of 6 months; HIV RNA concentrations should be observed closely during therapy.

IV. ANTIFUNGAL THERAPY

A. Amphotericin B (Fungizone, Abelcet, Amphotec, AmBisome)
   1. Mechanism of action
      a. Binds to ergosterol in the fungal cell membrane, altering membrane permeability and causing cell lysis
   2. Spectrum of activity
      a. In vitro
         i. *Candida, Blastomyces dermatitidis, Coccidioides immitis, Cryptococcus neoformans,* Paracoccidioides, *Histoplasma capsulatum, Sporothrix, Aspergillus,* mucormycoses
      b. Clinical use
         i. Cryptococcal meningitis
         ii. Systemic fungal infections caused by sensitive fungi
         iii. Limited use clinically with newer antifungals
   3. Adverse effects
      a. Renal toxicity (glomerular and tubular)
         i. Glomerular filtration rate decreases by about 40% within 2 weeks and usually stabilizes at 20%–60% of normal.
         ii. In general, reversible unless total dose is more than 4–5 g
         iii. Manifestations: renal tubular acidosis, urine casts, azotemia, oliguria, magnesium and potassium wasting
         iv. Prevention:
            (a) Correct salt depletion—3 L of normal saline for 24 hours or 500 mL of normal saline before and after amphotericin dose
            (b) Avoid diuretics and liberalize salt intake—risk/benefit with other disease states
      b. Thrombophlebitis
         i. Prevention
            (a) Dilute to 0.1 mg/mL and infuse for at least 4 hours; a faster infusion (i.e., 45 minutes to 2 hours) may be tolerated.
            (b) Use a central site.
            (c) Adding heparin may decrease phlebitis.
      c. Anemia
      d. Fever/chills
         i. Mechanism: Amphotericin B induces prostaglandin synthesis.
         ii. Premedications:
            (a) Hydrocortisone—25 mg intravenously before the dose or in the bottle significantly decreases fever and chills (higher doses are not significantly better)

iii. Ibuprofen (10 mg/kg up to 600 mg 30 minutes before infusion) – Significantly more fever/chills in placebo (87%) than in ibuprofen group (48%)
iv. Acetylsalicylic acid, acetaminophen, diphenhydramine—never shown to be effective (but not specifically studied)
   e. Treatment:
      i. Meperidine 50 mg—stops reaction within 30 minutes (mean = 10.8 minutes)
      ii. If the patient consistently needs meperidine, then prophylactic doses may be appropriate.
4. Dosing
   a. Test dose of 1 mg (in 25–50 mL of 5% dextrose in distilled water [D5W]) or aliquot of initial dose) for 20–30 minutes
   b. If tolerated, prepare dose to a concentration of 0.1 mg/mL in D5W (amphotericin B potency not affected by light [for 24 hours]).
   c. Start therapy with 0.25 mg/kg (some suggest 5–10 mg) administered for 4–6 hours.
   d. Increase gradually to desired milligram per kilogram concentration (i.e., 5- to 10-mg increments).
   e. May increase rapidly in fulminant infections or immunocompromised patients
   f. Amphotericin can be given on alternate days by doubling the daily dose to a maximum of 1.5 mg/kg.
5. Liposomal amphotericin
   a. Liposomal formulations are designed to maintain therapeutic efficacy, but they diminish renal- and infusion-related toxicity.

	Amphotericin B	Abelcet	Amphotec	AmBisome
Liposome Type		Multilamellar vesicle with ribbonlike structure	Colloidal dispersion in aqueous solution (disk-shaped bilayer)	Unilamellar liposome
Dose	1 mg/kg/day	5 mg/kg/day for 2 hours	3–4 mg/kg/day for 3–4 hours	3–5 mg/kg/day
Test dose	Yes	None	Yes	None
Chills/rigors (%)	54–56	18	77	18
Fever (%)	44–47	14	55	17
Nephrotoxicity (%)	34–47	28	8	19
Hypokalemia (%)	12–29	5	26	7
Hypomagnesemia (%)	11–26	NA	6	20

   b. Mostly taken up by macrophages in the lung, liver, spleen, bone marrow, and circulating monocytes
   c. Liposomes target fungi cell membranes much more than human cell membranes.
   d. Amphotericin dissociates from the liposome over time, decreasing its toxicity (only free drug is toxic).
   e. Primary use in patients with aspergillosis who cannot tolerate amphotericin B
   f. Potential use for invasive candidiasis

B. Azole Antifungals
   1. Mechanism of action
      a. Inhibits the synthesis of ergosterol, a component of the fungal cell membrane, vital for normal growth

2. Ketoconazole (Nizoral)
   a. Spectrum of activity
      i. In vitro
         (a) *Candida* species, *Blastomyces*, histoplasmosis, Paracoccidioides, *Sporothrix*, dermatophytes
      ii. Clinical use
         (a) Histoplasmosis, superficial *Candida* and other infections, blastomycosis, paracoccidioidomycosis
   b. Adverse effects
      i. Nausea, abdominal pain, headache, rash
      ii. Adrenal insufficiency, decreased libido, impotence, gynecomastia, menstrual irregularities (inhibits steroidogenesis)
      iii. Increased liver function tests, potential fulminate hepatitis
   c. Drug interactions (CYP3A4 substrate and inhibitor)
      i. Antacids, H_2-blockers, proton pump inhibitors, didanosine (gastrointestinal absorption)
      ii. Rifampin (decreases ketoconazole concentrations)
      iii. Cyclosporine
      iv. Phenytoin
      v. Warfarin
      vi. Methylprednisolone, midazolam, alprazolam, simvastatin, lovastatin
      vii. Protease inhibitors
   d. Dosing
      i. 200–400 mg/day
3. Fluconazole (Diflucan)
   a. Spectrum of activity
      i. In vitro
         (a) *Candida* species (poor activity against *C. glabrata* and no activity against *C. krusei*), *Cryptococcus, Blastomyces,* histoplasmosis, dermatophytes
      ii. Clinical use
         (a) Cryptococcal meningitis
         (b) *Candida* infections (primarily *C. albicans* and *C. parapsilosis*)
   b. Pharmacokinetics
      i. Well absorbed orally (F = 100%)—also available intravenously
      ii. Half-life is about 30 hours—primarily eliminated unchanged in the urine
   c. Adverse effects
      i. Nausea, abdominal pain, headache
      ii. Increased liver function tests
   d. Drug interactions (CYP3A4 inhibitor at more than 400 mg/day and CYP2C9 inhibitor at lower doses)
      i. Cyclosporine
      ii. Phenytoin
      iii. Warfarin
   e. Dosing
      i. Oral candidiasis—100–200 mg/day
      ii. Esophageal candidiasis—200 mg/day
      iii. Invasive candidiasis—400–800 mg/day
      iv. Acute cryptococcal meningitis—400 mg/day
      v. Cryptococcal meningitis prophylaxis—200 mg/day

4. Itraconazole (Sporanox)
   a. Spectrum of activity
      i. In vitro
         (a) *Candida* species (usually just *C. albicans*), *Cryptococcus, Aspergillus, Blastomyces,* histoplasmosis, dermatophytes
      ii. Clinical use
         (a) Onychomycosis
         (b) Histoplasmosis
         (c) *Aspergillus*
   b. Pharmacokinetics
      i. Oral absorption about 55% when given with food—also available intravenously
      ii. Half-life is about 20 hours—extensively metabolized—hydroxyitraconazole is active
   c. Adverse effects
      i. Nausea, abdominal pain, headache, rash
      ii. Increased liver function tests, potential fulminate hepatitis
   d. Drug interactions (CYP3A4 inhibitor at more than 400 mg/day and CYP2C9 inhibitor at lower doses)
      i. Antacids, H2-blockers, proton pump inhibitors, didanosine (gastrointestinal absorption)
      ii. Cyclosporine
      iii. Digoxin (decreases digoxin volume of distribution)
      iv. Phenytoin
      v. Warfarin
      vi. Protease inhibitors
      vii. HMG CoA (3-hydroxy-3-methylglutaryl coenzyme A) reductase inhibitors
   e. Dosing
      i. 200 mg/day
5. Voriconazole (Vfend)
   a. Spectrum of activity
      i. In vitro
         (a) *Candida* species, *Aspergillus, Fusarium, Scedosporium*
      ii. Clinical use
         (a) Resistant *Candida* infections (especially *C. glabrata* and *C. krusei*)
         (b) *Aspergillus*
   b. Pharmacokinetics
      i. Oral absorption about 95%—also available intravenously
      ii. Half-life is about 6 hours—extensively metabolized—CYP (2C9, 3A4, 2C19)
   c. Adverse effects
      i. Abnormal vision 30% (abnormal vision, color changes, photophobia). Short-term (20–30 minutes) effects on retina. Dose related. Not studied for more than 28 days of therapy
      ii. Increased liver function tests, rash, nausea
   d. Drug interactions (CYP3A4 inhibitor and substrate; see table)
   e. Dosing
      Aspergillosis: loading dose = 6 mg/kg 2 times intravenously (infuse for 2 hours); minimum dose = 4 mg/kg every 12 hours intravenously (infuse for 2 hours)
      200 mg every 12 hours orally if more than 40 kg and 100 mg every 12 hours orally if less than 40 kg (note: oral doses may be increased to 300 mg every 12 hours and 150 mg every 12 hours, respectively, if necessary)

Candida: 200 mg every 12 hours
  i. For patients who are receiving phenytoin, increase dose to 5 mg/kg every 12 hours intravenously or 200–400 mg every 12 hours orally.
  ii. Dose reduction for moderate-severe cirrhosis: after loading dose, decrease dose by 50% in Child-Pugh class A/B—no information for patients in Child-Pugh class C
  iii. No adjustment of the oral dose for renal insufficiency; patients with creatinine clearance less than 50 mL/minute should not receive the intravenous product because of accumulation of the intravenous vehicle sulfobutylether-β-cyclodextrin

Table 11. Drug Interactions Reported with Voriconazole

Drug	Effect	Recommendation
Rifampin (CYP inducer)	↓ Voriconazole	Coadministration contraindicated
Rifabutin (CYP inducer)	↓ Voriconazole, ↑ rifabutin	Coadministration contraindicated
Carbamazepine (CYP inducer)	↓ Voriconazole	Coadministration contraindicated
Barbiturates, long acting (CYP inducers)	↓ Voriconazole	Coadministration contraindicated
Pimozide (CYP3A4 substrate)	↑ Pimozide, ↑ risk QT prolongation	Coadministration contraindicated
Quinidine (CYP3A4 substrate)	↑ Quinidine, ↑ risk QT prolongation	Coadministration contraindicated
Ergot alkaloids	↑ Ergot alkaloids, ↑ risk ergotism	Coadministration contraindicated
Sirolimus (CYP3A4 substrate)	↑ Sirolimus	Coadministration contraindicated
Cyclosporine (CYP3A4 substrate)	↑ Cyclosporine	Reduce cyclosporine dose by half when initiating voriconazole. Monitor levels closely. Increase cyclosporine dose as necessary when voriconazole is discontinued
Tacrolimus (CYP3A4 substrate)	↑ Tacrolimus	Reduce tacrolimus dose to one-third of initial dose when initiating voriconazole. Monitor levels closely. Increase tacrolimus dose as necessary when voriconazole is discontinued
Omeprazole (CYP2C19 inhibitor, CYP2C19 and CYP3A4 substrate)	↑ Voriconazole, ↑ omeprazole	In patients receiving omeprazole doses ≥ 40 mg, reduce the omeprazole dose by half
Warfarin (CYP2C9 substrate)	↑ Warfarin, PT	Closely monitor PT/INR and adjust warfarin dose as needed

CYP = cytochrome P450; INR = international normalized ratio; PT = prothrombin time.

  6. Posaconazole (Noxafil)
     a. Spectrum of activity
        i. In vitro
           (a) *Candida* species, *Cryptococcus, Trichosporon, Aspergillus, Fusarium*
        ii. Clinical use
           (a) *Candida* infections
           (b) Aspergillosis
           (c) Zygomycoses
           (d) Fusariosis

b. Pharmacokinetics
      i. Oral absorption enhanced by a high-fat meal—no intravenous formulation
      ii. Half-life is about 24–30 hours—primarily eliminated unchanged in the feces
   c. Adverse effects
      i. Nausea, vomiting, diarrhea
      ii. Increased liver function tests, rash, hypokalemia, thrombocytopenia
      iii. Q-Tc interval prolongation
   d. Drug interactions – CYP3A4 inhibitor
   e. Dosing
      Oropharyngeal candidiasis: loading dose = 200 mg; then 100 mg/day
      Refractory oropharyngeal candidiasis: 400 mg 2 times/day
      Prophylaxis of invasive fungal infections in neutropenic and graft-versus-host disease patients: 200 mg 3 times/day

C. Echinocandins
   1. Mechanism of action
      a. Inhibits the synthesis of 1,3-β-D-glucan, an essential component of the fungal cell wall
   2. Caspofungin (Cancidas), Micafungin (Mycamine), Anidulafungin (Eraxis)
      a. Spectrum of activity
         i. In vitro
            (a) *Candida* species (weak against *C. parapsilosis*), *Aspergillus*
         ii. Clinical use
            (a) *Candida:* fungemia, intra-abdominal abscesses, peritonitis, and pleural space infections
            (b) Esophageal candidiasis
            (c) Invasive aspergillosis (refractory or intolerant of other therapies)
      b. Pharmacokinetics
         i. Only available intravenously
         ii. Half-life of about 1–2 days—caspofungin and micafungin hepatically metabolized; anidulafungin chemically degraded in the blood
      c. Adverse effects
         i. Infusion site–related reactions, headache, gastrointestinal symptoms
      d. Drug interactions
         i. Caspofungin: Avoid concomitant use with cyclosporine or tacrolimus.
         ii. Micafungin: Avoid concomitant sirolimus or nifedipine.
         iii. Anidulafungin: none
      e. Dosing
         i. Caspofungin—70 mg once intravenously, followed by 50 mg/day intravenously
         ii. Micafungin—150 mg/day
         iii. Anidulafungin—200 mg once intravenously, followed by 100 mg/day intravenously

REFERENCES

Human Immunodeficiency Virus
1. Panel on Antiretroviral Guidelines for Adults and Adolescents. Guidelines for the use of antiretroviral agents in HIV-1-infected adults and adolescents. Department of Health and Human Services. December 1, 2009; 1–161. Available at *www.aidsinfo.nih.gov/ContentFiles/AdultandAdolescentGL.pdf*. Accessed December 15, 2009.
2. Hammer SM, Eron JJ, Reiss P, et al. Antiretroviral treatment for adult HIV infection: 2008 recommendations of the International AIDS Society – USA Panel. JAMA 2008;300:555–70.
3. Perinatal HIV Guidelines Working Group. Public Health Service Task Force recommendations for use of antiretroviral drugs in pregnant HIV-infected women for maternal health and interventions to reduce perinatal HIV transmission in the United States. April 29, 2009; 1–90. Available at *aidsinfo.nih.gov/ContentFiles/PerinatalGL.pdf*. Accessed September 28, 2009.
4. Centers for Disease Control and Prevention. Updated U.S Public Health Service guidelines for the management of occupational exposures to HIV and recommendations for postexposure prophylaxis. MMWR 2005;54(No. RR-9):1-17. Updated at *aidsinfo.nih.gov/guidelines*. Accessed September 28, 2009.
5. See also *www.medscape.com/hiv* for more information on HIV, antiretroviral therapy, and drug interactions. Accessed September 28, 2009.

Opportunistic Infections in Patients with HIV
1. Centers for Disease Control and Prevention. Guidelines for prevention and treatment of opportunistic infections in HIV-infected adults and adolescents. MMWR 2009;58(No. RR-4):1–207. Updated at *aidsinfo.nih.gov/guidelines*. Accessed September 28, 2009.
2. Centers for Disease Control and Prevention. Guidelines for prevention and treatment of opportunistic infections among HIV-exposed and HIV-infected children. MMWR 2009;58(No. RR-11):1–166. Updated at *aidsinfo.nih.gov/guidelines*. Accessed September 28, 2009.

Tuberculosis
1. American Thoracic Society/Centers for Disease Control and Prevention/Infectious Diseases Society of America: treatment of tuberculosis. Am J Respir Crit Care Med 2003;167:603–62.
2. Havlir DV, Barnes PF. Tuberculosis in patients with human immunodeficiency virus infection. N Engl J Med 1999;340:367–73.
3. Small PM, Fujiwara PI. Management of tuberculosis in the United States. N Engl J Med 2001;345:189–200.
4. Targeted tuberculin testing and treatment of latent tuberculosis infection. Am J Respir Crit Care Med 2000;161:S221–47.
5. Jasmer RM, Nahid P, Hopewell PC. Latent tuberculosis infection. N Engl J Med 2002;347:1860–6.

ANSWERS AND EXPLANATIONS TO PATIENT CASES

1. Answer D
The patient should be treated at this time; potent combination antiretroviral therapy should be initiated when CD_4 counts fall below 350/mm^3. The combination therapy of tenofovir, emtricitabine, and atazanavir-ritonavir is a preferred initial therapeutic regimen. Monotherapy is not indicated for HIV. Although therapy with zidovudine-lamivudine and nevirapine is an acceptable alternative, it should not be first-line therapy.

2. Answer D
A change in potent combination antiretroviral therapy should be made when the viral load becomes detectable after a period of levels below detection. Some clinicians would wait and monitor the patient closely if the viral load increased to 10,000 copies/mL. However, these patients generally will require changes in therapy in the future. Resistance testing should be completed to optimize therapy. Without knowledge of resistance patterns, the best change is to initiate an entirely new regimen of abacavir, lamivudine, and fosamprenavir-ritonavir because changing all three agents simultaneously limits the possibility of resistance occurring quickly to the new regimen. In general, changes of only one drug in a regimen should be made only for intolerance. If the virus is resistant to the combination regimen, changing only one drug will simply lead to resistance to the new antiviral; moreover, changing only one drug is the equivalent of monotherapy. Ideally, any new regimen should have at least two fully active drugs.

3. Answer C
A patient taking fosamprenavir-ritonavir should be monitored for endocrine disturbances (e.g., hyperglycemia, fat redistribution, lipid abnormalities) because all protease inhibitors can cause endocrine disturbances. Because fosamprenavir-ritonavir does not cause peripheral neuropathy (although ddI, ddC, and d4T do), fosamprenavir-ritonavir does not need to be monitored. Drug interaction with drugs metabolized by CYP1A2 is not of concern because fosamprenavir is an inhibitor of CYP3A4, and ritonavir is an inhibitor of CYP 2D6 and 3A4. Fosamprenavir does not cause nephrolithiasis; thus, the patient does not need to be monitored for this (although a patient taking indinavir does).

4. Answer A
When the CD_4 count decreases to 135/mm^3, the patient should receive primary prophylactic treatment against PCP (CD_4 count less than 200/mm^3). Primary prophylaxis is necessary for MAC when the CD_4 count is less than 50/mm^3. For CMV, patients with CD_4 counts less than 50/mm^3 should receive regular funduscopic examinations. In general, primary prophylaxis is not used for cryptococcal meningitis.

5. Answer C
Although pentamidine would be an appropriate therapeutic option for a patient who is HIV positive with PCP, the optimal empiric therapy is TMP/SMZ intravenously with adjuvant prednisone therapy for 21 days. Although TMP/SMZ is the drug of choice for PCP, adjuvant prednisone therapy is indicated because the patient's A-a gradient is 55, and the patient's partial pressure of oxygen is less than 70. Atovaquone is indicated only for patients with mild to moderate PCP who cannot tolerate TMP/SMZ. This patient does not meet this criterion.

6. Answer B
Patients with cryptococcal meningitis should always receive secondary prophylaxis. One of the principles of treating AIDS-related illnesses is that the infections are rarely curable, and generally, long-term preventable therapy is required. Weekly amphotericin B has been studied for secondary prophylaxis, but fluconazole is the best agent for secondary prophylaxis. The agents that are effective for PCP prophylaxis have no activity against *Cryptococcus*.

7. Answer D
Maintenance therapy for cryptococcal meningitis with fluconazole can be discontinued when the CD_4 count increases to greater than 100–200/mm^3 for 6 months or longer after potent combination antiretroviral therapy. Because G.H.'s CD_4 counts have been greater than 200/mm^3 for at least 6 months, maintenance therapy can be discontinued.

8. Answer B
For the treatment of MAC, azithromycin plus EMB for at least 12 months is the best therapeutic combination and includes one of the newer macrolides and a second agent (EMB is usually the preferred second agent). Therapy may be discontinued after 12 months if CD_4 counts increase with potent combination antiretroviral therapy and if the patient is asymptomatic. Clarithromycin plus EMB for 2 weeks, followed by maintenance with clarithromycin alone, is incorrect because there is

no induction therapy followed by maintenance monotherapy for MAC. A therapeutic regimen of clarithromycin plus INH is not the best because isoniazid has no activity against MAC. Although EMB plus rifabutin has activity against MAC, the current recommendations are that all therapeutic regimens include either azithromycin or clarithromycin; therefore, the EMB plus rifabutin regimen is not the treatment of choice.

9. Answer B

This patient, who is positive for HIV infection, receives a new diagnosis of CMV retinitis and should receive foscarnet intravenously for treatment. Acyclovir does not have activity against CMV, whereas ganciclovir (and valganciclovir) and cidofovir can cause neutropenia, and this patient is at increased risk because of concomitant therapy with zidovudine and pyrimethamine-sulfadiazine.

10. Answer D

A patient with an induration of greater than 15 mm after a PPD skin test for TB needs to be evaluated for treatment. Because J.M.'s PPD skin test was negative last year, he is considered a recent converter and needs to be treated. He would also need to be treated if there were patients with TB at the long-term care facility. The booster effect is a phenomenon associated with an initial small reaction causing immunologic stimulation, followed by a larger reaction with a subsequent test. J.M. had an initial large reaction (18-mm induration). Age is not a factor to consider in treating latent TB. Initiating INH 300 mg/day orally for 6 months is the best recommendation for managing J.M.'s positive PPD.

11. Answer C

R.J. should have his HIV medications altered (RIF will induce the metabolism of fosamprenavir and ritonavir). He should not receive a protease inhibitor (except for full-dose ritonavir) or an NNRTI (except for efavirenz) with RIF. Patients who are HIV positive should be initiated on four drugs for TB, and fosamprenavir should not be used with RIF. Isoniazid, rifabutin, PZA, and EMB, with a lower dose of rifabutin, is the best recommendation; it includes the four drugs for TB and a lower dose of rifabutin (because of fosamprenavir-ritonavir inhibition). The fosamprenavir-ritonavir dose does not need to be changed when adding rifabutin.

12. Answer C

For R.J., only the rifamycin and INH need to be continued after 2 months of therapy with the four drugs for TB. The regimen can be simplified to a rifamycin and INH after 2 months, but the recommended total treatment duration is 6 months. The concentrations of HIV RNA should be monitored closely because of potential alterations in drug concentrations of the protease inhibitor.

ANSWERS AND EXPLANATIONS TO SELF-ASSESSMENT QUESTIONS

1. Answer: D
Transmission of HIV to a child is decreased if the mother's viral load is decreased. The benefits of therapy far outweigh the risk. A potent combination antiretroviral therapy that includes zidovudine throughout the pregnancy is the most appropriate therapeutic regimen for an asymptomatic patient with HIV who is pregnant (even in the first trimester) and has a low CD_4 count. [Intrapartum] zidovudine 300 [mg is given during pregnancy, followed by] the baby for 6 [weeks post-partum to decrease transmission. Other] antiretroviral [regimens for the patient's low CD_4 count include single-drug therapy] with nevirapine at the [time of delivery if viral load and CD_4 suppression as much as combination therapy throughout pregnancy is indicated] during their [pregnancy.]

[2. Answer: ...]
[...indinavir can cause... patients should be told to talk... combination therapy... problems with antiretrovirals... indinavir inhibits... an NRTI, not a protease inhibitor... telling the patient to cut back on products is incorrect... and many protease inhibitors are recommended... tenofovir and emtricitabine... neuropathy is incorrect... drugs is associated with] that adverse effect.

3. Answer: B
There are many other reasons to change antiretroviral therapy in addition to clinical deterioration. These include an inability to decrease viral load to undetectable levels, the detection of virus after initial suppression to undetectable levels, a failure to increase the CD_4 count by 50–100 cells/mm³ during the first year of therapy, and a failure to increase the CD_4 count above 350 cells/mm³ while on therapy. If there is a question of ineffective antiretroviral therapy, single drugs should be changed only with caution (consider changing the entire regimen). Resistance does not occur more commonly with emtricitabine than with other antiretroviral agents.

4. Answer: D
A change in therapy is indicated for the patient taking potent combination antiretroviral therapy and experiencing hyperglycemia, fat redistribution, and lipid abnormalities. Although adding lipid-lowering agents may be indicated to lower cardiovascular risks, simvastatin should not be used with lopinavir or ritonavir because of the drug interaction (increased simvastatin concentrations lead to increased risk of myalgias). Pravastatin is a better choice (although it may decrease ritonavir concentrations). Although adding an insulin-sensitizing agent may be indicated, pioglitazone should not be used with lopinavir or ritonavir because of the drug interaction (increased pioglitazone concentrations and potential induction of protease inhibitor metabolism by pioglitazone). Changing agents is a good solution, but NRTIs do not cause endocrine abnormalities, so changing from the nucleoside RTI zidovudine to the nucleotide RTI tenofovir will not improve the symptoms. At this time, changing agents (if possible) to an effective regimen that does not cause endocrine disturbances is the best option. Because protease inhibitors most commonly cause endocrine disturbances, changing to an NNRTI-based regimen is best.

5. Answer: D
The current recommended regimen for treating cryptococcal meningitis in patients positive for HIV is amphotericin B 0.7 mg/kg/day plus flucytosine 25 mg/kg every 6 hours for 2 weeks, followed by fluconazole 400 mg/day. Fluconazole alone is recommended only for mild to moderate cryptococcal meningitis, and the dose should be 400 mg/day. Studies have shown that early mortality is greater with fluconazole alone than with amphotericin B alone. When amphotericin B is used alone for cryptococcal meningitis, the dose should be 0.7 mg/kg/day, not 0.3 mg/kg/day. The flucytosine dose of 37.5 mg/kg every 6 hours is high and is especially prone to cause bone marrow suppression in patients who are HIV positive.

6. Answer: C

The number of patients needed to treat with INH over RIF to prevent one progression to active disease is 200 = 1/(0.008 − 0.003). The only information needed is the absolute risk in both groups (which is provided).

7. Answer: D

Pyrimethamine plus clindamycin and leucovorin for 6 weeks is the correct choice for the treatment of toxoplasmosis in a patient who is HIV positive and taking dapsone for PCP prophylaxis (but taking no antiretroviral agents). Atovaquone is not first-line therapy, although data support its effectiveness in combination with sulfadiazine or pyrimethamine; TMP/SMX is not effective for treatment or secondary prophylaxis of toxoplasmosis. Pyrimethamine and sulfadiazine are the first-line agents for toxoplasmosis; however, leucovorin should always be used with pyrimethamine to prevent myelosuppression.

8. Answer: B

To achieve flucytosine peak concentrations between 50 and 100 mcg/mL (assuming a trough concentration of 25 mcg/mL, every-6-hour dosing, and 100% bioavailability; flucytosine volume of distribution = 0.7 L/kg; half-life = 3 hours), the concentration needs to be changed by 25–75 mcg/mL. Using the equation $\Delta C_p = dose/V_d$, a dose of 12.5 mg/kg would increase the concentration only 17.8 mcg/mL. A dose of 75 mg/kg would increase the concentration by 107 mcg/mL, whereas a dose of 150 mg/kg would increase the concentration by 214 mcg/mL. The correct dose is 37.5 mg/kg because it would increase the concentration by 53.6 mcg/mL.

9. Answer: B

Because the patient is symptomatic and her sputum is acid-fast bacillus positive, she should be treated for an active TB infection. Isoniazid, RIF, PZA, and EMB for 2 months, followed by INH and RIF for 4 more months, is the recommended therapy for active TB. Patients should be initiated on at least three antibiotics for the first 2 months. Although fluoroquinolones have some activity against TB, their use as first-line monotherapy is inappropriate.

10. Answer: C

Data are continuous and probably normally distributed (given the large population of 350 patients in the study); therefore, a parametric test is indicated. The t-test is the best parametric test for comparing two groups. Although an analysis of variance is a parametric test, it is used to compare more than two groups. A chi-square test is used to compare proportions between two groups. The end points in this study are continuous and, therefore, should not be compared using this statistical test. The Wilcoxon rank sum test is a nonparametric analog to the t-test.

NEPHROLOGY

EDWARD F. FOOTE, PHARM.D., BCPS, FCCP

WILKES UNIVERSITY
WILKES-BARRE, PENNSYLVANIA

NEPHROLOGY

EDWARD F. FOOTE, PHARM.D., BCPS, FCCP

WILKES UNIVERSITY
WILKES-BARRE, PENNSYLVANIA

Learning Objectives:

1. Categorize acute kidney injury (AKI) as prerenal, intrinsic, or postrenal, based on patient history, physical examination, and laboratory values.

2. List risk factors for AKI and formulate strategies to decrease risk of AKI in specific patient populations.

3. Identify an appropriate approach to the management of AKI.

4. Identify medications and medication classes associated with acute and chronic kidney damage.

5. Discuss factors that determine the efficiency of dialysis of drugs.

6. Identify the stage of chronic kidney disease (CKD) based on patient history, physical examination, and laboratory values.

7. List risk factors for the progression of CKD and formulate strategies to slow the progression of CKD.

8. Describe the common complications of CKD.

9. Develop a care plan to manage the common complications observed in patients with CKD (e.g., anemia, secondary hyperthyroidism).

Self-Assessment Questions:
Answers to these questions may be found at the end of this chapter.

1. A.M. is a 75-year-old man who presents to your institution complaining of abdominal pain and dizziness. He has a brief history of gastroenteritis and has not eaten or drunk anything for 24 hours. His blood pressure (BP) reading while sitting is 120/80 mm Hg, which drops to 90/60 mm Hg when standing. His pulse rate is 90 beats/minute. His CHEM-7 profile shows sodium (Na) 135 mEq/L; chloride (Cl) 108 mEq/L; potassium (K) 4.7 mEq/L; CO_2 26 mEq/L; blood urea nitrogen (BUN) 40 mg/dL; serum creatinine (SCr) 1.5 mg/dL; and glucose 188 mg/dL. He has no known drug allergies. His weight is 92.5 kg, and his height is 6'1". Which one of the following is best approach to treat this patient?

    A. Administer furosemide 40 mg intravenously × 1.
    B. Insert Foley catheter to check for residual urine.
    C. Administer fluid bolus (1000 mL of normal saline solution).
    D. Administer Humalog insulin 3 units subcutaneously.

2. F.D. is a 44-year-old man admitted with gram-negative bacteremia. He receives 4 days of parenteral aminoglycoside therapy and develops acute tubular necrosis (ATN). Antibiotic therapy is adjusted based on culture and sensitivity results. Which one of the following is the urinalysis most likely to show?

    A. BUN/SCr ratio greater than 20:1; urine Na less than 10 mOsm/L; fractional excretion of sodium (FENa) less than 1%; specific gravity more than 1.018; hyaline casts.
    B. BUN/SCr ratio greater than 20:1; urine Na more than 20 mOsm/L; FENa more than 3%; specific gravity 1.010; no casts visible.
    C. BUN/SCr ratio 10–15:1; urine Na more than 40 mOsm/L; FENa more than 1%; specific gravity less than 1.015; muddy casts.
    D. BUN/SCr ratio 10–15:1; urine Na less than 10 mOsm/L; FENa less than 1%; specific gravity more than 1.018; muddy casts.

3. W.C. is a patient with chronic kidney disease (CKD) stage 4 (estimated creatinine clearance [CrCl] of 25 mL/minute). The patient has a diagnosis of gram-positive bacteremia, which is susceptible only to drug X. There are no published reports on how to adjust the dose of drug X in patients with diminished kidney function. Review of the drug X package insert shows that it has significant renal elimination, with 40% excreted unchanged in the urine. The usual dose for drug X is 600 mg/day intravenously and is provided as 100 mg/mL in a 6-mL vial. How many milliliters of drug X should be given to W.C.?

    A. 4.
    B. 4.5.
    C. 3.6.
    D. 5.5.

4. D.Z. is a 45-year-old patient with a long history of cancer. He has long-standing malnutrition and is well below his ideal body weight. He is to be dosed on carboplatin, in which an accurate estimate of kidney function is critical. Which one of the following is the best method for assessing kidney function in this patient?

    A. Cockcroft-Gault.
    B. Modification of diet in renal disease (MDRD).
    C. 24-hour collection of urine.
    D. Iothalamate study.

5. M.M.R., a 59-year-old patient who has had end-stage renal disease (ESRD) for 10 years, is maintained on chronic hemodialysis (HD). He has a history of hypertension, coronary artery disease (CAD), mild congestive heart failure (CHF), and type 2 diabetes mellitus. Medications are as follows: epoetin 10,000 units 3 times weekly at dialysis; Nephrocaps one daily; atorvastatin 20 mg/day; insulin; and calcium acetate 2 tablets 3 times/day with meals. Laboratory values are as follows: hemoglobin 9.2 g/L, parathyroid hormone (PTH) 300 pg/mL, Na 140, K 4.9, Cr 7.0, calcium 9 mg/dL, albumin 3.5 g/L, and Phos 4.8 mg/dL. He has ferritin 80 and % saturation 14. The red blood cell count (RBC) indices (mean corpuscular volume [MCV], mean corpuscular hemoglobin count [MCHC]) are normal. His white blood cell count (WBC) is normal. He is afebrile. Which of the following is the best approach to managing anemia in this patient?

   A. Increase epoetin.
   B. Add oral iron.
   C. Add intravenous iron.
   D. Maintain current regimen, patient at goal.

6. Q.R.S. is a 60-year-old (72 kg) patient in the intensive care unit. He suffered a myocardial infarction about 1 week ago with secondary heart failure. He now has pneumonia. He has been hypotensive for the past 5 days. Before his admission 1 week ago, he had an SCr of 1.0 mg/dL. His medical history is significant for diabetes mellitus and hypertension. His urine output has been steadily declining for the past 3 days, despite adequate hydration. He made only 700 mL of urine during the past 24 hours. His medications since surgery include intravenous dobutamine, nitroglycerin, and cefazolin. Yesterday, his BUN/SCr was 32 and 3.1 mg/dL; today, it is 41 and 3.9 mg/dL. His urine osmolality is 290 mOsm/kg. His urine Na is 40 mEq/L, and there are tubular cellular casts in his urine. Which one of the following is the most likely renal diagnosis?

   A. Prerenal azotemia.
   B. ATN.
   C. Acute interstitial nephritis (AIN).
   D. Hemodynamic/functional-mediated acute kidney injury (AKI).

7. You are evaluating a study comparing epoetin and darbepoetin regarding their efficacy on mean hemoglobin concentrations. Both drugs are initiated at the recommended dose, and the hemoglobin concentration is checked at 4 weeks. There are 50 patients in each group. The mean hemoglobin in the epoetin group is 12.1 g/L, and in the darbepoetin group, it is 12.2 g/L. Which one of the following statistical tests is best for this comparison?

   A. A paired t-test.
   B. An independent (unpaired) t-test.
   C. An analysis of variance.
   D. A chi-square test.

Patient Cases for AKI

1. H.D. is a 48-year-old African American man (70 kg) admitted to the intensive care unit after an acute myocardial infarction. His medical history is significant for type 2 diabetes mellitus diagnosed 1 year ago and for hypertension and tobacco use. His current medications are metformin 500 mg orally 2 times/day; amlodipine 5 mg/day orally; nicotine patch 14 mg/day applied each morning; and naproxen 500 mg/day orally. Before admission, his kidney function was normal (SCr 1.0. mg/dL); however, during the past 24 hours, it has declined (BUN 20 mg/dL, SCr 2.1 mg/dL). His urine demonstrates muddy casts. The patient is anuric. His current BP is 120/80 mm Hg. Which one of the following is the best assessment of H.D.'s kidney function?

    A. 26.2 mL/minute (CrCl using Cockcroft-Gault).
    B. 44 mL/minute/1.73 m^2 (glomerular filtration rate [GFR] using abbreviated MDRD).
    C. 23.1 mL/minute/70 kg (CrCl using the Brater equation).
    D. Assume CrCl less than 10 mL/minute.

2. Which one of the following represents the most likely cause of kidney dysfunction in this patient?

    A. Prerenal.
    B. Intrinsic.
    C. Postrenal.
    D. Functional.

3. Which of the following medications is best to discontinue at this time?

    A. Amlodipine.
    B. Naproxen.
    C. Metformin and amlodipine.
    D. Metformin and naproxen.

I. ACUTE KIDNEY INJURY (ACUTE RENAL FAILURE)

A. Definitions and Background
  1. Acute kidney injury is defined as an acute decrease in kidney function (GFR) over a period of hours, days, or even weeks. Associated with an accumulation of waste products and (usually) volume
      a. Definitions vary. A commonly used definition is an increase in an SCr of 0.5 mg/dL or greater or a decrease of 25% or greater in the GFR of patients with previous normal kidney function OR an increase of 1 mg/dL or greater in SCr in patients with CKD. Also defined based on urine output (less than 0.5 mL/kg/hour for at least 6 hours). The Acute Kidney Injury Network (AKIN): an abrupt (48 hours) absolute increase in SCr of more than 0.3 mg/dL or a 50% increase in baseline OR urine output less than 0.5 mL/kg/hour for more than 6 hours. The AKIN has recommended a classification/staging for AKI, but it is not widely used.
      b. Common complications include fluid overload as well as acid-base and electrolyte abnormalities.
      c. Urine output classification
          i. Anuric: less than 50 mL/24 hours—associated with worse outcomes
          ii. Oliguric: 50–500 mL/24 hours
          iii. Nonoliguric: more than 500 mL/24 hours—associated with better patient outcomes. Easier to manage because of fewer problems with volume overload

2. Community-acquired AKI
   a. Low incidence (0.02%) in otherwise healthy patients. As high as 13% in patients with CKD
   b. Usually has a very high survival rate (70%–95%)
   c. Single insult to the kidney, often drug induced
   d. Often reversible
3. Hospital-acquired AKI
   a. Has a moderate incidence (2%–5%) and moderate survival rate (30%-50%)
   b. Single or multifocal insults to the kidney
   c. Can still be reversible
4. Intensive care unit–acquired AKI: a high incidence (6%-23%) and a low survival rate (10%-30%)
5. Estimating GFR in AKI
   a. Difficult because commonly used equations (Cockcroft-Gault and MDRD) are not appropriate (need stable SCr)
   b. Equations by Brater and Jeliffe are probably more accurate than Cockcroft-Gault but have not been rigorously tested.

B. Risk Factors Associated with AKI
   1. Volume depletion—vomiting, diarrhea, poor fluid intake, fever, diuretic use. Effective volume depletion –CHF, liver disease with ascites
   2. Preexisting CKD
   3. Use of nephrotoxic agents/medications (intravenous radiographic contrast, aminoglycosides, amphotericin, nonsteroidal anti-inflammatory drugs [NSAIDs] and cyclooxygenase-2 [COX-2] inhibitors, angiotensin-converting enzyme inhibitors [ACEIs] and angiotensin II receptor blockers [ARBs], cyclosporine, and tacrolimus)
   4. Obstruction of the urinary tract

C. Classifications of AKI (Table 1)
   1. Prerenal azotemia
      a. Initially, the kidney is undamaged.
      b. Characterized by hypoperfusion to the kidney
         i. Systemic hypoperfusion: hemorrhage, volume depletion, drugs, CHF
         ii. Isolated kidney hypoperfusion: renal artery stenosis, emboli
      c. Urinalysis will initially be normal (no sediment) but concentrated.
      d. Physical examination: hypotension, volume depletion
   2. Functional AKI
      a. Kidney is undamaged. Often "lumped" with prerenal in classification
      b. Caused by reduced glomerular hydrostatic pressure
      c. In general, medication related (cyclosporine, ACEIs and ARBs, and NSAIDs). Seen in patients with underlying effective bloodflow (patients with CHF, patients with liver disease, and elderly patients) who cannot compensate for alterations in afferent/efferent tone. Concentrated urine
      d. Small increases in SCr (less than 1 mg/dL) after initiation of ACEI/ARB are acceptable.
   3. Intrinsic renal failure
      a. Kidney is damaged. Damage can be linked to structure involved: small blood vessels, glomeruli, renal tubules, and interstitium.
      b. Most common cause is ATN. Others include AIN, vasculitis, and acute glomerulonephritis.
      c. Urinalysis will reflect damage. Urine generally not concentrated

d. Physical examination: normotensive, euvolemic, or hypervolemic; check for signs of allergic reactions or embolic phenomenon
e. History: identifiable insult, drug use, infections
4. Postrenal failure
    a. Kidney is initially undamaged. Bladder outlet obstruction is the most common cause of postrenal AKI. Lower urinary tract obstruction may be due to calculi. Ureteric obstructions may be because of clots or intraluminal obstructions. Extrarenal compression can also cause postrenal disease. Increased intraluminal pressure upstream of the obstruction will result in damage if obstruction is not relieved.
    b. Urinalysis may be nonspecific.
    c. Physical examination: distended bladder, enlarged prostate
    d. History: trauma, benign prostatic hypertrophy, cancers

Table 1. Classifications of Acute Kidney Injury

	Prerenal and Functional	**Intrinsic (ATN and AIN)**	**Postrenal**
History/presentation	Volume depletion Renal artery stenosis CHF Hypercalcemia NSAID/ACEI use Cyclosporin	Long-standing renal hypoperfusion Nephrotoxins (e.g., contrast or antibiotics) Vasculitis Glomerulonephritis	Kidney stones BPH Cancers
Physical examination	Hypotension Dehydration Petechia if thrombotic Ascites	Rash, fever (with AIN)	Distended bladder Enlarged prostate
Serum BUN/SCr ratio	> 20:1	15:1	15:1
Urine concentrated?	Yes Low urine Na (< 20 mEq/L) Low FENa (< 1) High urine osmolarity	No Urine Na >40 mEq/L FENa > 2 Low urine osmolarity	No Urine Na > 40 mEq/L FENa > 2 Low urine osmolarity
Urine sediment	Normal	Muddy-brown granular casts; tubular epithelial casts	Variable, may be normal
Urinary WBC	Negative	2–4+	Variable
Urinary RBC	Negative	2–4+	1+
Proteinuria	Negative	Positive	Negative

ACEI = angiotensin-converting enzyme inhibitor; AIN = acute interstitial nephritis; BPH = benign prostatic hypertrophy; BUN = blood urea nitrogen; CHF = congestive heart failure; FENa = fractional excretion of sodium; GFR = glomerular filtration rate; NSAID = nonsteroidal anti-inflammatory drug; SCr = serum creatinine; RBC = red blood cell (count); WBC = white blood cell (count).

D. Prevention of AKI
1. Avoid nephrotoxic drugs when possible.
2. Ensure adequate hydration (2 L/day). If intravenous, 0.9% sodium chloride (NaCl) is preferred.
3. Patient education
4. Avoid dopamine, fenoldopam, diuretics
5. Drug therapies to decrease incidence of contrast-induced nephropathy—see drug nephrotoxicity section

E. Treatment and Management of Established AKI
1. Prerenal azotemia: correct primary hemodynamics
   a. Normal saline if volume depleted
   b. Pressure management if needed
   c. Blood products if needed
2. Postrenal azotemia: relieve obstruction. Early diagnosis is important. Consult urology and/or radiology.
3. Intrinsic: no specific therapy universally effective
   a. Eliminate the causative hemodynamic abnormality or toxin.
   b. Avoid additional insults.
   c. Prevent and treat complications.
      i. Fluid management
         (a) Maintain kidney perfusion and production of urine. Consider fluid bolus.
         (b) Diuretic therapy: Consider loop diuretics for patients who are oliguric and euvolemic or hypervolemic.
            (1) Give intravenously.
               (A) Furosemide intermittent therapy: 40-80 mg intravenously every 6-8 hours. May increase bolus dose up to 400 mg if no response
               (B) Furosemide continuous infusion: 40-80 mg intravenous bolus and then 10-20 mg/hour intravenously
            (2) Continuous intravenous therapy and/or combination with thiazide-like diuretics may decrease resistance.
         (c) Dopamine therapy. Renal dose dopamine (1-2 mcg/kg/minute) causes renal and mesenteric vasodilatation and can increase urinary output. Not proven to improve resolution of kidney failure or improve survival. Not recommended
      ii. Acidosis
         (a) Restrict dietary protein (less than 0.5 g/kg/day of high-quality protein).
         (b) Sodium bicarbonate to maintain HCO_3 more than 15 mEq/L and arterial pH more than 7.2
         (c) Dialysis
      iii. Electrolyte and nutrition abnormalities—supportive. See Fluid, Electrolyte, and Nutrition section.
4. Renal replacement therapy—indications
   a. Volume overload unresponsive to diuretics
   b. Uremia
   c. Life threatening electrolyte imbalance
   d. Refractory acidosis

Patient Cases for Drug-Induced Kidney Damage

4. E.P. is a 67-year-old man referred to cardiology for intermittent chest pain. The patient has a history significant for CKD, type 2 diabetes mellitus, and hypertension. His home medications include enalapril, hydrochlorothiazide, and pioglitazone. Laboratory values include SCr 1.8 mg/dL, glucose 189 mg/dL, hemoglobin 12 mg/dL, and hematocrit 36%. His physical examination is normal. The plan is to undergo elective cardiac catheterization. Which one of the following choices best characterizes the risk factors for developing contrast-induced nephropathy in this patient?

    A. CKD and diabetes.
    B. CKD, diabetes, anemia, and enalapril.
    C. Diabetes, anemia, and age.
    D. Diabetes.

5. The physician plans to start 0.9% normal saline for hydration. Which one of the following best represents the optimal time to start the intravenous infusion in relation to the timing of the procedure?

    A. 24 hours prior.
    B. 12 hours prior.
    C. 2 hours prior.
    D. Immediately prior.

6. In addition to intravenous fluid, which one of the following therapies is best to use in E.P. to decrease his likelihood of developing contrast-induced nephropathy?

    A. Fenoldopam.
    B. Acetylcysteine.
    C. Ascorbic acid.
    D. Hemofiltration.

II. DRUG-INDUCED KIDNEY DAMAGE

A. Introduction: Drugs are responsible for kidney damage through multiple mechanisms. Evaluate potential drug-induced nephropathy based on the period of ingestion, patient risk factors, and propensity of the suspected agent to cause kidney damage.
   1. Definitions vary. Increase in SCr of 0.5 mg/dL or more or decrease of 25% or more in GFR in patients with previous normal kidney function OR an increase of 1 mg/dL or more in SCr in patients with CKD
   2. Risk factors
      a. History of CKD
      b. Increased age
   3. Epidemiology
      a. 7% of all drug toxicities
      b. 18%-27% of AKI in hospitals
      c. 1%-5% of NSAID users in community
      d. Most implicated medications: aminoglycosides, NSAIDs, ACEIs, contrast dye, amphotericin

4. Kidney at risk of toxicity because:
    a. High exposure to toxin: Kidney receives 20%-25% cardiac output.
    b. Autoregulation and specialized bloodflow through glomerulus
    c. High intrarenal drug metabolism
    d. Tubular transport processes
    e. Concentration of solutes (i.e., toxins) in tubules
    f. High-energy requirements of tubule epithelial cells
    g. Urine acidification
5. Pseudo–drug-induced nephropathy
    a. Drugs that inhibit Cr tubular secretion: triamterene; cimetidine
    b. Drugs that increase BUN: corticosteroids; tetracycline
    c. Drugs that interfere with Cr assay: cefoxitin and other cephalosporins

B. Acute Tubular Necrosis
  1. Most common drug-induced kidney disease in the inpatient setting
  2. Aminoglycoside nephrotoxicity
      a. Incidence of 1.7%–58% of patients
      b. Pathogenesis
          i. Caused by proximal tubular damage leading to obstruction of the lumen
          ii. Cationic charge of drug leads to binding to tubular epithelial cells and uptake into those cells.
          iii. Accumulation of phospholipids and toxicity
      c. Presentation
          i. Gradual rise in SCr concentrations and decrease in GFR after about 6–10 days of therapy
          ii. Patients usually have nonoliguric kidney failure.
          iii. Wasting of K^+ and Mg^{2+} may occur.
      d. Risk factors
          i. Related to dosing: large total cumulative dose, prolonged therapy, trough concentration exceeding 2 mg/L, recent previous aminoglycoside therapy
          ii. Concurrent use of other nephrotoxins (cyclosporine, amphotericin B, and diuretics)
          iii. Patient related—preexisting kidney disease/damage, increased age, poor nutrition, shock, gram-negative bacteremia, liver disease, hypoalbuminemia, obstructive jaundice, dehydration, and K/Mg deficiencies
      e. Prevention
          i. Avoid in high-risk patients.
          ii. Maintain adequate hydration.
          iii. Limit the total cumulative aminoglycoside dose.
          iv. Avoid other nephrotoxins.
          v. Use extended-interval (once daily) dosing.
  3. Radiographic contrast media nephrotoxicity (intravenous contrast). Consists of isoosmolar (300 mOsm/kg), low osmolar (780–800 mOsm/kg), and high-osmolar (more than 1000 mOsm/kg) agents. Also categorized as ionic versus nonionic
      a. Incidence
          i. Third leading cause of inpatient AKI
          ii. Less than 2% and up to 50% of patients, depending on risk
          iii. Incidence increases as risk increases.
          iv. Associated with a high (34%) in-hospital mortality rate

b. Pathogenesis
    i. Direct tubular toxicity due to reactive oxygen species
    ii. Also may cause renal ischemia (prerenal picture from volume depletion) due to intrarenal hemodynamic alterations. Most contrast agents are hyperosmolar (more than 900 mOsm/kg), which leads to an osmotic diuresis and dehydration. Some contrast agents also cause systemic hypotension on injection and renal vasoconstriction.
c. Presentation
    i. Initial transient osmotic diuresis, followed by tubular proteinuria
    ii. Serum creatinine rises and peaks after about 2–5 days.
    iii. Fifty percent of patients develop oliguria, and some will require dialysis.
d. Risk factors for toxicity
    i. Preexisting kidney disease (SCr more than 1.5 mg/dL or CrCl less than 60 mL/minute)
    ii. Diabetes
    iii. Volume depletion
    iv. Age older than 75 years
    v. Anemia (hematocrit less than 39% men, less than 36% women)
    vi. Conditions with decreased bloodflow to the kidney (e.g., CHF)
    vii. Hypotension
    viii. Other nephrotoxins
    ix. Large doses of contrast (more than 140 mL) and/or hyperosmolar contrast agents
e. Prevention
    i. Hydration. Oral or intravenous. Begin 6–12 hours before procedure. Maintain urine output greater than 150 mL/hour. The addition of sodium bicarbonate is widely used, but there are conflicting data on efficacy.
    ii. Use an alternative imagining study if possible.
    iii. Discontinue nephrotoxic agents.
    iv. Use low-osmolar or iso-osmolar contrast agents in patients at risk (more expensive).
    v. Medications used to prevent contrast-induced nephropathy:
        (a) Acetylcysteine—antioxidant and vasodilatory mechanism. Accumulation of glutathione takes time and so may not be as effective in emergency cases. Various dosing recommendations
        (b) Ascorbic acid—antioxidant. One large study showed benefit when used immediately before. Not confirmed. Give ascorbic acid 3 g before procedure and 2 g 2 times/day × two doses after procedure. May have role in emergency cases
        (c) Theophylline-aminophylline—Avoid.
        (d) Fenoldopam—Avoid, given the CONTRAST (Controlled Multicenter Trial Evaluating Fenoldopam Mesylate for the Prevention of Contrast-Induced Nephropathy) trial, which showed no benefit on contrast-induced nephropathy and an increased incidence of hypotension.
        (e) Others not worth mentioning
f. Joint Commission on Accreditation of Healthcare Organizations
    i. Treated as a medication
    ii. Subject to all the standards for medication management in a health system

g. Nephrogenic systemic fibrosis also known as nephrogenic fibrosing dermopathy
   i. Rare. Associated with gadolinium-based agents used in high doses for magnetic resonance angiogram
   ii. Occurs in patients with moderate CKD to ESRD given contrast. Systemic acidosis seems to be a risk factor.
   iii. Onset 2–18 days after exposure
   iv. Presents as burning, itching, swelling/hardening/tightening of skin, skin patches, spots on eyes, joint stiffness, and muscle weakness
   v. Can cause organ damage. Deaths have occurred.
4. Cisplatin and carboplatin nephrotoxicity
   a. Incidence: 6%–13% with appropriate dosing and administration
   b. Pathogenesis – complex. Direct tubular toxin
   c. Presentation
      i. Serum creatinine peaks 10–12 days after starting therapy but may continue to rise with subsequent cycles of therapy.
      ii. Renal Mg wasting is common (may be severe with central nervous system symptoms) and may be accompanied by hypokalemia and hypocalcemia.
      iii. May result in irreversible kidney damage
   d. Risk factors for toxicity: multiple courses of cisplatin, patient age, dehydration, concurrent nephrotoxins, kidney irradiation, alcohol abuse
   e. Prevention
      i. Avoid concurrent nephrotoxins.
      ii. Use smallest dose possible, and decrease frequency of administration.
      iii. Aggressive intravenous hydration: 1–4 L within 24 hours of high-dose cisplatin or carboplatin
      iv. Amifostine: cisplatin-chelating agent. Should be considered in patients at risk of nephrotoxicity
5. Amphotericin B nephrotoxicity
   a. Incidence
      i. Increases as cumulative dose increases
      ii. Approaches 80% with cumulative doses of 4 g or more
   b. Pathogenesis
      i. Direct proximal and distal tubular toxicity
      ii. Arterial vasoconstriction
   c. Presentation
      i. Manifests after 2–3 g
      ii. Loss of tubular function leads to electrolyte wasting (especially K^+, Na^+, and Mg^{2+}) and distal tubular acidosis.
      iii. Patients may require substantial K^+ and Mg^{2+} replacement.
      iv. Serum creatinine increases and GFR decreases because of a decrease in kidney bloodflow from vasoconstriction caused by amphotericin.
   d. Risk factors for toxicity: existing kidney dysfunction, high average daily doses, diuretic use, volume depletion, concomitant nephrotoxins, rapid infusion
   e. Prevention
      i. Avoid other nephrotoxins (especially cyclosporine), and limit the total cumulative dose.
      ii. Intravenous hydration with at least 1 L/day of 0.9% NaCl before each dose
      iii. Use a liposomal product in high-risk patients.

C. Hemodynamically Mediated Kidney Failure
1. Results from a decrease in intraglomerular pressure through the vasoconstriction of afferent arterioles or the vasodilation of efferent arterioles
2. Angiotensin-converting enzyme inhibitors and ARBs
   a. Pathogenesis
      i. Vasodilation of the efferent arteriole
      ii. Leads to a decrease in glomerular hydrostatic pressure and a resultant decrease in GFR
   b. Presentation
      i. Exerts a predictable dose-related reduction in GFR
      ii. Serum creatinine is usually expected to rise by up to 30%.
          Usually occurs within 2–5 days
          Usually stabilizes in 2–3 weeks
          Increases greater than 30% may be detrimental.
          Usually reversible on drug discontinuation
   c. Risk factors for toxicity: patients with bilateral (unilateral with a solitary kidney) renal artery stenosis, decreased effective kidney bloodflow (CHF, cirrhosis), preexisting kidney disease, and volume depletion
   d. Prevention
      i. Initiate therapy with low doses of short-acting agents and gradually titrate upward.
      ii. Switch to long-acting agents once tolerance is established.
      iii. Initially, monitor kidney function and SCr concentrations often.
           Daily for inpatients
           Weekly for outpatients
      iv. Avoid use of concomitant diuretics, if possible, during therapy initiation.
3. Nonsteroidal anti-inflammatory drugs
   a. Incidence: Estimates indicate that 500,000–2.5 million people develop NSAID-induced nephrotoxicity annually in the United States.
   b. Pathogenesis
      i. Vasodilatory prostaglandins help maintain glomerular hydrostatic pressure by afferent arteriolar dilation, especially in times of decreased kidney bloodflow.
      ii. Administration of an NSAID in the setting of decreased kidney perfusion reduces this compensatory mechanism by decreasing the production of prostaglandins, resulting in afferent vasoconstriction and reduced glomerular bloodflow.
   c. Presentation
      i. Can occur within days of starting therapy
      ii. Patients generally have low urine volume and Na and an increase in BUN, SCr, K^+, edema, and weight.
   d. Risk factors for toxicity: preexisting kidney disease, systemic lupus erythematosus, high plasma renin activity (e.g., CHF, hepatic disease), diuretic therapy, atherosclerotic disease, and advanced age
   e. Prevention
      i. Use therapies other than NSAIDs when appropriate (e.g., acetaminophen for osteoarthritis).
      ii. Sulindac is a potent NSAID that may affect prostaglandin synthesis in the kidney to a lesser extent than other NSAIDs.
      iii. Question the utility of COX-2–specific inhibitors. They have not been found to prevent kidney dysfunction, and they increase cardiovascular complications.
   f. If NSAID-induced AKI is suspected, discontinue drug and give supportive care. Recovery is usually rapid.

4. Cyclosporine and tacrolimus
   a. Incidence
      i. The 5-year risk of developing CKD after transplantation of a nonrenal organ ranges from 7% to 21%.
      ii. The occurrence of kidney failure in the transplant patient population has a fourfold increased risk of death.
   b. Pathogenesis
      i. Results from a dose-related hemodynamic mechanism
      ii. Causes vasoconstriction of afferent arterioles through possible increased activity of various vasoconstrictors (thromboxane A_2, endothelin, sympathetic nervous system) or decreased activity of vasodilators (nitric oxide, prostacyclin)
      iii. Increased vasoconstriction from angiotensin II may also contribute.
      iv. Effects usually resolve with dose reduction.
   c. Presentation
      i. Can occur within days of starting therapy
      ii. Serum creatinine rises and GFR decreases.
      iii. Patients often have hypertension, hyperkalemia, and hypomagnesemia.
      iv. A biopsy is often needed for kidney transplant patients to distinguish this from acute allograft rejection.
   d. Risk factors for toxicity: increased age, high initial cyclosporine dose, kidney graft rejection, hypotension, infection, and concomitant nephrotoxins
   e. Prevention
      i. Monitor serum cyclosporine and tacrolimus concentrations closely.
      ii. Use lower doses in combination with other nonnephrotoxic immunosuppressants.
      iii. Calcium channel blockers may help antagonize the vasoconstrictor effects of cyclosporine by dilating afferent arterioles.

D. Tubulointerstitial Disease
   1. Involves the renal tubules and the surrounding interstitium
   2. Onset can be acute or chronic
      a. Acute onset generally involves interstitial inflammatory cell infiltrates, rapid loss of kidney function, and systemic symptoms (i.e., fever and rash).
      b. Chronic onset shows interstitial fibrosis, slow decline in kidney function, and no systemic symptoms.
   3. Acute allergic interstitial nephritis
      a. Cause of up to 3% of all cases of AKI. Results from an allergic hypersensitivity reaction that affects the interstitium of the kidney
      b. Many medications and medication classes can cause this type of kidney failure. The most commonly implicated are the β-lactams and the NSAIDs (although the presentations are different).
         i. Penicillins: Classic presentation of acute allergic interstitial nephritis. Signs/symptoms occur about 1–2 weeks after initiation of therapy and include fever, maculopapular rash, eosinophilia, pyuria, hematuria, and proteinuria. Eosinophiluria may also be present.
         ii. Nonsteroidal anti-inflammatory drugs: Onset, much more delayed, typically begins about 6 months into therapy. Usually occurs in elderly patients on chronic NSAID therapy. Patients usually do not have systemic symptoms.
      c. Kidney biopsy may be needed to confirm diagnosis.
      d. Treatment includes discontinuing the offending agent and possibly initiating steroid therapy.

4. Chronic interstitial nephritis
   a. Often progressive and irreversible
   b. Lithium
      i. Toxicity results from a dose-related decrease in response to an antidiuretic hormone.
      ii. Acute kidney injury from lithium usually occurs during acute lithium intoxication. Patients become dehydrated secondary to nephrogenic diabetes insipidus. There is also direct damage to the proximal and distal tubules.
      iii. Risks include elevated serum concentrations and repeated episodes of AKI from lithium toxicity.
      iv. Prevention is accomplished by maintaining lowest serum lithium concentrations possible, avoiding dehydration, and monitoring kidney function closely.
   c. Cyclosporine: Presents later in therapy (about 6–12 months) than hemodynamically mediated toxicity
5. Papillary necrosis
   a. Form of chronic interstitial nephritis affecting the papillae, causing necrosis of the collecting ducts
   b. Results from the long-term use of analgesics
      i. "Classic" example was with products that contained phenacetin
      ii. Occurs more often with combination products
      iii. Products containing caffeine may also pose an increased risk.
   c. Evolves slowly as time progresses
   d. Affects women more often than men
   e. Difficult to diagnose and much controversy remains regarding risk, prevention, and cause

E. Obstructive Nephropathy
   1. Results from obstruction of the flow of urine after glomerular filtration
   2. Renal tubular obstruction
      a. Caused by intratubular precipitation of tissue degradation products or precipitation of drugs or their metabolites
         i. Tissue degradation products
            Uric acid intratubular precipitation after tumor lysis following chemotherapy
            Drug-induced rhabdomyolysis leading to intratubular precipitation of myoglobin
            Results in rapid decline in kidney function with resultant oliguric or anuric kidney failure
         ii. Drug precipitation
            Sulfonamides, methotrexate, acyclovir, ascorbic acid
            Can be diagnosed by observing needlelike crystals in leukocytes found on urinalysis
      b. Prevention includes pretreatment hydration, maintenance of high urinary volume, and alkalinization of the urine.
   3. Extrarenal urinary tract obstruction
      a. Benign prostatic hypertrophy can be worsened by anticholinergics.
      b. Bladder outlet or ureteral obstruction from fibrosis after cyclophosphamide for hemorrhagic cystitis
   4. Nephrolithiasis
      a. Usually does not affect GFR and so does not have the classic signs/symptoms of nephrotoxicity
      b. A few medications contribute to the formation of kidney stones: triamterene, sulfadiazine, indinavir, and ephedrine derivatives.

F. Glomerular Disease
   1. Proteinuria is the hallmark sign of glomerular failure and may occur with or without a decrease in GFR.
   2. A few distinct drugs can cause glomerular failure.
      a. Nonsteroidal anti-inflammatory drugs: associated with acute allergic interstitial nephritis
      b. Heroin: can be caused by direct toxicity or toxicity from additives or infection from injection. End-stage renal disease develops in most cases.
      c. Parenteral gold: results from immune complex formation along glomerular capillary loops

---

Patient Cases for CKD

7. P.P. is a 55-year-old African American patient with type 2 diabetes mellitus, hypertension, hyperlipidemia, and CAD. He denies alcohol use but does smoke cigarettes (1 pack/day). His medications include glyburide 5 mg/day, atenolol 50 mg/day, and a multi-multiple vitamin. At your pharmacy, his BP is 149/92 mm Hg. He reports poor diabetes control. A 24-hour urine collection reveals 0.4 g of albumin and a CrCl of 80 mL/minute. Which of the following represents the stage of this patient's kidney disease?

   A. Stage 2.
   B. Stage 3.
   C. Stage 4.
   D. Stage 5.

8. Assuming that nonpharmacologic approaches have been maximized, which one of the following actions is best for P.P. to limit the progression of his kidney disease?

   A. Add nifedipine.
   B. Add diltiazem.
   C. Add enalapril.
   D. Increase atenolol.

III. CHRONIC KIDNEY DISEASE

A. Background
   1. Kidney disease is an underreported and undertreated problem in the United States. In 1984, there were fewer than 100,000 people with end-stage kidney disease requiring dialysis. At the end of 2006, there were more than 500,000 patients with ESRD in the United States (about 354,000 were on maintenance dialysis, and the remainder had functioning transplant grafts).
   2. There is also an increase in the number of people with earlier stages of kidney disease. It is estimated that 10.9% of adults in United States have CKD.
   3. The National Kidney Foundation Kidney Disease Outcome Quality Initiative Advisory Board recommends a definition of CKD and staging guidelines.
      a. Definition
         i. Kidney damage for more than 3 months, as defined by structural or functional abnormality of the kidney, with or without decreased GFR, manifested by either pathologic abnormalities or markers of kidney damage, including abnormalities in the composition of blood or urine or abnormalities in imaging tests
         ii. Glomerular filtration rate less than 60 mL/minute/1.73 m^2 for 3 months, with or without kidney damage

b. Stages of CKD
   i. Stage 1 kidney damage with normal or increased GFR (90 or more mL/minute/1.73 m²)
   ii. Stage 2 kidney damage with mild decrease in GFR (60–89 mL/minute/1.73 m²)
   iii. Stage 3 moderate decrease in GFR (30–59 mL/minute/1.73 m²)
   iv. Stage 4 severe decrease in GFR (15–29 mL/minute/1.73 m²)
   v. Stage 5 kidney failure (less than 15 mL/minute/1.73 m² or on dialysis

[handwritten note: add "T" if transplant eg. Stage 2T]

B. Etiology
   1. Diabetes (40% of new cases of ESRD in the United States)
   2. Hypertension (25% of new cases)
   3. Glomerulonephritis (10%)
   4. Others—urinary tract disease, polycystic kidney disease, lupus, analgesic nephropathy, unknown

C. Risk Factors
   1. Susceptibility (associated with an increased risk, but not proved to cause CKD): Advanced age, reduced kidney mass, low birth weight, racial/ethnic minority, family history, low income or education, systemic inflammation, and dyslipidemia. Mostly not modifiable
   2. Initiation (directly cause CKD): diabetes, hypertension, autoimmune disease, polycystic kidney diseases, and drug toxicity. Modifiable by drug therapy
   3. Progression (result in faster decline in kidney function): hyperglycemia, elevated BP, proteinuria, and smoking

D. Albuminuria/Proteinuria
   1. Marker of kidney damage, progression factor, and cardiovascular risk factor. Can be classified as follows
      a. Normal: albumin excretion less than 30 mg/24 hours
      b. Microalbuminuria: 30-300 mg/24 hours
      c. Macroalbuminuria: (overt proteinuria) more than 300 mg/24 hours
      d. Nephrotic range proteinuria: more than 3 g/24 hours
   2. Assessment for proteinuria - most commonly assessed by measurement of urinary albumin-creatinine ratio.
      a. Spot urine: Untimed sample is adequate for adults and children (screening test).

E. Assessment of Kidney Function
   1. Serum creatinine
      a. Avoid use as the sole assessment of kidney function.
      b. Dependent on age, sex, weight, and muscle mass
      c. Many laboratories use "standardized" Cr traceable to IDMS (isotope dilution mass spectrometry). This will alter calculations (Cockcroft-Gault and MDRD). Make sure you know if the Cr is standardized.
   2. Measurement of GFR. Inulin, iothalamate, and others are not routinely used.
   3. Measurement of CrCl through urine collection
      a. Reserve for vegetarians, patients with low muscle mass, patients with amputations, and patients needing dietary assessment, as well as when documenting need to start dialysis.
      b. Urine collection will give a better estimate in patients with very low muscle mass. In most cases, equations will overestimate kidney function because Cr concentrations will be low in patients with very low muscle mass.
   4. Calculated using Cockcroft-Gault (mL/minute CrCl) – overestimates GFR
      $[(140 - \text{age}) \times \text{body weight}]/[\text{SCr} \times 72] \times (0.85 \text{ if female})$

5. Estimated GFR with MDRD study data
   a. Estimated GFR (mL/minute/1.73 m^2) in patients with known CKD (less than 90 mL/minute)
   b. Abbreviated MDRD formula correlates well with the original MDRD formula, simpler to use GFR (mL/minute/1.73 m^2) = $186 \times SCr^{-1.154} \times age^{-0.203} \times (0.742$ if female$) \times (1.21$ if African American$)$. This equation and an adjusted equation for use with standardized creatinine are available at *www.nkdep.nih.gov* or *www.kidney.org*.
   c. CKD-EPI (Chronic Kidney Disease Epidemiology Collaboration) equation. Alternative equation to estimate GFR. See *www.kidney.org*.
6. For children, Schwartz and Counahan-Barratt formulas

F. Diabetic Nephropathy
   1. Pathogenesis
      a. Hypertension (systemic and intraglomerular)
      b. Glycosylation of glomerular proteins
      c. Genetic links
   2. Diagnosis
      a. Long history of diabetes
      b. Proteinuria
      c. Retinopathy (suggests microvascular disease)
   3. Monitoring
      a. Type I—Begin annual monitoring for microalbuminuria 5 years after diagnosis.
      b. Type II—Begin annual monitoring for proteinuria immediately (do not know how long they have had diabetes mellitus).
   4. Management/slowing progression
      a. Aggressive BP management
         i. Target BP in patients with diabetes and CKD is less than 130/80 mm Hg.
         ii. ACEI's and ARBs are preferred (often in combination with a diuretic) and should be used with any degree of proteinuria, even if the patient is not hypertensive.
         iii. Calcium channel blockers (nondihydropyridine) are second line to ACE/ARBs. Data are emerging for combined therapy.
      b. Intensive blood glucose control. Glycosylated hemoglobin less than 7%. Less aggressive with more advanced CKD
      c. Protein restriction—There are insufficient data in diabetes. Patients should avoid high-protein diets.

G. Nondiabetic Nephropathy
   1. Manage hypertension. If proteinuric and hypertensive, use ACE and ARB.
   2. Minimize protein in diet. Controversial. May slow progression based on MDRD study but may also impair nutrition

H. Other Guidelines to Slow Progression
   1. Manage hyperlipidemia. Follow National Cholesterol Education Program guidelines. Goal is low-density lipoprotein less than 100. Statins are first line.
   2. Stop smoking.

Patient Cases for Renal Replacement Therapy

9. R.R. is a 70-year-old man being assessed for HD access. He has a history of diabetes mellitus and hypertension but is otherwise healthy. Which of the following dialysis accesses has the lowest rate of complications and longest life span?
    A. Subclavian catheter.
    B. Tenckhoff catheter.
    C. Arteriovenous graft.
    D. Arteriovenous fistula.

10. W.Y. is a chronic HD patient who experiences intradialytic hypotension. After nonpharmacologic approaches have been maximized, which one of the following medications is best to manage his low BP?
    A. Levocarnitine.
    B. NaCl tablets.
    C. Fludrocortisone.
    D. Midodrine.

IV. RENAL REPLACEMENT THERAPY

A. Indications for Renal Replacement Therapy
   A – acidosis (not responsive to bicarbonate)
   E – electrolyte abnormality (hyperkalemia; hyperphosphatemia)
   I – intoxication (boric acid; ethylene glycol; lithium; methanol; phenobarbital; salicylate; theophylline)
   O – fluid overload (symptomatic [pulmonary edema])
   U – uremia (pericarditis and weight loss)

B. Two Primary Modes of Dialysis
   i. Hemodialysis—most common modality
   ii. Peritoneal dialysis

C. Hemodialysis (intermittent for ESRD)
   1. Access
      a. Arteriovenous fistula—preferred access!
         i. Natural, formed by anastomosis of artery and vein
         ii. Lowest incidence of infection and thrombosis, lowest cost, longest survival
         iii. Takes weeks/months to "mature"
      b. Arteriovenous graft
         i. Synthetic (polytetrafluoroethylene)
         ii. Often used in patients with vascular disease
      c. Catheters
         i. Commonly used if permanent access not available
         ii. Problems include high infection and thrombosis rates. Low bloodflows lead to inadequate dialysis.
   2. Dialysis membranes
      a. Conventional—not used much anymore. Small pores. Made of cuprophane
      b. High flux and high efficiency—large pores. Can remove drugs that were impermeable to standard membranes (vancomycin). Large amounts of fluid removal (ultrafiltrate)

3. Adequacy
   a. Kt/V—unitless parameter. K = clearance, t = time on dialysis, and V = volume of distribution of urea. Kidney Disease Outcomes Quality Initiative set goal of 1.2 or more.
   b. URR—urea reduction ratio. URR = BUN post/BUN pre × 100%. Goal is URR greater than 65%
4. Common complications of HD
   a. Intradialytic
      i. Hypotension—primarily related to fluid removal. Common in people who are elderly and people with diabetes mellitus. Tx: limit fluid gains between sessions; give normal or hypertonic saline, midodrine. Less well-studied agents include fludrocortisone, selective serotonin reuptake inhibitors
      ii. Cramps—vitamin E or quinine (controversial because of adverse effect profile)
      iii. Nausea/vomiting
      iv. Headache/chest pain/back pain
   b. Vascular access complications—most common with catheters
      i. Infection—*S. aureus*. Need to treat aggressively. May need to pull catheter
      ii. Thrombosis—suspected with low bloodflows. Oral antiplatelets for prevention not used because of lack of efficacy. Can treat with alteplase 1 mg per lumen
5. Factors that affect efficiency of HD
   a. Type of dialyzer used (changes in membrane surface area and pore size)
   b. Length of therapy
   c. Dialysis flow rate
   d. Bloodflow rate
   e. Development of polarized protein layer on the filter surface

D. Continuous HD for AKI
   1. CAVH/CVVH (continuous arteriovenous hemofiltration/continuous veno-venous hemofiltration). Removes fluid and solutes by dialysis. CAVH differs from CVVH because "VV" access requires an in-line pump. Used primarily when fluid removal is most important
   2. CVVHD/CAVHD. "D" is dialysate, which flows in countercurrent to bloodflow. Fluid and solute removal are greater with this procedure. Used when there is a need for fluid removal and better solute clearance

E. Peritoneal Dialysis
   1. Peritoneal dialysis membrane is 1-2 m^2 (approximates the body surface area) and consists of the vascular wall, the interstitium, the mesothelium, and the adjacent fluid films. From 1.5 to 3 L of peritoneal dialysate fluid may be instilled in the peritoneum (fill), allowed to dwell for a specified time, and then drained.
   2. Solutes and fluid diffuse across the peritoneal membrane.
   3. Peritoneal dialysis is usually not used to treat AKI in adults.
   4. Peritonitis
      a. Infection of the peritoneal cavity. Patient technique and population variables influence the rate of infection. Elderly patients or those with diabetes have a higher infection rate. Peritonitis is a major cause of failure of peritoneal dialysis.
      b. Treatment
         i. Most common gram-positive organisms include *Staphylococcus epidermis*, *S. aureus*, and streptococci. Most common gram-negative organisms include *Escherichia coli* and *Pseudomonas aeruginosa*.
         ii. Empiric treatment should cover gram-positive and gram-negative bacteria. Adjust as needed.

5. Types of peritoneal dialysis
   a. Continuous ambulatory peritoneal dialysis. Classic. Requires mechanical process, which requires multiple manual changes throughout the day. Can be interruptive to daytime routine
   b. Automated peritoneal dialysis. Many variants exist, but continuous cycling peritoneal dialysis is the most common. Patient undergoes multiple exchanges during sleep by a cycling machine. May have one or two dwells during day. Minimizes potential contamination. Lowest incidence of peritonitis

---

Patient Cases

11. R.T. is a 60-year-old HD patient who has had ESRD for 10 years. His HD access is a left arteriovenous fistula. He has a history of hypertension, CAD, mild CHF, type 2 diabetes mellitus, and seizure disorder. Medications: epoetin 14,000 units 3 times/week at dialysis; multivitamins (Nephrocaps) once daily; atorvastatin 20 mg/day; insulin; calcium acetate 2 tablets 3 times/day with meals; phenytoin 300 mg/day; and intravenous iron 100 mg/month. Laboratory values: hemoglobin 10.2 g/L; iPTH (immunoassay for parathyroid hormone) 800 pg/mL; Na 140; K 4.9; Cr 7.0; calcium 9 mg/dL; albumin 2.5 g/L; and Phos 7.8 mg/dL. Ferritin is 200, and transferrin saturation is 32%. The RBC indices (MCV, MCHC are normal. His WBC is normal. He is afebrile. Which one of the following is most likely contributing to relative epoetin resistance in this patient?
    A. Iron deficiency.
    B. Hyperparathyroidism.
    C. Phenytoin therapy.
    D. Infection.

12. In addition to diet modification and emphasizing adherence, which one of the following is the best approach to managing this patient's hyperparathyroidism and renal osteodystrophy?
    A. Increase calcium acetate.
    B. Change calcium acetate to sevelamer and add cinacalcet.
    C. Hold calcium acetate and add intravenous vitamin D analog.
    D. Add intravenous vitamin D analog.

V. COMPLICATIONS OF CKD

A. Anemia
   1. In CKD, anemia is generally treated with a hemoglobin concentration of less than 11 g/dL. Several factors are responsible for anemia in CKD: decreased erythropoietin production (most important), shorter life span of RBCs, blood loss during dialysis, iron deficiency, anemia of chronic disease, and renal osteodystrophy.
   2. Prevalence: Twenty-six percent of patients with a GFR greater than 60 mL/minute have anemia versus 75% of patients with a GFR less than 15 mL/minute.
   3. Signs and symptoms. Symptoms of anemia of CKD are similar to anemia associated with other causes.

4. Treatment—Treatment of anemia in CKD can decrease morbidity/mortality, reduce left ventricular hypertrophy, increase exercise tolerance, and increase quality of life. Some studies have suggested that treatment to high hemoglobin concentrations (greater than 13 g/dL) increases cardiovascular events. Most recently, TREAT (Trial to Reduce Cardiovascular Events with Aranesp Therapy) failed to show a benefit in outcomes but was associated with increased stroke. (NEJM 2009;361.)
   a. Anemia work-up—Initiate evaluation when CrCl is less than 60 mL/minute or hemoglobin is less than 11 g/dL.
      i. Hemoglobin/hematocrit
      ii. Mean corpuscular volume
      iii. Reticulocyte count
      iv. Iron studies
         Transferrin saturation (total iron/total iron-binding capacity)—assesses available iron
         Ferritin—measures stored iron
      v. Stool guaiac
   b. Erythropoietic receptor agonists
      i. Goal is to achieve target hemoglobin more than 11 g/dL. The most recent Kidney Disease Outcome Quality Initiative guidelines warn against intentionally increasing the hemoglobin more than 13 g/dL. (*Note:* The "old" target was 11–12 g/dL, and many sites still use this goal.) Because of concern about high hemoglobin concentrations, the 2007 update to the guidelines suggests a goal of 11–12 g/dL and the avoidance of a hemoglobin concentration greater than 13 g/dL.
      ii. Epoetin-α
         (a) Same molecular structure as human erythropoietin (recombinant DNA technology)
         (b) Binds to and activates erythropoietin receptor
         (c) Administered subcutaneously or intravenously
      iii. Darbepoetin-α
         (a) Molecular structure of human erythropoietin has been modified from 3 N-linked carbohydrate chains to 5 N-linked carbohydrate chains; increased duration of activity. The advantage is less-frequent dosing.
         (b) Binds to and activates erythropoietin receptor
         (c) May be administered subcutaneously or intravenously. Initial dose 0.45 mcg/kg/week; typically 40 mcg
      iv. Erythropoietic receptor agonist dose adjustment is based on hemoglobin response.
         (a) Adjustment parameters are the same for epoetin-α and darbepoetin-α.
         (b) Dosage adjustments upward should not be made more often than every 4 weeks. In general, dose adjustments are made in 25% intervals.
      v. Erythropoietic receptor agonist monitoring
         (a) Hemoglobin concentrations initially every 1–2 weeks and then every 2–4 weeks when stable
         (b) Monitor BP because it may rise (treat as necessary).
         (c) Iron stores
            (1) Ferritin: HD target is 200–500, and peritoneal dialysis/CKD target is 100–500.
            (2) Transferrin saturation target is greater than 20% (upper limit of 50% removed from recent guidelines)

vi. Common causes of inadequate response to erythropoietic receptor agonist therapy:
   (a) Iron deficiency is the most common cause of erythropoietin resistance. Increased use of intravenous iron products has reduced this problem, however.
   (b) Other causes in patients with adequate iron stores (the first three are the most common):
      (1) Infection/inflammation
      (2) Chronic blood loss
      (3) Osteitis fibrosa
      (4) Aluminum toxicity
      (5) Hemoglobinopathies
      (6) Folate or vitamin B_{12} deficiency
      (7) Multiple myeloma
      (8) Malnutrition
      (9) Hemolysis
      (10) Vitamin C deficiency
   vii. ESA's now under FDA's Risk Evaluation and Mitigation Strategy (REMS) program.
c. Iron therapy
   i. Most patients with CKD who are receiving erythropoietic therapy require parenteral iron therapy to meet needs (increased requirements, decreased oral absorption).
   ii. For adult patients who undergo dialysis, an empiric 1000-mg dose is usually given, and equations are rarely used.
   iii. Follow transferrin saturation and ferritin as noted during erythropoietic therapy.
   iv. Four commercial iron preparations are approved in the United States (Table 2).
   v. Oral iron not recommended in CKD patients on HD.

Table 2. Iron Therapy

	Iron Dextran	**Ferric Gluconate**	**Iron Sucrose**	**Ferumoxytol**
Replacement therapy %TSAT < 20% and ferritin < 100–200 mg/dL	IVP: 100 m IV 3 times/week during HD for 10 doses (1 g) IVPB: 500–1000 mg in 250 mL of NSS infused for at least 1 hour (option for non-HD patients)	125 mg IV 3 times/week during HD for 8 doses (1 g)	100 mg IV 3 times/week during HD for 10 doses (1 g) For nondialysis CKD, 200 mg IV × 5 doses	510 mg at up to 30 mg/second followed by a second 510 mg IV 3–8 days later (all CKD)
Maintenance therapy (iron stores in goal)	25-100 mg/week IV × 10 weeks	31.25-125 mg/week IV × 10 weeks	25-100 mg/week IV × 10 weeks	N/A
Iron overload %TSAT > 50% and/or ferritin > 500	Hold therapy	Hold therapy	Hold therapy	Hold therapy
Initial test dose	Yes; 25-mg one-time test dose	No	No	No

CKD = chronic kidney disease; HD = hemodialysis; IV = intravenous; IVP = IV push; IVPB = IV piggyback; N/A = not applicable; NSS = normal saline solution; TSAT = transferrin saturation.

B. Renal Osteodystrophy and Secondary Hyperparathyroidism
   1. Pathophysiology: Calcium and phosphorous homeostasis is complex, involving the interplay of hormones affecting the bone, gastrointestinal tract, kidneys, and PTH. Process may begin as early as GFR 60 mL/minute. The most important driving force behind the process is hyperphosphatemia! Nephron loss: decreased production of 1,25 dihydroxyvitamin D3 and phosphate retention. Increased phosphorous concentrations cause 1) an inhibition of vitamin D activation, reducing absorption of calcium in the gut; 2) a decrease in ionized (free) calcium concentrations; and 3) direct stimulation of PTH secretion. Elevated PTH concentrations cause decreased reabsorption of phosphorus and increased reabsorption of calcium in the proximal tube. This adaptive mechanism is lost as the GFR falls below 30 mL/minute. Important: Calcium is not well absorbed through the gut at this point, and calcium concentrations are maintained by increased bone resorption through elevated PTH. Unabated calcium loss from the bone results in renal osteodystrophy.
   2. Prevalence
      a. Major cause of morbidity and mortality in patients undergoing dialysis
      b. Very common
   3. Signs and symptoms
      a. Insidious onset: Patients may complain of fatigue and musculoskeletal and gastrointestinal pain; calcification may be visible on radiography; bone pain and fractures can occur if progression is left untreated.
      b. Laboratory abnormalities
         i. Phosphorus
         ii. Corrected calcium
         iii. Intact PTH
   4. Treatment
      a. Goals of therapy—Table 3

Table 3.

KDOQI Guidelines for Calcium, Phosphorus, CaxPO4 Product, and PTH in CKD Stages 3–5			
	CKD Stage 3	CKD Stage 4	CKD Stage 5
Calcium (mg/dL)[a]	Normal	Normal	8.4–9.5
Phosphorus (mg/dL)	2.7–4.6	2.7–4.6	3.5–5.5
Ca × PO4 product	< 55	< 55	< 55
PTH (pg/mL)	35–70	70–110	150–300

[a]Use corrected calcium = serum calcium + (0.8 × [4.0 − patient albumin]).
CKD = chronic kidney disease; KDOQI = Kidney Disease Outcomes Quality Initiative; PTH = parathyroid hormone.

   b. Nondrug therapy
      i. Dietary phosphorus restriction 800-1200 mg/day in stage 3 CKD or higher
      ii. Dialysis removes various amounts of phosphorus depending on treatment modalities but, by itself, is insufficient to maintain Phos balances in most patients.
      iii. Parathyroidectomy. Reserved for patients with unresponsive hyperparathyroidism
   c. Drug therapy
      i. Phosphate binders: Take with meals to bind phosphorus in the gut; products from different groups may be used together for additive effect.
         (a) Aluminum-containing phosphate binders (aluminum hydroxide, aluminum carbonate, and sucralfate). Effectively lowers phosphorus concentrations. In general, avoid. Not used as often because of aluminum toxicity (adynamic bone disease, encephalopathy, and erythropoietin resistance)

(b) Calcium-containing phosphate binders (calcium carbonate and calcium acetate)
   (1) Widely used phosphate binder. Calcium binders are initial binder of choice for stage 3 and 4 CKD. Calcium (or non-ionic binders) are considered initial binder of choice in stage 5 CKD. Carbonate salt is relatively inexpensive.
   (2) Carbonate is also used to treat hypocalcemia, which sometimes occurs in patients with CKD, and can decrease metabolic acidosis.
   (3) Calcium acetate: 667-mg capsule contains 167 mg of elemental calcium. Better binder than carbonate, so less calcium given
   (4) Use may be limited by development of hypercalcemia.
   (5) Total elemental calcium per day is 2000 mg/day (1500-mg binder; 500-mg diet)
(c) Sevelamer: a nonabsorbable phosphate binder
   (1) Effectively binds phosphorus
   (2) As with calcium, considered primary therapy in CKD stage 5. In particular, consider if calcium-phosphorus product is greater than 55 mg^2/dL^2 or calcium intake exceeds recommended dose with calcium-containing binders.
   (3) Decreases low-density lipoprotein cholesterol and increases high-density lipoprotein cholesterol
   (4) Hypocalcemia may occur if sevelamer is sole phosphate binder. Metabolic acidosis may worsen with sevelamer HCl.
   (5) Available as sevelamer HCl (Renagel) and sevelamer carbonate (Renvela)
(d) Lanthanum carbonate:
   (1) As effective as aluminum in phosphate-binding capability. Not widely used but indications similar to sevelamer
   (2) Tasteless, chewable wafer
   (3) Consider using if calcium × phosphorus product is more than 55 mg^2/dL^2.

ii. Vitamin D analogs: Suppress PTH synthesis and reduce PTH concentrations; therapy is limited by resultant hypercalcemia, hyperphosphatemia, and elevated calcium-phosphorus product. Products include calcitriol, doxercalciferol, and paricalcitol.
   (a) Calcitriol, the pharmacologically active form of 1,2 hydroxyvitamin D3, is U.S. Food and Drug Administration (FDA) label approved for the management of hypocalcemia and the prevention and treatment of secondary hyperparathyroidism
      (1) Oral and parenteral formulations
      (2) Does not require hepatic or renal activation
      (3) Low-dose daily oral therapy reduces hypocalcemia but does not reduce PTH concentrations significantly.
      (4) High incidence of hypercalcemia limiting PTH suppression
      (5) Dose adjustment at 4-week intervals
   (b) Paricalcitol: vitamin D analog; FDA label approved for the treatment and prevention of secondary hyperparathyroidism
      (1) Parenteral and oral formulation
      (2) Does not require hepatic or renal activation
      (3) Lower incidence of hypercalcemia (decreased mobilization of calcium from the bone and decreased absorption of calcium from the gut)
   (c) Doxercalciferol: vitamin D analog; FDA label approved for the treatment and prevention of secondary hyperparathyroidism

(1) Parenteral and oral formulation
(2) Prodrug, requires hepatic activation; may have more physiologic levels
(3) Lower incidence of hypercalcemia (decreased mobilization of calcium from the bone and decreased absorption of calcium from the gut)
  iii. Cinacalcet HCl: A calcimimetic that attaches to the calcium receptor on the parathyroid gland and increases the sensitivity of receptors to serum calcium concentrations, thus reducing PTH. Especially useful in patients with high calcium/phosphate concentrations and high PTH concentrations when vitamin D analogs cannot be used
    (a) The initial dose is 30 mg, irrespective of patient PTH concentration.
    (b) Monitor serum calcium every 1-2 weeks (risk of hypocalcemia is about 5%); do not start therapy if serum calcium is less than 8.4 mg/dL.
    (c) Can be used in patients irrespective of phosphate binder or vitamin D analog use
    (d) Caution in patients with seizure disorder (hypocalcemia may exacerbate)
    (e) Adverse effects are nausea (30%) and diarrhea (20%).
    (f) Cytochrome P450 2D6 metabolism: Dose reductions in drugs with narrow therapeutic indexes may be required (flecainide, tricyclic antidepressants, and thioridazine).
    (g) Ketoconazole increases cinacalcet concentrations up to 2-fold.

Patient Case for Dose Adjustments in Kidney Disease

13. P.P. is a 40-year-old dialysis patient with a history of grand mal seizures. He takes phenytoin 300 mg/day. His albumin concentration is 3.0 g/L. His total phenytoin concentration is 5.0 mg/dL. Which one of the following is the best interpretation of the phenytoin concentrations?
    A. The concentration is subtherapeutic, and a dose increase is warranted.
    B. The concentration is therapeutic, and no dosage adjustment is needed.
    C. The concentration is toxic, and a dose reduction is needed.
    D. The level is not interpretable.

VI. DOSAGE ADJUSTMENTS IN KIDNEY DISEASE

A. Dosages of many drugs will require adjustment to prevent toxicity in patients with CKD; adjustment strategies will vary, depending on whether the patient is receiving renal replacement therapy and, if so, the type of renal replacement therapy. The National Kidney Disease Education Program (NKDEP) of the NIH/NIDDK suggests that either estimated GFR (eGFR) or eCrCl can be used for drug dosing. If using eGFR in very large or small patients should multiply the eGFR by the actual BSA to obtain eGFR in ml/min.
B. Pharmacokinetic Principles Can Guide Therapy Adjustments.
  1. Absorption
    a. Oral absorption can be decreased.
      i. Nausea and vomiting
      ii. Increased gastric pH (uremia)
      iii. Edema
      iv. Physical binding of drugs to phosphate binders

2. Distribution
   a. Changes in concentrations of highly protein-bound and highly water-soluble drugs occur as extracellular fluid status changes.
   b. Acidic and neutral protein-bound drugs are displaced by toxin buildup. Other mechanisms include conformational changes of plasma protein–binding site. Phenytoin is a classic example. The "normal" free fraction of phenytoin is 10%. Can increase to as high as 25% with kidney disease and/or hypoalbuminemia.
      i. Hypoalbuminemia correction
         Concentration adjusted = concentration measured/[(0.2 × measured albumin) + 0.1]
      ii. Renal failure adjustment
         Concentration adjusted = concentration measured/[(0.1 × measured albumin) + 0.1]
      iii. Patients will have lower total concentrations despite having adequate free concentrations. (Increased free fraction)
      iv. Dosage adjustment of phenytoin not needed, just a different approach to evaluating concentrations
3. Metabolism. Variable changes can occur with uremia. Metabolites can accumulate.
4. Excretion – Decreased

C. Pharmacodynamic Changes Can Also Occur. (Example: Patients with CKD can be more sensitive to benzodiazepines.)

D. General Recommendations:
   1. Patient history and clinical data
   2. Estimate CrCl (Jeliffe or Brater in AKI; Cockcroft-Gault in stable kidney function).
   3. Identify medications that require modification (Table 4).

Table 4. Dose Adjustments in Decreased Kidney Function

Agent	Dose Adjustment
Antibiotics	Almost all antibiotics will require dosage adjustment (exceptions: cloxacillin, clindamycin, linezolid, metronidazole, and macrolides)
Cardiac medications	Atenolol, ACEIs, digoxin, nadolol, sotalol; avoid potassium-sparing diuretics if CrCl < 30 mL/minute
Lipid-lowering therapy	Clofibrate, fenofibrate, statins
Narcotics	Codeine, avoid meperidine; other agents may also accumulate
Antipsychotic/antiepileptic agents	Chloral hydrate, gabapentin, lithium, paroxetine, primidone, topiramate, trazodone, vigabatrin
Hypoglycemic agents	Acarbose, chlorpropamide, glyburide, glipizide, insulins, and metformin
Antiretrovirals	Individualize therapy: monitor CD_4 counts, viral load, and adverse effects (agents requiring dose adjustment: lamivudine, adefovir, didanosine, stavudine, tenofovir, zalcitabine, and zidovudine)
Miscellaneous	Allopurinol, colchicine, H_2-receptor antagonists, diclofenac, ketorolac, and terbutaline

ACEIs = angiotensin-converting enzyme inhibitors; CrCl = creatinine clearance.

4. Calculate drug doses individualized for the patient.
    a. Published data
    b. Rowland-Tozer estimate
        i. $Q = 1 - [Fe(1 - KF)]$
        ii. Q = kinetic parameter or drug dose adjustment factor
        iii. Fe = fraction of drug excreted unchanged in the urine
        iv. KF = ratio of patients' CrCl to normal (120 mL/minute)
5. Monitor patient (e.g., kidney function; clinical parameters) and drug concentration (if applicable).
6. Revise regimen as appropriate.

E. Drug Dosing in HD
    1. Dosing changes in HD patients may be necessary because of accumulation due to kidney failure AND/OR because the procedure may remove the drug from the circulation.
    2. Drug-related factors affecting drug removal during dialysis:
        a. Molecular weight—With high-flux membranes, larger molecules (such as vancomycin) can be removed.
        b. Water soluble—nonsoluble drugs not likely removed
        c. Protein binding—Because albumin cannot pass through membranes, protein-bound drugs cannot either.
        d. Volume of distribution—Drugs with a small V_d (less than 1 L/kg) available in central circulation for removal. Large V_ds cannot be removed (digoxin and tricyclic antidepressants), even if the protein binding is very low.
    3. Procedure-related factors affecting drug removal
        a. Type of dialyzer—high flux widely used now
        b. Bloodflow rate. Increased rates will increase delivery and maintain gradient across membrane.
        c. Duration of dialysis session
        d. Dialysate flow rate. High rates of flow will increase removal by maintaining the gradient across membranes.

REFERENCES

National Kidney Foundation's Kidney Disease Outcome Quality Initiative

1. Go to *www.kidney.org/professionals/*.

National Kidney Disease Education Program

1. Go to *www.nkdep.nih.gov/*.

Acute Kidney Injury

1. Hilton R. Acute kidney injury [review]. BMJ 2006;333:786–90.
2. Ympa YP, Sakr Y, Reinhart K, Vincent JL. Has mortality from acute kidney injury decreased? A systematic review of the literature. Am J Med 2005;118:827–32.
3. Dager W, Spencer A. Acute renal failure. In: DiPiro JT, Talbert RL, Yee GC, et al., eds. Pharmacotherapy: A Pathophysiologic Approach, 7th ed. New York: McGraw-Hill, 2008:723–43.
4. Stamatakis MK. Acute renal failure. In: Chisholm-Burns MA, Wells BG, Schwinghammer TL, et al., eds. Pharmacotherapy: Principles and Practice. New York: McGraw-Hill, 2007:chapter 22.
5. Mehta RL, Kellum JA, Shah SV, et al. Acute kidney injury network: report of an initiative to improve outcomes in acute kidney injury. Crit Care 2007;11:R31.

Drug-Induced Kidney Damage

1. Nolin TD, Himmelfarb J. Drug-induced kidney disease. In: DiPiro JT, Talbert RL, Yee GC, et al., eds. Pharmacotherapy: A Pathophysiologic Approach, 7th ed. New York: McGraw-Hill, 2008:795–810.
2. Schweiger MJ, Chambers CE, Davidson CJ, et al. Prevention of contrast induced nephropathy: recommendations for the high risk patient undergoing cardiovascular procedures. Catheter Cardiovasc Interv 2007;69:135–40.

Chronic Kidney Disease

1. Joy MS, Ksirsagar A, Franceshini N. Chronic kidney disease: progression-modifying therapies. In: DiPiro JT, Talbert RL, Yee GC, et al., eds. Pharmacotherapy: A Pathophysiologic Approach, 7th ed. New York: McGraw-Hill, 2008:745–64.
2. Hudson JQ. Chronic kidney disease: management of complications. In: DiPiro JT, Talbert RL, Yee GC, et al., eds. Pharmacotherapy: A Pathophysiologic Approach, 7th ed. New York: McGraw-Hill, 2008:765–92.
3. Schonder KS. Chronic and end-stage renal disease. In: Chisholm-Burns MA, Wells BG, Schwinghammer TL, et al., eds. Pharmacotherapy: Principles and Practice. New York: McGraw-Hill, 2007:chapter 23.
4. National Kidney Foundations. KDOQI. Clinical Practice Guidelines and Clinical Practice Recommendations for Diabetes and Chronic Kidney Disease. Am J Kidney Dis 49:S1-S180, 2007 (suppl 2).

Renal Replacement Therapy

1. Foote EF, Manly HJ. Hemodialysis and peritoneal dialysis In: DiPiro JT, Talbert RL, Yee GC, et al., eds. Pharmacotherapy: A Pathophysiologic Approach, 7th ed. New York: McGraw-Hill, 2008:793–4.
2. Piraino P, Bailie GR, Bernardini J, et al. Peritoneal dialysis-related infections recommendations: 2005 update. Perit Dial Int 2005;25:107–31.

Complications of CKD

1. Pharmacotherapy specialists should be aware of the National Kidney Foundation Kidney Disease Outcome Quality Initiative Web site. Available at *http://www.kidney.org/professionals/kdoqi/guidelines.cfm*. Accessed February 21, 2007.
2. Hudson JQ. Chronic kidney disease: management of complications. In: DiPiro JT, Talbert RL, Yee GC, et al., eds. Pharmacotherapy: A Pathophysiologic Approach, 7th ed. New York: McGraw-Hill, 2008:765–92.
3. Schonder KS. Chronic and end-stage renal disease. In: Chisholm-Burns MA, Wells BG, Schwinghammer TL, et al., eds. Pharmacotherapy: Principles and Practice. New York: McGraw-Hill, 2007:chapter 23.

Drug Therapy Adjustment in CKD

1. Kappel J, Calissi P. Nephrology: 3. Safe drug prescribing for patients with renal insufficiency. Can Med Assoc J 2002;166:473–7.

2. Matzke GR, Frye RF. Drug therapy individualization for patients with renal insufficiency. In: DiPiro JT, Talbert RL, Yee GC, et al., eds. Pharmacotherapy: A Pathophysiologic Approach, 7th ed. New York: McGraw-Hill, 2008:833–44.
3. Chronic Kidney Disease and Drug Dosing. Information for Providers. 2010 http://www.nkdep.nih.gov/professionals/drug-dosing-information.htm

ANSWERS AND EXPLANATIONS TO PATIENT CASES

1. Answer: D
Estimating CrCl in a patient with unstable kidney function is difficult. The Jeliffe or Brater equation has been recommended as preferable to other equations. In this case, the patient is anuric; hence, a CrCl (GFR) of 10 mL/minute or less (Answer D) should be assumed. Answer A (Cockcroft-Gault) is inappropriate because Cockcroft-Gault should only be used with stable kidney function. The use of MDRD (Answer B) in unstable kidney function is also inappropriate. Although Answer C, the Brater equation, may be used, it would still overestimate kidney function in this patient because the patient is anuric.

2. Answer: B
This patient very likely has ATN, which is a type of intrinsic renal failure (Answer B). The rapid rise in SCr, the BUN/Cr ratio of about 10, and the muddy casts all point to ATN. There is no evidence of prerenal causes (hypotension, volume depletion) (Answer A). Naproxen is associated with functional AKI, but the urine in these patients is bland without casts. Answer C is incorrect because there is no evidence of obstruction in this patient.

3. Answer: D
One of the strategies in the management of AKI is to remove potentially nephrotoxic drugs. It is common to see the following orders for patients in AKI: no ACEIs, ARBs, NSAIDs, or intravenous contrast. It is also important to remove (or reduce the dose of) agents that are cleared renally. Metformin, which accumulates in decreased kidney function with an increased risk of lactic acidosis, should be temporarily discontinued at this time. Because the patient is normotensive, there is no compelling need to discontinue the amlodipine. Review the drug therapy of patients with AKI, removing unnecessary agents and correcting doses for decreased kidney function.

4. Answer: B
The most important risk factors for contrast-induced nephropathy include the presence of CKD in a patient with diabetes. In men, a hematocrit less than 39% is also a risk factor. Enalapril may worsen the effects of contrast. The cutoff for age to be a risk factor is 75 years.

5. Answer: B
It is recommended to start intravenous normal saline 6–12 hours before the procedure. Answers C and D would likely not allow enough time for adequate hydration and diuresis. Answer A is reasonable, but there is no compelling reason to start that early, and this may prolong the hospital stay. Some recent data with sodium bicarbonate intravenously show benefit with a more narrow start time (2 hours).

6. Answer: B
Much data have published on the use of oral acetylcysteine in the prevention of contrast-induced nephropathy. Although many of the studies were observational, the low risk of the product has made it the standard of care in this situation. Fenoldopam (Answer A) should not be used based on the results of the CONTRAST trial. There are some data with ascorbic acid (Answer C), but they are limited. Hemofiltration (Answer D) has also been studied but is not generally recommended because of the questionable benefits and the real risk of complications.

7. Answer: A
He is currently at stage 2 CKD (GFR 60–89 mL/minute/1.73 m^2), which can be calculated by use of the MDRD formulae or Cockcroft-Gault. The five stages correlate from mild kidney damage (stage 1) to kidney failure (stage 5).

8. Answer: C
Based on his long history of diabetes and overt proteinuria, this patient likely has diabetic nephropathy. Progression will be accelerated by smoking, poor diabetes control, and poor BP control. In patients with diabetes, a target hemoglobin A$_{1c}$ of less than 7 g/dL is associated with a decrease in the rate of disease progression. Blood pressure control less than 130/80 mm Hg in patients also decreases the progression of kidney disease. The standard of care in patients with diabetic nephropathy is ACEIs (or ARBs). A nondihydropyridine (Answer B) might be initiated in patients who cannot tolerate ACE or ARB therapy. Dihydropyridine therapy (Answer A) is not recommended in diabetic nephropathy because of conflicting literature on its efficacy. An increase in atenolol (Answer D) might control BP, but inhibition of the renin-angiotensin system is still the best answer.

9. Answer: D

A native arteriovenous fistula is the preferred access for chronic HD. If an arteriovenous fistula cannot be constructed, a synthetic arteriovenous graft (Answer C) is considered second line. A subclavian catheter (Answer A) is a poor choice because of the increased risk of infection and thrombosis and because of the poor bloodflows obtained through a catheter. A Tenckhoff catheter (Answer B) is incorrect because this is a catheter for peritoneal dialysis.

10. Answer: D

The most well-studied medication is midodrine, an α_1-agonist. Levocarnitine (Answer A) has been tried, but there are limited data on its benefit. Fludrocortisone (Answer B) is a synthetic mineralocorticoid, which is used for hypotension in other situations; however, the primary mechanism is due to Na and water restriction in the kidney; hence, this medication is less likely to work. Sodium chloride tablets (Answer B) would not work acutely and should generally be avoided.

11. Answer: B

Hyperparathyroidism is associated with epoetin resistance in HD patients (Answer B). Although iron deficiency is the most common cause of epoetin deficiency, the laboratory results in this patient do not indicate iron deficiency (Answer A). Phenytoin therapy (Answer C) has been associated with anemia in other patient populations but not in HD patients. Infection (Answer D) and inflammation are very common causes of epoetin deficiency in patients on HD, but there is nothing in this patient's presentation to suggest an infectious or inflammatory process.

12. Answer: B

D.W. requires treatment for his elevated iPTH (800 pg/dL), which puts him at high risk of renal osteodystrophy. He has high serum phosphorous and calcium. The corrected calcium is 10.2 mg/dL, and the calcium × phosphorus factor is 80 mg^2/dL^2. The goal/target Ca × Phos factor in stage 5 CKD is less than 55 mg^2/dL^2. Current binder therapy is contributing to calcium exposure; therefore, calcium acetate should be discontinued and sevelamer, initiated. Cinacalcet will lower iPTH and potentially serum calcium. Answer A is incorrect because increasing the calcium acetate may worsen the hypercalcemia. Answer C is incorrect for two reasons. First, the patient needs some type of phosphate binder; second, intravenous vitamin D analogs can worsen hypercalcemia and are not very effective in reducing elevated iPTH in the presence of hyperphosphatemia.

Answer D is incorrect because intravenous vitamin D analogs can worsen hypercalcemia and are not very effective in reducing elevated iPTH in the presence of hyperphosphatemia.

13. Answer: B

The presence of kidney failure and low albumin results in an increased free fraction of phenytoin. Using the correction equation results in a corrected level of 12.5, which is therapeutic. A free phenytoin concentration can also be drawn.

ANSWERS AND EXPLANATIONS TO SELF-ASSESSMENT QUESTIONS

1. Answer: C
Initial treatment of AKI requires the identification and reversal (if possible) of the insult to the kidney. A.M.'s symptoms and presentation is consistent with pre-renal azotemia because of volume depletion, so fluid administration would be the best choice in this case. There is no suggestion of obstruction (distended abdomen, history of benign prostatic hypertrophy). Diuretic administration would not be appropriate because it would worsen his volume depletion and probably further impair his kidney function. Fluid management is critical to managing AKI, requiring a careful assessment of the patient. Although A.M.'s glucose concentration is elevated, insulin is not required at this point.

2. Answer: C
F.D. has intrinsic azotemia, resulting in damage to the kidneys. Aminoglycosides can cause direct damage to the tubules. The BUN/SCr ratio is normal (an increased BUN/SCr ratio reflecting hypovolemia is common in prerenal azotemia). Decreased urinary Na less than 20 mOsmol/L is also a marker of hypovolemia. Fractional excretion of Na additionally distinguishes prerenal and intrinsic renal damage. A low FENa (less than 1%) in an oliguric patient suggests tubular function is still intact. A FENa of 1%–2% is commonly seen in intrinsic renal failure. The specific gravity is normal in intrinsic renal failure. Elevated specific gravity greater than 1.018 is seen in prerenal failure, reflecting concentrated urine due to hypovolemia. Cellular debris is often present in intrinsic renal failure because of renal tubular cell death/damage.

3. Answer: A
Application of the Rowland-Tozer equation yields the following calculation:
$Q = 1 - [Fe(1 - KF)]$
$Q = 1 - [0.4(1 - 25/120)]$
$Q = 1 - [0.4(0.79)]$
$Q = 1 - 0.32$
$Q = 0.68$ or 68% of usual dose
Drug X usual dose = 600 mg
Formulation = 100 mg/mL in a 6-mL vial
Adjusted dose = 408 mg
Four milliliters would provide 400 mg of drug X.

4. Answer: C
In most cases, either the Cockcroft-Gault OR the MDRD equation is appropriate (and best) to assess kidney function. However, this patient has muscle wasting; hence, equations will overestimate. An iothalamate study will measure GFR, but it is not used clinically.

5. Answer: C
This patient is not at goal for hemoglobin. Iron studies indicate the patient is iron-deficient. Although a trial of oral iron might be indicated in CKD stages I–IV, HD patients should be given intravenous iron as first line.

6. Answer: B
The BUN/SCr ratio, urine osmolality, and presence of urinary casts all point to ATN. Prerenal and functional AKI look similar in urinalysis. Classically, AIN has eosinophils in the urine.

7. Answer: B
An unpaired/independent t-test is the most appropriate. There is no reason to think these continuous data will not be normally distributed. There are only two groups (otherwise, an analysis of variance would be needed with an appropriate post hoc test).

GASTROINTESTINAL DISORDERS

BRIAN A. HEMSTREET, PHARM.D., BCPS

UNIVERSITY OF COLORADO DENVER
SCHOOL OF PHARMACY
AURORA, COLORADO

GASTROINTESTINAL DISORDERS

BRIAN A. HEMSTREET, PHARM.D., BCPS

UNIVERSITY OF COLORADO DENVER
SCHOOL OF PHARMACY
AURORA, COLORADO

Learning Objectives:

1. Review and apply national guideline treatment strategies to the following gastrointestinal (GI) disorders: gastroesophageal reflux disease (GERD), peptic ulcer disease, ulcerative colitis (UC), Crohn's disease, viral hepatitis, alcoholic liver disease, and upper GI bleeding.

2. Recommend appropriate pharmacologic and non-pharmacologic interventions for the treatment of GERD.

3. Differentiate between clinical signs, symptoms, risk factors, and treatment of both *Helicobacter pylori*– and nonsteroidal anti-inflammatory drug (NSAID)-associated peptic ulcer disease.

4. Discuss the role of pharmacologic intervention in the treatment of nonvariceal upper GI bleeding.

5. Review the clinical differences in signs, symptoms, and treatment of Crohn's disease and UC.

6. Identify the common manifestations of alcoholic liver disease and their treatment.

7. Review the treatment of both acute and chronic viral hepatitis.

8. Recognize pertinent information for educating patients and prescribers regarding the appropriate use of pharmacologic agents for various GI disorders.

9. Understand commonly encountered statistical tests and concepts using GI disorders as examples.

Self-Assessment Questions:

Answers to these questions may be found at the end of this chapter.

1. A 58-year-old African American man presents with a 2-month history of burning epigastric pain and intermittent difficulty swallowing. The pain is not relieved by positional changes or by eating, and he has tried over-the-counter (OTC) antacids with minimal relief. He takes amlodipine 5 mg/day for hypertension and ibuprofen for occasional back pain. Which one of the following is best for this patient?

   A. Initiate famotidine 20 mg/day.
   B. Refer for possible endoscopic evaluation.
   C. Initiate omeprazole 20 mg 2 times/day.
   D. Change amlodipine to hydrochlorothiazide.

2. A 50-year-old woman is seen today in the clinic for complaints of severe pain related to the swelling of three of her metacarpophalangeal joints on each hand, as well as the swelling of her right wrist. She is unable to write or perform her usual household activities. Radiograms of these joints reveal bony decalcifications and erosions. A serum rheumatoid factor is obtained, which is elevated. Her medical history includes type 2 diabetes mellitus, hypertension, and dyslipidemia. Her medications include metformin 1000 mg 2 times/day, glyburide 10 mg/day, metoprolol 100 mg 2 times/day, aspirin 81 mg/day, and rosuvastatin 5 mg/day. The primary care provider would like to initiate systemic anti-inflammatory therapy for this patient's rheumatoid arthritis with high-dose nonsteroidal anti-inflammatory drug (NSAID) therapy; however, the primary care provider is worried about potential gastrointestinal (GI) toxicity. Which one of the following regimens is best for treating this patient's pain while minimizing the risk of GI toxicity?

   A. Celecoxib 400 mg 2 times/day.
   B. Indomethacin plus ranitidine.
   C. Naproxen plus omeprazole.
   D. Piroxicam plus misoprostol.

3. A 68-year-old Hispanic man is assessed in the emergency department for a 36-hour history of black, tarry stools; dizziness; confusion; and vomiting a substance resembling coffee grounds. He has a medical history of osteoarthritis, hypertension, myocardial infarction in 1996 and 1998, and seasonal allergies. He has been taking naproxen 500 mg 2 times/day for 4 years, metoprolol 100 mg 2 times/day, aspirin 325 mg/day, and loratadine 10 mg/day. Nasogastric aspiration is positive for blood, and subsequent endoscopy reveals a 3-cm antral ulcer with a visible vessel. The vessel is obliterated using an epinephrine solution, and a rapid urease test is negative for *Helicobacter pylori*. Which one of the following recommendations is best for this patient?

   A. Intravenous ranitidine 50 mg/hour for 5 days.
   B. Sucralfate 1 g 4 times/day by nasogastric tube.
   C. Oral lansoprazole 15 mg/day by nasogastric tube.
   D. Pantoprazole 80 mg intravenous bolus, followed by an 8-mg/hour infusion.

4. A 38-year-old white woman presents with an 8-week history of new-onset cramping abdominal pain together with two to four bloody stools per day. She has a medical history of urinary tract infection and reports an allergy to "sulfa"-containing medications (shortness of breath). Colonoscopy reveals diffuse superficial colonic inflammation consistent with

ulcerative colitis (UC). The inflammation is continuous and extends to the hepatic flexure. Which one of the following drug therapies is best?

A. Sulfasalazine 4 g/day.
B. Hydrocortisone enema 100 mg every night.
C. 6-mercaptopurine (6-MP) 75 mg/day.
D. Mesalamine (Asacol) 1.6 g orally 3 times/day.

5. A 45-year-old African American man with a history of alcoholic cirrhosis (Child-Pugh class B) was seen in the clinic today for follow-up. He was recently referred for screening endoscopy, which revealed several large esophageal varices. He has no history of bleeding; 1 month ago, propranolol 10 mg orally 3 times/day was initiated. At that time, his vital signs included temperature 98.7°F, pulse rate (PR) 85 beats/minute, respiratory rate (RR) 15, and blood pressure (BP) 130/80 mm Hg. At his evaluation today, he seems to be tolerating the propranolol and has no new complaints. His vital signs now include temperature 98.6°F, PR 79 beats/minute, RR 14, and BP 128/78 mm Hg. Which one of the following is the best course of action?

A. Continue current therapy with close follow-up in 4 weeks.
B. Increase propranolol to 20 mg orally 3 times/day.
C. Add isosorbide dinitrate 10 mg orally 3 times/day.
D. Change propranolol to atenolol 25 mg orally once daily.

6. A new stool antigen test to detect *H. pylori* was tested in 1000 patients with suspected peptic ulcer disease, and 865 had a positive result. All patients also had undergone a concomitant endoscopy with biopsy and culture as the gold standard comparative test, and 900 had a positive result. Of these 900 patients with confirmed disease, only 850 also have a positive result with the new stool antigen test. Based on these results, what is the sensitivity and specificity of the new stool antigen test?

A. Sensitivity 82%, specificity 86%.
B. Sensitivity 85%, specificity 97%.
C. Sensitivity 94%, specificity 85%.
D. Sensitivity 96%, specificity 90%.

7. A 50-year-old Asian woman is seeking advice regarding a recent possible exposure to hepatitis A virus (HAV). She saw on the local news report that a chef at a local restaurant where she had eaten about 3 weeks ago had active HAV. Having heard that HAV could be transmitted through food, she would like to know what her options are. She has not previously received the HAV vaccine. Which one of the following is the best recommendation for this patient?

A. Initiate HAV vaccine.
B. Administer HAV immune globulin.
C. Continue to observe the patient for symptoms.
D. Initiate HAV vaccine and immune globulin.

8. A 47-year-old woman with a history of alcoholic cirrhosis (Child-Pugh class C) was admitted to the hospital with nausea, abdominal pain, and fever. Physical examination reveals a distended abdomen with shifting dullness, a positive fluid wave, and the presence of diffuse rebound tenderness. She also has 1+ lower-extremity edema. Current medications include furosemide 80 mg 2 times/day and spironolactone 200 mg once daily. A diagnostic paracentesis reveals turbid ascitic fluid, which was sent for culture. Laboratory analysis of the fluid revealed an albumin concentration of 0.9 g/dL and presence of 1000 white blood cell (count) (WBC)/mm^3 (45% polymorphonuclear neutrophils). Serum laboratory studies reveal a serum creatinine of 0.5 mg/dL, aspartate aminotransferase (AST) 60 IU/mL, alanine aminotransferase (ALT) 20 IU/mL, serum albumin 2.5 g/dL, and total bilirubin 3.2 mg/dL. Which one of the following is the best course of action?

A. Initiate intravenous albumin and await culture results.
B. Initiate intravenous vancomycin plus tobramycin.
C. Initiate intravenous cefotaxime plus albumin therapy.
D. Initiate oral trimethoprim-sulfamethoxazole double strength.

9. A 50-year-old, 80-kg man with a history of intravenous drug abuse and chronic hepatitis C (HCV) (genotype 2) was initiated on pegylated interferon (PEG-IFN) 180 mcg subcutaneously and ribavirin 400 mg orally 2 times/day 2 weeks ago. He returns to the clinic today with complaints of fatigue, scleral icterus, and pallor. There is no clinical evidence of bleeding. Laboratory values reveal the following: hematocrit 31% (baseline 39%), total bilirubin 3.2 mg/dL (indirect 2.7 mg/dL, direct 0.5 mg/dL), AST 150 IU/mL (baseline 300 IU/mL), ALT 180 IU/mL (baseline 400 IU/mL), serum creatinine 0.7 mg/dL, HCV RNA 1×10^6 IU/mL (baseline 2.3×10^6 copies/mL), WBC 7800/mm^3, and platelet count 160,000/mm^3. Which one of the following is most likely the cause of this patient's current symptoms?

A. Worsening of his liver disease secondary to inadequate treatment.
B. An adverse effect secondary to treatment with PEG-IFN.

C. Systemic manifestations of chronic HCV disease.
D. An adverse effect secondary to treatment with ribavirin.

10. A 35-year-old man with a history of Crohn's disease is in the clinic today with a chief complaint of mucopurulent drainage from an erythematous region on his abdomen. Examination reveals a moderate-size enterocutaneous fistula in the left upper abdominal area. He takes mesalamine (Pentasa) 250 mg 4 capsules 3 times/day and azathioprine 150 mg/day. His physician wishes to prescribe infliximab. Which one of the following recommendations is best when initiating infliximab therapy?

A. Rule out tuberculosis by purified protein derivative or QuantiFERON-TB test.
B. Administer a test dose before the initial infusion.
C. Admit to the hospital for administration of all doses.
D. Obtain an echocardiogram to assess cardiac function.

I. GASTROESOPHAGEAL REFLUX DISEASE

A. Definition
 1. "A condition which develops when reflux of stomach contents causes troublesome symptoms and/or complications." This newer definition is based on the Montreal classification (Am J Gastroenterol 2006;101:1900–20) and is used as the basis for the recent American Gastroenterological Association (AGA) guidelines (Gastroenterology 2008;135:1383–91).
    a. Strength of guideline evidence is rated grade A, B, C, D, or insufficient, and quality is rated good, fair, or poor.
    b. Nonerosive reflux disease is not included as a classification in these new guidelines.
 2. Definition subdivides gastroesophageal reflex disease (GERD) into the following categories:
    a. Esophageal syndromes
       i. Symptomatic syndromes
          (A) Typical reflux syndrome
          (B) Reflux chest pain syndrome (presents similarly to cardiac chest pain)
       ii. Syndromes with esophageal injury
          (A) Reflux esophagitis
          (B) Reflux stricture
          (C) Barrett's esophagus
          (D) Adenocarcinoma
    b. Extraesophageal syndromes
       i. Established association
          (A) Reflux cough
          (B) Reflux laryngitis
          (C) Reflux asthma
          (D) Reflux dental erosions
       ii. Proposed association
          (A) Sinusitis
          (B) Pulmonary fibrosis
          (C) Pharyngitis
          (D) Recurrent otitis media
 3. Symptoms
    a. Patients ultimately decide how troublesome symptoms are based on interference with normal daily activities or well-being.
    b. Typical symptoms: Heartburn (pyrosis), regurgitation, acidic taste in the mouth
    c. Extraesophageal symptoms (formerly referred to as atypical): Chronic cough, asthma-like symptoms, recurrent sore throat, laryngitis/hoarseness, dental enamel loss, and noncardiac chest pain; sinusitis/pneumonia/bronchitis/otitis media are less common atypical symptoms.
    d. Alarm symptoms: Dysphagia (*troublesome dysphagia* is the preferred term in the new guidelines), odynophagia, bleeding, weight loss, choking, chest pain, and epigastric mass. These symptoms warrant immediate referral for more invasive testing.
    e. Aggravating factors: Recumbency (gravity), increased intra-abdominal pressure, reduced gastric motility, decreased lower esophageal sphincter (LES) tone, and direct mucosal irritation
    f. Long-term complications: Esophageal erosion, strictures/obstruction, Barrett's esophagus;, and reduction in patient's quality of life (Aliment Pharmacol Ther 2003;18:767–76)

B. Diagnosis
   1. Symptoms
      a. Patient description of classic GERD symptoms, such as pyrosis, is often enough to consider it an initial diagnosis; invasive testing is therefore not indicated in uncomplicated cases.
      b. The AGA guidelines state that it is reasonable to assume a diagnosis of GERD in patients who respond to initial acid-suppressive therapy, particularly proton pump inhibitors (PPIs).
      c. Symptoms do not predict the degree of esophagitis or complications secondary to GERD, if present.
      d. Patients presenting with extraesophageal symptoms should be reviewed on a case-by-case basis to consider the need for referral or alternative/invasive testing.
      e. Cardiac etiologies (ischemic) should be considered and explored before arriving at a diagnosis of reflux chest pain syndrome.
   2. Endoscopy (See recent guidelines on endoscopy in GERD. Gastroenterology 2006;131:1315–36.)
      a. Considered the technique of choice to identify Barrett esophagus (with biopsy) or complications of GERD; findings of typical symptoms in association with endoscopic mucosal changes are about 97% specific for the diagnosis of GERD; however, most patients with typical/atypical symptoms will have normal-appearing esophageal mucosa on endoscopy. Biopsies should be performed in areas of suspected metaplasia, dysplasia, or malignancy.
      b. Used in patients older than 45 years, those presenting with alarm symptoms (particularly troublesome dysphagia), and those refractory to initial treatment, as well as a preoperative assessment or possibly when extraesophageal symptoms are present (Grade B)
      c. Routine endoscopy to assess disease progression is not recommended (Grade D).
      d. Routine screening for Barrett esophagus in patients 50 years or older with more than 5–10 years of heartburn is not recommended (Evidence Grade: Insufficient).
   3. Manometry
      a. Used to evaluate peristaltic function of the esophagus in patients with normal endoscopic findings
      b. Should be used before pH testing to rule out esophageal motility disorders and to help localize the LES for subsequent pH testing (Grade B)
   4. pH testing (See recent review in Aliment Pharmacol Ther 2005;22(Suppl 3):2–9.)
      a. The main outcome measure of esophageal pH monitoring is the percentage of time the pH value is less than 4 in a 24-hour period.
      b. Ambulatory pH testing is useful in the following clinical situations:
         i. Patients with no mucosal changes on endoscopy and normal manometry who have continued symptoms (both typical and atypical) (Grade B)
         ii. Patients who are refractory to therapeutic doses of appropriate pharmacologic agents
         iii. Monitoring of reflux control in patients with continued symptoms on drug therapy
      c. Sensitivity/specificity of 96% reported
      d. The PPIs should be withheld for 7 days before pH testing, if possible, for most accurate results.

5. Role of *H. pylori* testing and eradication is controversial in patients presenting with GERD symptoms; should be assessed based on patient presentation and risk factors for gastric cancer. A 4-week trial of a twice-daily PPI can be considered for patients suspected of having reflux chest pain syndrome before manometry or pH testing (Grade A). Reported sensitivity and specificity of a short course of PPIs are 80% and 74% for diagnosing reflux chest pain syndrome.

C. Treatment Strategies for GERD
   1. Nonpharmacologic interventions/lifestyle modifications are unlikely to control symptoms in most patients. The AGA guidelines cite insufficient evidence to advocate lifestyle modifications for all patients, but rather, they advocate use in targeted populations. Thus, the following lifestyle modifications should be implemented only for the patient populations specified.
      a. Dietary modifications in patients whose *symptoms are associated with certain foods or drinks*
         i. Avoid aggravating foods/beverages; some may reduce LES pressure (alcohol, caffeine, chocolate, citrus juices, garlic, onions, peppermint/spearmint) or cause direct irritation (spicy foods, tomato juice, coffee).
         ii. Reduce fat intake (high-fat meals slow gastric emptying) and portion size.
         iii. Avoid eating 2–3 hours before bedtime.
         iv. Remain upright after meals.
      b. Weight loss *for overweight or obese patients* (Grade B)
      c. Reduce/discontinue nicotine use *in patients who use tobacco products* (affects LES).
      d. Elevate the head of the bed (6–8 in.) *if reflux is associated with recumbency* (Grade B).
      e. Avoid tight-fitting clothing (decreases intra-abdominal pressure).
      f. *Avoid medications that may reduce LES pressure*, delay gastric emptying, or cause direct irritation: α-Adrenergic antagonists, anticholinergics, benzodiazepines, calcium channel blockers, estrogen, nitrates, opiates, tricyclic antidepressants, theophylline, NSAIDs, and aspirin.
   2. Pharmacologic therapies
      a. Initial treatment will depend on severity, frequency, and duration of symptoms.
         i. "Step-down" treatment: Starting with maximal therapy, such as therapeutic doses of PPIs, is always appropriate as a first-line strategy in patients with documented esophageal erosion.
         Advantages: Rapid symptom relief, avoidance of over-investigation
         Disadvantages: Potential overtreatment, higher drug cost, increase potential of adverse effects
         ii. "Step-up" treatment: Starting with lower-dose OTC products
            Advantages: Avoids overtreatment, lower initial drug cost
            Disadvantages: Potential undertreatment (partial symptom relief), may take longer for symptom control, may lead to over-investigation
      b. American Gastroenterological Association guideline recommendations (Gastroenterology 2008;135:1383–91)
         i. Empiric drug therapy is appropriate for patients with uncomplicated heartburn.
         ii. Use of antisecretory drugs for patients with esophageal GERD symptoms, with or without esophagitis, is strongly recommended (Grade A).

iii. Proton pump inhibitors are more effective than histamine$_2$-receptor antagonists (H$_2$RAs), which are, in turn, better than placebo for patients with esophageal GERD symptoms.
iv. All PPIs are similar in efficacy when used for patients with esophageal GERD symptoms. Selection of drugs is based on adverse effects, onset of action, and prescription plan coverage. For instance, changing to an alternative PPI or lowering the dose if a patient experiences adverse effects is a reasonable approach.
v. Data are weak to support using PPIs or H$_2$RAs above standard doses. However, twice-daily dosing of PPIs is appropriate in patients who continue to have symptoms on once-daily PPI therapy (Grade B).
vi. Rapid-acting drugs should be used for patients who wish to take the drug in response to symptoms. Antacids are the fastest-acting agents available and may be combined with both PPIs and H$_2$RAs. Proton pump inhibitors and H$_2$RAs are more effective for preventing heartburn.
vii. Maintenance therapy is appropriate for patients with esophagitis in whom PPIs have been effective (Grade A). Titration to the lowest effective dose is recommended. Most patients with nonerosive disease will continue on maintenance therapy if they initially respond, but it may not be possible to titrate them down to on-demand therapy. On-demand therapy is not appropriate for patients with erosive esophagitis.
viii. Dosing PPIs less than once daily as maintenance therapy is ineffective for patients who initially had erosive esophagitis (Grade D).
ix. No evidence of improved efficacy by adding a bedtime dose of H$_2$RA to twice-daily PPI therapy (Evidence Grade: Insufficient)
x. Data are weak to support use of PPIs in patients with extraesophageal symptoms.
c. American Gastroenterological Association guideline recommendations for the management of extraesophageal symptoms
i. The presence of extraesophageal GERD syndromes in the absence of esophageal GERD syndromes is rare. Chronic cough, laryngitis, and asthma all have definite associations with GERD.
ii. Evidence is fair (Grade B) for use of once- or twice-daily PPI therapy for patients with an extraesophageal syndrome and a *concomitant* esophageal GERD syndrome (Grade B). A 2-month trial of twice-daily PPI therapy would be an appropriate therapy for these patients.
iii. Evidence is Grade D for the use of once- or twice-daily PPI therapy in patients with an extraesophageal syndrome *in the absence of* an esophageal GERD syndrome (Grade D).
iv. Evidence is insufficient to recommend once- or twice-daily PPI therapy for patients with suspected reflux cough syndrome.
d. Pharmacologic agents
i. Antacids
(A) Calcium-, aluminum-, and magnesium-based products are available OTC in a wide variety of formulations (capsules, tablets, chewable tablets, and suspensions).
(B) Neutralize acid and raise intragastric pH results in decreased activation of pepsinogen and increased LES pressure; rapid onset of action, but short duration, necessitating frequent dosing

(C) Some products (Gaviscon) contain the anti-refluxant alginic acid, which forms a viscous layer on top of gastric contents to act as a barrier to reflux (variable added efficacy).
(D) Used as first-line therapy for intermittent (less than 2 times/week) symptoms or as breakthrough therapy for those on PPI/H$_2$RA therapy; not appropriate for healing established esophageal erosions
(E) Adverse reactions: Constipation (aluminum), diarrhea (magnesium), accumulation of aluminum/magnesium in renal disease with repeated dosing
(F) Drug interactions: Chelation (fluoroquinolones, tetracyclines), reduced absorption because of increases in pH (ketoconazole, itraconazole, iron, atazanavir, delavirdine, indinavir, nelfinavir) or increases in absorption leading to potential toxicity (raltegravir, saquinavir)

ii. Histamine$_2$-receptor antagonists
(A) Reversibly inhibit histamine$_2$-receptors on the parietal cell
(B) All agents available as prescription and OTC products; a variety of formulations available; generics exist for all prescription products

Table 1.

Agent	Oral OTC Formulations	Oral Prescription Formulations
Ranitidine (Zantac)	75-mg tablet 150-mg tablet	150-mg tablets/EFFERdose tablets/granules 300-mg tablet 15 mg/mL of syrup
Cimetidine (Tagamet)	200-mg tablet	300-, 400-, 800-mg tablets 300 mg/5 mL solution
Nizatidine (Axid)	75-mg tablet	150-mg/300-mg capsules 15 mg/mL solution
Famotidine (Pepcid)	10-mg tablets, gelatin capsules, chewable tablets 20-mg tablets	20-mg/40-mg tablets 20-mg/40-mg rapidly disintegrating tablet 40 mg/5 mL suspension
Pepcid Complete	10 mg + 800 mg of calcium carbonate + 165 mg of magnesium hydroxide chewable tablets	

OTC = over the counter.

(C) Over-the-counter H$_2$RA products may be used for on-demand therapy for intermittent mild-moderate GERD symptoms; preventive dosing before meals or exercise is also possible for all agents. Higher prescription doses are often required for more severe symptoms or for maintenance dosing. Prolonged use may result in the development of tolerance and reduced efficacy (tachyphylaxis).
(D) Therapy with H$_2$RAs is less efficacious than therapy with PPIs in healing erosive esophagitis.
(E) Adverse effects: Most are well tolerated. Central nervous system (CNS) effects, such as headache, dizziness, fatigue, somnolence, and confusion, are the most common. Elderly patients and those with reduced renal function are more at risk. Prolonged cimetidine use is associated with rare development of gynecomastia.

(F) Drug interactions: May affect absorption of drugs dependent on lower gastric pH, such as ketoconazole, itraconazole, iron, atazanavir, delavirdine, indinavir, and nelfinavir, or increases in absorption leading to potential toxicity (raltegravir, saquinavir). Cimetidine also inhibits cytochrome P450 (CYP) enzymes 1A2, 2C9, 2D6, and 3A4. Warfarin, theophylline, and other agents metabolized by these enzymes may be affected. Cimetidine may also compete with medications and creatinine for tubular secretion in the kidney.

iii. Proton pump inhibitors

(A) Irreversibly inhibit the final step in gastric acid secretion; greater degree of acid suppression achieved and typically longer duration of action than H_2RAs

(B) Most effective agents for short- and long-term management of GERD, as well as for management of erosive disease (Aliment Pharmacol Ther 2003:18:559–68)

(C) Most costly agents: Omeprazole and lansoprazole now available as a generic prescription-strength product and OTC. The OTC products are considered safe and effective for intermittent short-term (2 weeks) use in patients with typical heartburn symptoms. Long-term use of OTC products should be discussed with prescriber to prevent loss of follow-up or to assess for potential undertreatment (Digestion 2009;80:226–34). Pantoprazole, lansoprazole, and esomeprazole are available in intravenous formulations.

(D) Most effective when taken orally before meals; for divided dosing, give evening dose before evening meal instead of at bedtime

Table 2.

Product	Dosage Forms
Esomeprazole (Nexium)	Delayed-release capsule (20 mg/40 mg) IV solution (20- and 40-mg vials) Delayed-release oral suspension (10-, 20-, 40-mg packets)
Omeprazole (Prilosec) Prilosec OTC Zegerid Zegerid OTC	Delayed-release capsule (10 mg/20 mg/40 mg) Delayed-release 20-mg tablet (magnesium salt) Immediate-release powder for oral suspension (20- and 40-mg packets); sodium bicarbonate buffer = 460 mg of Na^+/dose (two 20-mg packets are not equivalent to one 40-mg packet) Zegerid OTC 20 mg immediate-release capsules with sodium bicarbonate (1100 mg/capsule)
Lansoprazole (Prevacid) Lansoprazole (Prevacid 24HR)	Prevacid 24HR 15-mg delayed-release capsule Delayed-release capsule (15 mg/30 mg) Delayed-release oral suspension (15 mg/30 mg) Delayed-release orally disintegrating tablet (15 mg/30 mg) IV solution (30 mg/vial)
Rabeprazole (AcipHex)	Delayed-release enteric-coated tablet (20 mg/40 mg)
Pantoprazole (Protonix)	Delayed-release tablet (20 mg/40 mg) IV solution (40 mg/vial)
Dexlansoprazole (Kapidex)	Delayed-release capsule (30 mg/60 mg)

IV = intravenous; Na = sodium; OTC = over the counter.

(E) Alternative administration

Table 3.

Product	Alternative Administration Technique
Omeprazole (Prilosec) Esomeprazole (Nexium) Zegerid	• Open capsules; mix with applesauce/juice • Simplified omeprazole suspension; contents dissolved in bicarbonate (NG/OG) • Open esomeprazole capsules and mix with 60 mL of water by NG tube or dissolve oral suspension in 15 mL of water and administer by NG tube; IV bolus or continuous infusion • Zegerid mix packet with 20 mL of water in syringe (NG)
Lansoprazole (Prevacid)	• Open capsules; mix with applesauce, ENSURE, cottage cheese, pudding, yogurt, or strained pears or 60 mL of tomato/orange/apple juice • Open capsules + 40 mL of apple juice (NG/OG) • Simplified lansoprazole suspension; contents dissolved in bicarbonate (NG/OG) • DO NOT use oral suspension for NG/OG; mix packet with 30 mL of water and swallow • Orally disintegrating tablet by oral syringe: use 4 mL for 15 mg or 10 mL for 30 mg • Orally disintegrating tablet by NG tube (> 8 French): same preparation as for oral syringe • IV (bolus or continuous infusion)
Rabeprazole (AcipHex)	• DO NOT CRUSH
Pantoprazole (Protonix)	• DO NOT CRUSH • IV (bolus or continuous infusion) • Pantoprazole suspension (bicarbonate) (Am J Health Syst Pharm 2003;60:1324–9)
Dexlansoprazole (Kapidex)	• Open capsules and sprinkle on applesauce

IV = intravenous; NG = nasogastric; OG = orogastric.

(F) Adverse reactions: Overall, well tolerated; possible adverse effects include headache, dizziness, nausea, diarrhea, and constipation. Long-term use is not associated with significant increases in endocrine neoplasia or symptomatic vitamin B_{12} deficiency.
- ✓ A cohort study of 364,683 users of both PPIs and H_2RAs found an elevated risk of community-acquired pneumonia with these agents. The adjusted relative risk of pneumonia was 1.89 (95% confidence interval [CI], 1.36–2.62) with PPI use and 1.63 (95% CI, 1.07–2.48) for H_2RA use. Patients at risk of community-acquired pneumonia include the immunocompromised, the elderly, children, and those with asthma or chronic obstructive pulmonary disease. Acid suppression should be used for these patients only if necessary and only at the lowest possible dose (JAMA 2004;292:1955–60).
- ✓ A recent large prospective cohort study of hospitalized patients revealed an increased risk of hospital-acquired pneumonia in nonventilated patients who were prescribed PPIs (OR = 1.3; 95% CI, 1.1–1.4) (JAMA 2009;301:2120–8).

- ✓ Another recent study revealed a higher incidence of hip fracture in patients receiving higher doses of PPIs for longer durations (OR = 1.44; 95% CI, 1.3–1.59) (JAMA 2006;296:2947–53). This may be attributable to reductions in the absorption of calcium in patients receiving potent acid suppression or, possibly, interference with osteoclast function.
  - ➢ The 2008 AGA guidelines cite insufficient evidence to recommend bone density screening or calcium supplementation because of PPI use. Screening for osteoporosis in populations at risk, such as the elderly, is recommended regardless of PPI use.
- ✓ Other studies have revealed an association of overgrowth of *Clostridium difficile* in patients receiving PPIs, particularly in the hospital setting. Odds ratios (ORs) were reported as 2.1 (95% CI, 1.33–2.25) (J Hosp Infect 2003;54:243–5, CMAJ 2004;171:33–8).
- (G) Drug interactions: Drugs with pH-dependent absorption (ketoconazole, itraconazole, protease inhibitors, etc.); omeprazole inhibits the metabolism of diazepam through CYP2C19. Recent data suggest reduced effectiveness of clopidogrel through CYP2C19-mediated inhibition of conversion to active metabolite by omeprazole and esomeprazole. Recommendations are to avoid omeprazole, esomeprazole, and cimetidine (CYP effects, also) in patients receiving clopidogrel. See U.S. Food and Drug Administration (FDA) letter at *www.fda.gov/Safety/MedWatch/SafetyInformation/SafetyAlertsforHumanMedicalProducts/ucm190848.htm*.

iv. Promotility agents
   (A) Guidelines recommend against the use of metoclopramide as adjunctive therapy or monotherapy in patients with both esophageal and extraesophageal symptoms because the risk of adverse effects (EPS [extrapyramidal side effects] or tardive dyskinesia) outweighs the benefit (Grade D).
   (B) Work though cholinergic mechanisms to facilitate increased gastric emptying.
   (C) Metoclopramide: Dopamine antagonist; needs to be dosed several times a day; associated with many adverse effects such dizziness, fatigue, somnolence, drowsiness, extrapyramidal symptoms, and hyperprolactinemia. New 5- and 10-mg orally disintegrating tablet formulation (metoclopramide [Metozolv ODT]) is now available. Indications for GERD and diabetic gastroparesis.
   (D) Bethanechol: Cholinergic agonist; poorly tolerated because of adverse effects such as diarrhea, blurred vision, and abdominal cramping; may also increase gastric acid production
   (E) Cisapride: Available only on a restricted basis for patients whose other therapies have failed; cisapride was withdrawn from the market initially because of cardiac arrhythmia (torsades de pointes) when used in combination with drugs inhibiting CYP3A4

v. Surgical therapy
   (A) Proton pump inhibitor therapy should be tried before surgical intervention because of better safety (Grade A).
   (B) Antireflux surgery such as fundoplication remains a viable option for maintenance therapy of GERD; typically used in patients unresponsive to or intolerant of medical therapy (Grade A)

(C) A study showed increases in cardiovascular (CV) mortality in a veteran population treated with antireflux surgery versus medical therapy as a long-term treatment option (JAMA 2001;285:2331–8). However, although patients had fewer GERD symptoms after surgery, most were not able to discontinue medical therapy completely.

(D) Antireflux surgery can be considered for patients with extraesophageal GERD syndromes if symptoms persist despite PPI therapy (Grade C).

(E) Antireflux surgery is not recommended for patients who are well controlled on medical therapy or for prevention of Barrett's esophagus (Grade D).

Patient Case

1. A 75-year-old man with a 3-year history of severe GERD symptoms and Parkinson's disease has been taking lansoprazole 30 mg 2 times/day for 5 months. He has initiated proper nonpharmacologic measures, including elevating the head of his bed, reducing fat intake and portion size, avoiding tight-fitting clothes, and losing weight. Because he continues to have daily heartburn symptoms, he is referred for endoscopy, which reveals normal-appearing mucosa and no structural abnormalities. Which one of the following is the best course of action for this patient?
   A. Add metoclopramide 10 mg 4 times/day and reassess in 3 months.
   B. Educate about the proper use of lansoprazole and refer for manometry.
   C. Add metoclopramide 10 mg 4 times/day and refer for surgical intervention.
   D. Add famotidine 20 mg/day at bedtime and reassess in 4 months.

II. PEPTIC ULCER DISEASE

A. Classification of Peptic Ulcer Disease
   1. Duodenal ulcer
      a. Common causes: *H. pylori* infection (95%), NSAIDs, low-dose aspirin
      b. Uncommon causes: Zollinger-Ellison syndrome, hypercalcemia, granulomatous diseases, neoplasia, infections (cytomegalovirus, herpes simplex, tuberculosis), ectopic pancreatic tissue
      c. Clinical signs/symptoms: Epigastric pain, possibly worse at night; often, pain occurs 1–3 hours after a meal and may be relieved by eating. Pain may also be episodic. Associated symptoms may include heartburn, belching, a bloated feeling, nausea, and anorexia.
   2. Gastric ulcer:
      a. Common causes: NSAIDs, *H. pylori* infection
      b. Uncommon causes: Crohn's disease, infections (cytomegalovirus, herpes simplex)
      c. Clinical signs/symptoms: Epigastric pain, which is often made worse by eating; associated symptoms may include heartburn, belching, a bloated feeling, nausea, and anorexia

3. Patients at risk of NSAID-Induced GI toxicity (Am J Gastroenterol 2009;104:728–38)

Table 4.

Category	Risk Factors
High risk	1. History of complicated ulcer 2. Several (> 2) risk factors 3. Concomitant use of corticosteroids, anticoagulants, or antiplatelet drugs
Moderate risk (1 or 2 risk factors)	1. Age > 65 years 2. High-dose NSAID therapy 3. History of uncomplicated ulcer 4. Concurrent use of aspirin (including low dose), corticosteroids, or anticoagulants
Low risk	No risk factors

GI = gastrointestinal; NSAID = nonsteroidal anti-inflammatory drug.

    a. Some NSAIDs such as ibuprofen, diclofenac, and nabumetone are intrinsically less toxic to the GI tract than naproxen, which is considered moderate risk. Other agents, such as piroxicam or ketorolac, are considered high-risk drugs.
    b. Duration of NSAID use (higher risk in first 3 months). Presence of chronic debilitating disorders such rheumatoid arthritis or CV disease may also contribute to the increased GI toxicity of NSAIDs, but these are not generally considered independent risk factors.
    c. *H. pylori* infection is thought to confer additive risk of GI toxicity in NSAID users.
4. Diagnosis
    a. Symptom presentation
    b. Testing for *H. pylori* infection: Practitioners must be willing to treat if testing is positive because *H. pylori* is a known carcinogen.
        i. Testing is indicated for patients with active ulcer disease, history of peptic ulcer disease, or gastric mucosa-associated lymphoid tissue lymphoma.
        ii. The test-and-treat strategy for identifying *H. pylori*–positive patients is also acceptable for patients with uninvestigated dyspepsia who have no alarm symptoms and are younger than 55 years (Am J Gastroenterol 2007;102:1808–25).
    c. Diagnostic tests for *H. pylori* infection (Aliment Pharmacol Ther 2003;16(Suppl 1):16–23)
        i. Invasive (endoscopic)
            (A) Histology: 90%–95% sensitive, 98%–99% specific, subject to sampling error
            (B) Rapid urease tests (CLOtest, Hpfast, and PyloriTek): Detect the presence of ammonia (NH_3) on a sample generated by *H. pylori* urease activity; 80%–95% sensitive, 95%–100% specific. False negatives may result from a partially treated infection, GI bleeding, achlorhydria, or use of PPIs, H_2RAs, or bismuth. Patients should discontinue antisecretory agents for at least 1 week before test is performed.
            (C) Culture: Costly, time-consuming, and technically difficult, although 100% specific
        ii. Noninvasive
            (A) Serologic tests (QuickVue *H. pylori* gII, FlexSure HP): Detect immunoglobulin G to *H. pylori* in the serum by ELISA (enzyme-linked immunosorbent assay); 85% sensitive, 79% specific. Cannot distinguish between active infection and

past exposure. Because antibodies persist for long periods after eradication, cannot use to test for eradication after treatment. Newly available tests will detect the presence of *cagA* or *vacA* antibodies.

(B) Urea breath test (BreathTek UBT, PYtest): Detects the exhalation of radioactive CO_2 after the ingestion of ^{13}C- or ^{14}C-radiolabeled urea. *H. pylori* hydrolysis of the radiolabeled urea results in CO_2 production; 97% sensitive, 95% specific. Used to make a diagnosis and to test for eradication. Recent use of antibiotics or PPIs may result in false negatives in up to 40% of patients. Patients should discontinue antisecretory agents or antibiotics at least 2 weeks before or 4 weeks after treatment before test is performed.

(C) Stool antigen tests (Premier Platinum HpSA, ImmunoCard STAT! HpSA): Polyclonal or monoclonal antibody tests that detect the presence of *H. pylori* in the stool; 88%–92% sensitive, 87% specific. Can be used to make a diagnosis and to confirm eradication. Recent use of bismuth, antibiotics, or PPIs may also result in false negatives. Patients should discontinue antisecretory agents or antibiotics at least 2 weeks before or 4 weeks after treatment before the test is performed.

5. Treatment of *H. pylori*–associated ulcers (Am J Gastroenterol 2007;102:1808–25)
   a. General recommendations, based on the American College of Gastroenterology (ACG) guidelines, are to include an antisecretory agent (preferably a PPI) plus at least two antibiotics (clarithromycin and amoxicillin or metronidazole) in the eradication regimen. *H. pylori* eradication has been shown to have a relative risk reduction of 54% for duodenal ulcer recurrence and a 38% relative risk reduction for gastric ulcer recurrence (Cochrane Database Syst Rev 2006;(2):CD003840. DOI: 10.1002/14651858.CD003840.pub4).
   b. Therapy duration is 7–14 days depending on the regimen chosen. The ACG states that 14 days is preferred. Most regimens last 10 days.
   c. Follow-up testing for eradication should be performed in patients with a history of ulcer complication, gastric mucosa-associated lymphoid tissue lymphoma, early gastric cancer, or recurrence of symptoms.
   d. Urea breath tests or stool antigen tests are preferred for confirming eradication (should wait at least 4 weeks after treatment for both).
   e. Quadruple-based therapy with bismuth subsalicylate, metronidazole, tetracycline, and PPI can be used for 14 days as initial therapy if triple-based therapy fails or if the patient has an intolerance or allergy to components of the triple-drug therapy. Use of Pylera, a quadruple-based therapy formulated with tetracycline, bismuth, and metronidazole in 1 capsule, received FDA label approval in 2007. This product contains bismuth subcitrate salt rather than subsalicylate salt.
   f. Sequential therapy is a relatively new type of treatment in which a PPI and amoxicillin are given first for the first 5 days, followed by a PPI, clarithromycin, and tinidazole for an additional 5 days. This therapy requires further validation before widespread use will be accepted.
   g. A bismuth-based quadruple therapy for 14 days or a levofloxacin-based triple therapy for 10 days can be used in patients whose initial regimens as salvage therapy have failed.

Table 5. *H. pylori* Treatment Regimens[a,b]

Regimen	Duration (days)	Efficacy (%)[c]
Lansoprazole 30 mg BID + amoxicillin 1000 mg BID + clarithromycin 500 mg BID	10–14	81–86
Esomeprazole 40 mg once daily + amoxicillin 1000 mg BID + clarithromycin 500 mg BID	10–14	70–85
Omeprazole 20 mg BID + amoxicillin 1000 mg BID + clarithromycin 500 mg BID	10–14	70–85
Rabeprazole 20 mg PO BID + amoxicillin 1000 mg BID + clarithromycin 500 mg BID	7	70–85
Bismuth subsalicylate 525 mg QID + metronidazole 500 mg TID + tetracycline 500 mg QID + PPI BID	14	75–90
Bismuth subcitrate 420 mg + tetracycline 375 mg + metronidazole 375 mg[d] + PPI BID	10	85–92
PPI + amoxicillin 1 g BID for 5 days; then PPI, clarithromycin 500 mg BID + tinidazole 500 mg BID for 5 days	10 (5 each treatment)	> 90

[a]Pantoprazole does not have an FDA-approved indication for *H. pylori* eradication; however, 40 mg BID could be substituted in any of the 10- to 14-day regimens.
[b]Metronidazole 500 mg BID can be substituted for amoxicillin or clarithromycin in patients with penicillin or macrolide allergy for the triple-drug regimens. Treat for 14 days in this situation.
[c]Rates based on intention to treat.
[d]Triple-capsule formulation.
BID = 2 times/day; FDA = U.S. Food and Drug Administration; PO = orally; PPI = proton pump inhibitor; QID = 4 times/day; TID = 3 times/day.

    6. Primary prevention of NSAID-induced ulcers (ACG guidelines. Am J Gastroenterol 2009;104:728–38)
        a. Implement risk factor modification.
        b. Test and treat for *H. pylori* if patient is beginning long-term NSAID therapy.
        c. Determine level of GI-related risk (low, medium, high) using table in section IIA3.
        d. Based on association of increased risk of CV events with NSAID use, patient's CV risk should be determined as well.
            i. The ACG guidelines define *high CV risk as patients who require low-dose aspirin for prevention of cardiac events.* Naproxen is the one NSAID that does not appear to increase risk of CV events; therefore, its use is preferred in patients with CV risk factors (Am J Gastroenterol 2009;104:728–38).

Table 6. Preventive Strategies Based on Risk of NSAID-Related GI Complications and CV Risk

If low CV risk and:
• Low GI risk[a] → NSAID (lowest dose of least ulcerogenic agent)
• Moderate GI risk[b] → NSAID + PPI or misoprostol
• High GI risk[c] → COX-2 inhibitor + PPI or misoprostol
If *high CV risk (requirement for low-dose aspirin)* and:
• Low GI risk[a] → Naproxen + PPI or misoprostol
• Moderate GI risk[b] → Naproxen + PPI or misoprostol
• High GI risk[c] → Avoid NSAIDs or COX-2 inhibitors

[a]No risk factors.
[b]1 or 2 risk factors present.
[c]Positive history of ulcer complication or several (more than 2) risk factors or use of steroids and anticoagulants.
COX-2 = cyclooxygenase-2; CV = cardiovascular; GI = gastrointestinal; NSAID = nonsteroidal anti-inflammatory drug; PPI = proton pump inhibitor.

e. Misoprostol (Cytotec) should be given at full doses (800 mcg/day in divided doses); however, this therapy is poorly tolerated because of excessive nausea, vomiting, diarrhea, and abdominal cramping.
f. Concomitant use of antiplatelet agents and NSAIDs: Recent guidelines from a consensus cardiology and GI group (ACCF/ACG/AHQ) (Circulation 2008;118:1894–909)
   i. Need for antiplatelet therapy should first be evaluated.
   ii. If antiplatelet therapy is deemed necessary, then assess for the presence of GI risk factors (see A3 above). These guidelines also cite dyspepsia or GERD symptoms as risk factors.
   iii. Test and treat for *H. pylori* in patients with a history of a nonbleeding ulcer and in those with a history of an ulcer-related complication. Eradicating *H. pylori* before beginning chronic antiplatelet therapy is optimal.
   iv. Proton pump inhibitors are the preferred gastroprotective agents for both the treatment and prevention of aspirin- and NSAID-associated GI injury.
   v. Gastroprotective therapy should be prescribed for patients with GI risk factors who require the use of any NSAID (including OTC and COX-2 inhibitors) in conjunction with cardiac-dose aspirin.
   vi. Gastroprotective therapy should be prescribed for patients with GI risk factors who require preventive doses of aspirin. Aspirin doses greater than 81 mg/day should not be used in patients with GI risk factors during the chronic phase of aspirin therapy.
   vii. Proton pump inhibitors should be prescribed for patients receiving concomitant aspirin and anticoagulant therapy (unfractionated heparin, low-molecular-weight heparin, and warfarin).
   viii. A target international normalized ratio (INR) of 2.0–2.5 should be used in patients for whom warfarin is added to concomitant aspirin and clopidogrel therapy. The combination of both aspirin and clopidogrel with warfarin should only be used when benefit outweighs risk.
   ix. Clopidogrel is not recommended as a substitute for patients with recurrent ulcer bleeding. Aspirin plus a PPI is superior to clopidogrel.
   x. The health care provider who decides to discontinue aspirin therapy in patients with acute bleeding episodes should weigh the risks of subsequent GI or cardiac events.
   xi. For patients receiving dual antiplatelet therapy (aspirin plus clopidogrel) who require elective endoscopy (particularly colonoscopy and polypectomy), consider deferring if patient is at high risk of cardiac events. Elective endoscopy should be deferred for 1 year after the placement of drug-eluting stents.
7. Treatment/secondary prevention of NSAID-induced ulcers (Am J Gastroenterol 1998;93:2037–46, Aliment Pharmacol Ther 2004;19:197–208)
   a. Risk factor modification
   b. Discontinue/lower dose of NSAID if possible.
      i. Ulcers will heal with appropriate treatment, but it may take longer with continued NSAID use.
   c. Test for *H. pylori* and treat if present.
   d. Drug therapy
      i. Proton pump inhibitors: Drugs of choice for healing and secondary prevention of NSAID-induced ulcers (N Engl J Med 1998;338:719–26, N Engl J Med 1998;338:727–34)

ii. Misoprostol: Appears to be as effective as PPIs for healing/secondary prevention (N Engl J Med 1998;338:727–34); however, it necessitates several doses per day and is poorly tolerated because of the high incidence of diarrhea and abdominal pain
iii. Cyclooxygenase inhibitors: Celecoxib was recently shown to have rates of ulcer recurrence and bleeding comparable with a diclofenac plus omeprazole combination; use of celecoxib may be limited by its recent association with CV effects (N Engl J Med 2002;347:2104–11). Use is uncertain in combination with low-dose aspirin for secondary prevention of GI events.
iv. Combination of COX-2 inhibitor and PPI is not well studied but may be considered in high-risk patients such as the elderly, especially if they are receiving aspirin plus steroids or warfarin or have a history of a recent complicated GI event and require continued NSAID or aspirin use.
v. The H_2RAs: Inferior to misoprostol and PPIs in healing and preventing recurrence
vi. Clopidogrel is not recommended as a substitute in patients with recurrent ulcer bleeding. Aspirin plus a PPI is superior to clopidogrel (Circulation 2008;118:1894–909).

e. Cardiovascular safety of COX-2 inhibitors and NSAIDs
i. The main theory underlying the development of excess thrombotic events with COX-2 inhibitor use is that by reducing COX-2–mediated prostacyclin production, the prothrombic prostaglandin thromboxane A_2 continues to be produced by COX-1, leading to the development of a prothrombic state. The degree of development of these events does not appear to be equal across the class of COX-2 inhibitors.
ii. Data regarding the development of CV events with the chronic use of COX-2 inhibitors and nonselective NSAIDs led to the withdrawal of rofecoxib from the U.S. market in September 2004 and of valdecoxib in 2005.
iii. Guidelines for appropriate use and safety of NSAIDs, aspirin, and COX-2 inhibitors have been published by both the American Heart Association (Circulation 2007;115:1634–42) and a multidisciplinary clinical group (Clin Gastroenterol Hepatol 2006;4:1082–9).
iv. Rofecoxib 50 mg/day was first associated with a significant increase in myocardial infarction in the VIGOR trial compared with naproxen (0.4% vs. 0.1%; 95% CI, 0.1–0.6) (N Engl J Med 2000;343:1520–8). In the recent APPROVe trial, 25 mg/day used for preventing colonic polyps was associated with a 2-fold increase (relative risk = 1.92, 95% CI, 1.19–3.11) in stroke and myocardial infarction during an 18-month period. This study was the driving force behind the withdrawal of rofecoxib (N Engl J Med 2005;352:1092–102).
v. Celecoxib was not associated with increases in CV events until the APC trial for cancer prevention was halted in December 2004. Daily doses of 400 mg and 800 mg of celecoxib conferred a 2.5- and 3.4-fold higher risk of fatal and nonfatal myocardial infarction, which suggests a dose-related response for this toxicity (N Engl J Med 2005;352:1071–80).
vi. Valdecoxib has also been associated with the development of excess thrombotic events after use in patients undergoing coronary artery bypass surgery. This agent was voluntarily withdrawn from the market in 2005 (J Thorac Cardiovasc Surg 2003;125:1481–92).
vii. A stepped approach is recommended for patients with CV disease or risk factors for ischemic heart disease who require analgesic treatment of musculoskeletal symptoms based on recommendations from the American Heart Association (Circulation 2007;115:1634–42).

1. Consider using acetaminophen, aspirin, tramadol, or short-term narcotics first.
2. Nonacetylated salicylates can be considered next.
3. Non–COX-2-selective NSAIDS can be used next, followed by NSAIDs with some COX-2 activity. Use the lowest dose possible to control symptoms.
4. The COX-2 inhibitors should be reserved as last line. In patients at increased risk of thromboembolic events, coadministration with aspirin and a PPI may be considered.
5. Routinely monitor BP, renal function, and signs of edema or GI bleeding.

viii. Methods to reduce CV risk such as tobacco cessation, BP and lipid control, and glucose control are recommended for NSAID users but have not been proved to reduce NSAID-associated CV risk. In patients for whom the risk of GI bleeding outweighs CV risk, lower-risk NSAIDs such as ibuprofen, etodolac, diclofenac, or celecoxib should be used. In patients for whom CV risk outweighs the risk of GI bleeding, COX-2 inhibitors should be avoided. Limit the dose and therapy duration if possible (Clin Gastroenterol Hepatol 2006;4:1082–9).

ix. An FDA article also reviews the effects of ibuprofen on the attenuation of aspirin's antiplatelet effects (*www.fda.gov/cder/drug/infopage/ibuprofen/science_paper.htm*).

(A) The American Heart Association (Circulation 2007;115:1634–42) recommends that ibuprofen be taken at least 30 minutes after or 8 hours before the ingestion of immediate-release low-dose aspirin to prevent this interaction.

Gastrointestinal Disorders

Patient Cases

2. A 68-year-old woman referred to a gastroenterologist complains of intermittent upper abdominal pain with anemia and heme-positive stools. She has a history of type 2 diabetes mellitus with peripheral neuropathy and hypertension. She reports no known drug allergies and takes metformin 1000 mg 2 times/day, aspirin 325 mg/day, lisinopril 20 mg once daily, and gabapentin 1000 mg 3 times/day. In addition, she reports using OTC ketoprofen daily for the past 2 months secondary to uncontrolled pain. Her colonoscopy is negative, but her endoscopy reveals a 1-cm gastric ulcer with an intact clot. A rapid urease test (CLO) performed on the ulcer biopsy specimen is negative. Which one of the following treatments is best for this patient's ulcer?

   A. Ranitidine 150 mg 2 times/day for 4 weeks.
   B. Lansoprazole 30 mg 2 times/day plus amoxicillin 1000 mg 2 times/day plus clarithromycin 500 mg 2 times/day for 10 days.
   C. Lansoprazole 30 mg/day for 8 weeks.
   D. Misoprostol 200 mcg 4 times/day for 8 weeks.

3. A 42-year-old man is in the clinic with the chief complaint of sharp epigastric pain for the past 6 weeks. He states that the pain is often worse with eating and that it is present at least 5 days/week. He states that although he initially tried OTC antacids with some relief, the pain returns about 3 hours after each dose. He does not currently take any other medications. He reports an allergy to penicillin, which, he states, gives him a severe rash. His practitioner is concerned about a potential peptic ulcer and tests him for *H. pylori* using a urea breath test, the result of which is positive. Which one of the following treatments for *H. pylori* would be best?

   A. Amoxicillin 1 g 2 times/day plus clarithromycin 500 mg 2 times/day plus omeprazole 20 mg 2 times/day for 10 days.
   B. Cephalexin 1 g 2 times/day plus clarithromycin 500 mg 2 times/day plus omeprazole 20 mg 2 times/day for 10 days.
   C. Bismuth subsalicylate 525 mg 4 times/day plus tetracycline 500 mg 4 times/day plus metronidazole 500 mg 3 times/day plus omeprazole 20 mg 2 times/day for 14 days.
   D. Levofloxacin 500 mg once daily plus metronidazole 500 mg 2 times/day plus omeprazole 20 mg 2 times/day for 5 days.

III. UPPER GI BLEEDING

A. Background
   1. Prevalence: 170 cases/100,000 adults
      a. Associated annual costs are about $750 million.
      b. Mortality is 6%–10%.

B. Causes of Upper GI Bleeding
   1. Peptic ulcer disease (40%–70%)
      a. Nonsteroidal anti-inflammatory drugs and low-dose aspirin use
      b. *H. pylori*
   2. Esophagitis
   3. Erosive disease
   4. Esophageal varices
   5. Mallory-Weiss tear
   6. Neoplasm
   7. Stress ulcers (critically ill patients)

C. Clinical Symptoms and Presentation
1. Hematemesis or "coffee-ground" emesis
2. Hematochezia
3. Nausea, vomiting
4. Melena
5. Shock (tachycardia, clammy skin)
6. Hypotension
7. Associated organ dysfunction (renal/hepatic/cardiac/cerebral hypoperfusion)

Table 7. Clinical Predictors of Death Associated with Nonvariceal UGIB (Ann Intern Med 2003;139:843–57)

Advanced age (> 75 years highest risk)	Red blood on rectal examination
Shock/hypotension	Elevated serum urea
> 1 comorbid condition	Serum creatinine > 150 micromoles/L (1.7 mg/dL)
Continued bleeding/rebleeding	Elevated aminotransferases
Blood in gastric aspirate	Sepsis
Hematemesis	Onset of bleeding during hospitalization for other causes

UGIB = upper gastrointestinal bleeding.

D. Predictors of Persistent or Recurrent Upper GI Bleeding

Table 8.

Age > 65 years	Initial hemoglobin < 10 g/dL or hematocrit < 30%
Shock (systolic blood pressure < 100 mm Hg)	Coagulopathy
Comorbid illness	Endoscopic findings:
Erratic mental status	Active bleeding on endoscopy
Ongoing bleeding	Presence of high-risk stigmata
Red blood on rectal examination	Clot
Melena	Ulcer size ≥ 2 cm
Blood in gastric aspirate	Gastric or duodenal ulcer
Hematemesis	Location of ulcer on superior or posterior wall

GI = gastrointestinal.

E. Management of Nonvariceal Upper GI Bleeding
1. Volume resuscitation and hemodynamic stabilization
   a. Placement of one or two large-bore intravenous catheters
   b. Replacement with crystalloid such as 0.9% normal saline is preferred; colloids, such as blood, can be given after initial resuscitation to maintain a hemoglobin concentration of 8–10 g/dL
2. Risk stratification
   a. Clinical signs/symptoms
   b. Placement of nasogastric tube for aspiration
   c. Endoscopy (within 24 hours if possible)
   d. Assessment of comorbid illnesses (liver disease, coagulopathies, cardiac status)
3. Endoscopic therapy
   a. Endoscopic therapy associated with reductions in rebleeding, need for surgery, and mortality
   b. Observation of low-risk stigmata (clean-based ulcer or a nonprotuberant-pigmented dot in an ulcer bed) is not an indication for hemostatic therapy.

c. Clots visible in an ulcer bed should be irrigated with treatment of underlying lesions.
d. The presence of high-risk stigmata warrants immediate hemostatic therapy.
4. Endoscopic strategies
   a. The combination of injection and coaptive therapy is the most efficacious approach.
   b. The use of either technique plus pharmacotherapy is superior to monotherapy.
   c. Sclerotherapy: No single solution for injection is superior to another.
      i. Epinephrine with or without ethanolamine
      ii. Cyanoacrylate
      iii. Thrombin
      iv. Sodium tetradecyl sulfate
      v. Polidocanol
   d. Thermal coaptive therapy: No single method is superior to another.
      i. Heater probe thermocoagulation
      ii. Multipolar electrocoagulation
      iii. Laser coagulation (not often used because of cost)
      iv. Argon plasma coagulation
5. Pharmacotherapeutic management of nonvariceal upper GI bleeding (Ann Intern Med 2003;139:843–57)
   a. Treatment guidelines apply to NSAID-induced ulcers as well.
   b. Remove medications that are contributing to bleeding (NSAIDs, etc.).
   c. Proton pump inhibitor therapy
      i. Bolus 80 mg plus continuous infusion of 8 mg/hour for 72 hours after endoscopic therapy
      ii. Intravenous pantoprazole, lansoprazole, or esomeprazole can be used; most data are with intravenous omeprazole (used in Europe).
      iii. Associated with substantial decreases in rebleeding (and surgery in some cases) versus H_2RAs; no reductions in mortality observed
   d. Use of H_2RAs or somatostatin-octreotide is NOT recommended.
   e. High-dose PPI therapy can also be considered in patients awaiting endoscopy; route of administration is possibly intravenous for high-risk patients and oral for low-risk patients.
   f. Test for *H. pylori* and treat if results are positive.
   g. Assess the need for continued secondary prevention with PPI therapy.

Patient Case
4. A newly available NSAID was designed to reduce the incidence of adverse GI events compared with traditional NSAIDs. A large retrospective cohort study compares the incidence of ulceration and bleeding associated with the use of this new NSAID with that of ibuprofen and naproxen. The results indicate that the new agent is associated with no statistically or clinically significant reduction in ulceration or bleeding with chronic use compared with ibuprofen and naproxen. The investigators of the study argue that the lack of difference in safety is because the drug is being promoted as safer; therefore, most patients receiving it are at a much higher baseline risk of NSAID-induced ulceration and bleeding. If this phenomenon did indeed affect the study results, it would be consistent with which one of the following potential sources of bias?
   A. Recall bias.
   B. Misclassification bias.
   C. Interviewer bias.
   D. Channeling bias.

IV. INFLAMMATORY BOWEL DISEASE

A. Background
1. Inflammatory bowel disease includes both Ulcerative Colitis (UC) and Crohn's disease. In some instances, UC may not be distinguishable from Crohn's disease. This is referred to as indeterminate or intermediate colitis.
2. Pathophysiology: Continuing inflammation of the GI mucosa; exact cause is unknown, but it is thought that the inflammation is secondary to an antigen-driven response
3. Contributing factors
   a. Defects in the intestinal epithelial barrier and immune system
   b. Genetic: Definite genetic association; first-degree relatives of affected patients have a 4–20 times higher risk of developing inflammatory bowel disease
   c. Environmental
      i. NSAIDs: Worsen inflammatory bowel disease, most likely secondary to alteration of epithelial barrier
      ii. Smoking: Worsens Crohn's disease; however, is associated with improvement in UC symptoms
      iii. Luminal bacteria: Endogenous intestinal bacteria thought to be highly involved in stimulating the intestinal inflammatory response observed in inflammatory bowel disease
      iv. Dietary: Dietary antigens may also contribute to ongoing inflammation.
   d. Various proinflammatory cytokines, including interleukin-1, interleukin-6, and tumor necrosis factor, release and contribute to the ongoing inflammatory process.

B. Clinical Features
1. Presenting symptoms common to both diseases include fever, abdominal pain, diarrhea (may be bloody, watery, or mucopurulent), rectal bleeding, and weight loss. Symptoms may vary depending on disease location.

Table 9.

Clinical Findings	Ulcerative Colitis	Crohn's Disease
Bowel involvement	Confined to rectum and colon Terminal ileal involvement (backwash ileitis) occurs in a minority of patients	May be anywhere from mouth to anus (66% of cases located in ileum)
Perianal involvement	Unlikely	Yes
Depth of ulceration	Superficial	May extend to submucosa or deeper
Continuous inflammation	Very common	Rarely, a patchy, "cobblestone" appearance
Histology	Nontransmural, crypt abscesses	Transmural lesions Granulomas
Fistula/perforation/strictures	No	Yes
Development of toxic megacolon	Yes	No
Malabsorption or malnutrition	Rare	Yes, often vitamin deficiencies; possible growth retardation in children
Risk factor for colorectal cancer	Yes	Uncommon
Pseudopolyps	Common	Fairly uncommon

2. Systemic manifestations
   a. Both UC and Crohn's disease may present with concurrent systemic manifestations.
   b. Hepatobiliary: Primary sclerosing cholangitis, cholangiocarcinoma, hepatitis/cirrhosis, cholelithiasis, steatosis
   c. Rheumatologic arthritis, sacroiliitis, ankylosing spondylitis
   d. Dermatologic: Erythema nodosum, aphthous ulcers, pyoderma gangrenosum
   e. Ocular: Iritis/uveitis, episcleritis
3. Gauging clinical severity
   a. Ulcerative colitis (based on Truelove and Witts criteria)

Table 10.

Mild	Severe	Fulminant
➢ < 4 stools/day (±blood)	➢ > 6 stools/day with blood	➢ > 10 stools/day with continuous blood
➢ No fever, anemia, or tachycardia	➢ Temp > 99.5°F	➢ Temp > 99.5°F
➢ Normal ESR	➢ PR > 90	➢ PR > 90
	➢ ESR > 30	➢ ESR > 30
	➢ Hb < 75% of normal	➢ Transfusions required
	➢ Abdominal tenderness	➢ Abdominal pain
	➢ Bowel wall edema	➢ Dilated colon

ESR = erythrocyte sedimentation rate; Hb = hemoglobin; PR = pulse rate; Temp = temperature.

   b. Crohn's disease (recent guidelines: Am J Gastroenterol 2009;104:465–83)
   Mild-Moderate:
   • Tolerates oral administration; absence of fever, dehydration, and abdominal tenderness; less than 10% weight loss
   Moderate-Severe:
   • Failed treatment for mild-moderate
   • Above symptoms usually present; possibly anemia, nausea/vomiting, considerable weight loss
   Severe-Fulminant:
   • No response to outpatient steroids; high temperature/abdominal pain, persistent vomiting
   • Possible obstruction, abscess, cachexia, rebound tenderness
4. General management considerations
   a. Rule out possible infectious causes of bloody diarrhea in patients with acute symptoms.
   b. Most patients will receive colonoscopy to confirm diagnosis and extent of disease.
   c. Surgery is a viable option when complications (abscess, fistula, perforation) occur or when fulminant disease is unresponsive to medical treatment.
   d. Distribution and severity of disease will dictate the initial choice of therapeutic agents.
   e. Most patients will require maintenance therapy because of the high incidence of relapse after induction therapy; the relapse rate is 35%–80% at 2 years for Crohn's disease and 50%–70% at 1 year for UC (Am J Gastroenterol 2003;98(Suppl):S6–S17).

C. Medical Management of Inflammatory Bowel Disease
   a. Adjunctive therapies
      i. Use with caution in active disease because reduction in motility may precipitate toxic megacolon.

- b. Loperamide (Imodium)
    - i. May be useful for proctitis/diarrhea; 2 mg after each loose stool (16 mg/day maximum)
- c. Antispasmodics
    - i. Dicyclomine (Bentyl), 10–40 mg orally 4 times/day
    - ii. Propantheline (Pro-Banthine), 7.5–15 mg orally 3 times/day
    - iii. Hyoscyamine (Levsin), 0.125–0.25 mg orally/slow release every 4 hours as needed
- d. Cholestyramine (Questran)
    - i. Possibly for bile salt–induced diarrhea after ileal resection

D. Medications Used to Treat Inflammatory Bowel Disease
   - a. Treatment is selected on the basis of disease location and severity.
   - b. Aminosalicylates
     - i. Used for both induction and maintenance of remission
     - ii. Sulfasalazine: Prototype agent (Azulfidine, Azulfidine-EN)
       - (A) The drug is cleaved by colonic bacteria to the active portion (5-aminosalicylate) and the inactive carrier molecule sulfapyridine.
       - (B) Efficacy is best in colonic disease owing to colonic activation of drug. Toxicity may be dose related as well as related to the sulfapyridine portion.
       - (C) Dose-related adverse effects: GI disturbance, headache, arthralgia, folate malabsorption
       - (D) Idiosyncratic adverse effects: Rash, fever, pneumonitis, hepatotoxicity, bone marrow suppression, hemolytic anemia, pancreatitis, decreased sperm production in men
       - (E) Avoid in patients with a sulfa allergy.
       - (F) Doses are 4–6 g/day for induction and 2–4 g/day for maintenance; available as immediate-release and enteric-coated products. Doses should be titrated beginning at 500–1000 mg once or twice daily to avoid adverse effects.
     - iii. 5-Aminosalicylates (non-sulfa containing)
       - (A) In general, better tolerated than sulfasalazine; considered first line in mild-moderate UC and Crohn disease
       - (B) Product selection will depend on location of disease.
       - (C) Olsalazine is associated with secretory diarrhea in up to 25% of patients.

Table 11.

Drug	Trade Name	Formulation	Strength	Daily Dosage Range (g)	Site of Action
Mesalamine[a]	Rowasa	Enema	4 g/60 mL	4	Rectum Terminal colon
	Asacol Asacol HD	Delayed-release resin	400 mg 800 mg	1.6–4.8	Distal ileum Colon
	Canasa	Suppository	1000 mg	1	Rectum
	Pentasa	Microgranular-coated tablet	250 mg	2–4	Small bowel Colon
	Lialda	MMX delayed-release tablet	1.2 g	2.4–4.8 (once daily)	Colon
	Apriso	INTELLICOR delayed- and extended-release capsule	0.375 g	0.375–1.5 (once daily)	Colon
Olsalazine	Dipentum	Dimer of mesalamine (capsule)	250 mg	1–3	Colon
Balsalazide	Colazal	Capsule	750 mg	2–6.75	Colon

[a] Generic mesalamine enema now available.

- c. Corticosteroids
    - i. Work quickly to suppress inflammation during acute flares
    - ii. No role for maintenance therapy; however, more than 50% of patients with severe disease may become steroid-dependent
    - iii. Budesonide is about 15 times more potent than prednisone; because of its high first-pass metabolism, allow a 2-week overlap when changing from prednisone to budesonide to prevent adrenal insufficiency. Formulated to release in the terminal ileum and treats only terminal ileal/ascending colonic disease
    - iv. Adverse effects (systemic therapy) are adrenal suppression, glucose intolerance, hypertension, sodium/water retention, osteoporosis, cataracts, and impaired wound healing.

Table 12.

Route	Agents	Dose	Comments
Oral	Prednisone Prednisolone	20–60 mg/day	Taper ASAP
	Budesonide (Entocort EC)	9 mg/day PO; then 6 mg/day PO 2 weeks before discontinuing	Minimal absorption indicated for mild-moderate active CD involving terminal ileum or ascending colon.
IV	Hydrocortisone	100 mg every 8 hours	7- to 10-day course; change to PO when gut is functional
	Methylprednisolone	15–48 mg/day	
Topical (rectal)	Cortenema (100 mg/60 mL)	100 mg HS	Hydrocortisone-based products
	Cortifoam (90 mg/applicator)	90 mg/day BID	Used for patients with distal disease
	Anucort-HC 25 mg Proctocort 30 mg	25–50 mg PR BID	Suppositories, use for proctitis

ASAP = as soon as possible; BID = 2 times/day; HS = every night; IV = intravenous; PO = by mouth; PR = rectally.

d. Immunomodulators
   i. 6-Mercaptopurine (Purinethol or 6-MP), azathioprine (Imuran, Azasan; prodrug of 6-MP), or methotrexate
   ii. Doses: Azathioprine 2–2.5 mg/kg/day, 6-MP 1–1.5 mg/kg/day, methotrexate 15–25 mg/week intramuscularly (Crohn's disease only)
   iii. Indicated only for maintenance because of its long onset of action (3–15 months)
   iv. Use may result in a steroid-sparing effect.
   v. Azathioprine and 6-MP are metabolized by enzyme thiopurine methyltransferase; reduced expression of thiopurine methyltransferase may result in slower metabolism and increased toxicity. Thiopurine methyltransferase activity should be determined before initiating therapy.
   vi. Adverse reactions: Azathioprine and 6-MP: pancreatitis (3%–15%), bone marrow suppression, nausea, diarrhea, rash, possible hepatotoxicity. Methotrexate: Bone marrow suppression, nausea, diarrhea, rash, pulmonary toxicity, hepatotoxicity
e. Infliximab (Remicade)
   i. Chimeric monoclonal antibody versus tumor necrosis factor
   ii. Indicated for both Crohn's disease and UC
      (A) Moderate-severe active disease
      (B) Fistulizing Crohn's disease
      (C) Maintenance of moderate-severe disease
   iii. Available as intravenous injection only; very expensive
   iv. Studies of patients whose conventional therapy failed; response is about 40%–80%
   v. Dosing:
      (A) Moderate-severe active disease or fistulizing disease: 5 mg/kg as single dose, followed by 5 mg/kg at 2 and 6 weeks; then every 8 weeks as maintenance. Patients losing response over time may be treated with a 10-mg/kg dose (maintenance dosing in Crohn's disease based on results of the ACCENT trial: Lancet 2002;359:1541–9).
   vi. Adverse reactions:
      (A) Infusion related: Hypotension, fever, chills, urticaria, pruritus; infuse over at least 2 hours (may pretreat with acetaminophen and/or antihistamine)
      (B) Delayed hypersensitivity: May be associated with fever, rash, myalgia, headache, or sore throat 3–10 days after administration
      (C) Infection: Use is associated with the reactivation of latent infections (bacterial, including disseminated tuberculosis, fungal, sepsis); do not give to patients with active infections. Patients should have ruled out tuberculosis before initiating any biologic agents.
      (D) Heart failure exacerbations: Contraindicated in New York Heart Association class III/IV heart failure; do not exceed 5-mg/kg dose in other patients with chronic heart failure (Ann Intern Med 2003;138:807–11)
      (E) Antibody induction: Up to 50% of patients may develop antinuclear antibodies; 19% may develop anti–double-stranded DNA antibodies.
      (F) Bone marrow suppression (pancytopenia)
      (G) Lymphoma: Rare, but patients with Crohn's disease or rheumatologic arthritis may be at a several-fold increased risk of development
      (H) Hepatitis (reactivation of hepatitis B virus [HBV], autoimmune hepatitis); discontinue use if liver function tests rise to more than 5 times the upper limit of normal
      (I) Vasculitis with CNS involvement

f. Adalimumab (Humira)
   i. Fully humanized antibody to tumor necrosis factor alpha; therefore, theoretically, no development of antibodies
   ii. Indicated for both induction and maintenance therapy for moderate-severe active Crohn's disease in patients unresponsive to conventional therapy; also indicated for patients who no longer respond to infliximab
   iii. Dosing
      (A) Induction: 160 mg subcutaneously on day 1 (given as four separate 40-mg injections) or two 40-mg/day injections for 2 consecutive days, followed by 80 mg subcutaneously 2 weeks later (day 15). Then, can decrease dose to 40 mg subcutaneously every 2 weeks starting on day 29 of therapy
   iv. Efficacy
      (A) Complete remission rates at week 4 range from 21% to 54% (Am J Gastroenterol 2005;100:75–9, Gastroenterology 2006;130:323–32, Ann Intern Med 2007;146:829–38).
      (B) Efficacy rates for maintenance therapy range from 56% to 79% at week 4 to 36% to 46% at week 56 (Gastroenterology 2007;132:52–65, Gut 2007;56:1232–9)
   v. The adverse effect profile of adalimumab is similar to infliximab, except for the development of antibodies to adalimumab.
g. Certolizumab (Cimzia)
   i. Humanized monoclonal antibody fragment linked to PEG, with murine-complimentary determining regions
   ii. Indicated for both induction and maintenance therapy for moderate-severe active Crohn's disease in patients unresponsive to conventional therapy
   iii. Dosing
      (A) Induction: 400 mg subcutaneously; then 400 mg subcutaneously at weeks 2 and 4; maintenance dose is 400 mg subcutaneously every 4 weeks
   iv. Efficacy
      (A) Patients with a C-reactive protein concentration greater than 10 mg/L have the best response. Up to 37% response at 6 weeks versus 26% for placebo (p=0.04) (N Engl J Med 2007;357:228–38)
      (B) Up to 62% of patients with initial response and a C-reactive protein concentration greater than 10 mg/L may be maintained in remission at 26 weeks (N Engl J Med 2007;357:239–50).
   v. Certolizumab adverse effect profile is similar to infliximab and adalimumab.
h. Natalizumab (Tysabri)
   i. Humanized monoclonal antibody that antagonizes integrin heterodimers and inhibits α_4 integrin-mediated leukocyte adhesion
   ii. Indicated for inducing and maintaining clinical response and remission in adult patients with moderate-severe active Crohn's disease who have had an inadequate response to, or are unable to tolerate, conventional therapies and inhibitors of tumor necrosis factor alpha
   iii. Dosing
      (A) All patients must be enrolled in the TOUCH program before dispensing the drug because of its association with progressive multifocal leukoencephalopathy.
      (B) Induction and maintenance doses are both 300 mg intravenously every 4 weeks. If no effect after 12 weeks or inability to discontinue steroids within 6 months of beginning therapy, treatment should be discontinued

iv. Efficacy
   (A) The ENACT 1 and 2 trials (N Engl J Med 2005;353:1912–25) showed similar results for natalizumab and placebo at 10 weeks (56% vs. 49%; p=0.05). However, those who initially responded had rates of sustained response (61% vs. 28%; p=0.001) at week 36.
   (B) Discontinue if no response is observed by week 12 of treatment.
   (C) May also improve quality of life in patients who initially respond after 48 weeks of treatment (Am J Gastroenterol 2007;102:2737–46)
v. Safety
   (A) Natalizumab is associated with the development of progressive multifocal leukoencephalopathy. Monitor for mental status changes while on treatment. Consider MRI (magnetic resonance imaging) and lumbar puncture if mental status changes or weakness is observed.
   (B) Potential for hepatotoxicity; monitor for jaundice or other signs of liver disease
   (C) Increased risk of infection
   (D) Infusion-related reactions: Observe patient for 1 hour after infusion.
   (E) The drug should not be used in combination with inhibitors of tumor necrosis factor alpha or immunosuppressants.

2. Medical management of UC: Treatment is selected on the basis of disease location and severity (Am J Gastroenterol 2004;99:1371–85, Gastroenterology 2006;130:940–87, Inflamm Bowel Dis 2006;12:979–94).
   a. Guideline definitions of UC distribution:
      i. Distal disease: Distal to splenic flexure (may use oral/systemic or topical (rectal) therapy)
      ii. Extensive disease: Proximal to splenic flexure (requires systemic/oral therapy)
   b. Mild-moderate distal disease
      i. First-line therapy: Topical (enema/suppository) aminosalicylates are preferred and are superior to oral aminosalicylates and topical corticosteroids.
      ii. Patients refractory to oral aminosalicylates or topical corticosteroids may respond to mesalamine enemas or suppositories.
      iii. Oral mesalamine plus topical mesalamine can be considered, and may be, more effective compared with either alone (Inflamm Bowel Dis 2006;12:979–94).
      iv. Patients refractory to the above agents may require 40–60 mg of oral prednisone.
      v. Maintenance
         (A) Mesalamine suppositories (1 g rectally every day or 1 g 3 times/week) are effective for maintaining remission in patients with proctitis.
         (B) Mesalamine enemas (2–4 g/day) are effective for maintaining remission in patients with distal disease extending to the splenic flexure.
         (C) Oral treatment with sulfasalazine (2–4 g/day), mesalamine (1.5–4.8 g/day), or balsalazide (6.75 g/day) is also effective.
         (D) Topical steroids have no role in maintenance therapy.
         (E) Nicotine replacement (15–25 mg/day transdermally) may improve symptoms as an adjunctive therapy. Effects seem to be most beneficial in ex-smokers.
   c. Mild-moderate active extensive disease
      i. First-line therapy: Oral sulfasalazine (4–6 g/day) or an alternative aminosalicylate at a dose equivalent to 4.8 g/day of mesalamine
         (A) May consider combined oral and topical therapy for patients with distal disease
      ii. Infliximab may be used for moderate active disease at an initial dose of 5 mg/kg intravenously, followed by subsequent doses at 2 and 6 weeks.

iii. Patients refractory to the above agents may require oral corticosteroids (40–60 mg prednisone).
iv. Patients refractory to oral corticosteroids can be treated with azathioprine or 6-MP.
v. Maintenance
   (A) Aminosalicylates are the preferred agents for maintenance of remission.
   (B) Patients should not be treated with chronic steroids for maintenance therapy.
   (C) Azathioprine or 6-MP are effective steroid-sparing agents for maintenance of remission; can be used in combination with aminosalicylates
   (D) Infliximab may be given for maintenance of moderate disease at a dose of 5 mg/kg every 8 weeks.
d. Severe disease
   i. Patients with severe symptoms refractory to oral/topical aminosalicylates or corticosteroids should be treated with a 7- to 10-day course of intravenous corticosteroids (300 mg of hydrocortisone or 60 mg/day of methylprednisolone equivalent).
   ii. Infliximab may be used for severe active disease at an initial dose of 5 mg/kg intravenously, followed by doses at 2 and 6 weeks; maintenance doses of 5 mg/kg every 8 weeks may be used after treatment of active disease.
   iii. Antibiotics, particularly metronidazole, have mixed results in the treatment of active UC, but they may be used in severe colonic disease or for patients with pouchitis (Dig Dis Sci 2007;52:2920–5).
   iv. Patients refractory to intravenous corticosteroids are candidates for intravenous cyclosporine (4 mg/kg/day target concentration of 350–500 ng/mL), followed by oral therapy at 8 mg/kg/day with a target concentration of 200–350 ng/mL if initial response to intravenous cyclosporine is attained.
   v. Patients refractory to the above are candidates for colectomy.
   vi. Patients with toxic megacolon should undergo bowel decompression, treatment with broad-spectrum antibiotics, and possibly colectomy.
3. Medical management of Crohn's disease
   a. Treatment is selected on the basis of disease location and severity. General adult guidelines: Am J Gastroenterol 2009;104:465–83; perianal disease guidelines: Gastroenterology 2003;125:1503–7)
   b. Mild-moderate active disease
      i. First line for ileal, ileocolonic, or colonic disease:
         (A) Oral aminosalicylate (mesalamine 3.2–4 g/day or sulfasalazine–6 g/day). Commonly used but generally considered minimally effective
         (B) Budesonide 9 mg/day is preferred for terminal ileal and/or ascending colonic disease.
         (C) Metronidazole 10–20 mg/kg/day may be used in patients not responding to oral aminosalicylates but is generally more effective in perianal disease.
         (D) Ciprofloxacin 1 g/day is considered as effective as mesalamine (generally second line) but is usually more effective in perianal disease, typically in combination with metronidazole.
   c. Moderate-severe disease
      i. Corticosteroids (prednisone 40–60 mg/day or budesonide 9 mg/day if terminal ileal involvement) until resolution of symptoms and resumption of weight gain
      ii. Infliximab 5 mg/kg is an alternative first-line treatment (improvement in up to 80% of patients). Infliximab may be combined with azathioprine in patients whose therapy with aminosalicylates and corticosteroids has failed and who are naïve to biologic agents.

iii. Certolizumab 400 mg subcutaneously, and then 400 mg subcutaneously at weeks 2 and 4, or adalimumab 160 mg subcutaneously initially, followed by 80 mg subcutaneously 2 weeks later, may also be considered for use as an alternative therapy for moderate to severe disease, particularly in patients with C-reactive protein values greater than 10 mg/L.
iv. Adalimumab may be reserved for patients who no longer respond to infliximab therapy because they developed antibodies to infliximab.
v. Natalizumab 300 mg intravenously every 4 weeks may be considered for patients who did not respond to any other conventional medical therapy.
vi. Methotrexate maintenance therapy (25 mg/week intramuscularly or subcutaneously) is effective in patients whose active disease has responded to intramuscular methotrexate and who have steroid-dependent or steroid-refractory disease.

d. Severe-fulminant disease
   i. Severe symptoms despite oral corticosteroids or infliximab therapy
   ii. Assess need for surgical intervention (mass, obstruction, and abscess).
   iii. Administer intravenous corticosteroids (40–60 mg of prednisone equivalent).
   iv. Parenteral nutrition may be needed after 5–7 days.
   v. Possibly use intravenous cyclosporine or tacrolimus if steroids fail.

e. Maintenance therapy
   i. No role for long-term corticosteroid use, but budesonide may be used for up to 6 months in patients with mild-moderate disease having ileal involvement.
   ii. Azathioprine/6-MP can be used after induction with corticosteroids or infliximab (steroid-naïve patients).
   iii. Azathioprine/6-MP or mesalamine (more than 3 g/day) may also be used after surgical resection to prevent recurrence.
   iv. Infliximab 5 mg/kg at 0, 2, and 6 weeks and then every 8 weeks; adalimumab 40 mg subcutaneously every other week (starting on day 29 of therapy); or certolizumab 400 mg subcutaneously once monthly may be considered.
   v. Natalizumab 300 mg intravenously every 4 weeks may be considered for patients who did not respond to any other conventional medical therapy.
   vi. Methotrexate intramuscularly 25 mg for up to 16 weeks, followed by 15 mg/week intramuscularly, is effective for patients with chronic active disease.

f. Perianal disease
   i. Simple perianal fistulas
      (A) Antibiotics: Metronidazole or ciprofloxacin
      (B) Azathioprine/6-MP
      (C) Infliximab, adalimumab, or certolizumab
   ii. Complex perianal fistulas
      (A) Infliximab, adalimumab, or certolizumab
      (B) Antibiotics: Metronidazole or/and ciprofloxacin (mainly as adjunctive therapy in this case)
      (C) Azathioprine/6-MP or methotrexate
      (D) Cyclosporine or tacrolimus

Patient Case

5. A 35-year-old man with UC affecting most of his colon (pancolitis) has been taking balsalazide 6.75 g/day for 2 years and prednisone 40 mg/day for 1 year. When the physician decreases the dose of prednisone below 40 mg, the patient experiences fever, abdominal pain, and five or six bloody bowel movements a day. Which one of the following modifications to his drug regimen is best?
   A. Change balsalazide to sulfasalazine 6 g/day.
   B. Initiate therapy with methotrexate 25 mg intramuscularly once weekly.
   C. Initiate infliximab and attempt to taper the prednisone for several weeks.
   D. Add mesalamine suppository 1000 mg rectally once daily.

6. A 25-year-old woman presents to the emergency department with a 2-day history of cramping abdominal pain, fever, fatigue, and 10–12 bloody stools a day. She has had Crohn's disease for 5 years; typically, she is maintained on mesalamine (Pentasa) 250 mg 4 capsules 2 times/day. On admission, her vital signs include temperature 101°F, PR 110 beats/minute, RR 18 breaths/minute, and BP 118/68 mm Hg. Which one of the following therapeutic choices is best?
   A. Increase the dose of mesalamine (Pentasa) to 4 g/day.
   B. Administer cyclosporine 4 mg/hour by continuous infusion.
   C. Obtain a surgery consult for immediate colectomy.
   D. Administer hydrocortisone 100 mg intravenously every 8 hours.

V. COMPLICATIONS OF LIVER DISEASE

Scoring Systems for Severity of Liver Disease

Table 13. Child-Pugh Classification of the Severity of Cirrhosis (Br J Surg 1973;60:646–9)[a]

Variable	Score		
	1 point	2 points	3 points
Encephalopathy	Absent	Mild-moderate	Severe to coma
Ascites	Absent	Slight	Moderate
Bilirubin (mg/dL)	< 2	2–3	> 3
Albumin (g/L)	> 3.5	2.8–3.5	< 2.8
Prothrombin time (seconds above normal)	1–4	4–6	> 6

[a]Class A = total score of 5 or 6; class B = total score of 7–9; class C = total score more than 10.

Table 14. Model for End-Stage Liver Disease (MELD) (Hepatology 2007;45:797–805)

Version	Calculation	Comment
Original	9.57 × loge(creatinine) + 3.78 × loge(total bilirubin) + 11.2 × loge(INR) + 6.43	• Score ranges from 6 to 40 • Higher number indicates more severe disease • Used to predict mortality and prioritize patients for liver transplantation
MELD-Na	MELD − Na − [0.025 × MELD × (140 − Na)] + 140	• Incorporates sodium • May better discriminate risk of death
UNOS modification	Original MELD equation with limits set on laboratory values that are entered	• Lower end of laboratory values for SCr, bilirubin, and INR are set at 1 with a maximum of 4 • If two or more dialysis treatments within the prior week or 24 hours of CVVHD within the prior week, SCr concentration automatically set to 4.0 mg/dL

MELD Score Calculators. Available at www.mayoclinic.org/meld/mayomodel5.html.
CVVHD = continuous venovenous hemodialysis; INR = international normalized ratio; Na = nationwide; SCr = serum creatinine; UNOS = United Network for Organ Sharing.

A. Ascites
 1. Definition: Free fluid in the abdominal cavity secondary to increased resistance within the liver (forces lymphatic drainage into the abdominal cavity) and reduced osmotic pressure within the bloodstream (hypoalbuminemia); develops at a 5-year cumulative rate of 30% in compensated liver disease
 2. Clinical features: Protuberant abdomen, shifting dullness, fluid wave, bulging flanks, abdominal pain
 3. Diagnosis
  a. Clinical features: Abdominal ultrasound, paracentesis. Can use serum ascites albumin gradient, calculated by subtracting the ascites albumin concentration from the serum albumin concentration; a value greater than 1.1 indicates ascites secondary to portal hypertension
 4. Treatment (Hepatology 2009;49:2087–107)
  a. Attainment of negative sodium balance
   i. Dietary sodium restriction (less than 2000 mg/day), fluid restriction to less than 1.5 L/day if serum sodium is less than 120–125 mmol/L
   ii. Goal is excretion greater than 78 mmol/day of sodium. A random "spot" urine sodium concentration greater than the potassium concentration (ratio greater than 1) correlates with a 24-hour sodium excretion of greater than 78 mmol/day with 90% accuracy. Diuretics
    (A) Patients with minimal fluid overload may be treated with spironolactone alone (doses up to 400 mg/day); however, a combination of furosemide and spironolactone is preferable as initial therapy in most patients.
    (B) When used in combination, a ratio of 40 mg of furosemide to every 100 mg of spironolactone is an appropriate starting regimen. Amiloride 10–40 mg/day may be substituted for spironolactone in patients who develop tender gynecomastia.
    (C) If tense ascites is present, may use large volume paracentesis. Administer albumin at a dose of 6–8 g/L of asctic fluid removed (if > 5 L is removed at one time).
   iii. No upper limit of weight loss if massive edema is present, 0.5 kg/day in patients without edema

iv. The goal is to achieve 78 mmol or more urinary sodium excretions per day with diuretics.
v. Monitor for electrolyte imbalances, renal impairment, and gynecomastia (spironolactone).
b. Discontinue drugs associated with sodium/water retention such as NSAIDs.

B. Hepatic Encephalopathy
1. Definition: Disturbance in CNS function secondary to hepatic insufficiency, resulting in a broad range of neuropsychiatric manifestations
   a. Thought to be secondary to the accumulation of nitrogenous substances (mainly NH_3) arising from the gut; overall, NH_3 serum concentrations do not correlate well with mental status
   b. Other theories are related to the activation of γ-aminobutyric acid receptors by endogenous benzodiazepine-like substances, possible zinc deficiency, or altered cerebral metabolism.
2. Clinical features
   a. May result in acute encephalopathy with altered mental status and progress to coma if untreated; asterixis ("hand flap") is a classic physical finding
   b. May be precipitated by various factors including constipation, GI bleeding, infection, hypokalemia, dehydration, hypotension, and CNS-active drugs (benzodiazepines/narcotics)
3. Treatment (Am J Gastroenterol 2001;96:1968–76)
   a. Assess need for airway support and remove possible precipitating factors.
   b. Main treatments targeted at reducing the nitrogen load in the gut
   c. Lactulose
      i. Nonabsorbable disaccharide: Metabolized by colonic bacteria to acetic and lactic acid; NH_3 present in the GI lumen is reduced to ammonium ion (NH_4^+) through the reduction in pH ("ammonia trapping") and is therefore unable to diffuse back into the bloodstream. Lactulose may also alter bacterial metabolism, resulting in increased uptake of NH_3.
      ii. Dose: 45 mL orally every 1–2 hours until the patient has a loose bowel movement; then titrate to two or three loose bowel movements a day (typically 15–45 mL dose 2–3 times/day); may also administer as an enema (300 mL plus 700 mL of water retained for 1 hour). Powder formulation (KRISTALOSE) in 10- and 20-g packets that may be dissolved in 4 oz of water (10 g = 15 mL of traditional lactulose). This formulation is more palatable than the traditional syrup.
      iii. May be continued chronically for the prevention of recurrent encephalopathy
      iv. Flatulence, diarrhea, and abdominal cramping are common adverse effects.
   d. Antibiotics
      i. Targeted at reducing the number of intraluminal urease-producing bacteria that may be associated with excess NH_3 production
      ii. Neomycin (3–6 g/day × 1–2 weeks; then 1–2 g/day maintenance) or metronidazole (250 mg orally 2 times/day) may be used; neomycin is considered as effective as lactulose.
      iii. From 1% to 3% of neomycin is absorbed, so use caution with long-term use in patients having renal insufficiency; long-term metronidazole use may result in peripheral neuropathy.

iv. Rifaximin 400 mg orally 3 times/day is as effective as lactulose and other nonabsorbable antibiotics and may be better tolerated. Drug cost may be greater, but this may be offset by fewer hospitalizations and shorter lengths of stay (Pharmacotherapy 2008;28:1019–32).
   e. Other possible treatments
      i. Benzodiazepine antagonists such as flumazenil may be used in cases of suspected benzodiazepine overdose.
      ii. Zinc supplementation should used in patients with documented zinc deficiency.

C. Gastroesophageal Varices (Am J Gastroenterol 2009;104:1802–29)
   1. Background
      a. Resistance to bloodflow within the liver secondary to cirrhosis results in the development of portal hypertension. Collateral blood vessels (such as esophageal varices) are formed because of this increased resistance to bloodflow.
      b. Variceal hemorrhage may occur in around 25%–35% of patients with cirrhosis and varices; mortality rates are as high as 30%–50% per bleed; recurrence rates are as high as 70% within the first 6 months after an initial bleed.
   2. Management of acute variceal bleeding
      a. Fluid resuscitation and hemodynamic stabilization. Maintain hemoglobin concentration of about 8 g/dL. Administration of Fresh frozen plasma or platelet may be considered for patients with considerable coagulopathy.
      b. Endoscopy to assess the extent of disease with potential intervention
         i. Sclerotherapy: Effective in discontinuing bleeding in 80%–90% of patients; may be associated with complications such as perforation, ulceration, stricture, and bacteremia; possible sclerosing agents include ethanolamine and sodium tetradecyl sulfate
         ii. Endoscopic variceal band ligation may be used as an alternative to sclerotherapy; fewer complications
      c. Medical management of acute variceal bleeding
         i. Should be instituted after fluid resuscitation (before endoscopy, if possible)
         ii. Most therapies targeted at reducing splanchnic bloodflow and portal pressure; combination of endoscopic and vasoactive therapies most effective
         iii. Vasopressin: 0.2–0.4 unit/minute plus nitroglycerin 40–400 mcg/minute for 3–5 days
            (A) Vasopressin use results in splanchnic vasoconstriction; used less often secondary to need for both drugs and coronary vasoconstriction/hypertension with vasopressin (nitroglycerin attenuates these effects to some extent)
            (B) More adverse effects than octreotide, so overall, less preferable
         iv. Octreotide or somatostatin
            (A) Works possibly by preventing postprandial hyperemia, by reducing portal pressure (by reduced splanchnic bloodflow) through inhibitory effects on vasoactive peptides such as glucagon, or by a local vasoconstrictor effect
            (B) Preferred agents in combination with endoscopic interventions because of more favorable adverse effect profiles; main adverse effects include hyperglycemia and abdominal cramping (Digestion 1999;60(Suppl 2):31–41)
            (C) Dosing
               1. Octreotide: 50-mcg intravenous bolus; then 50 mcg/hour intravenously × 3–5 days
               2. Somatostatin: 250-mcg intravenous bolus; then 250–500 mcg/hour intravenously × 3–5 days

v. Nondrug measures to control bleeding
   (A) Typically used for medically unresponsive bleeding
   (B) Minnesota or Blakemore tube: Balloon compression applied directly to bleeding varices
   (C) Transjugular intrahepatic portosystemic shunt: Results in shunting of blood from the portal circulation; however, may be associated with complications such as bleeding and infection
   (D) Surgery
vi. Antibiotic therapy
   (A) The use of oral or intravenous prophylactic antibiotics in patients with cirrhosis with variceal bleeding has been shown to reduce short-term mortality; they should be prescribed (Hepatology 1999;29:1655–61).
   (B) Typical regimens include a fluoroquinolone (norfloxacin or ciprofloxacin) orally for 7 days. Intravenous therapy (ciprofloxacin) can be used if the oral route of administration is not an option. Ceftriaxone 1 g/day intravenously may be used if high rates of fluoroquinolone resistance are present.

d. Prevention of variceal bleeding
   i. Primary prophylaxis
      (A) A screening esophagogastroduodenoscopy (EGD) is recommended to evaluate for esophageal and gastric varices when the diagnosis of cirrhosis is made.
      (B) Pharmacologic therapy is not recommended to prevent the development of varices in patients with cirrhosis who have not yet developed varices.
      (C) Patients with small varices and no history of bleeding, but meeting the criteria for increased risk of bleeding (Child-Pugh class B or C, red wale marks on varices), should receive preventive drug therapy with nonselective β-blockers.
      (D) Nonselective β-blockers can be considered; however, the long-term benefit is unclear in patients with small varices and no history of bleeding but who DO NOT meet criteria for increased risk of bleeding.
      (E) Nonselective β-blockers are indicated in all patients with medium/large varices and no history of bleeding. Endoscopic variceal ligation can be used if nonselective β-blockers are contraindicated.
      (F) Mechanism of nonselective β-blockers: Blockade of $β_1$-receptors reduces cardiac output, whereas blockade of $β_2$-receptors prevents splanchnic vasodilation; unopposed $α_1$-mediated constriction of the splanchnic circulation also leads to reductions in portal pressure.
      (G) Therapy should aim for a PR of 55–60 beats/minute or a 25% reduction from baseline.
      (H) Nonselective β-blockers are associated with a significant reduction in the incidence of first bleed (OR = 0.54; 95% CI, 0.39–0.74) with a trend toward reduced mortality (Ann Intern Med 1992;117:59–70).
      (I) Long-acting nitrates (isosorbide mono- or dinitrate) should not be used for primary prophylaxis. These agents are believed to decrease intrahepatic resistance and are considered as effective as propranolol; however, there is an increased incidence of mortality in some studies when used as monotherapy.
      (J) Shunt surgery or endoscopic sclerotherapy should not be used for primary prophylaxis.

ii. Secondary prophylaxis
- (A) All patients with a history of variceal bleeding should receive secondary prophylaxis to prevent recurrent bleeding.
- (B) A combination of endoscopic variceal band ligation and nonselective β-blockers is considered the most effective regimen.
- (C) Nonselective β-blockers are associated with a 20% reduction in the incidence of variceal rebleeding (p<0.001; 11%–28%); reductions in mortality are minimal and not consistent among trials (Hepatology 1997;25:63–70); most studies are of patients with Child-Pugh class A or B cirrhosis; class C patients may not be able to tolerate β-blockers.
- (D) Combining nonselective β-blockers with nitrates leads to slightly better reductions in rebleeding rates; however, no added mortality benefit is observed, and there is a higher incidence of adverse effects with the combination.
- (E) Sclerotherapy is no longer recommended for secondary prophylaxis because endoscopic variceal ligation has been shown to be better with fewer complications.
- (F) The transjugular intrahepatic portosystemic shunt is very effective in preventing recurrent bleeding; however, it is associated with a 30%–40% incidence of encephalopathy; reserve for medically unresponsive patients.
- (G) Contraindications to nonselective β-blockers: asthma, insulin-dependent diabetes with frequent hypoglycemia, peripheral vascular disease
- (H) Adverse effects of nonselective β-blockers: light-headedness, fatigue, shortness of breath, sexual dysfunction, bradycardia
- (I) Adverse effects of EVL: transient dysphagia, chest discomfort

D. Spontaneous Bacterial Peritonitis (Hepatology 2009;49:2087–107)
1. Background
   a. Definition: Infection of previously sterile ascitic fluid without an apparent intra-abdominal source. Spontaneous bacterial peritonitis (SBP) is considered a primary peritonitis as opposed to secondary.
   b. May be present in 10%–30% of hospitalized patients with cirrhosis and ascites
   c. Associated with 20%–40% of in-hospital mortality; poor prognosis after recovery, with 2-year survival after initial episode reported as about 30%
2. Pathophysiology
   a. Principal theory is seeding of the ascitic fluid from an episode of bacteremia.
   b. Because the bacteria usually present are enteric pathogens, they may enter the blood because of increases in gut permeability secondary to portal hypertension, suppression of hepatic reticuloendothelial cells, or translocation of the gut wall and dissemination through the mesenteric lymph system.
   c. Reduced opsonic activity of the ascitic fluid and alterations in neutrophil function may also be contributing factors.
   d. Enteric gram-negative pathogens are most commonly involved, and more than 90% of cases involve a single bacterial species.

Table 15. Most Commonly Isolated Bacteria Responsible for SBP

Gram-Negative Bacilli (50%)	Gram-Positive Bacilli (17%)
Escherichia coli – 37%	*Streptococcus pneumoniae* – 10%
Klebsiella spp. – 6%	Other streptococci – 6%
Other – 7%	*Staphylococcus aureus* – 1%

SBP = spontaneous bacterial peritonitis.

3. Clinical and laboratory features
    a. Clinical presentation may be variable, but common symptoms include fever, abdominal pain, nausea, vomiting, diarrhea, rebound tenderness, and exacerbation of encephalopathy; about 33% of patients may present with renal failure, which is associated with significant increases in mortality. Although GI bleeding and septic shock/hypotension occur, they are rare.
    b. Laboratory
        i. May see systemic leucocytosis or increases in serum creatinine
        ii. Abdominal paracentesis must be performed:
            (A) The presence of more than 250 polymorphonuclear cells/mm^3 is diagnostic for SBP.
            (B) Lactate dehydrogenase, glucose, and protein values may help distinguish from secondary peritonitis.
        iii. Blood cultures positive in 50%–70% of cases; ascitic fluid cultures positive in 67% of cases
        iv. Gram stain of ascitic fluid is typically low yield.
4. Treatment of acute SBP (Hepatology 2009;49:2087–107)
    a. Because of the high associated mortality, treatment should be initiated promptly in patients with clinical and laboratory features consistent with SBP.
    b. Up to 86% of ascetic fluid cultures may be negative if one dose of an antibiotic is given before cultures are drawn.
    c. Predictors of poor outcomes include bilirubin more than 8 mg/dL, albumin less than 2.5 g/dL, creatinine more than 2.1 mg/dL, hepatic encephalopathy, hepatorenal syndrome, and upper GI bleeding.
    d. Antibiotic therapy plus albumin if patient meets criteria for use (see below)
        i. Empiric therapy targeting enteric gram-negative organisms should be instituted.
        ii. Third-generation cephalosporins have been studied the most and are considered first line.
            (A) Cefotaxime (2 g every 8–12 hours) or ceftriaxone (2 g/day intravenously)
        iii. Other agents, such as fluoroquinolones, may be used.
        iv. Avoid aminoglycosides because of the high risk of renal failure in patients with cirrhosis and SBP.
        v. Treatment duration: 5–10 days; most studies suggest that a 5-day treatment period is as effective as a 10-day period
    e. Albumin
        i. Rationale: The hemodynamics of patients with cirrhosis reflect a state of intravascular hypovolemia and organ hypoperfusion; SBP is thought to enhance this effect, resulting in progressive renal hypoperfusion and precipitation of renal failure or hepatorenal syndrome.

ii. The regimen most commonly used is based on one study (N Engl J Med 1999;341:403–9).
   (A) Albumin dosing: 1.5 g/kg on admission; 1 g/kg on hospital day 3
   (B) In addition, should give antibiotic treatment; cefotaxime was used in this study
   (C) The incidence of renal failure was reduced to 10% versus 33% for placebo (p=0.002).
   (D) In-hospital mortality was 10% for albumin versus 29% for placebo (p=0.01).
   (E) Thirty-day mortality was reduced to 21% with albumin versus 41% for placebo (p=0.03).
   (F) Recent guidelines suggest <u>using this albumin regimen with antibiotics</u> if serum creatinine is more than 1 mg/dL, BUN more than 40 mg/dL, or total bilirubin more than 4 mg/dL (Hepatology 2009;49:2087–107)

5. Prevention (Hepatology 2009;49:2087–107)
   a. Prophylactic oral antibiotics are used to prevent SBP in high-risk patients to reduce the number of enteric organisms in the GI tract (GI decontamination), with the hope of reducing the chance of bacterial translocation.
   b. Antibiotic regimens are similar for both primary and secondary prevention:
      i. Fluoroquinolones: Norfloxacin or ciprofloxacin
      ii. Trimethoprim-sulfamethoxazole 1 double-strength tablet 5 times/week (Monday–Friday)
   c. Primary prevention
      i. For acute upper GI bleeding (7-day course during hospitalization only), give ceftriaxone or norfloxacin 400 mg 2 times/day.
      ii. May also consider for indefinite use in patients without GI bleeding if ascitic fluid protein concentration less than 1.5 g/dL and at least one of the following is present: serum creatinine more than 1.2 mg/dL, BUN more than 25 mg/dL, sodium less than 130 mg/dL, or Child-Pugh score more than 9 with bilirubin more than 3 mg/dL.
      iii. Use norfloxacin 400 mg once daily or trimethoprim-sulfamethoxazole.
   d. Secondary prevention
      i. All patients recovering from an initial episode of SBP should be treated with oral prophylactic antibiotics (norfloxacin or trimethoprim-sulfamethoxazole) indefinitely.
      ii. Consider for liver transplantation because 2-year survival is 25%–30% after recovery.

Gastrointestinal Disorders

Patient Case

7. A 56-year-old man with a history of Child-Pugh class B cirrhosis secondary to alcohol abuse, hypertension, low back pain, and chronic renal insufficiency is admitted with a 2-day history of confusion, disorientation, somnolence, and reduced oral intake. On examination, he is afebrile with abdominal tenderness, reduced reflexes, dry mucous membranes, and asterixis. Paracentesis is negative for infection. He takes oxycodone 10 mg every 4–6 hours, temazepam 15 mg at bedtime as needed, and propranolol 20 mg 3 times/day. Which one of the following recommendations is best for treating this patient's hepatic encephalopathy?

    A. Discontinue propranolol and initiate intravenous gentamicin.
    B. Initiate oral lactulose and discontinue oxycodone-temazepam.
    C. Initiate scheduled oxazepam for alcohol withdrawal prophylaxis.
    D. Initiate oral neomycin and discontinue propranolol-oxycodone.

8. A 36-year-old woman is admitted with a 36-hour history of hematemesis, fatigue, dizziness, and black, tarry stools. She has a history of alcohol abuse and cirrhosis, as well as a myocardial infarction 2 years ago. On evaluation, she is afebrile, disoriented, and orthostatic. She is administered intravenous fluids and sent for emergency endoscopy. Several large, actively bleeding, esophageal varices are identified and banded. In addition to endoscopic intervention, which one of the following pharmacologic interventions is best?

    A. Initiate nadolol 20 mg orally once daily × 3 days.
    B. Initiate vasopressin continuous infusion × 2 days.
    C. Initiate octreotide 50-mcg intravenous bolus; then 50-mcg/hour intravenous infusion.
    D. Initiate pantoprazole 80-mg bolus; then 8 mg/hour × 72 hours.

VI. VIRAL HEPATITIS

A. For all hepatitis virus infections, acute hepatitis is defined as infection for less than 6 months, whereas chronic infection is greater than 6 months.

B. Hepatitis A Virus
  1. Background
     a. An RNA virus that is associated with the development of self-limited hepatitis.
     b. Transmission occurs mainly through the fecal-oral route.
        i. Areas of poor sanitation; also associated flooding leading to increased spread
        ii. Foodborne: Shellfish, water, milk, vegetables
        iii. Person-to-person contact: Sexual, daycare, intravenous drug use, household, restaurant workers
     c. After exposure, incubation for 14–50 days takes place; patients may exhibit general, nonspecific symptoms such as nausea, vomiting, diarrhea, myalgia, fever, abdominal pain, and jaundice.
     d. Most patients have self-limited disease lasting less than 2 months; death of the hepatocyte results in elimination of the virus.
     e. Hepatitis A virus is associated with very low mortality (less than 1%) and is not associated with the development of chronic hepatitis. Fulminant hepatitis may occur in some instances.
  2. Diagnosis
     a. Clinical signs/symptoms such as nausea, abdominal pain, jaundice, fever malaise, or anorexia. Some patients may have mild asymptomatic disease.
     b. Recent possible exposures
     c. Laboratory data

Gastrointestinal Disorders

   i. Immunoglobulin M antibody to HAV (anti-HAV): Detectable in the serum 5–10 days before the onset of symptoms; once the infection clears, the immunoglobulin M antibody is replaced by immunoglobulin G antibodies during a 2- to 6-month period; these antibodies confer lifelong protective immunity against subsequent infection.
   ii. Elevation of aminotransferases
   d. Management of acute HAV infection is mainly supportive; avoid hepatotoxic medications, such as acetaminophen.
3. Preexposure prophylaxis
   a. Active (vaccination) or passive (immune globulin) prophylaxis can be used.
   b. Havrix (GlaxoSmithKline) and Vaqta (Merck) are the two available HAV vaccines; Twinrix is a combination HAV and HBV product (GlaxoSmithKline).
   c. Populations requiring preexposure prophylaxis with HAV vaccine
      i. All children older than 1 year
      ii. Children living in areas where rates of hepatitis are above twice the national average
      iii. People working in or traveling to countries with high or intermediate endemicity (may take up to 4 weeks for full protection)
      iv. Men who have sex with men
      v. Illegal drug users
      vi. Those with occupational risk of exposure (exposure to sewage)
      vii. Patients with chronic liver disease
      viii. Patients with clotting factor disorders
      ix. Optional: Food handlers, workers in institutions
   d. Populations requiring preexposure prophylaxis with HAV immune globulin
      i. Travelers to endemic countries
      ii. Children younger than 2 years (vaccine not approved for this age group)
      iii. Doses: 0.02 mL/kg intramuscularly (3 months coverage or more); 0.06 mL/kg intramuscularly (3–5 months of coverage); repeat every 5 months if travel or exposure is prolonged
4. Postexposure prophylaxis
   a. Immune globulin can be given at a dose of 0.02 mL/kg intramuscularly within 2 weeks of exposure. Hepatitis A vaccine may also be used. Efficacy approaches that of immune globulin, but it is recommended only in patients age 40 or younger.
   b. Offer to those not previously vaccinated in the following situations:
      i. Close personal contact with a documented infected person
      ii. Staff or attendees of daycare centers if one or more cases are recognized in children or employees or if cases are recognized in two or more households of attendees
      iii. Common source of exposures:
         (A) If a food handler receives a diagnosis of hepatitis A, vaccine or IG should be administered to other food handlers at the same establishment. Hepatitis A vaccine or IG administration to patrons typically is not indicated but may be considered if:
            (1) During the time the food handler was likely to be infectious, the food handler both directly handled uncooked or cooked food and had diarrhea or poor hygienic practices and (2) patrons can be identified and treated in 2 weeks or less after exposure.

(B) In settings where repeated exposures to HAV may have occurred, stronger consideration of hepatitis A vaccine or IG use could be warranted. In a common-source outbreak, postexposure prophylaxis should not be provided to exposed individuals after cases have begun to occur because the 2-week period after exposure during which IG or hepatitis A vaccine is known to be effective will have been exceeded.

C. Hepatitis B Virus
   1. Background
      a. Hepatitis B is a DNA virus; there are more than 350 million infected patients worldwide.
      b. Transmission routes
         i. Parenteral: Intravenous drug abuse, needlestick, transfusion, ear or body piercing
         ii. Bodily fluids: Saliva, semen, vaginal fluid
         iii. Sexual contact: Heterosexual and homosexual; prostitution
         iv. Perinatal: Mother to child at birth
      c. Associated with both acute and chronic disease
         i. Natural history of HBV is age-dependent.
            (A) Risk of developing chronic infection after an acute infection is 90% in neonates, 25%–30% in children younger than 5 years, and 10% in adults.
      d. Chronic infection with HBV increases the risk of developing hepatocellular carcinoma.
      e. Diagnosis
         i. Clinical signs and symptoms: Nausea, vomiting, diarrhea, myalgia, fever, abdominal pain, jaundice (30% may have no symptoms)
         ii. Serologic diagnosis
         iii. Combinations of serologic markers must be reviewed to distinguish acute from chronic infections.
         iv. Eight different HBV genotypes (A–H) exist. Routine genotype testing is not endorsed by the guidelines.

Table 16. Hepatitis B Serologies

Serologic Marker	Abbreviation	Comment
Surface antigen	HBsAg	First detectable serum antigen during acute infection; also present in chronic infection
Core antigen	HBcAg	Present early after cell damage during acute infection; typically unable to measure this in the serum
E antigen	HBeAg	Denotes ongoing active viral replication
Anti-surface antigen antibody	Anti-HBs	Confers protective immunity; present after recovery from acute infection or after vaccination
Anticore antigen antibody (IgG)	Anti-HBc	Appears at onset of symptoms Denotes prior exposure to HBV Cannot use to distinguish acute from chronic infection
Anti-E antibody	Anti-HBe	May indicate peak replication has passed
HBV B DNA	HBV DNA	Marker of active HBV replication

HBcAg = hepatitis B core antigen; HBeAg = hepatitis B early antigen; HBsAg = hepatitis B surface antigen; HBV = hepatitis B virus; IgG = immunoglobulin G.

(A) Most patients will have HBeAg positive disease.
(B) Hepatitis B early antigen–negative disease: Mutation in the precore or core promoter regions. These variants are known as "precore mutants"; these mutations do not allow monitoring of loss of E antigen as a clinical marker of suppressed replication. Monitor reduction in HBV DNA in these patients; patients infected with these variants also tend to have lower serum HBV DNA and more fluctuating liver function tests.
(C) Recent Centers for Disease Control and Prevention guidelines released for screening for HBV infection (MMWR 2008;57(RR08):1–20)
  (1) Serologic assay for HBV surface antigen should be the serologic screening test used for the following populations. Additional HBVs are needed in combination with HBV surface antigen for select populations as listed below.
    (a) People born in geographic regions with HBV surface antigen prevalence of more than 2% regardless of vaccination history
    (b) Men who have sex with men; also test for anti-HBc or anti-HBs
    (c) Past or current intravenous drug users; also test for anti-HBc or anti-HBs
    (d) Individuals receiving cytotoxic chemotherapy or immunosuppressive therapy related to organ transplantation or rheumatologic or GI disorders. In addition, test for anti-HBc or anti-HBs.
    (e) U.S.-born person not vaccinated as infant whose parents were born in regions with HBV endemicity more than 8%
    (f) People with elevated ALT/AST of unknown etiology
    (g) Donors of blood, plasma, organs, tissues, or semen. In addition, test for anti-HBc and HBV DNA.
    (h) Pregnant women (during each pregnancy, preferably in the first trimester)
    (i) Infants born to HBV surface antigen–positive mothers
    (j) Household, needlesharing, or sex contacts of individuals known to be HBsAg positive. In addition, test for anti-HBc or anti-HBs.
    (k) Individuals who are the sources of blood or bodily fluid for exposures that might require postexposure prophylaxis
    (l) Individuals who are human immunodeficiency virus (HIV) positive. In addition, test for anti-HBc or anti-HBs.
  vii. Clinical definitions

Table 17.

Chronic HBV Infection	Inactive HBV Carrier State
• HBsAg positive > 6 months • Serum HBV DNA 20,000 IU/mL (10^5 copies/mL), lower values 2000–20,000 IU/mL (10^4–10^5 copies/mL) are often observed in HBeAg-negative chronic hepatitis B • Persistent/intermittent elevation of AST/ALT • Chronic hepatitis and moderate-severe necroinflammation on biopsy	• HBsAg positive > 6 months • HBeAg negative, anti-HbeAg positive • Serum HBV DNA < 2000 IU/mL (10^4 copies/mL) • Persistently normal AST/ALT; absence of significant hepatitis on biopsy

ALT = alanine aminotransferase; AST = aspartate aminotransferase; HBcAg = hepatitis B core antigen; HBeAg = hepatitis B early antigen; HBsAg = hepatitis B surface antigen; HBV = hepatitis B virus; LFT = liver function test; ULN = upper limit of normal.

2. Treatment of chronic infection
    a. Treatment recommendations (Hepatology 2009;50:1–36)
        i. Patients who are HBeAg positive with elevated ALT concentrations and compensated liver disease should be observed for 3–6 months for spontaneous conversion from HBeAg positive to anti-HBeAg negative before initiating treatment. Antiviral treatment should be considered in patients whose ALT remains greater than 2 times the upper limit of normal and whose HBV DNA is more than 20,000 IU/mL.
        ii. Patients who are HBeAg negative with positive anti-HBe as well as normal ALT and HBV less than 2000 IU/mL should be monitored every 3 months for 1 year and then every 6–12 months if they remain in the inactive carrier state.
    b. Patients who meet the criteria for chronic infection as outlined previously should be treated. Choice of initial therapy is based on patient profile, prior treatments, and contraindications to drug therapy and medication/monitoring costs.
    c. Monitoring for efficacy should be based on the following responses:
        i. Biochemical: ↓ liver function tests to within the normal range
        ii. Virologic: ↓ HBV DNA to undetectable concentrations and loss of HBeAg if HBeAg positive
            (A) A primary nonresponse is considered a decrease in HBV DNA less than 2 log/mL after at least 24 weeks of therapy. Patients NOT meeting these criteria should receive an alternative treatment.
            (B) Response should be assessed by reductions in HBV DNA for HBeAg negative patients
3. Drug therapies
    a. Interferon alfa/pegylated interferon
        i. Cytokine with antiviral, antiproliferative, and immunomodulatory effects
        ii. Best predictors of response to treatment are high pretreatment ALT, low-serum HBV DNA, presence of active inflammation on biopsy, and acquisition of infection as an adult HBeAg-negative disease responds less favorably to IFN.
        iii. Dosing: Use traditional agents: HBeAg positive: typical dose is 5 MU/day subcutaneously × 16–24 weeks or 10 MU subcutaneously 3 times/week × 16–24 weeks; patients with HBeAg negative disease should be treated for 12 months. Use of PEG α-2a (Pegasys): 180 mcg subcutaneously once weekly × 48 weeks (duration is same for HBeAg antigen negative and positive disease)
        iv. In general, response to traditional IFN is poor; 37% loss of HBV surface antigen, 33% loss of HBV early antigen with 12–24 weeks of treatment; this equates to about 20% better than placebo. Some trials suggest that PEG-IFN has only slightly better efficacy in HBV early antigen–positive disease, with 25% loss of HBV DNA and 30% loss of HBV early antigen at 48 weeks. Adherence may be better based on less-frequent dosing.
        v. If a response is obtained, it is usually long lasting (more than 4–8 years).
        vi. Treatment with IFN typically results in an increase in ALT 4–8 weeks into treatment. This is an expected response; it should not be viewed as an adverse effect of therapy.

Table 18. Available INFα Products

Product	IFN Subtype	Route of Administration	Dosage Form(s)
Roferon A[1]	α-2a	SQ or IM	Single-dose vial (36 MU/mL) Multidose vial (18 MU/vial) Prefilled syringe (3, 6, 9 MU/0.5 mL)
Infergen	Acon-1	SQ	Single-dose vials 9 mcg (0.3 mL), 15 (0.5 mL)
Intron[1]	α-2b	SQ or IM	Powder, solution, multidose pen
PEG-Intron	PEG α-2b	SQ	Single-dose vials (2 mL) + diluent 50, 80, 120, 150 mcg/0.5 mL Single-use REDIPEN 50, 80, 120, 150 mcg/0.5 mL
Pegasys[1]	PEG α-2a	SQ	Single-dose vial (1 mL) 180 mcg/mL Prefilled 180 mcg syringes (4/pack)

[1] Preferred for HBV.

IM = intramuscular; INFα = interferon alfa; PEG = pegylated; SQ = subcutaneous.

      vii. Adverse effects
         (A) Interferon is associated with many serious adverse effects.
            (1) Bone marrow suppression (J Clin Gastroenterol 2005;39:S9–S13)
                (a) Leukopenia: May use filgrastim (granulocyte colony-stimulating factor) for support
                (b) Thrombocytopenia: Minimal data with oprelvekin (interleukin-11). Not used because of many adverse effects including pulmonary hypertension
         (B) Predisposition to infections
         (C) Central nervous system: Depression, psychosis, anxiety, insomnia, seizures. Adverse CNS effects occur in 22%–31% of patients.
         (D) Flulike symptoms (tolerance usually develops after a few weeks)
         (E) Anorexia, alopecia, thyroid dysfunction, neuropathy
         (F) Exacerbation of underlying autoimmune disorders (i.e., thyroid)
         (G) Ischemic/hemorrhagic cerebrovascular disorders
         (H) Serious hypersensitivity and rash formation
         (I) Manufacturers give recommendations for dose reductions in patients who develop bone marrow suppression and depression while on therapy.
         (J) Contraindicated in patients with a history of current psychosis, severe depression, neutropenia, thrombocytopenia, symptomatic heart disease, decompensated liver disease, and uncontrolled seizures; also, use caution in patients with autoimmune disorders
    b. Reverse transcriptase inhibitors
      i. In general, lamivudine and telbivudine are not preferred as first-line therapies because of high rates of resistance.
      ii. All reverse transcriptase inhibitors carry a black box warning for the development of lactic acidosis and severe hepatomegaly with steatosis, Monitor for worsening liver function tests, and periodically assess renal function. Female and obese patients are at higher risk.
      iii. Lamivudine (Epivir-HBV)

(A) Reduces HBV DNA by 3–4 log
(B) Dose: 100 mg/day orally (tablets or solution) for at least 1 year (HBeAg negative and positive); dose is 150 mg orally 2 times/day for patients with HIV coinfection; doses require adjustment for reduced renal function
(C) Efficacy: 17%–32% loss of HBV early antigen and 41%–72% normalization of ALT at 52 weeks; may be used for INF failures and patients with decompensated liver disease
(D) Toxicity: Well tolerated (headache, nausea, vomiting, fatigue), rare lactic acidosis
(E) Resistance: Prolonged use is associated with development of mutations in the YMDD sequence of the HBV polymerase (20% at 1 year, 70% at 4 years). Risk factors for lamivudine resistance include elevated pretherapy HBV DNA or ALT, male sex, increased body mass index, previous exposure to lamivudine or famciclovir, and inadequate suppression on HBV DNA after 6 months of treatment.
(F) Therapy discontinuation is often accompanied by rebound liver function test elevations; viral breakthrough may also be evident during treatment.

iv. Adefovir (Hepsera)
(A) Reduces HBV DNA by 2–4 log
(B) Indicated in HBeAg positive and negative disease, as well as in decompensated liver disease; also effective in lamivudine-resistant YMDD mutants and IFN failures
(C) Dose: 10 mg orally every day for at least 1 year HBeAg negative and –positive disease)
(D) Efficacy: Up to 72% normalization of ALT and 12% loss of HBeAg at 48 weeks
(E) Toxicity: Renal dysfunction (3%), headache, nausea, vomiting, fatigue, rare lactic acidosis
(F) Therapy discontinuation is often accompanied by rebound liver function test elevations; viral breakthrough may also be evident during treatment. Resistance reported as 29% at 5 years

v. Entecavir (Baraclude)
(A) Indicated for HBeAg negative and positive patients with persistently elevated AST/ALT or histologically active disease. Effective in lamivudine-resistant YMDD mutants
(B) Reduces HBV DNA by up to 6.86 log in HBeAg positive naïve patients and by 5.2 log in HBeAg negative patients or those with lamivudine resistance
(C) Dose: 0.5 mg orally once daily for individuals older than 16 years and nucleoside naïve; 1 mg orally once daily for patients older than 16 years with HBV viremia while receiving lamivudine or in lamivudine-resistant HBV
(D) Dose adjustments required for renal impairment
(E) Toxicity: Similar to lamivudine with headache, cough, upper respiratory infection, abdominal pain; possibly fewer ALT flares. Rare lactic acidosis. Resistance reported as similar to 1% at 5 years.

vi. Telbivudine (Tyzeka)
(A) Indicated for HBeAg negative and positive patients with persistently elevated AST/ALT or histologically active disease
(B) Not effective in lamivudine-resistant YMDD mutants
(C) A direct comparison with lamivudine (GLOBE trial) showed greater efficacy in both HBeAg negative and positive patients.

(D) Reduces HBV DNA by up to 6.45 log in HBeAg positive naïve patients and by 5.2 log in HBeAg negative patients
(E) Dose: 600 mg orally once daily. Dose adjustments required for renal impairment
(F) Toxicity: Similar to lamivudine; small incidence of myopathy. Creatine kinase elevations greater than 7 × upper limit of normal 9% for telbivudine versus 3% with lamivudine in the GLOBE study. Rare lactic acidosis. Resistance reported as 25% at 2 years

vii. Tenofovir (Viread)
(A) Nucleotide analog, formulated as tenofovir disoproxil fumarate indicated for chronic HBV infection
(B) Effective for lamivudine-resistant HBV
(C) A direct comparison with adefovir for 48 weeks showed greater viral suppression to less than 400 copies/mL plus histologic improvement for tenofovir compared with adefovir in HBeAg positive patients (66% vs. 12%; p<0.001) and HBeAg negative patients (71% vs. 49%; p<0.001) (N Engl J Med 2008;359:2442–55). Dose: 300 mg orally once daily. Dose adjustments required for renal impairment
(D) Toxicity: Overall, well tolerated. Headache, nausea, and nasopharyngitis most commonly reported. Potential renal toxicity, so periodic monitoring of serum creatinine recommended. Potential ALT flares on withdrawal. Rare lactic acidosis.

Table 19. Summary of Treatment Recommendations for Chronic HBV Infection in Adults

HBV Population	Preferred Treatment Options	Duration	Comments
HBeAg positive	Entecavir and tenofovir are preferred oral agents Use of the other oral reverse transcriptase inhibitors is possible but not preferred	Minimum of 1 year	• Preferred if contraindications or nonresponse to INFα
	INFα PEG INFα	16 weeks 48 weeks	• If contraindication or no response, use entecavir and tenofovir
HBeAg negative	Entecavir and tenofovir are preferred oral agents Use of the other oral reverse transcriptase inhibitors is possible but not preferred	> 1 year	• Preferred if contraindications or no response to INFα
	INFα PEG INFα	≥ 1 year	• If contraindication or nonresponse, use entecavir and tenofovir
Development of resistant HBV	<u>Lamivudine or telbivudine resistance:</u> add adefovir or tenofovir or change to entecavir <u>Adefovir resistance:</u> add lamivudine Entecavir resistance: change to tenofovir	N/A	• Confirm resistance with genotypic testing • Reinforce adherence to therapy

HBeAg = hepatitis B early antigen; HBV = hepatitis B virus; INFα = interferon alfa; N/A = not applicable; PEG = pegylated.

4. Preventive strategies
    a. Vaccination (preexposure)
        i. Indicated in the following groups:
            (A) All infants born to HBV surface antigen–negative mothers
            (B) Adolescents with high-risk behavior (intravenous drug abuse, multiple sex partners)
            (C) Workers with possible occupational risk of exposure
            (D) Staff and clients at institutions for the developmentally disabled
            (E) Hemodialysis patients
            (F) Patients receiving clotting factor concentrates
            (G) Household contacts and sex partners of infected patients
            (H) Adoptees from countries where HBV infection is endemic
            (I) International travelers (more than 6 months' travel in an endemic area, short-term travel if contact with blood in a medical setting is expected, or sexual contact with residents in areas of intermediate- to high-endemic disease); series of vaccinations started 6 months before travel

(J) Injection drug users
(K) Sexually active homosexual or bisexual men, as well as heterosexual men and women
(L) Patients seeking treatment of a sexually transmitted disease
(M) Inmates of long-term correctional facilities
(N) Patients with chronic HIV infection or chronic liver disease
(O) All other individuals seeking protection from HBV infection
  b. Available HBV vaccines (dose schedules vary by age)
     i. Dose schedules

Table 20.

Patient and Age Groups		Recombivax HB		Engerix-B		Schedule
		Dose (mcg)	Volume (mL)	Dose (mcg)	Volume (mL)	
Infants (< 1 year)		5	0.5	10	0.5	Most common schedule is 3 IM doses at 0, 1, and 6 months
Children (1–10 years)		5	0.5	10	0.5	
Adolescents	11–15 years	10	1	N/A	N/A	
	11–19 years	5	0.5	10	0.5	Variations in schedule may occur depending on age and medical history
Adults	≥ 20 years	10	1	20	1	
Hemodialysis patients and other immuno-compromised individuals	< 20 years	5	0.5	10	0.5	
	> 20 years	40	1	40	2	

IM = intramuscular; N/A = not applicable.

     ii. Obtain titers 1–2 months after third dose of the series for health care personnel.
     iii. Hepatitis B virus vaccines are available as combination products with HAV (Twinrix), DTP/IPV (Pediarix), and Hib (Comvax). Avoid Twinrix in patients with HIV.
  c. Postexposure prophylaxis
     i. Exposure may result in the need for HBV vaccine and/or immune globulin.
     ii. Doses of HBV immune globulin are 0.06 mL/kg intramuscularly and must be given within 7 days of exposure.
     iii. Patient populations requiring postexposure prophylaxis
        (A) Perinatal transmission
           (1) Children born to HBV surface antigen–positive mothers should receive vaccine plus HBV immune globulin within 12 hours of birth.
           (2) Children born to mothers with unknown HBV surface antigen status (but suspected) should receive vaccine within 12 hours of birth; testing should be performed on child and, if positive, HBV immune globulin should be administered within 1 week.
           (3) Infants weighing less than 2 kg at birth whose mothers are documented to be HBV surface antigen negative should receive the first dose of vaccine 1 month after birth or at hospital discharge, whichever comes first.
        (B) Sexual contact or household contact with an infected person: Should receive HBV immune globulin plus vaccine series if exposed person is previously unvaccinated

(C) Sexual contact or household contact with an HBV carrier: Should receive vaccine series if exposed person was previously unvaccinated

D. Hepatitis C Virus
  1. Background
     a. RNA virus: Six genotypes (50 subtypes)
        i. Genotype 1 (subtypes 1a, 1b, 1c) accounts for 70%–75% of infections in the United States.
        ii. Genotypes 2 (subtypes 2a, 2b, 2c) and 3 (3a, 3b) are common in the United States.
        iii. Genotype helps determine therapy duration and likelihood of responding to therapy.
     b. Leading cause of liver disease and liver transplantation in the United States; also, a common cause of hepatocellular carcinoma
     c. Viral replication occurs in the hepatocyte (virus is not directly cytopathic).
     d. Transmission: Mainly bloodborne (transfusion, intravenous drug abuse)
        i. High risk:
           (A) Transfusion, intravenous drug abuse abuse
        ii. Low risk:
           (A) Snorting cocaine or other drugs
           (B) Occupational exposure
           (C) Body piercing and acupuncture with un-sterilized needle
           (D) Tattooing
           (E) From pregnant mother to child
           (F) Nonsexual household contacts (rare)
           (G) Sharing razors and/or toothbrushes
           (H) Sexual transmission
     e. Associated with acute and chronic infection; after acute infection, most patients (60%–85%) will develop chronic infection
  2. Clinical features: About 30% of patients are asymptomatic.
     a. Acute infection: Symptoms present 4–12 weeks after exposure; most patients are asymptomatic and seldom progress to fulminant disease; those who develop symptoms have nonspecific findings such as malaise, weakness, anorexia, and jaundice.
     b. Chronic infection: Defined as the presence of viral RNA in the serum for 6 months or more
        i. May be associated with the long-term development of end-stage liver disease, cirrhosis, hepatocellular carcinoma
        ii. Progression to complications and end-stage liver disease may be accelerated by concurrent alcohol use and coinfection with HIV; younger females have slower progression.
     c. Extrahepatic manifestations: Rheumatoid symptoms, glomerulonephritis, cryoglobulinemia
  3. Diagnosis and monitoring
     a. Clinical signs/symptoms such as nausea, abdominal pain, jaundice, fever, malaise, or anorexia. Many patients have asymptomatic disease.
     b. Laboratory
        i. Serum anti-HCV antibodies: 99% sensitivity/specificity (enzyme immunoassays)
           (A) Used as an initial screening for HCV; presence of anti-HCV antibody does not confer protective immunity from subsequent infection
        ii. Serum HCV RNA

(A) Obtain in patients who test positive for anti-HCV antibodies.
(B) Quantitative: "Viral load" typically polymerase chain reaction reported in international units per milliliter; obtain for patients who will receive treatment; for use in monitoring treatment response. Preferred assays for diagnosis and monitoring of drug therapy
(C) Qualitative: Typically polymerase chain reaction; lower limit of detection of 50 IU/mL (equivalent to 100 copies/mL) preferred (specificity is about 98%); typically used to confirm diagnosis in patients who are HCV antibody positive. The AASLD guidelines state that there is no longer a need for qualitative assays. Quantitative assays are preferred.

Table 21. Definitions and Monitoring of Chronic HCV Treatment Based on HCV RNA

Parameter	Definition
Rapid virologic response (RVR)	Undetectable HCV RNA at week 4 of treatment
Early virologic response (EVR)	> 2-log reduction in HCV RNA compared with baseline or undetectable HCV RNA at 12 weeks
End of treatment response (ETR)	Undetectable HCV RNA at the end of a 24- or 48-week course depending on genotype
Sustained virologic response (SVR)	Undetectable HCV RNA 24 weeks after finishing treatment
Breakthrough	Reappearance of HCV RNA while on treatment
Relapse	Reappearance of HCV RNA after finishing a course of treatment
Nonresponder	Failure to clear HCV RNA from serum after 24 weeks of therapy
Null responder	Failure to decrease HCV RNA by < 2 log after 24 weeks of therapy
Partial responder	Decrease in HCV RNA by > 2 log after 24 weeks of therapy but HCV RNA still detectable

HCV = hepatitis C virus.

    iii. Liver biopsy: Consider if patient and health care provider wish to obtain information regarding fibrosis stage or prognostic purposes or to make a decision regarding treatment. Alanine aminotransferase: Nonspecific; may fluctuate with chronic disease (should decrease with treatment)
    iv. Genotyping: Genotype 1 is the most common genotype in the United States; it is also the least responsive to treatment; genotypes 2 and 3 comprise the other two most common genotypes in the United States.
    v. Treatment response is dependent on other factors such as race, age, or coinfection, among others.
4. Treatment
  a. Acute HCV infection
    i. Patients with acute HCV should be considered for INF-based therapy, preferably with PEG-INFα for 12–24 weeks. Adding ribavirin may be considered, but it is not clear that this improves sustained virologic response (SVR) rates.
    ii. Alternatively, treatment may be delayed for 8–12 weeks to assess for spontaneous resolution.
    iii. Main benefit of treatment is prevention of chronic infection.
  b. Chronic infection (Hepatology 2009;49:1335–64, 2009;39:1147–71)
    i. Therapy goal is to attain an SVR.

ii. Indications for the treatment of patients who are treatment naïve
   (A) Age older than 18 years and positive serum HCV RNA
   (B) Portal or bridging fibrosis with at least moderate inflammation/necrosis on biopsy
   (C) Compensated liver disease, acceptable hemoglobin (13 g/dL men, 12 g/dL women) and neutrophils (more than 1500/mm^3), serum creatinine less than 1.5 mg/dL
   (D) Willingness to be treated and to be adherent
   (E) No contraindications to therapy
iii. Difficult patient populations that require individualized therapy
   (A) Normal ALT (treatment dependent on genotype, degree of fibrosis, symptoms)
   (B) Liver biopsy indicating no or mild fibrosis
   (C) Advanced liver disease (fibrosis or decompensated cirrhosis)
   (D) Recurrence after liver transplantation
   (E) Patients younger than 18 years
   (F) Coinfection with HIV or HBV
   (G) Chronic kidney disease
   (H) Users of alcohol or illicit drugs who are willing to participate in substance abuse treatment programs
   (I) Nonresponder or relapser
iv. Contraindications to treatment of chronic HCV
   (A) Major uncontrolled depressive disorder
   (B) Solid-organ transplantation (renal, heart, lung)
   (C) Autoimmune hepatitis or other autoimmune conditions
   (D) Untreated thyroid disease
   (E) Pregnant or unwilling to adhere to adequate contraception
   (F) Severe concurrent medical disease (hypertension, heart failure, coronary heart disease, poorly controlled diabetes mellitus, chronic obstructive pulmonary disease)
   (G) Age younger than 2 years
   (H) Hypersensitivity to INF or ribavirin

c. Ribavirin in the treatment of HCV infection
   (A) Oral nucleoside analog
   (B) Available as 200-mg tablets (Copegus) or capsules (Rebetol) (generic now available)
   (C) Significant adverse effect profile
      (1) Hemolytic anemia: May occur in up to 10% of patients (usually within 1–2 weeks of initiating therapy): may worsen underlying cardiac disease; monitor complete blood cell count at baseline, 2 weeks, 4 weeks, and periodically thereafter. In patients with no cardiac history, decrease dose to 600 mg/day when hemoglobin drops to 10 g/dL or less, and discontinue when hemoglobin drops to 8.5 g/dL or less. In patients with a cardiac history, decrease dose to 600 mg/day if hemoglobin drops more than 2 g/dL in any 4-week period during treatment. Discontinue if hemoglobin drops to less than 12 g/dL 4 weeks after dose reduction. May use epoetin or darbepoetin to stimulate red blood cell production, improve anemia (J Clin Gastroenterol 2005;39:S9–S13), and sustain initial starting dose. Also need to confirm iron studies are normal and within range during treatment
      (2) Teratogenicity: Category X drug. Requires a negative pregnancy test at

baseline and every month up to 6 months after treatment, as well as the use of two forms of barrier contraception during treatment and for 6 months after treatment. Applies to women taking the drug and female partners of male patients taking ribavirin
- (3) Contraindicated in patients with creatinine clearance less than 50 mL/minute and underlying hemoglobinopathies
- (4) Other possible adverse events include pancreatitis, pulmonary dysfunction (dyspnea, pulmonary infiltrate, and pneumonitis), insomnia, and pruritus.
- d. Recommendations from AASLD guidelines for the treatment of chronic HCV infection
  - (A) First-line therapy: PEG-IFN plus ribavirin
  - (B) Efficacy: 42%–46% SVR for genotype 1; 76%–82% SVR for genotype 2 or 3
  - (C) Factors associated with increased response: Genotype other than 1, lower initial HCV RNA (less than 600,000 IU/mL), minimal fibrosis/inflammation on biopsy, lower body weight or surface area, and non–African Americans.
- ii. Dosing of HCV treatment regimens
  - (A) Pegylated interferon
    - (1) Pegasys: 180 mcg/week subcutaneously
    - (2) PEG-Intron: 1–1.5 mcg/kg/week subcutaneously
  - (B) Ribavirin (Rebetol or Copegus 200-mg tablets or capsules) generic products are now available as well.
    - (1) Genotype 1:
      - (a) Copegus with Pegasys: 1200 mg/day in two divided doses (more than 75 kg); 1000 mg/day in two divided doses (less than 75 kg/day)
      - (b) Rebetol with PEG-Intron: 800 mg/day if less than 65 kg, 1000 mg/day if 65–85 kg, 1200 mg/day for 85–105 kg, 1400 mg/day if more than 105 kg
    - (2) Genotype 2 or 3: 800 mg/day in two divided doses
  - (C) Treatment duration
    - (1) Genotype 1:
      - (a) If patients do not achieve an early virologic response (EVR), retest viral load at week 24. If HCV RNA is positive; then treatment should be discontinued; individualized treatment may be considered according to tolerability, severity of liver disease, and demonstration of virologic response.
      - (b) If patients have delayed viral clearance, as evidenced by an undetectable HCV RNA concentration between weeks 12 and 24, then extend therapy to 72 weeks.
      - (c) If EVR is attained, treatment should be continued for a total of 48 weeks; HCV RNA should be rechecked at 48 weeks (ETR) and then 24 weeks later for evidence of SVR.
    - (2) Genotypes 2 and 3:
      - (a) Treat for 24 weeks.
- iii. Retreatment with PEG-INF plus ribavirin is not recommended in patients who did not achieve an SVR after a prior full course of therapy.
- iv. Retreatment with PEG-IFN plus ribavirin may be considered for nonresponders or relapsers previously treated with an unmodified INF with or without ribavirin or PEG-INF monotherapy if they have bridging fibrosis or cirrhosis.
- e. Prevention of HCV
  - i. No vaccine or immune globulin available

ii. Risk factor modification
- (A) Intravenous drug abuse: Methadone maintenance, syringe exchange
- (B) Sexual contact: Appropriate barrier contraception
- (C) Avoid blood exposure: Occupational (universal precautions) or other contact, such as sharing toothbrushes or razors or receiving a tattoo
- (D) The HAV and HBV vaccine to prevent further progression of liver disease

Patient Cases

9. A 45-year-old woman with a history of intravenous drug abuse is seen in the clinic for evaluation of chronic HBV infection. Although she was given the HBV diagnosis 8 months ago, she has not yet received treatment for it. Laboratory values reported today include HbSAg positive, HbeAg positive, AST 650 IU/mL, ALT 850 IU/mL, HBV DNA 107,000 IU/mL, serum creatinine 0.9 mg/dL, INR 1.3, and albumin 3.9 g/dL. She has no evidence of ascites or encephalopathy. A liver biopsy has revealed severe necroinflammation and bridging fibrosis. Resistance testing indicates the presence of the YMDD mutation. Which of the following is the best course of action?

    A. Withhold drug therapy and recheck HBV DNA in 6 months.
    B. Initiate PEG-IFNα-2a plus ribavirin.
    C. Initiate lamivudine 100 mg/day.
    D. Initiate tenofovir 10 mg/day.

10. A new enzyme immunoassay for HCV RNA has a reported sensitivity of 95% and a specificity of 92%. If the prevalence of HCV in a cohort of 500 patients is 40%, which one of the following is the positive predictive value of this new test?

    A. 75%.
    B. 89%.
    C. 92%.
    D. 96%.

11. A 38-year-old white man is being treated with PEG-IFNα-2b 1.5 mcg/kg/week subcutaneously, as well as ribavirin 400 mg in the morning and 600 mg in the evening for chronic HCV (genotype 1). The patient, who weighs 75 kg, is in the clinic today for his 12-week treatment follow-up. Pretreatment laboratory values included AST 350 IU/mL, ALT 420 IU/mL, and HCV RNA 450,000 IU/mL. Today's laboratory values include AST 90 IU/mL, ALT 64 IU/mL, and HCV RNA 3500 IU/mL. Which of the following is the best course of action?

    A. Discontinue therapy and monitor for symptoms.
    B. Continue treatment for another 12 weeks.
    C. Decrease dose of ribavirin to 800 mg/day.
    D. Continue treatment for an additional 72 weeks.

REFERENCES

Gastroesophageal Reflux Disease

1. American Gastroenterological Association Institute. Medical position statement on the management of gastroesophageal reflux disease. Gastroenterology 2008;135:1383–91.
2. American Gastroenterological Association Institute. Technical review on the management of gastroesophageal reflux disease. Gastroenterology 2008;135:1392–413.
3. Devault KR, Castell DO. Updated guidelines for the diagnosis and treatment of gastroesophageal reflux disease. Am J Gastroenterol 2005;100:190–200.

Peptic Ulcer Disease

1. Chey WD, Wong BVY. American College of Gastroenterology guidelines for the management of *Helicobacter pylori* infection. Am J Gastroenterol 2007;102:1808–25.
2. Lanza FL, Chan FKL, Quigley EMM, et al. Guidelines for the prevention of NSAID-ulcer complications. Am J Gastroenterol 2009;104:728–38.
3. Wilcox CM, Allison J, Benzuly K, et al. Consensus development conference on the use of non-steroidal anti-inflammatory agents, including cyclooxygenase inhibitors and aspirin. Clin Gastroenterol Hepatol 2006;4:1082–9.
4. ACCF/ACG/AHA 2008 Expert consensus document on reducing the gastrointestinal risks of antiplatelet therapy and NSAID use. Circulation 2008;118:1894–909.

Upper GI Bleeding

1. Barkun A, Bardou M, Marshall JK. Consensus recommendations for managing patients with non-variceal upper gastrointestinal bleeding. Ann Intern Med 2003;139:843–57.
2. Zed PJ, Loewen PS, Slavik RS, Marra CA. Meta-analysis of proton-pump inhibitors in treatment of bleeding peptic ulcer. Ann Pharmacother 2001;35:1528–34.
3. Dallal HJ, Palmer KR. Upper gastrointestinal bleeding. BMJ 2001;323:1115–6.

Inflammatory Bowel Disease

1. Kornbluth A, Sachar DB. Ulcerative practice guidelines in adults (update): American College of Gastroenterology, Practice Parameters Committee. Am J Gastroenterol 2004;99:1371–85.
2. Lichtenstein GR, Hanauer SB, Sandborn WJ, and The Practice Parameters Committee of the American College of Gastroenterology. Management of Crohn's disease in adults. Am J Gastroenterol 2009;104:465–83.
3. American Gastroenterological Association Institute. Technical review on corticosteroids, immunomodulators, and infliximab in inflammatory bowel disease. Gastroenterology 2006;130:940–87.

Complications of Liver Disease

1. Garcia-Tsao G, Lim J; and Members of the Veterans Affairs Hepatitis C Resource Center Program. Management and treatment of patients with cirrhosis and portal hypertension: recommendations from the Department of Veterans Affairs Hepatitis C Resource Center Program and the National Hepatitis C. Am J Gastroenterol 2009;104:1802–29.
2. Runyon BA. Management of adult patients with ascites due to cirrhosis: an update. Hepatology 2009;49:2087–107.
3. Blei AT, Cordoba J. Hepatic encephalopathy. Am J Gastroenterol 2001;96:1968–76.

Viral Hepatitis

1. Update: Prevention of hepatitis A after exposure to hepatitis A virus and in international travelers. Updated recommendations of the Advisory Committee on Immunization Practices (ACIP). MMWR 2007;56:1080–4.
2. Lok A, McMahon BJ. Chronic hepatitis B: update 2009. Hepatology 2009;50:1–36.
3. Centers for Disease Control and Prevention. Updated U.S. Public Health Service guidelines for the management of occupational exposures to HBV, HCV, and HIV and recommendations for postexposure prophylaxis. MMWR 2001;50(RR11):1–52.

4. Centers for Disease Control and Prevention. A comprehensive immunization strategy to eliminate transmission of hepatitis B virus infection in the United States: recommendations of the Advisory Committee on Immunization Practices (ACIP). Part 1. Immunization of infants, children, and adolescents. MMWR 2005;54(RR16):1–23.

5. Centers for Disease Control and Prevention. A comprehensive immunization strategy to eliminate transmission of hepatitis B virus infection in the United States: recommendations of the Advisory Committee on Immunization Practices (ACIP). Part II. Immunization of adults. MMWR 2006;54(RR16):1–40.

6. Centers for Disease Control and Prevention. Recommendations for identification and public health management of persons with chronic hepatitis B virus infection. MMWR 2008;57(RR08):1–20.

7. Ghany MG, Strader DB, Thomas DL, Seef LB. Diagnosis, management, and treatment of hepatitis C: an update. Hepatology 2009;49:1335–64.

ANSWERS AND EXPLANATIONS TO PATIENT CASES

1. Answer B

Those who assess patients resistant to medical therapy should try to identify exacerbating drug and disease factors. Proper use of medications, such as PPIs, is a key factor in ensuring that medical therapy is maximized. Patients should be instructed to take PPIs 30 minutes before a meal and to take their evening dose before their evening meal rather than at bedtime. Endoscopic evaluation is appropriate for patients older than 45 years; however, many patients will have normal-appearing mucosa. For patients with normal-appearing mucosa and continued symptoms despite medical therapy, evaluation with manometry is useful to exclude potential esophageal motility disorders. Prokinetic agents facilitate gastric emptying; in the past, they have been cited as having efficacy similar to H_2RAs. Metoclopramide use is not recommended as adjunctive therapy or monotherapy because of the increased risk of adverse neurologic events, such as tardive dyskinesia, compared with the potential benefit, as evidenced by the Grade D attained in the most recent GERD treatment guidelines. Furthermore, use of dopamine antagonists, such as metoclopramide, should be avoided in patients with Parkinson disease because they may worsen symptoms and cause extrapyramidal adverse effects. Use of combined H_2RAs and PPI therapy most likely will not result in substantial added symptom relief and is not recommended in the GERD guidelines (Evidence Grade: Insufficient). Surgical intervention is an appropriate intervention in patients intolerant of, or not responding to, medical therapy with PPIs. Motility disorders are a relative contraindication to antireflux surgery, so this patient should be first invested using manometry and possible pH testing before surgical intervention.

2. Answer C

The two most common causes of peptic ulcer disease are *H. pylori* and NSAID use. This patient has a gastric ulcer with evidence of a clot (indicating recent bleeding) in the setting of multiple NSAID use (aspirin plus ketoprofen). In addition, she is older than 60 years, which is another risk factor for an NSAID-induced ulcer. This most likely is contributing to her upper GI complaints and anemia. The rapid urease test performed on the biopsy specimen is negative, indicating the absence of *H. pylori*. First, the patient should discontinue NSAID use. Continued NSAID use can markedly delay healing; therefore, it should only be continued if necessary. Healing of the ulcer should be facilitated by appropriate acid-suppressive therapy. Histamine$_2$-receptor antagonists, although effective in some instances, are less efficacious in the healing of gastric ulcers than PPIs, making Answer A incorrect. Because the patient has tested negative for *H. pylori,* use of an *H. pylori* eradication regimen is not required; therefore, Answer B is incorrect. Misoprostol, which is effective in preventing and healing ulcers, is not preferred secondary to the need for several daily doses, and it is very poorly tolerated because of a high incidence of abdominal pain, cramping, and diarrhea. The PPIs are the preferred drugs for healing NSAID-induced ulcers because of their excellent efficacy and favorable adverse effect profile, and they are better tolerated, making Answer C correct.

3. Answer C

The test-and-treat approach is appropriate in dyspeptic patients suspected of having *H. pylori* infections. Patients older than 45–55 years, or those with alarm features, should be referred for endoscopic evaluation to rule out the possibility of a more complicated disease. Ambulatory patients can be tested for *H. pylori* using various diagnostic approaches, such as the urea breath test. The eradication of *H. pylori* leads to high rates of ulcer healing and minimizes ulcer recurrence. According to treatment guidelines, eradication regimens for *H. pylori* infection should include at least two antibiotics plus an antisecretory agent given for 10–14 days. This can be accomplished with triple-drug therapies containing amoxicillin (or metronidazole) plus clarithromycin in addition to a PPI. Likewise, quadruple therapy with bismuth, tetracycline, metronidazole, and a PPI can be used first line in penicillin-allergic patients or as a second-line treatment of initial failures of triple-drug therapy. This patient requires treatment secondary to a positive test. Because he reports a penicillin allergy, Answer A would not be appropriate. Answer B would not be viable because cephalosporins are not recommended in *H. pylori* treatment regimens. Answer D would be incorrect because fluoroquinolone-based regimens should be reserved as salvage therapy for patients in whom triple and quadruple therapy has failed, making Answer C correct; quadruple therapy offers similar efficacy and is a viable option in penicillin-allergic patients. Patient adherence should be reinforced to maximize efficacy.

4. Answer D

Several different forms of bias exist that may adversely affect the validity or results of a trial. Errors in sampling or measurement, incorrect methodology in patient enrollment, or differences in patient populations studied in a trial are examples of areas of study design and conduction that may introduce bias. When evaluating drug literature, an important aspect of deciding whether the reported results are valid is to recognize important causes of bias. A retrospective cohort design typically uses medical records to evaluate events that occurred in the past after exposure to a drug. Recall bias pertains to study outcomes or events that patients are asked to recall, with results differing depending on the ability of patients to remember an event. For this study, objective documentation of ulceration or bleeding was performed to make comparisons between groups, eliminating patient recall as a potential bias. Misclassification bias is typically problematic in case-control studies, where patients may be entered in the case study group but not have had actual exposure to the drug in question, which would not be applicable in this case. Interviewer bias, also known as observer bias, is typically problematic in direct patient survey studies and pertains to variation in the way different investigators collect data within a trial. To eliminate this, everyone involved in data collection in a study should be appropriately trained in the same manner of data collection to maintain consistency. Again, because an objective measure of GI toxicity was recorded by endoscopy, the possibility of interviewer bias is minimized. Channeling bias is a form of allocation bias, in which medications with similar therapeutic indications are administered to patients with differing prognoses or risk levels. Should claims be made that a new drug introduced to a therapeutic class has particular advantages – in this case, a safer GI toxicity profile – then the chance that use will be channeled to high-risk patients is much greater. Given that the drug may be studied in higher-risk patients versus the comparator group, the development of more events in this newer drug group may mask potential differences in safety and cause these events to be attributed to drug-induced toxicity.

5. Answer C

This represents a "steroid-dependent" patient, as evidenced by the inability to withdraw prednisone without exacerbation of his disease. Corticosteroids have no role in the long-term maintenance of inflammatory bowel disease; however, many patients often become steroid-dependent. Initiating a maintenance drug such as infliximab or azathioprine that has steroid-sparing effects would be best. The onset of action is slow for azathioprine and may take 3–15 months to achieve full efficacy. Infliximab, which would work much faster, can be dosed intermittently by intravenous infusion. Changing aminosalicylates would be possible; however, balsalazide is as effective as sulfasalazine, with a lower incidence of adverse effects. Methotrexate has shown efficacy in active Crohn's disease, but not UC. Combination treatment with systemic and topical therapy (such as a suppository) is a more effective option for patients with distal disease who are experiencing severe rectal symptoms, as in ulcerative proctitis.

6. Answer D

This patient is experiencing a severe-to-fulminant flare of her Crohn's disease, as evidenced by more than 10 bloody bowel movements a day, fever, tachycardia, and abdominal pain. She takes maintenance doses of mesalamine at home. Given the acuity of her symptoms, she requires rapid suppression of her inflammation. Increasing the amount of aminosalicylate she takes to a remission dose would be appropriate if she had mild to moderate active disease. The next step in quickly suppressing inflammation would be to use corticosteroid therapy. Oral therapy would be preferred for moderate to severe disease; however, this patient most likely needs high-dose intravenous therapy with the equivalent of 300 mg/day of hydrocortisone for up to 7 days. Corticosteroids work fastest to suppress inflammation in patients with active disease. Attempts to taper after 7 days would be appropriate because corticosteroids have no role in maintenance therapy. Intravenous cyclosporine would be reserved for patients who have not responded to high-dose steroids, although surgical intervention would be preferred in patients for whom medical therapy has failed or for those with emergencies, such as toxic megacolon.

7. Answer B

Treatment of acute hepatic encephalopathy is targeted at reducing NH_3 and nitrogenous waste production from the GI tract, as well as removing potential precipitating factors. Options for reducing NH_3 production include oral lactulose or neomycin. Both are equally effective; however, lactulose 30–45 mL titrated to two or three loose bowel movements a day is generally preferred as first-line therapy. Given that the patient has underlying renal insufficiency, long-term use of oral neomycin, as well as short-term use of nephrotoxic agents such as gentamicin, should be avoided. Discontinuation of CNS-active agents, such as narcotics and benzodiazepines, should be attempted because they may precipitate and worsen encephalopathy. Narcotic use also contributes to constipation, which can precipitate encephalopathy. The patient may need benzodiazepine therapy for withdrawal; however, symptom-triggered therapy using a protocol such as the CIWA (Clinical Institute Withdrawal Assessment) scale is preferred. Propranolol, which may be used to prevent variceal bleeding and treat hypertension, should be discontinued only if it is thought to be contributing to the patient's altered mental status.

8. Answer C
Management of acute variceal bleeding should initially involve patient stabilization and fluid resuscitation. Endoscopic therapy in combination with pharmacologic therapy targeting reductions in portal pressure is the most effective strategy for acutely discontinuing bleeding and preventing rebleeding. The somatostatin analog octreotide administered as a continuous infusion for 5 days reduces portal pressures with minimal adverse effects in patients with variceal bleeding. Vasopressin is also effective in reducing portal pressure but is associated with peripheral vasoconstriction. Therefore, it should be given in combination with nitroglycerin. This patient has coronary artery disease, which also makes vasopressin less favorable to use. Nonselective β-blockers are used in the primary and secondary prevention of variceal bleeding and have no role in acute management. Initiating β-blocker therapy may worsen associated hypotension from blood loss. She would likely benefit from β-blocker therapy on discharge to prevent variceal rebleeding, as well as for post–myocardial infarction prevention. Acid suppression with an intravenous PPI is indicated in the setting of nonvariceal upper GI bleeding or possibly for stress ulcer prophylaxis in patients with contraindications to H_2RAs.

9. Answer D
This patient has evidence of chronic HBV infection based on elevations in ALT/AST, presence of HBV surface antigen, and high concentrations of circulating HBV DNA, as well as evidence of severe necroinflammation on biopsy. The patient has HBV early antigen positivity, and a YMDD mutation is present. She appears to have compensated liver disease based on her albumin, INR, and lack of ascites or encephalopathy. Given her persistently elevated liver function tests, biopsy results, and high viral load, she should receive treatment. Treatment with an oral reverse transcriptase inhibitor is preferred first-line therapy. Interferon and ribavirin are preferred for chronic HCV infection. Given that the patient has a lamivudine-resistant organism, as evidenced by the presence of the YMDD mutation, a drug therapy that treats lamivudine-resistant pathogens, such as adefovir, is recommended as initial therapy.

10. Answer B
Positive predictive value tells you the proportion of patients with a disease when the presence of the disease is indicated by a diagnostic test. It is affected by disease prevalence; thus, as disease prevalence falls, so will the positive predictive value of the test. Using the sensitivity, specificity, and prevalence, a 2 × 2 table can be constructed. The positive predictive value is calculated by dividing the true positives by the sum of the true and false positives. In this case, that would be 190/(190 + 24) × 100 = 89%.

Result	Infection	No Infection	Total
Positive	190	24	214
Negative	10	276	286
Total	200	300	500

11. Answer B
Response to therapy for HCV is monitored mainly by reductions in HCV RNA. Genotype 1 is the least responsive to treatment, and HCV viral RNA should be monitored at 12 weeks after therapy to assess the attainment of an EVR. Patients with genotype 1 achieving an EVR can be treated for a total of 48 weeks, with HCV RNA rechecked at 48 weeks to assess for the attainment of an ETR, and again 24 weeks after the treatment course for evidence of SVR. For genotype 1, therapy should be discontinued if patients do not meet the criteria for EVR at week 24. For this patient, the viral load should be repeated at week 24 and, if still positive, discontinue therapy. If undetectable at week 24, then continue therapy for a total of 72 weeks.

ANSWERS AND EXPLANATIONS TO SELF-ASSESSMENT QUESTIONS

1. Answer: B
This patient is exhibiting signs of dysphagia, an "alarm" symptom that may be associated with a more complicated case of GERD. The patient has tried antacids with minimal relief and has a history of NSAID use. The patient is older than 45 years, which increases his risk of developing gastric cancer. Therefore, the patient should be referred for endoscopic evaluation to rule out a more complicated disease. Using either H$_2$RAs or PPI as initial therapy would be appropriate if the patient did not respond to antacids; however, a twice-daily dosing of PPIs is not necessary as initial dosing. Changing medications that reduce LES, such as calcium channel antagonists, is an appropriate recommendation for reducing GERD symptoms; this should be considered after invasive testing is performed.

2. Answer: C
For patients beginning chronic NSAID therapy, a thorough assessment of patient- or drug-related factors that may predispose them to the development of GI toxicity is necessary. Likewise, evaluation of the patient's level of CV risk is necessary. Based on the use of low-dose aspirin for preventing CV events, this patient would be considered at high risk of CV events. Efforts to avoid GI toxicity should include the use of the least GI-toxic agent at the lowest effective therapeutic dose. A GI-protective agent should highly be considered to minimize NSAID-induced erosions and ulcers. Indomethacin and piroxicam are more likely to cause GI complications than naproxen. Use of COX-2 inhibitors is acceptable in patients with rheumatoid arthritis because these agents have been shown to reduce GI complications and effectively treat pain. However, in this case, the patient has CV risk factors including diabetes, hypertension, and dyslipidemia. Recent findings of increased CV events, especially with high doses of COX-2 inhibitors, would preclude their use. Therapy with an acid-suppressive agent is also an acceptable choice for GI prevention in users of nonselective NSAIDs. Proton pump inhibitors are effective for this indication. The H$_2$RAs are ineffective in preventing serious NSAID-induced GI complications. Misoprostol, although effective, is associated with a high incidence of diarrhea and abdominal pain, as well as the need for multiple daily dosing. Given that this patient is considered moderate risk of GI complications based on the use of aspirin and need for high-dose NSAIDs, the use of naproxen plus a PPI would be preferred according to the recent ACG guidelines.

3. Answer: D
This patient presents with signs and symptoms consistent with an NSAID-induced upper GI bleed. He has several risk factors for NSAID-induced GI bleeding, including age older than 60 years, use of aspirin, and long duration of NSAID use. Presence of underlying CV disease, although not a direct risk factor, may also contribute to increases in NSAID GI toxicity. He also has many criteria that place him at high risk of rebleeding. Based on the consensus recommendations for nonvariceal bleeding, he should receive an intravenous PPI by bolus and subsequent continuous infusion for 72 hours. Note that in the guidelines provided, it states that this therapeutic approach can be extrapolated to patients with NSAID-induced ulcers and bleeding, even though most of the data included in the guidelines are related to non–NSAID-induced causes of upper GI bleeding. He will then require treatment at an appropriate dose of an oral PPI for at least 8 weeks; after that, he should be assessed for possible continued prophylactic use. Histamine$_2$-receptor antagonists have been shown to be less efficacious for the treatment and prevention of rebleeding for NSAID-induced ulcers. Sucralfate has minimal efficacy in the setting of acute GI bleeding; more often, its use is in the prevention of stress-related mucosal damage in critically ill patients. Oral PPIs are effective in preventing and healing NSAID-induced ulcers; however, in this case, the dose of lansoprazole is inadequate for treatment. Oral PPIs should be used at an appropriate dose after intravenous therapy.

4. Answer: D
Based on presenting symptoms, this patient would most likely be classified in the mild to moderate active disease category. First-line therapy for active extensive disease would consist of an oral aminosalicylate at a dose equivalent to 4.8 g/day of mesalamine. A product such as Asacol is formulated to release mesalamine in the colon, which would be appropriate in this case. Sulfasalazine has reported efficacy for this indication and is activated in the colon; however, this patient reports a life-threatening allergy to sulfonamide-containing medications. Topical therapy with hydrocortisone enema would be appropriate if the patient had disease distal to the splenic flexure. Immune modulators such as 6-MP have a long onset of action (3–15 months) and are not appropriate for acute active disease.

5. Answer: B

Primary prophylaxis of bleeding should be instituted in patients with large varices and cirrhosis. Nonselective β-blockers are appropriate as first-line therapy. Therapy should be targeted to achieve a PR of 55 beats/minute or a 25% reduction from baseline. The patient has been taking propranolol for 1 month and has not met these goals. Because he is tolerating the propranolol, the dose should be increased, and he should be observed to reassess the need for further dosage adjustments. Adding a nitrate would result in an increased reduction in portal pressures; however, it has not been shown to improve mortality. Most patients experience an increased risk of adverse effects with this combination. Nonselective β-blockers are preferred over $β_1$-selective agents because antagonism of the $β_2$-receptor prevents splanchnic vasodilation.

6. Answer: C

The sensitivity of a test can be thought of as the proportion of patients with a disease who have a positive test, whereas specificity deals with the proportion of patients without the disease who have a negative test. Calculating these values is accomplished by establishing a 2 × 2 table representing the results of the test. The sensitivity can be calculated by dividing the number of patients having the disease using the new test who were also positive using a gold standard test (true positives) – which, in this case, is 850 – by the total number of patients receiving a diagnosis of having the disease using the gold standard, which in this case is 900. The 900 represents the true positives as well as the 50 patients with the disease but without the diagnosis of it according to the new test (false negatives). Specificity can be calculated by taking the total number of patients not having the disease using the gold standard who tested negative with the new test (true negatives = 85). Then, divide this by the number of patients who truly had no disease using the gold standard, 100, which incorporates the 15 patients who tested positive with the new test but truly had no disease (i.e., false positives).
Sensitivity = 850/(850 + 50) = 94%; specificity = 85/(85 + 15) = 85%

Result	Infection	No Infection	Total
Positive	850	15	865
Negative	50	85	135
Total	900	100	1000

7. Answer: C

Postexposure therapy for HAV may be offered to restaurant patrons if a food handler at a restaurant is documented to have HAV and is considered infectious while handling food. The most effective therapies for postexposure prophylaxis are administration of HAV immune globulin or vaccine. The efficacy of the vaccine approaches that of immune globulin but only in patients younger than 40 according to the Centers for Disease Control and Prevention guidelines. The timeframe for administration should be within 14 days of exposure; therefore, this patient does not meet the criteria for receiving HAV immune globulin or vaccine. She should be observed for signs and symptoms of active disease. Hepatitis A vaccine should be offered to patients as preexposure therapy if they are considered at risk of exposure to HAV. The combination of vaccine and immune globulin for postexposure therapy is unnecessary.

8. Answer: C

Patients with cirrhosis and ascites are at risk of developing SBP, an infection of the ascitic fluid usually caused by an enteric gram-negative organism. Typical signs of infection include fever, abdominal pain, nausea, and rebound tenderness. Diagnosis is based on clinical symptoms plus laboratory evidence. The laboratory diagnosis is by paracentesis, with identification of more than 250/mm^3 neutrophils (polymorphonuclear neutrophils) in the ascitic fluid. This patient's value is 450/mm^3. Should clinical and laboratory signs and symptoms be present, antibiotic therapy directed against enteric gram-negative bacteria should be initiated. Third-generation cephalosporins such as cefotaxime or ceftriaxone are preferred. Aminoglycosides should be avoided because of their potential to cause nephrotoxicity. Vancomycin should be reserved for resistant gram-positive organisms. In addition to antibiotic therapy, use of intravenous albumin reduces the incidence of renal failure and improves in-hospital and 30-day mortality. Use of oral antibiotics for the treatment of acute SBP is not well studied; however, an oral regimen, such as norfloxacin or trimethoprim-sulfamethoxazole daily, should be instituted and continued indefinitely after recovery to reduce the incidence of subsequent infections.

9. Answer: D

The treatment of chronic HCV is PEG-IFN in combination with ribavirin. Genotypes 2 and 3 respond well to therapy. Although this patient appears to be responding to treatment, as evidenced by reductions in aminotransferases and HCV RNA, the earliest that HCV RNA should be evaluated is 4 weeks, not 2 weeks. Interferon therapy is associated with many adverse effects, such as flulike symptoms, CNS effects, leukopenia, and thrombocytopenia. This patient does not appear to be experiencing these types of symptoms or those consistent with extrahepatic manifestations of HCV, such as glomerulonephritis or rheumatologic disorders. The patient does have evidence of hemolysis, including scleral icterus, rapid decline in hematocrit, fatigue, and elevated indirect bilirubin. This most likely represents hemolytic anemia secondary to ribavirin, which commonly occurs within the first 2 weeks of therapy. Furthermore, there is no evidence that the drop in hematocrit is secondary to bleeding.

10. Answer: A
Infliximab is an appropriate agent for the treatment of fistulizing Crohn's disease. Because of its effects on tumor necrosis factor, latent infections such as tuberculosis may become reactivated during therapy. Therefore, patients should have a purified protein derivative placed or a QuantiFERON-TB test to rule out underlying tubercular disease before initiating treatment. Although infliximab therapy is associated with infusion-related reactions, administration of a test dose is not routinely recommended. Infliximab may be administered in a clinic setting; it does not require admission to the hospital for monitoring. Infliximab therapy is associated with exacerbations of underlying heart failure and is contraindicated in patients with New York Heart Association class III or IV disease. This patient is young, with no history of heart failure, and does not exhibit the clinical signs of heart failure. Therefore, a baseline echocardiogram is not necessary to assess cardiac function.

ONCOLOGY SUPPORTIVE CARE

LINDA R. BRESSLER, PHARM.D., BCOP
UNIVERSITY OF ILLINOIS
CHICAGO, ILLINOIS

ONCOLOGY SUPPORTIVE CARE

LINDA R. BRESSLER, PHARM.D., BCOP
UNIVERSITY OF ILLINOIS
CHICAGO, ILLINOIS

Learning Objectives:

1. Identify, assess, and recommend appropriate pharmacotherapy for managing common complications of cancer chemotherapy, including nausea and vomiting; myelosuppression and the appropriate use of growth factors; infection; anemia and fatigue; cardiotoxicity; and extravasation injury.

2. Assess and recommend appropriate pharmacotherapy for managing cancer-related pain.

3. Assess and recommend appropriate pharmacotherapy for managing oncologic emergencies, including hypercalcemia, hyperuricemia, and spinal cord compression.

Self-Assessment Questions:

Answers to these questions may be found at the end of this chapter.

1. A 50-year-old man is in the clinic today to receive his third cycle of cyclophosphamide, doxorubicin, vincristine, prednisone, and rituximab for non-Hodgkin lymphoma. He is very anxious and complains of nausea and vomiting lasting for about 12 hours after his previous cycle of chemotherapy. The antiemetic regimen he received for his previous cycle of chemotherapy was granisetron × 1 dose plus dexamethasone × 1 dose administered 30 minutes before chemotherapy. Which one of the following regimens should he receive on day 1 of the next cycle of chemotherapy?
    A. Granisetron × 1 dose + dexamethasone × 1 dose administered 30 minutes before chemotherapy.
    B. Dolasetron × 1 dose + dexamethasone × 1 dose administered 30 minutes before chemotherapy.
    C. Palonosetron × 1 dose + dexamethasone × 1 dose, + lorazepam × 1 dose administered 30 minutes before chemotherapy.
    D. Metoclopramide × 1 dose + dexamethasone × 1 dose + aprepitant × 1 dose administered 30 minutes before chemotherapy.

2. A 65-year-old man with metastatic non–small cell lung cancer is brought to the clinic by his family because of alterations in his mental status. Pertinent laboratory values include a serum calcium concentration of 12.0 mg/dL and an albumin concentration of 2.0 g/dL. Which one of the following therapies is best for this patient's altered mental status?

    A. Calcitonin 4 units/kg every 12 hours.
    B. Furosemide 20 mg orally.
    C. Dexamethasone 10 mg orally 2 times/day.
    D. Zoledronic acid 4 mg intravenously.

3. A 20-year-old man was recently given a diagnosis of acute non–lymphocytic leukemia. His white blood cell (count) (WBC) is 35,000/mm^3, and he will receive chemotherapy tomorrow. Which one of the following is the best prevention strategy for tumor lysis syndrome?
    A. Hydration with 5% dextrose (D_5W), 1 L before chemotherapy, plus allopurinol 300 mg/day.
    B. Hydration with D_5W, 100 mL/hour starting at least 24 hours before chemotherapy, plus allopurinol 300 mg/day.
    C. Normal saline 100 mL/hour starting at least 24 hours before chemotherapy plus allopurinol 300 mg/day.
    D. Hydration with normal saline 100 mL/hour starting at least 24 hours before chemotherapy plus sodium bicarbonate 500 mg orally every 6 hours.

4. An 18-year-old man is about to begin chemotherapy for acute lymphoblastic leukemia. On today's complete blood cell count (CBC), his hemoglobin is 7 g/dL, and he complains of fatigue. Which one of the following is the correct treatment?
    A. Initiate epoetin.
    B. Transfuse with packed red blood cells (RBCs).
    C. Delay chemotherapy treatment until hemoglobin recovers.
    D. Reduce chemotherapy doses to prevent further decreases in hemoglobin.

5. A patient received her fourth cycle of chemotherapy with paclitaxel-carboplatin for ovarian cancer 12 days ago. She reports to the clinic today complaining of a temperature this morning of 103°F. Her CBC is WBC 500/mm^3; segmented neutrophils 55%; band neutrophils 5%; basophils 15%; eosinophils 5%; monocytes 15%; and platelet count 99,000/mm^3. She denies any signs and symptoms of infection. Her blood pressure (BP) is 115/60 mm Hg; pulse rate is 80 beats/minute; and respiratory rate is 15 breaths/minute. What is her absolute neutrophil count (ANC)?
    A. 275.
    B. 300.
    C. 25.
    D. 500.

6. Which one of the following is the correct course of action for the patient in the previous question?
   A. Admit to the hospital for intravenous antibiotic drugs.
   B. Treat as an outpatient with antibiotic drugs.
   C. Initiate a colony-stimulating factor (CSF).
   D. Discontinue chemotherapy.

7. Which one of the following statements about the above patient is correct?
   A. Based on her monocyte count, her neutropenia is expected to last for another week.
   B. This is a nadir neutrophil count, and neutrophils would be expected to start increasing soon.
   C. The elevated absolute eosinophil count indicates an allergic reaction to carboplatin.
   D. It is unusual for the ANC to be this low in the face of an elevated platelet count.

8. A 60-year-old man has head and neck cancer with extensive involvement of facial nerves. His pain medications include transdermal fentanyl 100 mcg/hour every 72 hours and oral morphine solution 40 mg every 4 hours. He is still having problems with neuropathic pain. Which one of the following treatments listed below is best to recommend?
   A. Begin gabapentin and decrease the dose of fentanyl.
   B. Increase the dose of fentanyl and increase the dose of morphine.
   C. Begin diazepam and increase the dose of fentanyl.
   D. Begin gabapentin and continue fentanyl and morphine.

9. A patient is receiving chemotherapy for limited-stage small cell lung carcinoma. After the third cycle of chemotherapy, she was hospitalized with febrile neutropenia. She recovered and is scheduled to receive the fourth cycle of chemotherapy today. Which one of the following statements is correct?
   A. The patient should receive filgrastim 250 mcg/m^2/day subcutaneously for 10 days.
   B. The patient should receive filgrastim 5 mcg/kg/day subcutaneously, starting today.
   C. The patient should receive pegfilgrastim 1 mg/day subcutaneously for 6 days.
   D. The patient should receive filgrastim 5 mcg/kg/day subcutaneously for 7 days, beginning tomorrow.

10. A 60-year-old woman with breast cancer is to begin chemotherapy with AC (doxorubicin and cyclophosphamide). Laboratory values today include sodium 140; potassium 3.8; glucose 100; serum creatinine 1.1; aspartate aminotransferase 6; alanine aminotransferase 35; and total bilirubin 2. Which one of the following statements is correct?
    A. The dose of doxorubicin should be decreased.
    B. The dose of cyclophosphamide should be decreased.
    C. Both chemotherapy drugs should be given at standard doses.
    D. Both chemotherapy drugs should be given at decreased doses.

11. Large cell lymphoma is considered intermediate (between indolent and highly aggressive) in tumor growth and biology. Large cell lymphoma is sensitive to chemotherapy and potentially curable. Metastatic colorectal cancer is considered slow growing. Although responses to chemotherapy commonly occur and chemotherapy can prolong survival (by months), metastatic colorectal cancer is not generally considered curable with chemotherapy. Based on these differences between large cell lymphoma and metastatic colorectal cancer, which one of the following statements is correct?
    A. Patients with large cell lymphoma should receive allopurinol beginning before the first cycle of chemotherapy because they are at an increased risk of developing tumor lysis syndrome.
    B. Patients with metastatic colorectal cancer should receive allopurinol beginning before the first cycle of chemotherapy because they are at an increased risk of developing tumor lysis syndrome.
    C. Patients with large cell lymphoma should receive pamidronate beginning before the first cycle of chemotherapy because they are at an increased risk of developing hypercalcemia.
    D. Patients with metastatic colorectal cancer should receive pamidronate beginning before the first cycle of chemotherapy because they are at an increased risk of developing hypercalcemia.

12. Consider the information provided above about large cell lymphoma and metastatic colorectal cancer. Patient 1 with large cell lymphoma is receiving CHOP-R (cyclophosphamide, doxorubicin [hydroxydaunomycin], vincristine [Oncovin], prednisone, and rituximab) chemotherapy. Patient 2 with metastatic colorectal cancer is receiving FOLFIRI (5-fluorouracil–leucovorin, irinotecan) chemotherapy. On the day cycle 2 is due, both patients have an ANC of 800/mm^3. Which one of the following statements is correct?

- A. Patient 1 should get chemotherapy to keep him on schedule because he has a curable disease.
- B. Patient 2 should get chemotherapy to keep him on schedule because he has a curable disease.
- C. The chemotherapy for patient 1 should be held for now, and he should receive filgrastim after the next time he has chemotherapy.
- D. The chemotherapy for patient 2 should be held for now, and he should receive filgrastim after the next time he has chemotherapy.

13. Sometimes, extravasation is not immediately evident when it occurs. Immediately after administering CHOP-R to patient 1 above, an extravasation is suspected. Which one of the following should be initiated?
    - A. Application of a warm pack for suspected extravasation of doxorubicin.
    - B. Application of a cold pack for suspected extravasation of vincristine.
    - C. Application of dimethyl sulfoxide and intravenous dexrazoxane for suspected extravasation of doxorubicin.
    - D. Application of sodium thiosulfate for suspected extravasation of cyclophosphamide.

I. ANTIEMETICS

A. Definitions
   1. Nausea is described as an awareness of discomfort that may or may not precede vomiting; nausea is accompanied by decreased gastric tone and decreased peristalsis.
   2. Retching is the labored movement of abdominal and thoracic muscles associated with vomiting.
   3. Vomiting (emesis) is the ejection or expulsion of gastric contents through the mouth.
      a. Acute vomiting is vomiting occurring 0-24 hours after chemotherapy administration.
      b. Delayed vomiting is vomiting occurring more than 24 hours after chemotherapy administration.
         i. The distinction between acute and delayed symptoms with regard to time of onset is somewhat arbitrary, and it becomes blurred when chemotherapy is administered for multiple days.
         ii. Delayed symptoms are best described with cisplatin, although they are commonly reported in association with other agents as well.
         iii. The importance of the distinction between acute and delayed (and anticipatory) symptoms is that they likely have different mechanisms and therefore different management strategies.
   4. Anticipatory vomiting (or nausea) is triggered by sights, smells, or sounds and is a conditioned response; it is more likely to occur in patients whose postchemotherapy nausea/vomiting has not been well controlled.

B. Risk Factors for Chemotherapy-Induced Nausea and Vomiting
   1. Patient factors
      a. Poor control of nausea and vomiting during previous cycles of chemotherapy
      b. Female sex
      c. Young age
      d. Possible protective role of alcohol
      e. History of motion sickness
      f. History of nausea or vomiting during pregnancy
   2. Emetogenicity of anticancer agents
      a. Several schemes for assessing emetogenicity have been proposed. Historically, emetogenic risk was classified as "none," "mild," "moderate," and "severe." In 1997, a classification proposing five levels of emetogenicity was published. More recently, the five levels were once again collapsed into three. Levels (e.g., low, moderate, high emetogenic risk) are defined by the percentage of patients expected to experience any emesis. Nausea is an important source of discomfort for patients, but emetogenic risk levels include only vomiting. High risk is arbitrarily defined as more than 90% risk of vomiting. Moderate risk includes many drugs and represents a broad range (30%–90% risk of vomiting). Low risk is less than 30% risk of vomiting. Cisplatin is the prototype high-risk agent. The combination of doxorubicin or epirubicin with cyclophosphamide (AC or EC) is also often considered high risk. Doxorubicin or epirubicin alone is considered moderate risk. Docetaxel is an example of an agent with a low risk of emetogenicity. Some agents cause almost no nausea or vomiting (e.g., bleomycin, vincristine).
   3. Radiation therapy can also cause nausea and vomiting. The incidence and severity of radiation-induced nausea and vomiting vary by site of radiation and size of radiation field. Radiation to the head and neck or to the extremities is considered mildly emetogenic;

radiation to the upper abdomen and pelvis and craniospinal radiation are considered moderately emetogenic; and total body irradiation, total nodal irradiation, and upper-half-body irradiation are considered highly emetogenic.

C. General Principles for Managing Chemotherapy-Induced Nausea and Vomiting and Radiation-Induced Nausea and Vomiting
1. Prevention is key. Prophylactic antiemetics should be administered before moderately or highly emetogenic agents and before moderately and highly emetogenic radiation. Vincristine and bleomycin given as single agents do not require prophylactic antiemetics.
2. Antiemetics should be scheduled for delayed nausea and vomiting for select chemotherapy regimens (e.g., cisplatin, AC) and should be available if prolonged acute symptoms or ineffective antiemetic prophylaxis occurs.
3. Begin with an appropriate antiemetic regimen based on the emetogenicity of the chemotherapy drug(s).
    a. Newer oral tyrosine kinase inhibitors (e.g., sorafenib, sunitinib) are associated with a low emetogenic risk but may cause intolerable symptoms because the drugs are administered for several weeks in a row or even continuously.
    b. Follow-up is also essential. Whatever the emetogenicity and antiemetic regimen, the response should guide the choice of antiemetic regimen for subsequent courses of therapy.
    c. Nausea and vomiting are distinct phenomena. Vomiting mechanisms are better understood and have been better studied. Most antiemetic studies incorporate vomiting primary end points, and in studies that evaluate nausea, nausea outcomes are generally worse than vomiting outcomes.
    d. The most common antiemetic regimen for highly emetogenic chemotherapy/radiation is the combination of a serotonin receptor antagonist and dexamethasone. The addition of a corticosteroid to a serotonin receptor antagonist for highly (or moderately) emetogenic anticancer therapy increases efficacy by 10%–20%.
    e. Aprepitant may be added to the above antiemetic regimen for highly emetogenic chemotherapy and/or to prevent delayed nausea and vomiting.
    f. The combination of metoclopramide and dexamethasone was the most common regimen to prevent delayed nausea and vomiting before the availability of aprepitant. This combination is still used when aprepitant has not been incorporated into the initial regimen for chemotherapy-induced nausea and vomiting.
    g. Single-agent phenothiazine, butyrophenone, or steroid are used for mildly to moderately emetogenic regimens and for "as-needed" use for prolonged symptoms (i.e., breakthrough symptoms).
    h. Cannabinoids are generally used after the failure of other regimens or to stimulate appetite.
    i. Agents whose primary indication is other than treatment of nausea and vomiting are being investigated. Clinically, these agents may be used for patients whose symptoms do not respond to "standard" antiemetics.

D. Antiemetics
1. Serotonin (5-HT$_3$) receptor antagonists (dolasetron, granisetron, ondansetron, and palonosetron)
    a. These drugs block serotonin receptors peripherally in the gastrointestinal tract and centrally in the medulla.
    b. The most common adverse events include headache and constipation, occurring in 10%–15% of patients.

     c. All drugs have similar efficacy (see below), and choice of drug is often based on cost and organizational contracts.
     d. Palonosetron is approved for the prevention of both acute and delayed chemotherapy-induced nausea and vomiting. It is reportedly distinct from the other serotonin receptor antagonists, based on receptor binding and half-life. Palonosetron is considered the preferred serotonin receptor antagonist in some national guidelines, but this is not universally accepted.
2. Corticosteroids (dexamethasone; methylprednisolone)
     a. Exact mechanism is unknown; thought to act by inhibiting prostaglandin synthesis in the cortex
     b. Adverse events associated with single doses and short courses of steroids are infrequent; they may include euphoria, anxiety, insomnia, increased appetite, and mild fluid retention; rapid intravenous administration may be associated with transient and intense perineal, vaginal, or anal burning.
     c. Dexamethasone has been studied more often in clinical trials than methylprednisolone.
3. Neurokinin-1 receptor antagonists (aprepitant or fosaprepitant)
     a. Aprepitant is approved for use in combination with other antiemetic drugs for preventing acute and delayed nausea and vomiting associated with initial and repeat courses of chemotherapy known to cause these problems, including high-dose cisplatin.
     b. Aprepitant improved the overall complete response (defined as no emetic episodes and no use of rescue therapy) by about 20% when added to a serotonin receptor antagonist and dexamethasone.
     c. Metabolized primarily by cytochrome P (CYP) 450 3A4 with minor metabolism by CYP1A2 and CYP2C19; the potential exists for drug interactions, including with dexamethasone
4. Benzamide analogs (metoclopramide)
     a. Metoclopramide may exert an antiemetic effect by blockade of dopamine receptors in the chemoreceptor trigger zone; stimulation of cholinergic activity in the gut, increasing (forward) gut motility; and antagonism of peripheral serotonin receptors in the intestines. These effects are dose related.
     b. Adverse events include mild sedation and diarrhea, as well as extrapyramidal reactions (e.g., dystonia, akathisia).
5. Phenothiazines (prochlorperazine, chlorpromazine)
     a. Phenothiazines block dopamine receptors in the chemoreceptor trigger zone.
     b. Common adverse events associated with this class of antiemetics include drowsiness, hypotension, akathisia, and dystonia.
     c. Chlorpromazine is often preferred in children because it is associated with fewer extrapyramidal reactions than prochlorperazine.
6. Butyrophenones (haloperidol, droperidol)
     a. The mechanism of action and activity of these two drugs are similar to the phenothiazines.
     b. They are at least as effective as the phenothiazines, and some studies indicate they are superior; they offer a different chemical structure that may bind differently to the dopamine receptor and offer an initial alternative when a phenothiazine fails.
     c. The most common adverse event is sedation; hypotension is less frequent than with the phenothiazines; extrapyramidal symptoms are also seen.
     d. The use of droperidol as an antiemetic has fallen out of favor because of the risk of QT prolongation or torsades de pointes.

7. Benzodiazepines (lorazepam)
    a. Lorazepam as a single agent has minimal antiemetic activity. However, several properties make lorazepam useful in combination with or as an adjunct to other antiemetics.
        i. Anterograde amnesia helps prevent anticipatory nausea and vomiting.
        ii. Relief of anxiety
        iii. Management of akathisia caused by phenothiazines, butyrophenones, or metoclopramide
    b. Adverse events include amnesia, sedation, hypotension, perceptual disturbances, and urinary incontinence. Note that amnesia and sedation may, in fact, be desirable.
8. Cannabinoids (dronabinol, nabilone)
    a. The existence of cannabinoid receptors has recently been discovered. Cannabinoid receptors may mediate at least some of the antiemetic activity of this class of agents. Additional antiemetic mechanisms that have been proposed include inhibition of prostaglandins and blockade of adrenergic activity.
    b. Adverse events include drowsiness, dizziness, euphoria, dysphoria, orthostatic hypotension, ataxia, hallucinations, and time disorientation. Appetite stimulation is also seen with cannabinoids and may, in fact, be desirable.

II. PAIN MANAGEMENT

A. Principles of Cancer Pain Management
    1. The oral route is preferred when available. Although the ratio of oral to parenteral potency of morphine is commonly noted to be 1:6, clinical observation of chronic morphine use indicates this ratio is closer to 1:3 (oral-to-parenteral potency) for all opioids.
    2. Choose the analgesic drug and dose to match the degree of pain suffered by the patient.
    3. Pain medications should always be administered on a scheduled basis, NOT AS NEEDED.
        a. It is always easier to prevent pain from recurring than to treat it once it has recurred.
        b. As-needed dosing should be used for breakthrough pain, which is pain that "breaks through" the regularly scheduled opioid; an immediate-release, short-acting opioid should always accompany a long-acting opioid.
    4. For persistent, severe pain, use a product with a long duration of action.

Patient Cases

1. A 60-year-old woman was recently given a diagnosis of advanced non–small cell lung cancer. She is going to begin treatment with cisplatin 100 mg/m^2 plus vinorelbine 30 mg/m^2. Which one of the following is an appropriate antiemetic regimen for preventing acute emesis?
    A. Aprepitant plus dolasetron plus dexamethasone.
    B. Aprepitant plus prochlorperazine plus dexamethasone.
    C. Aprepitant plus granisetron plus ondansetron.
    D. Lorazepam plus ondansetron plus metoclopramide.

2. Which one of the following is an appropriate regimen for delayed nauseas and vomiting?
    A. Aprepitant plus dexamethasone.
    B. Aprepitant plus metoclopramide.
    C. Ondansetron plus dexamethasone.
    D. Ondansetron plus lorazepam.

5. Before adding an additional drug or changing to another drug, maximize the dose and schedule of the current analgesic drug.
6. Provide drugs to prevent adverse events such as constipation and sedation.
7. Reevaluate pain and pain relief often, especially during the initiation of pain therapy; if more than two as-needed doses are required for breakthrough pain in a 24-hour period, consider modifying the regimen.
8. Use appropriate adjuvant analgesics and nondrug measures to maximize pain control.

B. Pain Rating Scales
1. Use pain assessment tools to evaluate pain intensity at baseline and to assess how well a pain medication regimen is working.
   a. Numeric rating scale of 0–10, with 0 = no pain and 10 = worst pain imaginable
   b. Pediatric patients: Faces-of-Pain Scale, poker-chip method
2. Because pain is subjective, it is best evaluated by the patient (i.e., not a caregiver and not the health professional).

C. Treatment of Pain—The Analgesic Ladder
1. For mild to moderate pain (pain rating of 1–3 on a 10-point scale)., the first step is a nonopioid analgesic drug: nonsteroidal anti-inflammatory drug (NSAID), aspirin, or acetaminophen (APAP)
2. For persistent or for moderate to severe pain (pain rating of 4–6 on the 10-point scale), add a weak opioid: codeine or hydrocodone, available in combination with nonopioid analgesic drugs.
3. For persistent or for severe pain (pain rating of 7–10 on the 10-point scale), replace the weak opioid with a strong opioid: morphine, oxycodone, or similar drug.

D. Nonopioid Analgesics
1. Mechanism: Act peripherally to inhibit the activity of prostaglandins in the pain pathway
2. There is a ceiling effect to the analgesia provided by NSAIDs.
3. Adverse events: Consider inhibition of platelet aggregation and the effects of inhibition of renal prostaglandins.
4. Remember, NSAIDs are generally used in addition to, not instead of, opioids.

E. Nonopioid-Opioid Combinations
1. Aspirin or APAP or ibuprofen plus codeine or hydrocodone or oxycodone are the most commonly used combinations.
2. Be aware of the risk of APAP overdose with these products. As with any combination product, dose escalation of one component necessitates escalation of the other(s). For patients requiring high doses, pure opioids are preferred.
3. Oxycodone-APAP is available in several strengths; however, the amount of APAP increases with increasing oxycodone.

F. Opioid Analgesics
1. Mechanism: Opioids act centrally in the brain (periaqueductal gray region) and at the level of the spinal cord (dorsal horn) at specific opioid receptors.
2. The opioids have no analgesic ceiling.
3. Morphine
   a. Morphine is the standard to which all other drugs are compared; opioids may differ in duration of action, relative potency, oral effectiveness, and adverse event profiles, but none is clinically superior to morphine.

b. Flexibility in dosage forms and administration routes: oral (sustained release [SR], immediate release), sublingual, intravenous, intrathecal/epidural, subcutaneous, and rectal
c. Long duration of action: SR products last 8–12 hours or, for some preparations, 24 hours.
d. Morphine is one of the most inexpensive opioids.
4. Oxycodone
   a. Available as a single drug (i.e., not in combination) in both a long-acting and short-acting formulation
   b. Excellent alternative to morphine
5. Fentanyl
   a. Fentanyl is available as a transdermal preparation, an oral transmucosal preparation, and a buccal tablet. Transmucosal and buccal fentanyl are used for breakthrough pain.
   b. Each transdermal patch provides sustained release of drug and can provide pain relief for 48–72 hours.
   c. Consider implications for dosing transdermal fentanyl in cachectic patients: The fentanyl initially forms a depot in subcutaneous tissue, and patients with little or no fat may not achieve pain relief.
   d. Slow onset, long elimination after patch application and removal, respectively
   e. Bioavailability is greater with buccal tablets than with the transmucosal preparation; thus, equivalent doses are higher for transmucosal and lower for buccal tablets.

G. Adverse Events
   1. Sedation: tolerance usually develops within several days; remember that more sedation may be expected in a patient who has been unable to sleep because of uncontrolled pain. For patients who do not develop tolerance to sedation and have good pain control, a dose reduction may be considered. If dose reduction compromises pain control, the addition of a stimulant (e.g., dextroamphetamine, methylphenidate) may be considered. Other central nervous system adverse events include dysphoria and hallucinations.
   2. Constipation is very common, and tolerance does NOT develop to this effect. Decreased intestinal peristalsis is caused by decreased intestinal tone; delayed gastric emptying may also occur. Regular use of stimulant laxatives is often required to manage constipation.
   3. Nausea and vomiting are common. As is seen with sedation, tolerance develops within about a week. Nausea and vomiting may have a vestibular component, developing as pain relief promotes increased mobility. Antivertigo agents (e.g., meclizine, dimenhydrinate) may be useful in managing the vestibular component. Nausea and vomiting may also occur because of stimulation of the chemoreceptor trigger zone. Drugs that block dopamine receptors (e.g., phenothiazines) provide relief of this component of nausea and vomiting until tolerance develops.
   4. Urinary retention/bladder spasm is more common in the elderly and in patients taking long-acting formulations.

H. Bisphosphonates
   1. Bisphosphonates have been shown to decrease pain and number of skeletal-related events in patients with breast cancer and multiple myeloma when given for 1 year. Skeletal-related events include pathological fracture, need for radiation therapy to bone, surgery to bone, and spinal cord compression.
   2. In 2000, the American Society of Clinical Oncology published initial guidelines for the use of bisphosphonates in breast cancer (updated in November 2003).

a. For patients with breast cancer who have evidence of bone metastases on plain radiographs, it is recommended they receive either pamidronate 90 mg delivered over 2 hours or zoledronic acid 4 mg over 15 minutes every 3–4 weeks.
b. Women with abnormal bone scan and abnormal computerized tomographic scan or magnetic resonance imaging showing bone destruction but a normal radiograph should also receive the above recommended bisphosphonates.
c. Using bisphosphonates in women who are asymptomatic and who have an abnormal bone scan with normal radiograph is not recommended.
d. Therapy should continue until there is evidence of a substantial decline in a patient's performance status.
e. Bisphosphonates may be used in combination with other pain therapies in patients with pain caused by osteolytic disease.
3. In 2002, the American Society of Clinical Oncology published guidelines for the use of bisphosphonates in multiple myeloma.
   a. Patients with lytic bone destruction seen on plain radiographs should receive either pamidronate 90 mg intravenously over at least 2 hours or zoledronic acid 4 mg over 15 minutes every 3–4 weeks.
   b. Therapy should continue until there is evidence of substantial decline in a patient's performance status.
   c. Patients with osteopenia but no radiologic evidence of bone metastases can receive bisphosphonates.
   d. Bisphosphonates are not recommended for the following groups of patients: patients with solitary plasmacytoma, smoldering or indolent myeloma, and monoclonal gammopathy of undetermined significance.
   e. Bisphosphonates may be used in patients with pain caused by osteolytic disease.
4. Adverse events associated with pamidronate or zoledronic acid include low-grade fevers, nausea, anorexia, vomiting, hypomagnesemia, hypocalcemia, hypokalemia, and nephrotoxicity.
   a. Serum creatinine should be monitored before each dose (see package insert for specific recommendations).
   b. Package insert recommends initiating patients on oral calcium 500 mg plus vitamin D 400 IU/day to prevent hypocalcemia.
   c. Numerous reports of osteonecrosis of the jaw occurring in patients receiving bisphosphonates have appeared in the literature. Osteonecrosis of the jaw most often follows a dental procedure or dental pathology. The long half-life of bisphosphonate in bone makes this adverse event difficult to prevent and manage. Patient education and education of dentists are important.

I. Adjuvant analgesics are drugs whose primary indication is other than pain; they are used to manage specific pain syndromes. Most often, adjuvant analgesics are used in addition to, rather than instead of, opioids.
   1. Antidepressants (e.g., amitriptyline) and anticonvulsants (e.g., gabapentin, carbamazepine) are used for neuropathic pain (e.g., phantom limb pain, nerve compression caused by tumor)
   2. Transdermal lidocaine is useful in localized neuropathic pain.
   3. Corticosteroids are useful in pain caused by nerve compression or inflammation, lymphedema, bone pain, or increased intracranial pressure.
   4. Benzodiazepines: diazepam, lorazepam: useful for muscle spasms; baclofen is another alternative for intractable muscle spasms

5. Strontium-89: radionuclide for treatment of bone pain caused by osteoblastic lesions; a single dose may provide relief for several weeks or even months; however, it is myelosuppressive
6. Nonsteroidal anti-inflammatory drugs are recommended for the treatment of pain caused by bone metastases. Prostaglandins sensitize nociceptors (pain receptors) to painful stimuli, thus providing a rationale for using NSAIDs.

III. TREATMENT OF FEBRILE NEUTROPENIA

A. Principles of Chemotherapy-Induced Bone Marrow Suppression
   1. Bone marrow suppression is the most common dose-limiting toxicity associated with traditional cytotoxic chemotherapy.
   2. White blood cell (count) = a normal range of $4.8–10.8 \times 10^3$ cells/mm^3 with a circulating life span of 6–12 hours; decreased WBC = neutropenia, leucopenia, or granulocytopenia; the risk is life-threatening infections; the risk increases with ANC less than 500/mm^3, and the risk is greatest with ANC less than 100/mm^3. Because neutrophils have the fastest turnover, the effects of cytotoxic chemotherapy are greatest on neutrophils (compared with platelets or RBCs).
      a. The nadir (usually described by the ANC) is the lowest value to which the blood count falls after cytotoxic chemotherapy. Usually occurs 10–14 days after chemotherapy administration, with counts usually recovering by 3–4 weeks after chemotherapy; exceptions include mitomycin and nitrosoureas (carmustine and lomustine), which have nadirs of 28–42 days after chemotherapy and recovery of neutrophils 6–8 weeks after treatment
      b. Absolute neutrophil count = WBC × % granulocytes or neutrophils (segmented neutrophils plus band neutrophils).
         Example: patient's WBC = 4.5×10^3 cells/mm^3 with 10% segmented neutrophils and 5% band neutrophils. What is the ANC? *4500 × (0.1 + 0.05) = 675.*
      c. To administer chemotherapy, a patient should have WBC greater than 3000/mm^3 OR ANC greater than 1500/mm^3 AND platelet count of 100,000/mm^3 or greater. These are general guidelines; some protocols specify different (lower) thresholds for administering chemotherapy; if cytopenia is attributable to disease in the bone marrow, chemotherapy (full dose) may cause improvement; some drugs are nonmyelosuppressive (e.g., vincristine, bleomycin, monoclonal antibodies).
      d. The potential curability of the disease influences what action will be taken during the next cycle of chemotherapy—either dose reduction of myelosuppressive chemotherapy or support with a CSF.
   3. Megakaryocytes (platelets) = a normal range of 140,000-440,000 cells/mm^3 with a circulating life span of 5–10 days; decreased platelet count = thrombocytopenia; the risk is bleeding; the risk is greatest with platelet count less than 10,000/mm^3
   4. Red blood cells = a normal range of $4.6–6.2 \times 10^6$ cells/mm^3 with a circulating life span of 120 days; decreased RBCs = anemia, with the potential for hypoxia, fatigue, and exacerbation of congestive heart failure
   5. Other factors affecting myelosuppression include previous chemotherapy, previous radiation therapy, and direct bone marrow involvement by tumor.

B. Neutropenia and Febrile Neutropenia
  1. The current version of the Infectious Diseases Society of America guidelines for the use of antibiotics in patients with cancer and neutropenia was issued in 2002. As of this writing, the next edition is scheduled for release in 2010.
  2. Neutropenia is defined as an ANC of 500/mm^3 or less or a count of less than 1000/mm^3 with a predicted decrease to less than 500/mm^3 during the next 48 hours.
  3. Febrile neutropenia is defined as neutropenia and a single oral temperature of 101°F or more or a temperature of 100.4°F or more for at least 1 hour.
  4. Neutropenic patients are at an increased risk of developing serious and life-threatening infections.
  5. The usual signs/symptoms of infection (e.g., abscess, pus, infiltrates on chest radiograph) are absent, with fever often being the only indicator. In addition, cultures are negative more often than not. Thus, prompt investigation and treatment of febrile neutropenia are essential.
  6. The initial assessment of patients with febrile neutropenia includes a risk assessment for complications/severe infection.
      a. Characteristics of low-risk neutropenia include ANC of 100/mm^3 or more and absolute monocyte count of 100/mm^3 or more; normal chest radiograph; almost normal renal and hepatic function; duration of neutropenia less than 7 days and resolution expected in less than 10 days; no intravenous access site or catheter site infection; early evidence of bone marrow recovery; malignancy in remission; peak oral temperature of less than 102°F; no neurologic or mental status changes; no appearance of illness; absence of abdominal pain; no comorbid complications (e.g., shock, hypoxia, pneumonia, other deep organ infection, vomiting, diarrhea).
      b. The Multinational Association for Supportive Care in Cancer has developed a scoring index to help identify patients with low-risk febrile neutropenia. Scores are assessed on the basis of factors such as those listed above.
      c. Febrile neutropenia that is considered at low risk of complications may be treated with either oral or intravenous antibiotics in an outpatient or inpatient setting.
      d. Patients with high-risk febrile neutropenia (i.e., patients who do not have low-risk characteristics as noted above) should receive intravenous antibiotics in the hospital.
  7. Considerations in the initial selection of an antibiotic include the potential infecting organism, potential site(s) and source of infection, local antimicrobial susceptibilities, organ dysfunction potentially affecting antibiotic clearance or toxicity, and drug allergy. The most common source of infection is endogenous flora, which could be gram-negative or gram-positive bacteria; the more prolonged the neutropenia (and the more prolonged the administration of antibacterial antibiotics), the greater chance of fungi playing a role in the infection.
  8. All patients should be reassessed after 3–5 days of antibiotic therapy, and antibiotics should be adjusted accordingly.

Patient Cases

3. A 45-year-old woman has metastatic breast cancer. The main sites of metastatic disease are regional lymph nodes and bone (several rib lesions). She complains of aching pain with occasional shooting pains. The latter are thought to be the result of nerve compression by enlarged lymph nodes. She has been taking oxycodone-APAP 5 mg 2 tablets every 4 hours and ibuprofen 400 mg every 8 hours. Her current pain rating is 8 on a scale of 10, and she states that her pain cannot be controlled. Which one of the following choices is best to manage her pain at this time?
    A. Increase oxycodone-APAP to 7.5 mg, 2 tablets every 4 hours.
    B. Increase oxycodone-APAP to 10 mg, 2 tablets every 4 hours.
    C. Discontinue ibuprofen and add morphine SR every 12 hours.
    D. Discontinue oxycodone-APAP and add morphine SR every 12 hours.

4. Which one of the following might be an additional change for this patient's pain regimen?
    A. Naproxen.
    B. Single-agent (single ingredient) APAP.
    C. Gabapentin.
    D. Baclofen.

IV. USE OF CSFs IN NEUTROPENIA AND FEBRILE NEUTROPENIA

A. Colony-stimulating factors enhance both the production and function of their target cells; three products are currently available in the United States: G-CSF (filgrastim); pegylated G-CSF (pegfilgrastim or PEG G-CSF); and GM-CSF (sargramostim).

B. Pegfilgrastim is approved for use in patients with nonmyeloid malignancies who are receiving myelosuppressive chemotherapy associated with a high incidence of febrile neutropenia.

C. G-CSF and GM-CSF have been proved to reduce the incidence, magnitude, and duration of neutropenia after chemotherapy and bone marrow transplantation.

D. Guidelines for the use of CSFs were established by the American Society of Clinical Oncology in 1994; the most recent update was published in 2006.

E. Colony-stimulating factors have been shown to reduce the incidence of febrile neutropenia by about 50%, and their use for primary prophylaxis is recommended with chemotherapy regimens associated with a 20% or greater risk of febrile neutropenia.
    1. The CSF and GM-CSF are given by daily subcutaneous injection.
    2. To date, no large trials have compared G-CSF and GM-CSF. Therefore, although it cannot be stated unequivocally that the two are therapeutically equivalent, they are often used interchangeably.
    3. Pegfilgrastim is given as a single 6-mg subcutaneous dose, generally administered 24 hours after chemotherapy.
    4. A single dose of pegfilgrastim is as effective as 11 daily doses of G-CSF 5 mcg/kg in reducing the frequency and duration of severe neutropenia, promoting neutrophil recovery, and reducing the frequency of febrile neutropenia.
    5. The choice of CSF (pegfilgrastim vs. filgrastim or sargramostim) should be based on the expected duration of neutropenia and the specific anticancer regimen (e.g., short courses of a daily CSF rather than one dose of pegfilgrastim with chemotherapy administered on a weekly schedule).

6. Adverse events associated with all three preparations appear similar; they include bone pain (most common) and fever.
7. The CSF should be initiated between 24 and 72 hours after the completion of chemotherapy.
8. The package literature recommends continued administration of G-CSF until the post-nadir ANC is greater than 10,000/mm^3; however, both G-CSF and GM-CSF are commonly discontinued when "adequate neutrophil recovery" is evident. To decrease cost without compromising patient outcome, many centers continue the CSF until ANC is greater than 2000–5000/mm^3. Note that the ANC will decrease about 50% per day after the CSF is discontinued if the marrow has not recovered (i.e., if the CSF is discontinued before the ANC nadir is reached).
9. Avoid the concomitant use of CSF in patients receiving chemotherapy and radiation therapy; the potential exists for worsening myelosuppression.

F. Refer to the American Society of Clinical Oncology Guidelines for the following indications: increasing chemotherapy dose intensity; using as adjuncts to progenitor-cell transplantation; administering to patients with myeloid malignancies; and using in pediatric populations

G. American Society of Clinical Oncology Guidelines for Secondary CSF Administration
    1. If chemotherapy administration has been delayed or the dose reduced because of prolonged neutropenia, then CSF use can be considered for subsequent chemotherapy cycles; administering a CSF in this setting is considered secondary prophylaxis.
    2. Dose reduction of chemotherapy should be considered the first option (i.e., instead of a CSF) after an episode of neutropenia in patients being treated with the intent to palliate (i.e., not a curative intent).

H. Use of CSFs for Treatment of Established Neutropenia
    1. Administering CSFs in patients who are neutropenic, but not febrile, is not recommended.
    2. Administering CSFs in patients who are neutropenic and febrile may be considered in the presence of risk factors for complications (e.g., ANC less than 100/mm^3, pneumonia, hypotension, multiorgan dysfunction, invasive fungal infection); CSFs may be used in addition to antibiotics to treat neutropenia in patients with these risk factors.

Patient Cases

5. A 50-year-old woman is receiving adjuvant chemotherapy for stage II breast cancer. She received her third cycle of doxorubicin and cyclophosphamide (AC) 10 days ago. Her CBC today includes WBC 600/mm^3, segmented neutrophils 60%, band neutrophils 10%, monocytes 12%, basophils 8%, and eosinophils 10%. Which one of the following represents this patient's ANC?
    A. 600/mm^3.
    B. 360/mm^3.
    C. 240/mm^3.
    D. 420/mm^3.

6. Based on this ANC, which one of the following statements is most correct?
    A. The patient should be initiated on a CSF.
    B. The patient should begin prophylactic treatment with either a quinolone antibiotic or trimethoprim-sulfamethoxazole.
    C. The patient, who is neutropenic, should be monitored closely for signs and symptoms of infection.
    D. Decrease the doses of doxorubicin and cyclophosphamide with the next cycle of treatment.

V. THROMBOCYTOPENIA

A. Defined as a platelet count less than 100,000/mm^3; however, the risk of bleeding is not substantially increased until the platelet count is 20,000 or less. Practices for platelet transfusion vary widely from institution to institution. Many institutions do not transfuse platelets until the patient becomes symptomatic (ecchymosis, petechiae, hemoptysis, or hematemesis). Other institutions will transfuse when the platelet count is 10,000/mm^3 or less, even in the absence of bleeding.

B. Oprelvekin (interleukin-11) is approved for the prevention of severe thrombocytopenia in patients undergoing chemotherapy for nonmyeloid malignancies.
   1. Oprelvekin is administered as a daily subcutaneous injection, beginning 6–24 hours after completion of myelosuppressive chemotherapy.
   2. Treatment is continued until a post-nadir platelet count of 50,000 cells/mm^3 or greater is achieved; dosing beyond 21 days is not recommended, and oprelvekin must be discontinued at least 2 days before (the next cycle of) chemotherapy.
   3. The current role of oprelvekin is to maintain the dose intensity of chemotherapy, although it is not nearly as widely used as the CSFs for neutrophils. A pharmacoeconomic analysis (from the payer's perspective) did not show oprelvekin to be a cost-saving strategy compared with routine platelet transfusions for patients with severe chemotherapy-induced thrombocytopenia.
   4. Common adverse events associated with oprelvekin include edema, shortness of breath, tachycardia, and conjunctival redness.

VI. ANEMIA/FATIGUE

A. Causes of Anemia and Fatigue in Adult Patients with Cancer
   1. Unmanaged pain or other symptoms can increase fatigue.
   2. Decreased RBC production because of anticancer therapy, either radiation or chemotherapy
   3. Decreased or inappropriate endogenous erythropoietin production or decreased responsiveness to endogenous erythropoietin
   4. Decreased body stores of vitamin B$_{12}$, iron, or folic acid
   5. Blood loss
   6. Although anemia can certainly contribute to or worsen fatigue, there are likely other (perhaps many) mechanisms of fatigue (e.g., cytokines) that are independent of hemoglobin concentration.

B. Principles of Anemia and Fatigue
   1. Fatigue is estimated to affect 60%-80% of all patients with cancer.
   2. Fatigue may be because of the disease or treatment.
   3. Fatigue can be assessed with a numeric rating scale, 0 = no fatigue and 10 = worst fatigue imaginable, or with any of several questionnaires (e.g., FACT-An).
   4. Drugs used in the treatment of anemia and fatigue
      a. Epoetin and darbepoetin alfa are approved for the treatment of chemotherapy-induced anemia, the end point of treatment being decreased need for transfusion.

b. In recent years, reports of a detrimental effect of erythropoiesis-stimulating proteins (e.g., increased deaths, poorer chemotherapy outcomes) have led to changes in the reimbursement for these agents and to changes in practice guidelines. Hemoglobin targets are lower than previously, and hemoglobin is carefully monitored.
c. It is important to distinguish between the use of these agents for chemotherapy-associated anemia and cancer-associated anemia. The latter is not an approved use.

Patient Case

7. A 45-year-old man is beginning his third cycle of chemotherapy for extensive-stage small cell lung cancer. At diagnosis, his hemoglobin was 10 g/dL; however, today, his hemoglobin is less than 10 g/dL. The patient complains of considerable fatigue that is interfering with his activities of daily living. Which one of the following statements is true?
   A. Treatment with epoetin should be considered.
   B. Treatment with darbepoetin should be considered when hemoglobin falls to less than 9 g/dL.
   C. Extensive-stage small cell lung cancer is an incurable disease, and erythropoiesis-stimulating proteins should not be used.
   D. The patient should not receive RBC transfusions because he is symptomatic.

VII. CHEMOPROTECTANTS

A. Properties of an Ideal Protectant Drug for Chemotherapy and Radiation-Induced Toxicities
   1. Easy to administer
   2. No adverse events
   3. Prevents all toxicities, including non–life threatening (alopecia) toxicities, irreversible morbidities (neuropathies, ototoxicity), and mortality (severe myelosuppression, cardiotoxicity)
   4. Does not interfere with the efficacy of the cancer treatment
   5. To date, no such drug has been identified.

B. Dexrazoxane
   1. The anthracyclines (daunorubicin, doxorubicin, idarubicin, and epirubicin) can cause cardiomyopathy that is related to the total lifetime cumulative dose.
   2. Dexrazoxane acts as an intracellular chelating agent; iron chelation leads to a decrease in anthracycline-induced free radical damage.
      a. Dexrazoxane is approved for use in patients with metastatic breast cancer. It may be considered for patients who have received 300 mg/m^2 or more of doxorubicin and who may benefit from continued doxorubicin, considering the patient's risk of cardiotoxicity with continued doxorubicin use.
      b. Dexrazoxane may increase the hematologic toxicity of chemotherapy.
      c. An early study suggested that dexrazoxane decreases the response rate to chemotherapy. More recent data suggest this is not the case, but dexrazoxane is still not indicated for patients with early (curable) breast cancer.
   3. Dexrazoxane has recently also been approved for use as an antidote for the extravasation of anthracycline chemotherapy.

C. Amifostine
   1. Amifostine is used to prevent nephrotoxicity from cisplatin.
   2. It is also used to decrease the incidence of both acute and late xerostomia in patients with head and neck cancer who are undergoing fractionated radiation therapy.
   3. Adverse events associated with amifostine include sneezing, allergic reactions, warm or flushed feeling, metallic taste in mouth during infusion, nausea and vomiting, and hypotension. The latter is the most clinically significant toxicity. Prevention of hypotension includes withholding antihypertensive medications, hydration, and close monitoring of BP.

D. Mesna (sodium-2-mercaptoethane sulfonate)
   1. The metabolite acrolein is produced from both cyclophosphamide and ifosfamide, and it has been implicated in sterile hemorrhagic cystitis.
   2. Mesna detoxifies acrolein by binding to the compound and preventing its interaction with host cells.
   3. Mesna is always used with ifosfamide and may be used with cyclophosphamide.
   4. Mesna may be given intravenously or orally. Several dosing schedules may be used. With any schedule, mesna must begin concurrently with or before ifosfamide or cyclophosphamide and end after ifosfamide or cyclophosphamide (i.e., mesna must be present in the bladder when acrolein is present in the bladder).

VIII. ONCOLOGY EMERGENCIES

A. Hypercalcemia
   1. The most common tumors associated with hypercalcemia are lung (metastatic non–small cell lung cancer > small cell lung cancer), breast, multiple myeloma, head and neck, renal cell, and non-Hodgkin lymphoma.
   2. Cancer-associated hypercalcemia results from increased bone resorption with calcium release into the extracellular fluid; in addition, renal clearance of calcium is decreased.
      a. Some tumors cause direct bone destruction, resulting in osteolytic hypercalcemia.
      b. Other tumors release parathyroid hormone–related protein (i.e., humoral hypercalcemia).
      c. Immobile patients are also at an increased risk of hypercalcemia because of increased resorption of calcium.
      d. Medications (e.g., hormonal therapy, thiazide diuretics) may precipitate or exacerbate hypercalcemia.
   3. Management of hypercalcemia
      a. Mild hypercalcemia (corrected calcium less than 12 mg/dL) may not require aggressive treatment. Hydration with normal saline followed by observation is an option in asymptomatic patients with chemotherapy-sensitive tumors (e.g., lymphoma, breast cancer).
      b. Moderate hypercalcemia (corrected calcium 12–14 mg/dL) requires basic treatment of clinical symptoms.
      c. Severe hypercalcemia (corrected calcium greater than 14 mg/dL; symptomatic) requires aggressive treatment.
         i. Hydration with normal saline about 3–6 L in 24 hours
         ii. Loop diuretics may be administered after volume status has been corrected or to prevent fluid overload during hydration.

iii. Thiazide diuretics are contraindicated in hypercalcemia because of the increase in renal tubular calcium absorption.
iv. Bisphosphonates bind to hydroxyapatite in calcified bone, which prevents dissolution by phosphatases and inhibits both normal and abnormal bone resorption. The onset of action is 3–4 days.
v. Calcitonin inhibits the effects of parathyroid hormone and has a rapid-onset (though short-lived) hypocalcemic effect.
vi. Steroids may be used to lower calcium in patients with steroid-responsive tumors (lymphoma and myeloma).
vii. Phosphate is reserved for patients who are both hypophosphatemic and hypercalcemic. Phosphate is seldom used because of the possibility of calcium and phosphate precipitation in soft tissue.
viii. Dialysis may be required in patients with hypercalcemia and renal failure.
ix. Cyclooxygenase inhibitors (e.g., indomethacin) may have some effect, but they should be used only in patients who have not responded to or tolerated other drugs.
4. In practice, concentrations for corrected calcium or ionized calcium may not always be monitored. If the total calcium is high and the clinical status is consistent with hypercalcemia, treatment may be initiated (or the progress of treatment monitored) without calculating or measuring corrected or ionized calcium.

B. Spinal Cord Compression
1. Signs and symptoms include back pain, weakness, paresthesias, and loss of bowel and bladder function.
2. Treatment consists of dexamethasone and radiation therapy or surgery.

C. Tumor Lysis Syndrome
1. Occurs secondary to the rapid cell death that follows the administration of chemotherapy in patients with leukemia or lymphoma or in patients with high tumor burdens from other diseases that are also highly chemosensitive
2. Manifestations include hyperuricemia, hyperkalemia, hyperphosphatemia, and secondary hypocalcemia. Uric acid may precipitate in the kidney and can lead to renal failure.
3. The primary management strategy is prevention with intravenous hydration and allopurinol.
4. Rasburicase is a recombinant urate oxidase that converts uric acid into allantoin, which is 5–10 times more soluble in urine than uric acid. Rasburicase should be considered for patients at high risk of developing tumor lysis syndrome, such as those with a serum uric acid concentration more than 10 mg/dL, large tumor burden, preexisting renal dysfunction, or inability to take allopurinol. The drug is expensive, and currently, it is not recommended for prophylaxis in all patients.

Patient Cases

8. A 38-year-old woman has recurrent Hodgkin lymphoma. Two years ago, she completed six cycles of ABVD chemotherapy (i.e., doxorubicin, bleomycin, vinblastine, and dacarbazine). Each cycle included doxorubicin 50 mg/m². Because her initial response to ABVD lasted for 2 years, the plan is to re-treat her with the same regimen. Which one of the following statements is the most correct?
    A. The patient has not reached the appropriate cumulative dose of doxorubicin to consider dexrazoxane.
    B. The patient has reached the appropriate cumulative dose of doxorubicin to consider dexrazoxane.
    C. The patient should not receive any more doxorubicin because she is at an increased risk of cardiotoxicity.
    D. The patient should not receive dexrazoxane because of the possibility of increased myelosuppression.

9. Which one of the following is the correct sequence for administering mesna and ifosfamide?
    A. Mesna before ifosfamide and then at 4 and 8 hours after ifosfamide.
    B. Ifosfamide before mesna and then at 4 and 8 hours after mesna.
    C. Mesna and ifosfamide beginning and ending at the same time.
    D. Mesna on day 1 and ifosfamide on days 2–5.

IX. MISCELLANEOUS ANTINEOPLASTIC PHARMACOTHERAPY

A. Leucovorin "rescue" may be used after methotrexate doses more than 100 mg/m²; in general, methotrexate doses greater than 500 mg/m² require leucovorin rescue.

B. Factors that increase the likelihood of methotrexate toxicity include renal dysfunction (causing delayed elimination), third-space fluid (e.g., pleural effusion, ascites), and administration of other drugs that may delay methotrexate elimination. Toxic reactions include mucous membrane toxicity (e.g., oral mucositis) and myelosuppression.

C. The dose of leucovorin depends on the methotrexate dose or level and the time since the completion of methotrexate. Methotrexate levels are usually obtained 24–48 hours after "intermediate" or "high" dose methotrexate, and leucovorin is continued until the methotrexate level falls to less than 0.1 mM (less than 1×10^{-7} M).

D. In contrast to its use with methotrexate, leucovorin is given in combination with 5-fluorouracil to enhance activity, not to "rescue" normal cells.

E. Extravasation Injuries
    1. A vesicant is an agent that, on extravasation, can cause tissue necrosis. Vesicant antineoplastic drugs include doxorubicin, daunorubicin, epirubicin, mechlorethamine, mitomycin, vincristine, vinblastine, vinorelbine, and streptozocin, ± oxaliplatin, ± paclitaxel.
    2. Anthracyclines cause the most severe tissue damage on extravasation.
    3. The literature generally recommends administering vesicants by intravenous injection rather than infusion, but some exceptions exist:
        a. Some institutional policies require infusions for every drug.
        b. Vincristine has been incorrectly administered by intrathecal injection with fatal consequences. Dilution of vincristine for administration as a short intravenous infusion has been recommended to prevent this error from occurring.
        c. Paclitaxel is administered as an infusion (1, 3, or 24 hours, depending on the protocol).

4. Management of extravasation
   a. Cold for doxorubicin, daunorubicin, and epirubicin
   b. Heat for vincristine, vinblastine, and vinorelbine
   c. Sodium thiosulfate for mechlorethamine
   d. Topical dimethyl sulfoxide has been recommended for anthracyclines. Its use is not as well established as the antidotes above. Hyaluronidase is recommended for vinca alkaloids, but hyaluronidase is of limited availability. Antidotes for mitomycin, streptozocin, paclitaxel, and oxaliplatin are not well documented in the literature.
   e. Dexrazoxane for doxorubicin, daunorubicin, idarubicin and epirubicin
   f. Many institutions do not allow the administration of vesicants through a peripheral vein, but rather, require that vesicants be administered through a central line with a venous access device. Although administering vesicants through a central line minimizes the likelihood of an extravasation injury, extravasation may still occur. The management of extravasation is intended for suspected or actual extravasation from a peripheral or central vein.

F. Management of Diarrhea
   1. Intensive loperamide therapy using doses higher than the recommended dose was initially described for irinotecan-induced diarrhea.
   2. Intensive antidiarrhea treatment is also used for other agents (e.g., 5-fluorouracil, epidermal growth factor receptor inhibitors)

G. Dose Adjustment for Organ Dysfunction
   1. Conflicting recommendations for dose adjustment have been reported. Many drugs have not been studied in patients with organ dysfunction.

   2. Dose adjustment for renal dysfunction may be considered for methotrexate, carboplatin, cisplatin etoposide, bleomycin, topotecan, and lenalidomide.

   3. Dose adjustment for hepatic dysfunction may be considered for doxorubicin, daunorubicin, vincristine, vinblastine, docetaxel, paclitaxel, and sorafenib.

Patient Case

10. A 40-year-old man is about to begin CHOP-R chemotherapy for large cell non-Hodgkin lymphoma. The patient asks how long the treatment will take and whether he can be treated as an outpatient. Which one of the following is the best answer?
    A. Administration of this regimen is expected to be complete in 1 hour, but because the regimen is highly emetogenic, it is usually given to patients while in the hospital.
    B. Administration of this regimen may take as long as 6 hours because the rituximab infusion rate is slowly increased, but the regimen is usually given to outpatients.
    C. Administration of this regimen may take as long as 6 hours because the vesicants doxorubicin and vincristine should be infused over several hours, but the regimen is usually given to outpatients.
    D. Administration of this regimen is expected to be complete in 1 hour, but because of the risk of tumor lysis syndrome, it is usually given to patients in the hospital.

REFERENCES

Antiemetics

1. National Comprehensive Cancer Network (NCCN). Clinical practice guidelines in oncology—antiemesis, version 4. 2009. http://www.nccn.org/professionals/physician_gls/f_guidelines.asp accessed February 3, 2010
2. Gralla RJ, Raftopoulos H. Progress in the control of chemotherapy-induced emesis: new agents and new studies. J Oncol Pract 2009;5:130–3.
3. Herrstedt J, Dombernowsky P. Anti-emetic therapy in cancer chemotherapy: current status. Basic Clin Pharmacol Toxicol 2007;101:143–50.
4. Naeim A, Dy SM, Lorenz KA, et al. Evidence-based recommendations for cancer nausea and vomiting. J Clin Oncol 2008;26:3903–10.
5. Hesketh PJ, Kris MG, Grunberg SM, et al. Proposal for classifying the acute emetogenicity of cancer chemotherapy. J Clin Oncol 1997;15:103–9.

Pain Management

1. U.S. Department of Health and Human Services Public Health Service Agency for Health Care Policy and Research (AHCPR). Clinical practice guideline, no. 9. Management of cancer pain. AHCPR Publication 94-0592, March 1994.
2. Foley KM. The treatment of cancer pain. N Engl J Med 1985;313:84–95.
3. Hillner BE, Ingle JN, Chlebowski RT, et al. American Society of Clinical Oncology 2003 update on the role of bisphosphonates and bone health issues in women with breast cancer. J Clin Oncol 2003;21:4042–57.
4. Berenson JR, Hillner BE, Kyle RA, et al. American Society of Clinical Oncology clinical practice guidelines: the role of bisphosphonates in multiple myeloma. J Clin Oncol 2002;20:3719–36.

Febrile Neutropenia/CSFs

1. Rolston KVI. The Infectious Diseases Society of America 2002 Guidelines for the Use of Antimicrobial Agents in Patients with Cancer and Neutropenia: salient features and comments. Clin Infect Dis 2004;39:S44–S48.
2. Hughes WT, Armstrong D, Bodey GP, et al. 2002 Guidelines for the use of antimicrobial agents in neutropenic patients with unexplained fever. Clin Infect Dis 2002;34:730–51.
3. Klastersky J, Paesmans M. Risk-adapted strategy for the management of febrile neutropenia in cancer patients. Support Care Cancer 2007;15:477–82.
4. Smith TJ, Khatcheressian J, Lyman GH, et al. 2006 Update of recommendations for the use of white blood cell growth factors: an evidence-based clinical practice guideline. J Clin Oncol 2006;24:1–19.

Thrombocytopenia

1. Adams VR, Brenner TL. Oprelvekin (Neumega). J Oncol Pharm Pract 1999;5:117–24.
2. Cantor SB, Elting LS, Hudson DV, Rubenstein EB. Pharmacoeconomic analysis of oprelvekin for secondary prophylaxis of thrombocytopenia for solid tumor patients receiving chemotherapy. Cancer 2003;97:3099–106.
3. Schiffer CA, Anderson KC, Bennett CL, et al. Platelet transfusions for patients with cancer: clinical practice guidelines of the American Society of Clinical Oncology. J Clin Oncol 2001;19:1519–38.

Anemia/Fatigue

1. National Comprehensive Cancer Network (NCCN). Practice guidelines in oncology—cancer- and chemotherapy-induced anemia, version 2. 2010. http://www.nccn.org/professionals/physician_gls/f_guidelines.asp accessed February 3, 2010

Chemoprotectants

1. Schuchter LM, Hensley ML, Meropol NJ, Winer EP. 2002 update of recommendations for the use of chemotherapy and radiotherapy protectants: clinical practice guidelines of the American Society of Clinical Oncology. J Clin Oncol 2002;20:2895–903.
2. Links M, Lewis C. Chemoprotectants: a review of their clinical pharmacology and therapeutic efficacy. Drugs 1999;57:293–308.
3. Bukowsi R. Cytoprotection in the treatment of pediatric cancer: review of current strategies in adults and their application to children. Med Pediatr Oncol 1999;32:124–34.

Oncology Emergencies

1. Abrahm JL. Management of pain and spinal cord compression in patients with advanced cancer. Ann Intern Med 1999;131:37–46.
2. Nicolin G. Paediatric update. Emergencies and their management. Eur J Cancer 2002;38:1365–77.
3. Nakshima L. Guidelines for the treatment of hypercalcemia associated with malignancy. J Oncol Pharm Pract 1997;3:31–7.
4. Brigden ML. Hematologic and oncologic emergencies. Doing the most good in the least time. Postgrad Med 2001;109:143–63.
5. Krimsky WS, Behrens RJ, Kerkvliet GJ. Oncology emergencies for the internist. Cleve Clin J Med 2002;69:209–22.
6. Holdsworth MT, Nguyen P. Role of iv. allopurinol and rasburicase in tumor lysis syndrome. Am J Health Syst Pharm 2003;60:2213–24.
7. Yim BT, Sims-McCallum RP, Chong PH. Rasburicase for the treatment and prevention of hyperuremia. Ann Pharmacother 2003;37:1047–54.

ANSWERS AND EXPLANATIONS TO PATIENT CASES

1. Answer: A
This is a highly emetogenic regimen, and it is associated with delayed nausea and vomiting. The best choice is a serotonin receptor antagonist with dexamethasone and aprepitant for prophylaxis against nausea and vomiting. Prochlorperazine is not effective against a highly emetogenic stimulus. Granisetron and ondansetron are both serotonin receptor antagonists, and no rationale exists for combining them. Lorazepam may be a useful addition, but it does not replace dexamethasone or aprepitant for highly emetogenic chemotherapy.

2. Answer: A
Aprepitant and dexamethasone should be continued after chemotherapy administration. Serotonin receptor antagonists are generally thought not to be effective in preventing delayed nausea and vomiting. Metoclopramide plus dexamethasone is also commonly used, but this combination was not one of the options.

3. Answer: D
The patient is taking oxycodone-APAP 5 mg/325 mg, which provides 60 mg of oxycodone per day and 3900 mg of APAP. We should not increase her current drugs because of concerns about APAP toxicity. If she is changed to a higher strength of the combination product, APAP toxicity is still a concern, which eliminates the choices of increasing to oxycodone-APAP 7.5 mg 2 tablets every 4 hours or oxycodone-APAP 10 mg 2 tablets every 4 hours. Adding SR morphine is a good option. Continuing the ibuprofen might be helpful for bone pain. Oxycodone-APAP, which is short acting, could be continued for breakthrough pain, but she is already getting a lot of APAP without good pain relief.

4. Answer: C
Gabapentin might help the neuropathic component (i.e., the shooting pains) of her pain. There is no point to adding APAP, and the case does not mention muscle spasms. She is already receiving an NSAID, so there is no need to add naproxen.

5. Answer: D
To calculate the ANC, multiply the WBC by the segmented neutrophils and the band neutrophils: $600/mm^3 \times (0.6 + 0.1) = 420/mm^3$.

6. Answer: C
The patient is neutropenic; however, she should not begin a CSF. Her ANC is greater than $100/mm^3$, and she does not have any signs/symptoms of active infection. Prophylactic treatment with antibiotic drugs is not necessary and can increase the risk of resistant organisms. At this time, the patient should be monitored for evidence of infection (e.g., she should be instructed to take her temperature and return to the clinic or emergency department if a single oral temperature of 101°F or more or 100.4°F or greater for at least 1 hour or if she develops any signs/symptoms of infection). Because the disease is potentially curable, doses should not be reduced on the next cycle.

7. Answer: A
Recent literature and subsequent changes in guidelines and CMS (Centers for Medicare and Medicaid Services) reimbursement suggest that an erythropoiesis-stimulating protein be considered when hemoglobin is less than 10 g/dL. Transfusion is also an option.

8. Answer: B
The patient has received a cumulative dose of 300 mg/m^2 of doxorubicin (50 mg/m^2 × 6 cycles). This is the appropriate cumulative dose of doxorubicin to consider dexrazoxane. She is at an increased risk of cardiotoxicity; however, dexrazoxane protects the heart from this toxicity. Dexrazoxane may increase the myelosuppression from chemotherapy, but that does not represent a contraindication.

9. Answer: A
Several different schedules of ifosfamide and mesna administration exist (e.g., ifosfamide short infusion followed by intermittent infusions of mesna and continuous infusion of both ifosfamide and mesna). But mesna should always be continued longer than ifosfamide.

10. Answer: B
The CHOP-R regimen is commonly given in the outpatient setting. Cyclophosphamide, doxorubicin, and vincristine can all be administered by intravenous bolus injection or short intravenous infusion. Rituximab is a chimeric monoclonal antibody, and infusion reactions are often observed with rituximab administration. Although some protocols specify infusion for 1 hour, the usual recommended infusion schedule for rituximab involves

increasing the rate by 50 mg/hour every 30 minutes (100 mg/hour every 30 minutes for doses after the first dose) and slowing the rate if a reaction occurs. Administering the usual dose of 375 mg/m^2 can therefore take as long as 6 hours (or more) for the initial infusion.

ANSWERS AND EXPLANATIONS TO SELF-ASSESSMENT QUESTIONS

1. Answer: C
Patients who have had poor control of nausea and vomiting on previous cycles of chemotherapy are at an increased risk of anticipatory emesis. Anxious patients are also at an increased risk of chemotherapy-induced nausea and vomiting. Benzodiazepines help decrease anxiety and, by causing anterograde amnesia, may minimize anticipatory symptoms. Although it is not clear that patients who do not respond to one serotonin receptor antagonist will respond to another, a change in regimen is needed. Substituting dolasetron for the granisetron would be acceptable, but the addition of lorazepam is essential. Palonosetron is the preferred serotonin receptor antagonist in some guidelines, but this is not universally agreed on. For this patient, the palonosetron option also includes lorazepam. Metoclopramide is another option, but an effective dose might be difficult to administer orally (especially as tablets), and again, the addition of lorazepam would be preferred over the addition of aprepitant in this patient.

2. Answer: D
This patient's altered mental status is most likely because of hypercalcemia. The corrected calcium is 13.6 mg/dL. Corrected calcium concentrations more than 12 g/dL should be treated with a bisphosphonate (either pamidronate or zoledronic acid) in addition to hydration with normal saline. Furosemide may be required during hydration, but not before hydration, because the patient is likely dehydrated. This patient does not require rapid reversal of hypercalcemia; hence, calcitonin is not needed. Dexamethasone may be used in patients with lymphoma or myeloma, but it will have no effect on metastatic non–small cell lung cancer.

3. Answer: C
The patient is at risk of tumor lysis syndrome because he has a chemosensitive tumor and a high tumor burden (WBC). Prevention is the key in tumor lysis syndrome and includes adequate saline hydration and the use of allopurinol. Dextrose 5% is not an appropriate intravenous fluid for hydration because it does not contain saline. The value of alkalinization with sodium bicarbonate is somewhat controversial, and alkalinization is not a replacement for allopurinol.

4. Answer: B
This anemia is not attributable to treatment because chemotherapy has not yet begun. Epoetin and darbepoetin are only indicated for chemotherapy-associated anemia. Chemotherapy should not be delayed, nor should chemotherapy doses be reduced in the setting of a potentially curable malignancy. Therefore, the patient should be transfused with packed RBCs.

5. Answer: B
$(55\% + 5\%) \times 500 = 300$

6. Answer: A
The patient is neutropenic (ANC 300/mm^3). Temperature of 103°F places the febrile neutropenia outside the definition of low-risk febrile neutropenia. Therefore, the patient should be hospitalized for intravenous antibiotics and an infection work-up. She does not have any of the appropriate reasons to administer CSFs (i.e., documented pneumonia, hypotension, sepsis syndrome, or fungal infection). Her chemotherapy may need to be delayed, but it should be continued. She should receive a CSF with the next cycle of chemotherapy.

7. Answer: B
Febrile neutropenia developed at the time of the expected neutrophil nadir—12 days after chemotherapy. Marrow recovery would be expected to follow. The percent eosinophils may be slightly elevated, but the absolute count is low. The platelet count is also low, not elevated. Neutrophils are often affected by myelosuppressive chemotherapy to a greater degree than platelets.

8. Answer: D
Opioids may provide some relief from neuropathic pain, but often, the response to opioids is less than optimal. In general, higher doses of opioids provide greater pain relief; thus, increasing the dose of fentanyl and morphine is an option for this patient. But this assumes that a lower dose previously provided some benefit. Nothing in the history suggests that the patient is deriving much, if any, benefit at the present opioid doses. Adjuvant analgesic drugs, including tricyclic antidepressants and anticonvulsants, are used to help manage neuropathic pain. Gabapentin, with a relatively good adverse event profile, is a reasonable option. Note, however, that adjuvant analgesic drugs should not be given to decrease the opioid dose or discontinue the use of opioid drugs. (It may be possible to decrease the dose later if gabapentin provides adequate pain relief.) Diazepam is more effective for muscle spasms than for neuropathic pain, and this option also included decreasing the fentanyl dose at the same time the new drug was initiated.

9. Answer: D
Limited-stage small cell lung cancer is potentially curable; therefore, the patient should continue on the planned doses of chemotherapy. The correct dose of filgrastim is 5 mcg/kg/day subcutaneously, not 250 mcg/m² (this is the dose for sargramostim). The correct dose for pegfilgrastim is a single 6-mg injection. Filgrastim should not be given on the same day as chemotherapy; therefore, Answer D is correct.

10. Answer: A
Doxorubicin undergoes hepatic clearance, and there are recommendations for dosage reduction based on bilirubin. There is no reason to reduce the dose of cyclophosphamide.

11. Answer: A
Large cell lymphoma is faster growing and more chemosensitive than metastatic colorectal cancer. Thus, patients with large cell lymphoma are more likely to develop hyperuricemia or tumor lysis syndrome from rapid cell turnover, both before treatment and after chemotherapy. Hypercalcemia is not a common complication of either of these diseases. Some aggressive lymphomas may be associated with hypercalcemia, but pamidronate is used to treat, not prevent, this complication.

12. Answer: C
Neither patient should undergo chemotherapy with an ANC of 800/mm³. Both can be treated when neutropenia resolves (likely within 1 week). It is important to keep patient 1 on schedule because his disease is potentially curable; therefore, patient 1 should receive filgrastim after the next chemotherapy treatment to prevent another dose delay. When patient 2 resumes chemotherapy, his doses can be decreased to prevent a recurrence of neutropenia. The dose decrease is not likely to have a substantially negative effect on the treatment outcome because the goal of treatment is usually not cure.

13. Answer: C
Injury after extravasation of an anthracycline is potentially the most severe. Thus, when the recommended antidotes for different vesicants conflict (e.g., heat vs. cold), treatment should be directed at the anthracycline. Dexrazoxane is now indicated for doxorubicin extravasation. Cold rather than heat would also be appropriate. Cyclophosphamide is not considered a vesicant.

MEN'S AND WOMEN'S HEALTH

SHAREEN Y. EL-IBIARY, PHARM.D., BCPS
MIDWESTERN UNIVERSITY COLLEGE OF PHARMACY - GLENDALE
GLENDALE, ARIZONA

MEN'S AND WOMEN'S HEALTH

SHAREEN Y. EL-IBIARY, PHARM.D., BCPS
MIDWESTERN UNIVERSITY COLLEGE OF PHARMACY - GLENDALE
GLENDALE, ARIZONA

Learning Objectives:

1. Recommend appropriate treatment options for patients with osteoporosis, menopausal symptoms, and sexual dysfunction.

2. Identify drugs that are considered safe and unsafe in pregnancy and lactation.

3. Modify contraceptive regimens based on estrogen- and progestin-related adverse effects or drug interactions.

4. Devise a pharmacotherapeutic plan for appropriate contraceptive use, misused contraceptive methods, and use of emergency contraception.

5. Identify the common sexually transmitted diseases and recommend appropriate pharmacotherapy.

Self-Assessment Questions:

Answers to these questions may be found at the end of this chapter.

1. J.L. is a 63-year-old white man who drinks alcohol daily, smokes 1 pack/day, and has a sedentary lifestyle. He drinks four glasses of whole milk daily. He is 5'7" and weighs 190 lb (86.4 kg). His bone mineral density (BMD) T-score is −1.9 at the hip and −2.5 at the spine. Which one of the following statements is correct?
   A. Normal BMD of the hip and spine.
   B. Osteopenia of the hip and spine.
   C. Osteoporosis of the spine and osteopenia of the hip.
   D. Osteoporosis in men is defined when a fracture has occurred.

2. Which one of the following treatments is best for J.L.?
   A. Recommend continuation of milk consumption for calcium and vitamin D, quit smoking, and begin weight-bearing exercise.
   B. Take risedronate, continue milk consumption, quit smoking, and begin weight-bearing exercise.
   C. Take raloxifene, quit smoking, and begin weight-bearing exercise.
   D. Use teriparatide, continue milk consumption, and quit smoking.

3. A 28-year-old woman who is 5'4" and weighs 130 lb (59 kg) has a history of two deep venous thromboses (DVTs) but is otherwise healthy; she is seeking to become pregnant. She currently takes warfarin 2 mg orally daily. Which of the following is the best recommendation for this patient?
   A. Discontinue anticoagulation therapy because it consists of category X medications.
   B. Continue current warfarin dose to prevent clots during pregnancy.
   C. Discontinue warfarin and start enoxaparin 40 mg subcutaneously daily until she is pregnant and continue through pregnancy.
   D. Discontinue warfarin, start enoxaparin 40 mg subcutaneously daily until she is 12 weeks pregnant, and then restart warfarin.

4. K.B. is a 53-year-old postmenopausal woman suffering from severe hot flashes that have not resolved with venlafaxine 75 mg orally daily. She is otherwise healthy with no history of cancer and no surgeries. She is given conjugated estrogen 0.625 mg orally daily. Which of the following statements below is best for K.B.?
   A. No other drug is required; estrogen alone is sufficient for hot flashes.
   B. Medroxyprogesterone acetate should be added to decrease the risk of endometrial cancer.
   C. No other drug is required because K.B., otherwise healthy, should continue on venlafaxine.
   D. Medroxyprogesterone acetate should be added to decrease the risk of stroke.

5. C.B. is a 23-year-old woman initiated on Ortho-Novum 7/7/7 four months ago for contraception. She was recently prescribed erythromycin for acne. Which one of the following drug interactions may occur with Ortho-Novum 7/7/7 and erythromycin?
   A. The effectiveness of the oral contraceptive (OC) may be increased.
   B. The effectiveness of the OC may be decreased.
   C. The effectiveness of erythromycin may be increased.
   D. The effectiveness of erythromycin may be decreased.

6. A study compares the incidence of herpes simplex genital infections in patients receiving suppressive therapy with patients receiving acyclovir or famciclovir. After 1 year of follow-up, 27% in the acyclovir group and 24% in the famciclovir group experience a recurrent infection ($p<0.05$). Which one of the following represents how many patients (in 1 year) would need to be treated with famciclovir over acyclovir to prevent one recurrent infection?
   A. 3.
   B. 24.
   C. 34.
   D. There is insufficient information to calculate this number.

7. S.F. is a 36-year-old married woman with a history of DVT seeking contraception. She is 5'8" and weighs 202 lb (91 kg), with blood pressure (BP) today of 140/88 mm Hg; she denies smoking and alcohol use and states she would like to have children in a year or so. Which of the following is the best contraceptive agent for S.F.?

   A. Depo-Provera.
   B. Ortho-Evra.
   C. Nor-QD.
   D. Yasmin.

8. D.S. is a 43-year-old man who has difficulty maintaining an erection during intercourse. His medical history includes diabetes mellitus, hyperlipidemia, and hypertension. His drugs include aspirin, metformin, lovastatin, and hydrochlorothiazide. Blood pressure is 130/85 mm Hg, hemoglobin A_{1c} 6.2, total cholesterol 190, low-density lipoprotein (LDL) 102, high-density lipoprotein (HDL) 55, triglycerides 142, total testosterone concentration 998 ng/dL (reference range 270–1070 ng/dL), and free testosterone concentration 23 ng/dL (reference range 9–30 ng/dL). Which one of the following drugs should be initiated for his erectile dysfunction?

   A. Fluoxetine.
   B. Testosterone scrotal dermal patch.
   C. Sildenafil.
   D. Yohimbine.

9. A.R., a 42-year-old man, is an intravenous drug abuser who lives in and out of homeless shelters. He is taken to the emergency department by ambulance after experiencing paralysis on the right side of his body. The people at the shelter thought he might be having a stroke. In the emergency department, a laboratory profile was performed, which was positive for the Venereal Disease Research Laboratory (syphilis test) with 10 white blood cells (count) per cubic millimeter. R.L. has no known significant medical history (except for treatment of sexually transmitted disease [STD]), but he is allergic to penicillin (anaphylactic reaction). Which one of the following therapies is best for R.L.?

   A. Benzathine penicillin G 2.4 million units intramuscularly every week for 3 weeks after penicillin desensitization.
   B. Doxycycline 200 mg intravenously or orally every 12 hours for 6 weeks.
   C. Levofloxacin 250 mg intravenously × 1.
   D. Penicillin G 4 million units every 4 hours intravenously for 14 days after penicillin desensitization.

10. A prospective, double-blind study compared the effects of acyclovir versus valacyclovir in 350 patients with first-episode genital herpes. Which one of the following statistical tests should be used to compare the mean duration of time until the lesions healed?

    A. Analysis of variance (ANOVA).
    B. Chi-square test.
    C. Mann-Whitney U-test.
    D. Student t-test.

I. HORMONE THERAPY/MENOPAUSE

   A. Estrogen and Progestin Therapy
      1. Primary indication: treatment of moderate to severe menopause symptoms and osteoporosis treatment when others have failed
      2. Benefits and risks of estrogen and progestin therapy
         a. Benefits of estrogen
            i. Relieves genitourinary atrophy
               Thinning of hair of the mons and shrinkage of the labia minora
               Atrophy of vulva leads to pruritus and pain.
               Vaginal pH 4.5–5 → 6–8, creating a favorable environment for bacterial colonization
               Loss of lubrication → dyspareunia
               Recurrent episodes of urinary frequency and urgency with dysuria
            ii. Relieves vasomotor instability
               Occurs in 75%–85% of women
               Occurs usually within 12–24 months after the last menstrual period
               Increased skin temperature, nausea, dizziness, headache, palpitations, diaphoresis, night sweats
            iii. Osteoporosis: reduction of hip fractures by 25%; reduction of vertebral fractures by 50%. Estrogen reduces the rate of resorption but does not restore bone loss.
            iv. It was once thought to lower LDL cholesterol and increase HDL cholesterol; however, it was not shown to lower coronary heart disease based on the HERS (Heart and Estrogen/Progestin Replacement Study, JAMA 1998;280:605–13) or Women's Health Initiative (WHI; JAMA 2002;288:321–33) trial.
            v. Insomnia and fatigue
            vi. Mood changes
            vii. Sexual function
         b. Risks of estrogen
            i. Endometrial cancer by unopposed estrogen. Cancer is dependent on duration of estrogen use; cancer risk increases 8-fold for 10–20 years of estrogen use. Not recommended for use in women with a history of endometrial cancer
            ii. Breast cancer with unopposed estrogen: uncertain. May increase slightly (25%) among women who take estrogen for 10–20 years. Not recommended for use in women with a history of breast cancer
            iii. Increased risk of cardiovascular outcomes (See WHI trial.)
            iv. Adverse effects: bloating, headache, breast tenderness (5%–10%)
            v. Unpredictable uterine bleeding with unopposed estrogen (35%–40%)
         c. Benefits of progestin
            i. Decreased risk of estrogen-induced irregular bleeding, endometrial hyperplasia, and carcinoma
            ii. Protection against breast carcinoma
            iii. Enhancement of estrogen prophylaxis of osteoporosis
         d. Risks of progestin
            i. Adverse effects: bloating, weight gain, irritability, depression (dose related)
            ii. Unpredictable endometrial bleeding with continuous estrogen-progestin during first 8–12 months (30%–50%)

3. The WHI trial
   a. Conjugated estrogens and medroxyprogesterone acetate and cardiovascular outcomes (HERS trial, JAMA 1998;280:605–13)

   Table 1. Summary of WHI Outcomes

Risk or Benefit	Relative Risk	Absolute Risk Each Year
Heart attacks	1.29 or 29% ↑	7 more cases in 10,000 women
Breast cancer	1.26 or 26% ↑	8 more cases in 10,000 women
Strokes	1.41 or 41% ↑	8 more cases in 10,000 women
Blood clots	2.11 or 111% ↑	18 more cases in 10,000 women
Hip fractures	0.66 or 33% ↓	5 fewer cases in 10,000 women
Colon cancer	0.63 or 37% ↓	6 fewer cases in 10,000 women
Dementia	2.05 or 105% ↑	23 more cases in 10,000 women older than 65

   WHI = Women's Health Initiative.

   b. A longer duration of use leads to a greater decrease in relative hazards in nonfatal myocardial infarction (MI) and coronary heart disease death.
   c. Further information suggests increased risk of ovarian cancer and lung cancer (JAMA 2009;302:298–305, Lancet 2009;374:1243–51.)

Patient Case

1. N.I. is a 51-year-old woman complaining of hot flashes and vaginal irritation. She has tried exercise, diet, and antidepressants to help relieve her hot flashes but has been unsuccessful. She is otherwise healthy with no history of cancer and no surgeries. She states her hot flashes are interfering with her daily activities and wants to try hormone therapy. When counseling N.I. on the use of hormone therapy and explaining the WHI trial, which one of the following was proved statistically significant with conjugated estrogen and medroxyprogesterone acetate and should be mentioned to N.I.?
   A. Decreased risk of strokes.
   B. Decreased risk of MI.
   C. Increased risk of fractures.
   D. Increased risk of DVT.

---

4. Hormone regimens (Ann Intern Med 1992;117:1038–41)
   a. Unopposed estrogen
      i. Conjugated estrogen taken daily without interruption suggested for women with a hysterectomy to prevent endometrial cancer in women with a uterus
      ii. Transdermal estradiol patches in women intolerant of oral preparations
      iii. Therapy duration – lowest dose for least amount of time, check after 3 months to 1 year if asymptomatic; if symptoms recur, treat for an additional 3 months, best to keep less than 5 years of treatment
   b. Estrogen plus cyclic progestin
      i. Estrogen as above
      ii. Cyclic progestin such as medroxyprogesterone acetate 5–10 mg/day or the equivalent for 10–14 days/month
      iii. Similar to female cycle

        c. Estrogen plus continuous progestin
            i. Estrogen as above
            ii. Continuous progestin 2.5 mg/day or the equivalent without interruption
            iii. Irregular menstrual cycle for the first 8–12 months of hormone therapy
        d. Daily or intermittent
            i. Continuous estrogen daily
            ii. Three days on with progestin, 3 days off
            iii. Not used frequently
    5. Monitoring criteria
        a. Monthly: breast self-examination
        b. Annually: breast examination, mammography, pelvic examination
        c. Evaluation of vaginal bleeding
        d. Unopposed estrogen: any episode of vaginal bleeding unless the woman has had a normal assessment in the past 6 months
        e. Estrogen plus cyclic progestin: if bleeding occurs other than at the time of expected withdrawal bleeding
        f. Estrogen plus continuous progestin: if bleeding is heavier than normal, prolonged (longer than 10 days at a time), frequent (more often than monthly), or persists longer than 10 months after beginning therapy

Products and Dosing

Table 2. Oral Estrogen Products

Generic Name	Brand Name	Dosages Available (mg)
Conjugated estrogens	Premarin	0.3, 0.45, 0.625, 0.9, 1.25
Synthetic conjugated estrogens, A	Cenestin	0.3, 0.45, 0.625, 0.9, 1.25
Synthetic conjugated estrogens, B	Enjuvia	0.3, 0.45, 0.625, 0.9, 1.25
Estradiol acetate	Femtrace	0.45, 0.9, 1.8
17 beta-estradiol	Estrace	0.5, 1.0, 2.0
Esterified estrogens	Menest	0.3, 0.625, 1.25, 2.5
Estropipate	Ortho-Est	0.625, 1.25, 1.5

Table 3. Vaginal Estrogen Products

Formulation	Generic Name	Brand Name	Dose
Vaginal creams	Micronized estradiol (0.1 mg/g)	Estrace	Initial: 2–4 g/day for 1–2 weeks; then 1 g/day
	Conjugated estrogens (0.625 mg/g)	Premarin	0.5–2 g/day
Vaginal rings	17 beta-estradiol 7.5 mcg/day	Estring	One ring every 3 months
	Estradiol acetate 0.05 mg/day or 0.10 mg/day	Femring	
Vaginal tablet	Estradiol hemihydrate 25 mcg of estradiol/day	Vagifem	One vaginal tablet 2 times/week; then 1 tablet 2 times/week

Table 4. Transdermal Estrogen Products

Formulation	Brand Name	Estrogen Delivery (mg/day)	Dose
17 beta-estradiol matrix patch	Alora Climara Vivelle Vivelle Dot Esclim Menostar	0.025, 0.05, 0.075, 0.1 0.025, 0.0375, 0.05, 0.075, 0.1 0.05, 0.1 0.025, 0.0375, 0.05, 0.075, 0.1 0.025, 0.0375, 0.05, 0.075, 0.1 0.014	1 patch 2 times/week 1 patch weekly 1 patch 2 times/week 1 patch 2 times/week 1 patch 2 times/week 1 patch weekly
17 beta-estradiol reservoir patch	Estraderm	0.05, 0.1	1 patch 2 times/week
17 beta-estradiol topical emulsion	Estrasorb	0.05 for 2 packets	Apply 3.48 g/day to skin (2 packets)
17 beta-estradiol transdermal gel	EstroGel 0.06% Elestrin 0.06% Divigel 0.1%	0.035 0.0125 0.003, 0.009, 0.027	Apply 1.25 g/day (1 pump) Apply 0.87 g/day (1 pump) 0.25, 0.5, or 1 g of gel
17 beta-estradiol transdermal spray	Evamist	0.021	Initial 1 spray/day (0.021 mg) increasing to 2 or 3 sprays/day

Table 5. Combination Products

Formulation	Brand Name	Hormone Strengths	Dose
Conjugated estrogens/ medroxyprogesterone acetate	Prempro	0.625 mg estrogen with 2.5 or 5 mg of progestogen 0.3 or 0.45 mg of estrogen with 1.5 mg of progestogen	One daily
Conjugated estrogens/ medroxyprogesterone acetate	Premphase	0.625 mg of estrogen with 5 mg of progestogen	0.625 mg/day for 14 days; then 0.625 mg and 5 mg/day for 14 days
17 beta-estradiol/ norethindrone acetate	CombiPatch	0.05 mg of estrogen, 0.14 mg of progestogen 0.05 mg of estrogen, 0.25 mg of progestogen	One patch 2 times/week
17 beta-estradiol/ levonorgestrel	Climara Pro	0.045 mg of estrogen, 0.015 mg of progestogen	One patch weekly
17 beta-estradiol/ norgestimate	Prefest	1 mg of estrogen, 0.09 mg of progestogen	3 days of estrogen tablets only, 3 days of estrogen and progestogen
17 beta-estradiol/ norethindrone acetate	Activella	0.5 mg of estrogen, 0.1 mg of progestogen 1 mg of estrogen, 0.5 mg of progestogen	One daily
Ethinyl estradiol/ norethindrone acetate	Femhrt	2.5 mcg of estrogen, 0.5 mg of progestogen 5 mcg of estrogen, 1 mg of progestogen	One daily
17 beta-estradiol-drospirenone	Angeliq	1 mg of estrogen, 0.5 mg of progestogen	

Table 6. Progestin Products

Generic Name	Brand Name	Dosage Strengths
Medroxyprogesterone acetate	Provera	2.5-, 5-, 10-mg oral tablets
Norethindrone acetate	Aygestin	5-mg oral tablets
Norethindrone	Micronor, Nor-QD	0.35-mg oral tablets
Norgestrel	Ovrette	0.075-mg oral tablets
Progesterone in peanut oil	Prometrium	100-mg, 200-mg oral capsules
Levonorgestrel	Mirena	20 mcg/day released from intrauterine system
Progesterone gel	Prochieve 4%, 8%	45 mg/applicator vaginally, 90mg/applicator vaginally
Megestrol acetate	Megace	20-, 40-mg oral tablets

    B. Serotonin Reuptake Inhibitors – best for vasomotor symptoms
        1. Venlafaxine 75 mg orally every day (Loprinzi C, et al. Lancet 2000;356:2059–63)
        2. Fluoxetine 20 mg orally every day
        3. Paroxetine 20 mg orally every day
        4. Sertraline 100 mg orally every day

    C. Natural Products – some data for effectiveness
        1. Soy isoflavones – may still have adverse effects similar to conjugated estrogens
        2. Evening primrose oil – no solid evidence for use
        3. Black cohosh – some effectiveness for vasomotor symptoms
        4. Bioidentical hormones – may still have adverse effects similar to conjugated estrogens

    D. Others – used for vasomotor symptoms
        1. Clonidine
        2. Megestrol
        3. Gabapentin

II. OSTEOPOROSIS

    A. World Health Organization (WHO) Definitions
        1. Normal = BMD within 1 standard deviation (SD) of the young adult mean
        2. Osteopenia = BMD between −1 SD and −2.5 SD below the young adult mean
        3. Osteoporosis = BMD at least −2.5 SD

    B. Guidelines are based on 2003 American Association of Clinical Endocrinologists (AACE) Medical Guidelines for Clinical Practice for the Prevention and Treatment of Postmenopausal Osteoporosis, 2004 American College of Obstetricians and Gynecologists (ACOG) Clinical Management of Osteoporosis, 2006 North American Menopause Society (NAMS) Position Statement on the Management of Osteoporosis in Postmenopausal Women, and 2008 Clinician's Guide to Prevention and Treatment of Osteoporosis by the National Osteoporosis Foundation (NOF).
        1. Risk factors for osteoporotic fractures
            a. Female sex
            b. White race
            c. Poor nutrition, long-term low-calorie intake

d. Early menopause (before age 45) or prolonged premenopausal amenorrhea
e. Estrogen deficiency
f. Drugs: glucocorticoids, heparin, anticonvulsants, excessive levothyroxine, gonadotropin-releasing hormone agonists, lithium, cancer drugs
g. Low body mass index (BMI) or low weight
h. Family history of osteoporosis
i. Low calcium and vitamin D intake
j. Sedentary lifestyle, decreased mobility
k. Cigarette smoking
l. Alcoholism
m. Dementia
n. Impaired eyesight despite adequate correction
o. Previous fractures
p. History of falls

2. Recommendations
   a. Advise patient to avoid smoking and to consume only moderate amounts of alcohol.
   b. Encourage regular weight-bearing and muscle-strengthening exercise.
   c. Encourage adequate intake of calcium (at least 1200 mg/day) and vitamin D (800–1000 IU/day).
   d. Assessment
      i. Dual-energy x-ray absorptiometry (DXA)
      ii. Peripheral DXA
      iii. FRAX score
      iv. Quantitative computed tomography
   e. Recommended BMD testing
      i. All women 65 years and older (NAMS, ACOG, AACE), men older than 70 (NOF)
      ii. Men aged 50–70 years with risk factors or previous fractures
      iii. All postmenopausal women with medical causes of bone loss (NAMS)
      iv. Postmenopausal women younger than 65 years with at least one of the following:
         (a) Previous fracture after menopause other than skull, facial bone, angle, finger, and toe; thinness (body weight less than 127 lb or BMI less than 21 kg/m^2); history of hip fracture in a parent; current smoking) (NAMS)
         (b) With any risk factor listed in section B1 (ACOG)
         (c) Previous fracture not caused by severe trauma (AACE)
         (d) Thinness (body weight less than 127 lb), family history of spine or hip fracture (AACE)
   f. Initiation of drug therapy
      i. North American Menopause Society
         (a) If BMD T-score is below −2.5 in the absence of risk factors
         (b) If BMD T-score is below −2.0 to −2.5 with at least one of the following: previous fracture after menopause other than skull, facial bone, angle, finger, and toe; thinness (body weight less than 127 lb or BMI less than 21 kg/m^2); history of hip fracture in a parent) (NAMS)
         (c) All postmenopausal women who have had an osteoporotic vertebral fracture

ii. American College of Obstetricians and Gynecologists
   (a) If fragility or low-impact fracture
   (b) If BMD T-score is below −2.0 in the absence of risk factors
   (c) If BMD T-score is below −1.5 in the presence of one or more risk factors in section B1
iii. American Association of Clinical Endocrinologists
   (a) If low-trauma fracture
   (b) If BMD T-score is below −2.5 with no risk factors
   (c) If BMD T-score is below −1.5 with risk factors in section B1
   (d) If nonpharmacologic preventive measures are ineffective
iv. National Osteoporosis Foundation
   (a) A hip or vertebral fracture
   (b) BMD T-score is below −2.5 at femoral neck or spine excluding secondary causes
   (c) BMD T-score between −1.0 and −2.5 at femoral neck or spine and 10-year probability of hip fracture greater than 3% or 10-year probability of major osteoporosis-related fracture of greater than 20% based on the FRAX system
   g. Follow up on BMD-DXA every 2 years

C. Osteoporosis Treatments
   1. Selective estrogen receptor modulators
      a. Evista: raloxifene
      b. Indication: prevention and treatment of osteoporosis in postmenopausal women
      c. Mechanism: selective estrogen receptor modulator
         i. Reduction in resorption of bone
         ii. Decrease in overall bone turnover
         iii. Data suggest estrogen antagonist in uterine and breast tissue
      d. Efficacy:
         i. Reduces the risk of vertebral fractures; reduces vertebral fractures by 30%–50%
         ii. Lowers total cholesterol by 7% and LDL by 11%; does not reduce risk of coronary heart disease
      e. Adverse reactions:
         i. Hot flashes: 6%–25%
         ii. Leg cramps: 6%
      f. Dose: 60 mg/day orally
      g. Contraindications
         i. Pregnancy, nursing, pediatrics
         ii. History of venous thromboembolic events; greatest risk of venous thromboembolic events occurs during first 4 months
      h. Drug interactions
         i. Bile acid resins decreased raloxifene by 60%.
         ii. Warfarin's prothrombin time decreased by 10%.
         iii. Thyroid hormones—separate administration by 12 hours
   2. Bisphosphonates
      a. Alendronate (Fosamax), risedronate (Actonel), ibandronate (Boniva), zoledronic acid (Reclast)
      b. Inhibits normal and abnormal bone resorption; a selective inhibitor unlike etidronate (inhibitor of bone formation)
      c. First-line drug

d. Efficacy
   i. Reduces vertebral and non-vertebral fractures by 30%–50%
e. Adverse events (not dose-dependent):
   i. Gastrointestinal (GI) (comparable to etidronate): flatulence, acid regurgitation, esophageal ulcer, dysphasia, abdominal distention, gastritis
   ii. Miscellaneous: headache, musculoskeletal pain, rash
   iii. Laboratory values: Ca^{2+} decreases; phosphate decreases by first month. No more decreases during 3 years
   iv. Osteonecrosis of jaw. Most are associated with dental procedures. Most cases in patients with cancer after prolonged therapy. Intravenous administration has a greater risk than oral therapy.
f. Drug-food interactions – Wait at least 30 minutes after taking bisphosphonate before taking the above drugs or any food.
g. Dosage for osteoporosis:
   i. Alendronate: 10 mg/day with water 30 minutes before breakfast or 70 mg/week
   ii. Alendronate with vitamin D: 10 mg/day with water 30 minutes before breakfast or 70 mg/week
   iii. Risedronate: 5 mg/day or 35 mg/week
   iv. Risedronate with calcium: 5 mg/day or 35 mg/week
   v. Ibandronate: 2.5 mg/day or 150 mg once monthly orally waiting at least 60 minutes before eating, drinking, or taking another drug or 3 mg intravenously every 3 months
   vi. Zoledronic acid: 5 mg intravenously × 1 annually
h. Renal impairment
   i. Creatinine clearance = 35–60 mL/minute   No dosage change
   ii. Creatinine clearance less than 35 mL/minute Not recommended
3. Calcium
   a. Calcium intake

Table 6.

Age Group	Optimal Daily Intake of Calcium (mg)
19–50 years	1000
Older than 50 years	1200 according to ACOG, AACE 1500 for women not taking hormone therapy and all women older than 65 years according to the National Institutes of Health

AACE = American Association of Clinical Endocrinologists; ACOG = American College of Obstetricians and Gynecologists.

   b. Avoid doses higher than 2500 mg/day.
4. Vitamin D
   a. Promotes calcium reabsorption
   b. Dose = 800–1000 IU/day for those older than 50 years, 400–800 IU/day for those younger than 50 years
   c. Doses higher than 2000 IU/day may cause hypercalciuria or hypercalcemia.
   d. Goal level: 30 ng/mL in adults
5. Calcitonin-salmon (Miacalcin)
   a. Inhibition of bone resorption
   b. Indicated for osteoporosis treatment in women in postmenopause for at least 5 years
   c. Not a first-line drug. Useful for bone pain caused by vertebral compression fractures

d. Efficacy: Nasal calcitonin reduced the incidence of new vertebral fractures by 36%.
e. Adverse effects
   i. Nasal (10%–12%): rhinitis, epistaxis, irritation, nasal sores, dryness, tenderness
   ii. Other (3%–5%): backache, arthralgia, headache
f. Drug interactions: none
g. Dosage: 200 IU/day in one nostril, alternating nostrils daily
   200 IU nasally = 50–100 IU by injection
   200 IU per actuation, so one bottle will last about 2–3 weeks

6. Teriparatide (Forteo)
   a. Recombinant human parathyroid hormone regulates bone metabolism, intestinal calcium absorption, and renal tubular calcium and phosphate reabsorption.
   b. Efficacy:
      i. Reserved for treating women at high risk of fracture, including those with very low BMD (T-score worse than −3.0) and a previous vertebral fracture
      ii. Decreases vertebral fractures by 65% and non-vertebral fractures by 53%
   c. Contraindications: hypercalcemia, bone metastases, disorders that predispose women to bone tumors such as Paget disease
   d. Adverse effects: nausea, orthostatic hypotension
   e. Carcinogenicity: osteosarcoma in rats
   f. Drug interactions: Teriparatide increases calcium concentrations and may increase risk of digoxin toxicity.
   g. Dosage: 20 mcg/day subcutaneously

7. Denosumab (Prolia) – under consideration
   a. Inhibits osteoclast-mediated bone resorption, monoclonal antibody against RANKL (receptor activator of nuclear factor κ β ligand), cytokine essential for formation, function, survival of osteoclasts
   b. Administered subcutaneously every 6 months
   c. Efficacy
      i. Increased BMD hip (6%) and spine (9%)
      ii. Reduced spinal fracture risk by 68%, hip fracture risk by 40%
   d. Safety issues
      i. Possible opportunistic infections
      ii. U.S. Food and Drug Administration (FDA) panel requested additional data before approving for osteopenia/prevention.

8. Hormone therapy (estrogen and progestins, please see hormone therapy section above)

Patient Cases

2. C.A. is a 71-year-old white woman who rarely drinks alcohol, does not smoke, and exercises for 30 minutes 3 times/week. She takes calcium 500 mg/vitamin D 400 IU 3 times/day. She is 5'3″ and weighs 140 lb. Her BMD T-score is −1.8 at the hip and −2.6 at the spine. Which one of the following statements is the correct diagnosis for C.A.?
    A. Normal BMD of the spine.
    B. Osteopenia of the spine.
    C. Osteoporosis of the spine.
    D. Osteoporosis is defined when a fracture has occurred.

3. Which one of the following is the best treatment for C.A.?
    A. Teriparatide 20 mcg subcutaneously daily.
    B. Alendronate 70 mg PO every week.
    C. Miacalcin nasal spray 1 spray (200 IU) in one nostril daily.
    D. No additional therapy required; continue on calcium and vitamin D.

III. DRUGS IN PREGNANCY

A. Definitions and Overview
   1. Teratogen: drug or environmental agent that has the potential to cause abnormal fetal growth and development
   2. Teratogenicity: capability of producing congenital abnormalities
      a. Major or minor malformations
   3. Cause of defect
      a. Genetic predisposition 25%
      b. Drug 2%–3%
      c. Unknown 72%–73%
   4. Factors that influence
      a. Genotypes of mother and fetus
      b. Embryonic stage at exposure
      c. Dose of medication
      d. Simultaneous exposure to other drugs that may increase or decrease
      e. Timing of exposure
         i. One month before conception: folic acid 0.4 mg or more to prevent neural tube defects
         ii. Around time of conception and implantation
         iii. First 12–15 days postconception: If one cell is damaged, another can assume its function.
         iv. First 3 months: physical malformations
         v. Throughout pregnancy: functional and behavioral defects because brain development occurs throughout pregnancy
      f. Factors for placental transport
         i. Molecular weight of drug less than 400–600 Da cross placenta; most drugs weigh 250–400 Da
         ii. Degree of protein binding; lower in fetus, so more free-drug concentration
         iii. Maternal and fetal bloodflow usually equivalent; simple diffusion allows fetal drug concentration to be 50%–100% of maternal

iv. Metabolic activity of the placenta; excretion of medications by the fetus occurs in liver and placenta
5. Risk factor categories
   a. In 1983, the FDA required all new drugs to have a risk factor category.
   b. The FDA pregnancy risk categories

Table 7.

| A: Controlled studies in women fail to show risk |
| B: Animal studies indicate no risk |
| C: No available studies of women or animals |
| D: Positive evidence of fetal risk |
| X: Definite fetal risk in animals or women |

6. The FDA decides current pregnancy risk categories are not adequate; 2008 recommends that new labeling system be adapted that will include:
   a. Fetal risk summary
   b. Clinical considerations
   c. Data section
   d. Information for exposure registries
7. Factors to consider when initiating medications in pregnant women
   a. Risk-to-benefit ratio
   b. Is drug necessary?
   c. Most effective with least risk
   d. Lowest effective dose for shortest possible duration
   e. Health of mother without drug

B. Some Category D and X Drugs Known to Be Teratogens

Table 8.

Alcohol	Androgens
Anticonvulsants	Antineoplastics
Cocaine	Diethylstilbestrol
Vitamin A	Iodides
Isotretinoin	Lithium
Live vaccines	Methimazole
Penicillamine	Statins
Tetracyclines	Warfarin
Lead	Methotrexate
Mercury	Thalidomide
Angiotensin-converting enzyme inhibitors	

C. Common Category B and C Drugs

Table 9.

Acetaminophen	Cephalosporins
Corticosteroids	Docusate sodium
Erythromycin	Multivitamins
Narcotic analgesics	Penicillins
Phenothiazines	Thyroid hormones
Tricyclic antidepressants	

D. Drugs with Non-teratogenic Adverse Effects – Should Be Used with Caution

Table 10.

Antithyroid Drugs	Aminoglycosides
Aspirin	Barbiturates
Benzodiazepines	β-Blockers
Caffeine	Chloramphenicol
Diuretics	Isoniazid
Nicotine	Narcotic analgesics (chronic)
Oral hypoglycemics	NSAIDs
Propylthiouracil	Sulfonamides

NSAID = nonsteroidal anti-inflammatory drug.

E. Types of Adverse Effects After Fetal Drug Exposure

Table 11.

Low birth weight for gestational age	Cancer
Developmental delay/deficiency	Fetal death
Growth retardation	Hematologic abnormalities
Metabolic abnormalities	Renal dysfunction
Seizures	Sexual/reproductive dysfunction
Teratogenic abnormalities	Thyroid dysfunction
Withdrawal	

Patient Case

4. S.E. is a 28-year-old woman who is would like to get pregnant soon. Her medical history includes hypertension and allergies. Her medications include lisinopril, nasal saline spray, and folic acid. Which one of the following is best to treat her hypertension while she is pregnant or trying to conceive?
   A. Continue lisinopril.
   B. Discontinue lisinopril and all other medications.
   C. Discontinue lisinopril and start methyldopa.
   D. Continue lisinopril and add metoprolol.

IV. DRUGS IN LACTATION

A. Drugs That Decrease Milk Supply

Table 12.

Sympathomimetics	Nicotine
Levodopa	Bromocriptine
Ergot alkaloids	Pyridoxine
Monoamine oxidase inhibitors (MAOIs)	Androgens
Estrogen	

B. Drugs That Increase Milk Production (Galactorrhea)

Table 13.

Antipsychotics	Cimetidine
Metoclopramide	Reserpine
Amoxapine	Methyldopa

C. Ways to Minimize Effects of Drugs During Breastfeeding
   1. Short-term drug. Mother can pump and discard milk.
   2. Choose drugs with short half-lives.
   3. Administer drug immediately after a feeding or before a long sleep period.
   4. Consider whether the drug is given to neonates.

D. Drugs Contraindicated in Breastfeeding According to the American Academy of Pediatrics

Table 14.

Amphetamines	Bromocriptine
Cocaine	Ergotamine
Lithium	Nicotine
Antineoplastics	Drugs of abuse

E. Relatively Safe Agents During Lactation

Table 15.

Alcohol (in moderation)	Caffeine (in moderation [1 or 2 cups/day])
Analgesics	Laxatives
Anticonvulsants	Insulin
Antibiotics (penicillins, cephalosporins, erythromycins)	

V. COMPLICATIONS IN PREGNANCY

A. Conditions in Pregnancy
   1. Morning sickness
   2. Heartburn
   3. Constipation
   4. Hemorrhoids
   5. Headache
   6. Coagulation disorders
   7. Gestational diabetes mellitus
   8. Pregnancy-induced hypertension
   9. Preterm labor
   10. Induction of labor

B. Morning Sickness
   1. Nausea and vomiting associated with pregnancy
   2. Usually during first trimester
   3. Usually occurs on rising and diminishes as day progresses
   4. Cause: unknown
   5. Hyperemesis gravidarum: Severe nausea/vomiting leads to dehydration and malnutrition.
   6. Nonmedical treatment – first line
      a. Eat soda crackers.
      b. Keep stomach from becoming completely empty.
      c. Eat small, dry meals.
      d. Avoid spicy and odorous foods.
   7. Symptomatic treatment
      a. Phenothiazines
      b. Meclizine
      c. Cyclizine
      d. Dimenhydrinate
      e. Doxylamine
      f. Pyridoxine
      g. Ondansetron (category B)

C. Heartburn
   1. Occurs during latter half of pregnancy
   2. Cause: Enlarged uterus puts pressure on stomach, and esophageal sphincter relaxes.
   3. Nonmedical treatment
      a. Smaller, more-frequent meals
      b. Avoid food and liquids 3 hours before bed.
      c. Elevate head of bed with blocks.
   4. Symptomatic relief
      a. Antacids
         i. Magnesium hydroxide
         ii. Aluminum hydroxide
         iii. Calcium carbonate
      b. Sucralfate – not absorbed in GI tract
      c. Second line: hydrogen receptor antagonists
      d. Proton pump inhibitors

D. Constipation
   1. Cause: decreased peristalsis
   2. Increase high-fiber foods.
   3. Increase fluid intake to eight 8-oz glasses of water a day.
   4. Increase exercise.
   5. Symptomatic relief
      a. Bulk laxatives – not absorbed
      b. Surfactants
      c. Avoid mineral oil – impairs vitamin K absorption and could cause hypoprothrombinemia

E. Hemorrhoids
   1. Caused by constipation and increased venous pressure below uterus
   2. Correct constipation with stool softeners.
   3. Sitz baths
   4. External medications preferred
   5. Avoid topical anesthetics and steroids.

F. Headache
   1. Cause: hormone fluctuations
   2. Therapy
      a. Rest, ice packs
      b. Acetaminophen
   3. Drugs to avoid
      a. Aspirin and NSAIDs (near term)
      b. Triptans, ergotamine

G. Coagulation Disorders
   1. Anticoagulation necessary
      a. History of DVT
      b. Prosthetic heart valve
      c. Deficiencies of clotting factors
      d. Antiphospholipid antibodies
   2. Therapy
      a. Avoid warfarin.
      b. Heparin or low-molecular-weight heparin recommended

H. Gestational Diabetes Mellitus
   1. Insulin
      a. Regular (most studied)
      b. Neutral protamine Hagedorn (insulin)
      c. Lispro and aspart (category B drugs), starting to be used
   2. Sulfonylureas (glyburide) in patients unable to use insulin injections (not first line) N Engl J Med 2000 343:1134-8
   3. Metformin ongoing studies (not first line) N Engl J Med 2008 358:2003-15

I. Pregnancy-induced hypertension: hypertension occurring after 20 weeks' gestation
   1. Gestational hypertension: more than 140/90 mm Hg without proteinuria or pathologic edema
   2. Preeclampsia: hypertension plus proteinuria (300 mg or more every 24 hours)

3. Eclampsia: tonic-clonic seizures
4. Chronic hypertension: preexisting hypertension before 20 weeks' gestation
5. Chronic hypertension with superimposed preeclampsia: new-onset proteinuria after 20 weeks, sudden 2- to 3-fold increase in proteinuria, sudden increase in BP, increased aspartate transaminase–alanine transaminase, thrombocytopenia
6. Prevention
   a. Women at high risk of development, aspirin 60 mg beginning in weeks 24–28 until labor
7. Treatment
   a. Delivery if at term
   b. If not at term, get bedrest and monitor BP.
   c. Severe preeclamptic, parenteral magnesium sulfate to prevent seizures
   d. Methyldopa is first-line therapy.
   e. Alternatives: certain β-blockers, labetalol, calcium channel blockers
   f. Medications to avoid: angiotensin-converting enzyme (ACE) inhibitors, angiotensin II receptor blockers
   g. Parenteral antihypertensives: hydralazine, labetalol

J. Preterm Labor
   1. Definitions
      a. Term labor: between weeks 37 and 40
      b. Preterm labor: uterine contractions with cervical changes before week 37
   2. Nonpharmacologic treatment
      a. Inhibition of labor not usually attempted before week 20
      b. Bedrest, hydration, and sedation
   3. Tocolytic drugs (inhibit uterine contractions) especially if cervix dilated less than 4 cm and membranes intact
      a. β-Agonists
         i. Terbutaline: often used, intravenously, subcutaneously, orally
         ii. Adverse effects: hypotension, tachycardia, hypokalemia, tremor, nervous, angina, headache, hypoglycemia in patients with diabetes mellitus
      b. Magnesium sulfate
         i. Inhibits uterine activity by antagonism of calcium
         ii. Anticonvulsant in preeclampsia
         iii. Serum magnesium concentrations 6–8 mEq/L
         iv. May be drug of choice in patients with diabetes
      c. Prostaglandin synthetase inhibitors (NSAIDs)
         i. Prostaglandins are in amniotic fluid during labor/delivery but not during pregnancy.
         ii. Indomethacin: oral or rectal
         iii. Adverse effects: premature closure of ductus arteriosus, necrotizing enterocolitis, intracranial hemorrhage, renal dysfunction
         iv. Limit use to 72 hours.
      d. Calcium channel blockers
         i. Calcium necessary for muscle contraction
         ii. Nifedipine: typically used
         iii. Verapamil: large doses needed that mother usually cannot tolerate

K. Induction of Labor
   1. Induction indicated
      a. Severe maternal infection
      b. Uterine bleeding
      c. Preeclampsia/eclampsia
      d. Diabetes mellitus
      e. Macrosomia
      f. Maternal renal insufficiency
      g. Premature rupture of membranes after week 36
      h. Evidence of placental insufficiency
   2. Inducing agents
      a. Oxytocin
         i. Drug of choice
         ii. Intravenous
         iii. Adverse effects: uterine rupture, uteroplacental hypoperfusion, fetal distress from hypoxia
      b. Ergot alkaloids
         i. Not used to induce labor at term or late in pregnancy
         ii. Violent sustained uterine contractions
         iii. Used to terminate early pregnancy
         iv. Decrease postpartum or postabortion bleeding
         v. Oral and parenteral
      c. Prostaglandins
         i. Dinoprostone
         ii. Vaginal gel or insert
         iii. Applied to cervix
         iv. Adverse effect: hyperstimulation

VI. CONTRACEPTION

PRESCRIPTION CONTRACEPTION

Abbreviations Used

These are used interchangeably:
OC-Oral contraceptive
BC-Birth control
BCP-birth control pills

Others:
POP-Progestin-only pill
COC-Combination oral contraceptive
BUM-backup method
FSH-follicle-stimulating hormone
LH-luteinizing hormone

Progestins:
NEAC–norethindrone acetate
NE–norethindrone
LNG–levonorgestrel
DLNG–d-levonorgestrel
DSG–desogestrel
NG–norgestimate
MPA–medroxyprogesterone acetate
DMPA–depo-medroxyprogesterone acetate

Estrogen:
EE–ethinyl estradiol

A. Epidemiology
   1. About 49% of pregnancies are unintended in the United States, with around 26.5% of those resulting in abortions.
   2. According to National Center of Statistics reports, around 10.4 million women in 1995 were using an OC pill in the United States, 1.1 million were using injections, and 515,000 were using implants.

B. Physiology Review – Menstrual Cycle
   1. Follicular phase – Gonadotropin-releasing hormone stimulates release of follicle-stimulating hormone (FSH) and luteinizing hormone (LH), FSH stimulates estradiol secretion and stimulates follicles to develop; one in particular will become the dominant follicle; occurs in first half of cycle; later in follicular phase; LH causes an increase in androgen levels
   2. Ovulation – occurs midcycle; mature follicle ruptures; there is a surge in LH right before ovulation
   3. Luteal phase – Progesterone is the more dominant hormone in second half of cycle.
   4. Menses – Hormones have decreased, and withdrawal bleeding occurs if a woman does not become pregnant.

C. Properties Desired in Contraceptives
   1. Highly effective
   2. Prolonged duration of action
   3. Rapidly reversible

4. Privacy of use
5. Protection against STI
6. Easily accessible

D. Factors in Selecting Contraception
1. Effectiveness
   a. Theoretical
   b. Actual
2. Importance of not being pregnant
3. Likelihood and ability to adhere
4. Frequency of intercourse
5. Age
6. Cost and ability to pay
7. Adverse effects
8. Perceptions, misperceptions, risk/benefit
9. Concomitant drug use
10. Health status and habits

E. Methods of Birth Control
1. Abstinence
2. Male/female sterilization
3. Natural family planning
4. Spermicides
5. Barrier methods
   a. Diaphragm
   b. Condom
   c. Female condom
   d. Sponge
6. Hormonal contraception
   a. Combined contraceptives
      i. Combined oral contraceptive pill (COC)
      ii. Transdermal patch
      iii. Vaginal ring
   b. Progestin-only
      i. Progestin-only pill (POP or minipill)
      ii. Progestin-only injectable
   c. Implanted rods
7. Intrauterine device (IUD)
   a. Copper-T IUD
   b. Progestin-containing IUD

Focus on Combined Hormonal Contraceptives

Combined Hormonal Contraceptives contain both an estrogen and a progestin hormone.

A. Indications:
  1. FDA approved
     a. Prevent pregnancy
     b. Acne (Estrostep, Ortho Tri-Cyclen, YAZ)
     c. Premenstrual dysphoric disorder (YAZ)
  2. Off-label use
     a. Acne
     b. Hirsutism
     c. Cycle control
     d. Headaches
     e. Premenstrual syndrome
     f. Iron-deficiency anemia
     g. Relief of menstrual cramps

B. Components:
  1. Estrogen
     a. Types of estrogens available in products in the United States
        i. Ethinyl estradiol (in almost all products)
        ii. Mestranol (not used often)
     b. Pharmacologic actions of estrogen in contraceptives
        i. Feeds back to the pituitary, inhibiting FSH and ovulation
        ii. Increases aldosterone levels, results in increased sodium and water retention
        iii. Increases sex hormone binding globulin, which is produced in the liver and binds free androgens; this may result in clearing up hormone-mediated acne and unwanted facial hair/hirsutism in women
     c. Adverse effects owing to estrogen
        i. Nausea, vomiting
        ii. Bloating, edema
        iii. Irritability
        iv. Cyclic weight gain
        v. Cyclic headache
        vi. Hypertension
        vii. Breast fullness, tenderness
  2. Progestin
     a. Types of progestins available in products in the United States
        i. Norethindrone
        ii. Norethindrone acetate
        iii. Ethynodiol diacetate
        iv. Norgestrel
        v. Levonorgestrel
        vi. Desogestrel
        vii. Norgestimate
        viii. Etonogestrel
        ix. Drospirenone

b. Pharmacologic actions of progestins in contraceptives
   i. Feeds back to pituitary and helps inhibit ovulation (but not as much as estrogen)
   ii. Causes endometrial atrophy (thinning of uterus lining)
   iii. Thickens cervical mucus (inhibits sperm from traveling)
c. Adverse effects owing to progestin, androgenic adverse effects**
   i. Headaches
   ii. Increased appetite
   iii. Increased weight gain
   iv. Depression, fatigue
   v. Changes in libido
   vi. Hair loss, hirsutism**
   vii. Acne, oily skin**

C. Contraindications for Combined Hormonal Contraceptives
   1. The WHO medical eligibility criteria are separated into four categories:
      a. A condition for which there is no restriction for the use of the contraceptive method
      b. A condition in which the advantages of using the method generally outweigh the theoretical or proven risks
      c. A condition in which the theoretical or proven risks usually outweigh the advantages of using the method
      d. A condition that represents an unacceptable health risk if the contraceptive method is used
   2. Category 4 contraindications for combined hormonal contraceptives
      a. Breastfeeding less than 6 weeks postpartum
      b. Smoker 35 years and older
      c. Several risk factors for cardiovascular disease
      d. Blood pressure greater than 160/100 mm Hg
      e. Vascular disease
      f. Current DVT/pulmonary embolism or history of DVT/pulmonary embolism
      g. Complicated diabetes
      h. Presence of liver tumors, severe cirrhosis, or active viral hepatitis
      i. Major surgery with prolonged mobilization
      j. Known thrombogenic mutations
      k. Current/history of ischemic heart disease
      l. Stroke (history of cerebrovascular accident)
      m. Complicated valvular heart disease
      n. Migraine headache with aura
      o. Current breast cancer

D. Adverse Effects (see estrogen and progestin sections above for specific hormone-causing adverse effects)
   1. The main reason for discontinuation of contraceptives. Based on a 1998 study, discontinuation was attributable to:
      a. Bleeding irregularities – 32%
      b. Nausea – 19%
      c. Weight gain – 14%
      d. Mood swings – 14%
      e. Breast tenderness – 11%
      f. Headache – 11%

2. Management of adverse effects
   a. Breakthrough bleeding
      i. Select new birth control based on when bleeding occurs.
      ii. If early in the cycle, likely that there is not enough estrogen; select regimen with higher estrogen activity
      iii. If late in the cycle, likely that there is not enough progestin; select regimen with higher progestin activity
      iv. In general, if breakthrough bleeding occurs, best to select a regimen with higher estrogen and progestin activities
   b. Nausea
      i. Nausea is more likely related to estrogen component.
      ii. Suggest that the patient take the pill at night before bed.
      iii. Take pill with food.
      iv. If possible, try product for 3 months; nausea may subside.
   c. Acne
      i. Acne more likely related to androgenic properties of progestin
      ii. Select a product with lower androgenic activity.
      iii. Alternatively, select a product with higher estrogen activity.
3. Serious adverse effects (ACHES) (Hatcher et al.)
   a. **A**-Abdominal pain, could signal liver problems
   b. **C**-Chest pain, shortness of breath, coughing up blood, could signal blood clot in lung
   c. **H**-Headaches (severe), could signal stroke, blood clot
   d. **E**-Eye problems (blurred vision, flashing lights, blindness), could signal optic neuritis, stroke, clots
   e. **S**-Severe leg pain with or without swelling, could signal DVT

Patient Case

5. Y.G. is a 33-year-old woman initiated on Mircette 4 months ago for contraception. She has breakthrough bleeding at the start of her active pills that lasts a few days before resolving. The physician wants to change the OC. Which one of the following OCs on her formulary is best for the physician to prescribe?

Name of OC	Estrogen Property	Progestin Property	Androgen Property
Mircette (desogestrel 0.15 mg/EE 20 mcg)	Low	High	Low
Ortho-Cept (desogestrel 0.15 mg/EE 30 mcg)	Intermediate	High	Low
Alesse (levonorgestrel 0.1 mg/EE 20 mcg)	Low	Low	Low
Loestrin 21 (norethindrone acetate 1.5 mg/30 mcg)	Low	High	High

EE = ethinyl estradiol.

A. Continue on Mircette for another 3 months.
B. Change to Ortho-Cept.
C. Change to Loestrin 21.
D. Change to Alesse.

E. Drug Interactions
1. Increases effect of hormonal contraceptives
   a. Atorvastatin
2. Decreases effect of hormonal contraceptives
   a. Barbiturates
   b. Carbamazepine
   c. Felbamate
   d. Griseofulvin
   e. Modafinil
   f. Oxcarbazepine
   g. Phenytoin
   h. Protease inhibitors
   i. Rifamycins
   j. St. John's wort
3. Drugs that enhance hormonal contraceptive effects
   a. Antidepressants, tricyclic
   b. β-Blockers
   c. Caffeine
   d. Corticosteroids
   e. Cyclosporine
   f. Theophyllines
4. Questionable effects hormonal contraceptives may have on other drugs
   a. Anticoagulants – Hormonal contraceptives may increase certain clotting factors and reduce antithrombin III, so it is questionable whether hormonal contraceptives interfere with anticoagulants.
   b. Reported antibiotic cases in the literature: tetracycline, minocycline, erythromycin, penicillins, and cephalosporins; pharmacokinetic studies have not shown decreased OC steroid concentrations with tetracycline, doxycycline, ampicillin, metronidazole, quinolones, or fluconazole.
      i. Proposed mechanisms of drug interactions
         (a) Interference of absorption: Ethinyl estradiol is conjugated in liver, excreted in bile, hydrolyzed by intestinal bacteria, and reabsorbed as an active drug; non–liver enzyme–inducing antibiotics temporarily decrease colonic bacteria and inhibit enterohepatic circulation of ethinyl estradiol. Gut flora have recovered 3 weeks after the introduction of antibiotics.
         (b) Liver enzyme induction (rifampin and griseofulvin): The metabolism of progesterone and estrogen is accelerated.
         (c) Use alternative contraception for the length of antibiotic therapy plus 7 days after discontinuing antibiotic.

F. Types of Hormonal Contraceptives
1. Oral – Combined oral contraceptives
   a. Regimens of COCs
      i. Monophasic – same amount of hormone in pill every day except placebo pills
      ii. Biphasic – amount of hormone may change halfway through cycle
      iii. Triphasic – amount of hormone changes every week
      iv. Traditional – Progestin usually changes and estrogen stays the same.
      v. Estrophasic – estrogen changes

b. Dosing
   i. High estrogen – 50 mcg or higher (higher than 50 mcg not really used anymore)
   ii. Low-dose estrogen – less than 50–30 mcg (generally 30–35 mcg)
   iii. Very low-dose estrogen – less than 30 mcg (20–25 mcg)
c. Effectiveness – when taken every day at the same time every day 99.7% (perfect use), typical use (about 92%)[2]
d. Adherence – 68% continue after 1 year[2]
e. Start methods
   i. **Same-day start** – start taking an active pill the first day of menses
   ii. **Sunday start** – start taking an active pill the first Sunday after menses begins (use a backup method (BUM) for at least 7 days, most conservative for 1 month)
   iii. **Quick start** – start taking an active pill at the doctor's office or first of prescription, regardless of menstrual cycle day. Use a BUM for at least 7 days. Most conservative; use a BUM for 1 month. Menses will not begin until all the active pills have been taken.
   iv. **When switching pills from brand to brand**, start the new pack of pills after finishing the placebo pills from the old pack.
f. Counseling
   i. Proper use – Take one tablet once daily at the same time every day.
   ii. Adverse effects
      (a) See above
      (b) Adverse effects usually subside after 3 months, general recommendation is to stay on a brand for at least 3 months if adverse effects are not excessively bothersome.
   iii. Missed doses[5] – Missed COC pill means greater than 24 hours between doses. There are different thoughts on what to do about missed doses.
      (a) **Miss 1 pill:**
         Take as soon as remembered – no BUM
      (b) **Miss 2 pills if in week 1 or 2 of cycle:**
         Take 2 pills for 2 days plus BUM for 7 days (BUM = condoms, condoms plus spermicide, diaphragm, or no intercourse)
      (c) **Miss 2 pills in week 3 of cycle:**
         If day 1 starter, begin new pack that day plus BUM for 7 days
         If Sunday starter, take 1 pill daily until Sunday (no placebos); start new pack on Sunday plus BUM for 7 days
      (d) **Miss 3 pills in first 3 weeks:**
         If day 1 starter, begin new pack plus BUM for 7 days
         If Sunday starter, take 1 pill daily until Sunday (no placebos); start new pack on Sunday plus BUM for 7 days
      (e) **Miss placebos** – Just continue taking pills – No BUM!
      (f) **Alternative method** – If patient has had intercourse in the past 5 days, consider emergency contraception, and then instruct the patient to continue using her birth control until the end of the pack, plus 7 days of BUM.
      (g) **Other methods** – For dose of EE, if taking less than 30 mcg and missed 2 pills, treat as if she missed 3 pills.

g. Advantages and disadvantages

Table 16

Advantages	Disadvantages
• Effective	• No HIV/STI protection
• Safe	• Patient adherence
• Easy to use	• Expensive
• Reversible	• Adverse effects
• Menstrual cycle	• Circulatory complications
• Reduction of several cancers	• Menstrual cycle changes
• Decreased risk of benign breast tumors	• Sexual/psychological effects
• Improves acne	• Hepatocellular adenoma
• Sexual enjoyment	• Gallbladder disease
• Emergency contraception	• Drug interactions
• Transition therapy for perimenopause	

HIV = human immunodeficiency virus; STI = sexually transmitted infection.

2. Transdermal Patch
   a. Patch placed on skin, delivers 150 mcg of norelgestromin and 20 mcg of ethinyl estradiol daily (originally thought, now known that more than 35 mcg of oral tablet of ethinyl estradiol provided from patch)
   b. Effectiveness
      i. Similar to pills (8% failure rate for typical use, 0.3% for perfect use)[2]
      ii. Less effective in women weighing more than 198 lb, should not be used
   c. Adherence – better adherence rates than pill, especially in teens
   d. Counseling
      i. Proper use
         (a) Place patch on a dry, hairless area of upper arm, shoulder, abdomen, or buttocks. Should not be placed on the breast. Rotate site of patch each week.
         (b) One patch per week for 3 weeks; week 4 is patch free (menses will occur then)
      ii. Adverse effects
         (a) Higher incidence of blood clots
         (b) Site irritation from the patch
         (c) See adverse effects above
      iii. Missed doses
         (a) If patch is off for less than 24 hours, reapply patch, no BUM needed
         (b) If patch is off more than 24 hours, open a new patch, new day 1, must use BUM for first week of the new cycle

e. Advantages and disadvantages

Table 17.

Advantages	Disadvantages
• Efficacy • Adherence • User controlled • Readily reversible	• Site reactions • Patch detachment • Appearance, less privacy • Breast discomfort • Dysmenorrhea • Headache • Nausea • Questionable increased risk of blood clots

3. Vaginal ring
    a. Product inserted vaginally, delivers 15 mcg of ethinyl estradiol and 120 mcg of etonogestrel (active form of desogestrel) daily
    b. Effectiveness – similar to pills (8% failure rate for typical use, 0.3% for perfect use)[2]
    c. Adherence
        i. One study[6] found that 92.4% of women using a vaginal ring were adherent versus 75.4% using the COC pill.
        ii. A total of 1950 women aged 18–41 years, 13 cycles of use, 96% satisfied, 97% would recommend the ring[7]
        iii. Reasons for liking the ring:
            (a) "Not having to remember anything" (45%)
            (b) "Ease of use" (27%)
    d. Counseling
        i. Proper use
            (a) Insert vaginal ring into vagina and leave for 3 weeks. Week 4, remove ring and menses will occur.
            (b) Should not be removed during intercourse
            (c) May be worn with tampon if there is breakthrough bleeding
        ii. Missed doses – Inadvertent removal, expulsion, or prolonged ring-free interval[8]
            (a) If 3 hours or less, rinse with cool to lukewarm water and reinsert as soon as possible
            (b) If more than 3 hours, reinsert and use BUM until ring has been used continuously for 7 days
        iii. Adverse effects
            (a) Decreased libido (8%)
            (b) Breast tenderness (4%)
            (c) Device-related events (2.5%–5%)
            (d) Vaginal discomfort (2.5%)

(e) Irregular bleeding (1.5%–5%)

Table 18.

Advantages	Disadvantages
• Efficacy • Adherence • User controlled • Cycle control • Readily reversible • Privacy	• Adverse effects similar to other combined regimens • Vaginal discomfort • Potential partner awareness of ring

4. Extended regimens
   a. Three months – using active form of combined hormonal contraception for 3 months (results in menses every 3 months instead of once a month). Marketed product: Seasonale (ethinyl estradiol 30 mcg/levonorgestrel 150 mcg), Seasonique (ethinyl estradiol 30 mcg/levonorgestrel 150 mcg, ethinyl estradiol 10-mcg tablets instead of placebo pills), LoSeasonique (ethinyl estradiol 20 mcg/levonorgestrel 100 mcg, ethinyl estradiol 10-mcg tablets instead of placebo pills)
   b. One year – using active form of combined hormonal contraception for 1 year, product: Lybrel
   c. One year – vaginal ring, clinical trials

Progestin-only Contraceptives

Progestin-only contraceptives contain only a progestin agent with no estrogen.

A. Indications – those who cannot use or tolerate combined hormonal contraceptives
   1. History/current MI, stroke, DVT, cardiovascular disease
   2. Atrial fibrillation
   3. Blood pressure 160/100 mm Hg
   4. Smoker age 35
   5. Breast cancer within 5 years
   6. Active, symptomatic liver disease
   7. Benign or malignant liver tumors
   8. History of cholestasis because of BCPs
   9. Migraine headache with neurologic impairment
   10. Retinopathy or neuropathy because of diabetes
   11. Surgery within the past 4 weeks
   12. Breastfeeding

B. Components – one of the following progestins:
   1. Medroxyprogesterone acetate (Depo-Provera injectable/Depo-Provera subcutaneously)
   2. Norethindrone 0.35 mg (Micronor, Nor-QD)
   3. Norgestrel 0.075 mg (Ovrette)

C. Mechanisms of Action
   1. Thickens cervical mucus, prevents sperm movement

2. Thins uterus lining
3. Suppresses midcycle peak of LH and FSH, inhibits ovulation (not so much with oral progestin pills)

D. Contraindications
   1. Suspected or demonstrated pregnancy
   2. Active hepatitis, hepatic failure, jaundice
   3. Inability to absorb sex steroids from GI tract (i.e., active colitis)
   4. Concurrently taking medications that increase hepatic clearance (CYP450 inducers)
   5. If taking antibiotic, considered WHO category 1

E. Adverse Effects – See chart of progestin adverse effects above.

F. Types
   1. Oral
      a. Effectiveness – 8% failure rate (typical), 0.3% failure (perfect use)[2]
      b. Start methods – may start on any day or on first day of period. There are no hormone-free days with the POPs.
      c. Adverse effects – progestin related, see above
      d. Missed doses – Missed dose of POP means more than 3 hours; if a missed dose occurs, must use a BUM for 48 hours
      e. Advantages
         i. Efficacy
         ii. Decreased menstrual blood loss, cramps, pain
         iii. Readily reversible
         iv. Preferable in lactating women
      f. Disadvantages
         i. Progestin-related adverse effects (e.g., weight gain, acne)
         ii. Irregular menses
         iii. Adherence – short window of time for a missed pill
         iv. Low-dose progestin, patient may ovulate
         v. Fewer noncontraceptive benefits
   2. Depo-Provera injection
      a. A 1-mL crystalline suspension of 150 mg of depot medroxyprogesterone acetate (DMPA) injected intramuscularly into deltoid or gluteus maximus muscle every <u>11–13 weeks</u>
      b. Effectiveness[2]: Perfect use failure rate: 0.3%; typical use failure rate: 3%
      c. Start methods
         i. Preferred start: first 5 days of menses. No backup needed
         ii. Alternative start: any time in cycle if not pregnant. Use backup for 7 days.
         iii. Postpartum: may give injection before hospital discharge
         iv. Breastfeeding: may start immediately or wait 4–6 weeks
         v. Switching methods: any time patient not known to be pregnant. Use backup if necessary.
      d. Adverse effects:
         i. Progestin related (see above)
         ii. Progressive significant weight gain
         iii. Severe depression (rare)

iv. Black box warning – loss of bone, women who used DMPA for at least 5 years have significantly reduced BMD of lumbar spine and femoral neck, particularly after 15 years of use and if started before age 20
    (a) Effect is almost completely reversible, even after 4 years or more of DMPA use.
    (b) All women placed on DMPA should be taking sufficient calcium and exercising regularly.
  e. Missed doses – greater than 13 weeks between injections
  f. Patient Counseling
    i. Do not massage area for a few hours where shot was given.
    ii. Expect irregular bleeding/spotting in beginning – decreases over time
    iii. Take calcium if not achieving 1000–1200 mg/day through diet.
    iv. Return in 11–13 weeks for next injection. Use backup if ever more than 13 weeks.
    v. If ever changing from DMPA to another method, start method when next injection is due.
3. Depo subcutaneously – subcutaneous injection of 104 mg of DMPA, may facilitate women giving themselves Depo injections at home

Intrauterine Devices/Systems

A. Indications – to prevent pregnancy long term

B. Recommended for women who:
1. Have at least one child
2. Are in a mutually monogamous relationship
3. Have no history of pelvic inflammatory disease (PID) or ectopic pregnancy
4. Have heavy menses, cramps, anemia, or dysfunctional uterine bleeding
5. Women seeking long-term (2 years or more) pregnancy protection

C. Types
1. Copper (Copper-T)
  a. Copper IUD inserted by a health care professional into the uterus
  b. Mechanism of action
    i. Primary action: spermicide
    ii. Copper ions inhibit sperm motility and acrosomal enzyme activation so that sperm seldom reach fallopian tube and are unable to fertilize the ovum
    iii. Sterile inflammatory reaction created in endometrium phagocytizes sperm
    iv. Does not interfere with ovulation and is not an abortifacient
  c. Effectiveness: Perfect use failure rate: 0.6%; typical use failure rate: 0.8%[2]
  d. Contraindications specific to Copper-T
    i. Pregnancy
    ii. Women with current or recent (within 3 months) STI or woman at risk of STI
    iii. Uterus less than 6 cm or greater than 9 cm
    iv. Undiagnosed abnormal vaginal bleeding
    v. Active cervicitis or active pelvic infection
    vi. Known symptomatic actinomycosis
    vii. Recent endometritis (past 3 months)
    viii. Allergy to copper; Wilson disease

       ix. Uterine distortion or pathology affecting placement
       x. Known or suspected uterine or cervical cancer
       xi. Unresolved abnormal Papanicolaou test
       xii. Severe anemia (relative contraindication)
  e. Advantages and disadvantages

Table 19.

Advantages	Disadvantages
• Efficacy (long term)	• Monthly blood loss increased about 35%
• Adherence	• Dysmenorrhea
• Spontaneous sexual activity	• Spotting/cramping
• Readily reversible	• Expulsion
• Cost-effective	• Foreign body
• Patient satisfaction	• Increased risk of infection for 20 days after insertion

2. Progestogen (Mirena)
  a. Inserted into uterus by health care professional, stays in for up to 5 years, releases 20 mcg/day of levonorgestrel
  b. Mechanism of action
       i. Foreign object in uterus, prevents implantation
       ii. Progestin thickens cervical mucus, thins endometrium, and inhibits sperm motion.
  c. Contraindications[9]
       i. Pregnancy or suspicion of pregnancy
       ii. Congenital or acquired uterine anomaly
       iii. Acute/history of PID
       iv. Postpartum endometritis or infected abortion in the past 3 months
       v. Known or suspected uterine or cervical neoplasia
       vi. Unresolved abnormal Papanicolaou test
       vii. Genital bleeding of unknown etiology
       viii. Untreated acute cervicitis or vaginitis
       ix. Acute liver disease or liver tumor (benign or malignant)
       x. Woman or partner with several sexual partners
       xi. Conditions associated with increased susceptibility to infections with microorganisms (e.g., leukemia, AIDS [acquired immunodeficiency syndrome], intravenous drug abuse)
       xii. Genital actinomycosis
       xiii. A previously inserted IUD that has not been removed
       xiv. Hypersensitivity to any component of this product
       xv. Known or suspected carcinoma of the breast
       xvi. History of ectopic pregnancy or condition that would predispose to ectopic pregnancy

d. Advantages and disadvantages

Table 20.

Advantages	Disadvantages
• Efficacy (long term) • Adherence • Menorrhagia improves • Spontaneous sexual activity • Readily reversible	• Progestin-related adverse effects • Irregular menses • Expulsion • Increased risk of infection first 20 days after insertion • Foreign body

D. Patient Counseling
1. Strings of IUD will be outside the vaginal canal. Sometimes, trimmed strings are given to the patient to be able to check if IUD is still inserted.
2. Adverse effects – PAINS
    a. **P**– Period late; abnormal spotting or bleeding
    b. **A**– Abdominal pain, pain with intercourse
    c. **I**– Infection exposure (STI); abnormal vaginal discharge
    d. **N**– Not feeling well, fever, chills
    e. **S**– String missing, shorter or longer

Implants

A. Indications – long-term prevention of pregnancy

B. Components – etonogestrel, releases 60–70 mcg/day during weeks 5–6 and then decreases to 35–45 mcg/day by the end of the first year, 30–40 mcg/day after second year, and 25–30 mcg/day at the end of 3 years

C. Mechanism of action – a rod inserted in upper arm, 99% effective for up to 3 years, releases progestin etonogestrel, which acts similarly to other progestin-only contraceptives

D. Adverse Effects
1. Similar to progestin-related adverse effects
2. Site reactions, inflammation, hematoma, pain, redness at site (3.6%)
3. Difficulty removing rod, rod breaks, fibrosis (1.7%)

Patient Case

6. L.M., a 37-year-old woman, states she is going to get married soon and wants to begin taking BCPs for now; however, she would like to have children in a year or so. Medical history includes hypertension for 2 years and gastroesophageal reflux disease; she admits to two glasses of wine a week and smokes ½ pack/day. Her medications include hydrochlorothiazide 25 mg orally daily, Lotrel 5/20 (amlodipine-benazepril) orally daily, Prilosec 20 mg (omeprazole) orally daily, and occasional ibuprofen. She is 5'7" and weighs 210 lb (95 kg). Which one of the following contraceptive products should the physician prescribe?
    A. Ortho-Evra.
    B. YAZ.
    C. Micronor.
    D. Mirena.

Emergency Contraception

A. Definition: "A therapy for women who have had unprotected sexual intercourse, including sexual assault." ACOG definition (ACOG Practice Bulletin. Int J Gynecol Obstet 2002;78:191–8)

B. Mechanism of Hormonal Methods (Yuzpe and progestin-only)
   1. Inhibits ovulation
   2. Prevents fertilization
   3. Increases thickness of cervical mucus
   4. Prevents implantation
   5. Not considered an abortifacient by medical standards, does not disrupt an implanted fertilized egg

C. Indications
   1. Condom broke
   2. Misused contraceptive method (e.g., missed a pill, contraceptive patch fell off)
   3. Sexual assault
   4. Exposure to teratogen
   5. Unprotected intercourse within 120 hours

D. Timing: within 120 hours after unprotected intercourse; package insert for marketed products states 72 hours, but studies show up to 120 hours may still prevent pregnancy

E. Effectiveness: 57%–85%

F. Methods
   1. Yuzpe method
      a. High-dose estrogen plus progestin
      b. FDA-labeling approved doses (based on norgestrel/L-norgestrel)
         i. Ovral 2 tablets immediately; then 2 tablets 12 hours later
         ii. Levora, Low-Ogestrel, Cryselle, Lo/Ovral, Levlen, Nordette, Portia, Seasonale 4 tablets immediately; then 4 tablets 12 hours later
         iii. Trivora, Tri-Levlen, Triphasil (yellow pills only – 120 mcg of ethinyl estradiol) 4 tablets immediately; then 4 tablets 12 hours later
         iv. Alesse, Levlite, Lessina, Lutera, Aviane 5 tablets immediately; then 5 tablets 12 hours later
      c. Adverse effects
         i. Nausea: 30%–60%; vomiting: 33% with estrogen-containing emergency contraception (If vomiting within 2 hours of dose, repeat dose. May take with food or meclizine 50 mg prophylactically 30–60 minutes before each dose)
         ii. May notice changes in menstrual cycle
         iii. Breast tenderness, headache
   2. Progestin-only method
      a. Products
         i. Ovrette 20 tablets immediately; then 20 tablets 12 hours later
         ii. Plan B (2 tablets of levonorgestrel 0.75 mg)
            (a) Over-the-counter (OTC) 2006 for women 18 years and older, recent change to 17 years and older

            (b) Prescription for women younger than 18 years unless state allows pharmacist initiation
            (c) May take the 2 tablets at the same time or separated by 12–24 hours
        iii. Plan B One-Step (1 tablet of levonorgestrel 1.5 mg)
            (a) Over-the-counter for women 17 years and older
            (b) Prescription for women younger than 17 years unless state allows pharmacist initiation
    b. Adverse effects
        i. Nausea: 18%; vomiting: 4%
        ii. May notice changes in menstrual cycle
        iii. The WHO recommends using levonorgestrel only. A double-blind, randomized study of 2000 women showed levonorgestrel 750 mcg repeated 12 hours later prevented 85% of pregnancies versus the Yuzpe regimen (ethinyl estradiol 100 mcg/levonorgestrel 0.5 mg repeated 12 hours later), which prevented 57%. Less nausea and vomiting with levonorgestrel 750 mcg (Lancet 1998;352:428–33)
3. Copper IUD – may be used within 5 days of unprotected intercourse, requires in-office visit
4. RU-486 – may be used within 5 days of unprotected intercourse but will disrupt an established pregnancy; requires in-office visit

---

Patient Case

7. Monday morning, you receive a telephone call from a patient asking about BCPs. The patient visited her relatives in Michigan the past weekend and forgot to bring her Micronor, a progestin-only OC. The last pill she took was on Saturday morning. You tell the patient to continue taking the pills as usual. Which of the following will you tell the patient about alternative contraceptive methods?

A. These methods are not necessary.
B. These methods are necessary for 24 hours.
C. These methods are necessary for 48 hours.
D. These methods are necessary until her next menses.

VII. SEXUALLY TRANSMITTED DISEASES INCLUDING PELVIC INFLAMMATORY DISEASE, GYNECOLOGIC INFECTIONS

Patient Case

8. D.H. is a 21-year-old woman who presents to the clinic with genital itching and vesicles on her vulva. She is sexually active with one partner who has a history of herpes. Her partner does not always use a condom when they have sex. She is initiated on acyclovir for this initial herpes simplex infection. Which one of the following statements is accurate to tell Y.O. regarding treatment of her herpes infection?

   A. Treatment of the initial infection will decrease the risk of recurrent herpes infections.
   B. Treatment will shorten the duration of symptoms and infectivity of the initial infection.
   C. Treatment of the initial infection will decrease the severity of recurrent herpes infections.
   D. Treatment of the initial infection will prevent the virus from remaining latent in the dorsal root ganglia.

A. Herpes Simplex Virus (HSV) Infection
   1. Characteristics
      a. Types HSV-1 and HSV-2 can cause genital herpes.
      b. Diagnosed in at least 50 million people in the United States
      c. Treatment can partly control symptoms but does not affect the risk, frequency, or severity of recurrences after treatment is discontinued.
      d. Symptoms include itching, genital burning, vesicle formation, and ulcer formation.
      e. After the primary infection, the virus is latent in the sacral dorsal root ganglia.
      f. From 50% to 80% of patients have recurrent infections (generally less severe and of shorter duration).
   2. Diagnosis
      a. Culture
      b. Serologic testing
   3. Therapy
      a. Initial HSV infection
         i. Acyclovir 400 mg orally 3 times/day for 7–10 days
         ii. Acyclovir 200 mg orally 5 times/day for 7–10 days
         iii. Famciclovir 250 mg orally 3 times/day for 7–10 days
         iv. Valacyclovir 1 g orally 2 times/day for 7–10 days

Patient Case

9. D.H. returns to the clinic 10 months after her initial herpes infection. She is troubled by all of the recurrences she is having (seven to date). Which one of the following therapies is best to recommend?

   A. Valacyclovir 500 mg orally 2 times/day to be used for 5 days whenever she notices a recurrence beginning.
   B. Acyclovir 400 mg orally 3 times/day to be used for 10 days whenever she notices a recurrence beginning.
   C. Suppressive therapy with famciclovir 250 mg orally 3 times/day.
   D. Suppressive therapy with valacyclovir 500 mg/day orally.

- b. Recurrent HSV infection
  - i. If treatment is initiated within 1 day of lesion onset, patients with recurrent infections may benefit.
    - (a) Acyclovir 400 mg orally 3 times/day for 5 days
    - (b) Acyclovir 800 mg orally 3 times/day for 2 days
    - (c) Acyclovir 800 mg orally 2 times/day for 5 days
    - (d) Famciclovir 125 mg orally 2 times/day for 5 days
    - (e) Famciclovir 1000 mg 2 times/day for 1 day
    - (f) Valacyclovir 500 mg orally 2 times/day for 3 days
    - (g) Valacyclovir 1000 mg/day orally for 5 days
  - ii. Daily suppressive therapy recommended in patients with six or more episodes yearly (reassess annually the need for suppressive therapy)
    - (a) Acyclovir 400 mg orally 2 times/day
    - (b) Famciclovir 250 mg orally 2 times/day
    - (c) Valacyclovir 500 mg/day orally
    - (d) Valacyclovir 1000 mg/day orally
4. Herpes encephalitis
   - a. Characteristics
     - i. Primarily caused by HSV-1
     - ii. Spreads through neural routes during primary or recurrent infection
     - iii. Primarily temporal lobe involvement with eventual hemorrhagic encephalitis
     - iv. High mortality if untreated and frequent neurologic sequelae
   - b. Diagnosis
     - i. Signs and symptoms (nonspecific)
       - (a) Headache
       - (b) Fever
       - (c) Speech disorders and behavioral changes
       - (d) Focal seizures
     - ii. Cerebrospinal fluid analysis
       - (a) Moderate pleocytosis (generally lymphocytosis)
       - (b) Normal glucose and moderately elevated protein
     - iii. Brain biopsy (rarely performed)
   - c. Therapy
     - i. Acyclovir intravenously 5–10 mg/kg every 8 hours for 2–7 days, followed by oral antiviral therapy for at least 10 days of total therapy

B. Syphilis (*Treponema pallidum*)
  1. Diagnosis
     - a. Dark-field examination and direct fluorescent antibody stains of exudate for spirochetes
     - b. Nontreponemal (Venereal Disease Research Laboratory and rapid plasma reagin); detect serum concentrations of antibody to cardiolipin
     - c. Treponemal (fluorescent treponemal antibodies and *T. pallidum* particle agglutination test)—detect antibodies to *T. pallidum*
     - d. In general, perform a nontreponemal test for screening purposes and confirm with a treponemal test.
  2. Primary syphilis
     - a. From 10 to 90 days after exposure (mean = 21 days)
     - b. The primary symptom is the development of a chancre.

- c. The chancre resolves spontaneously in 2–6 weeks even without treatment.
- d. Recommended treatment
    - i. Benzathine penicillin G 2.4 million units intramuscularly in a single dose (adults)
    - ii. If penicillin allergy: doxycycline 100 mg 2 times/day or tetracycline 500 mg 4 times/day for 2 weeks
3. Secondary syphilis/early latent syphilis
    - a. From 4 to 10 weeks after exposure
    - b. Skin lesions: characteristically on the palms and soles
    - c. Latent phase begins when all symptoms have resolved.
    - d. Recommended treatment
        - i. Benzathine penicillin G 2.4 million units intramuscularly in a single dose
        - ii. If penicillin allergy: doxycycline 100 mg 2 times/day **or** tetracycline 500 mg 4 times/day for 2 weeks
4. Late latent syphilis (more than 1 year in duration) or unknown duration
    - a. Recommended treatment
        - i. Benzathine penicillin G 2.4 million units intramuscularly every week for 3 weeks
        - ii. If penicillin allergy: doxycycline 100 mg 2 times/day **or** tetracycline 500 mg 4 times/day for 4 weeks
5. Tertiary syphilis
    - a. Infectious granulomas and cardiovascular effects: aortic insufficiency and aortitis
    - b. Recommended treatment
        - i. Benzathine penicillin G 2.4 million units intramuscularly every week for 3 weeks (total dose 7.2 million units)
        - ii. If penicillin allergy: doxycycline 100 mg 2 times/day **or** tetracycline 500 mg 4 times/day for 4 weeks
6. Neurosyphilis
    - a. Recommended treatment
        - i. Aqueous crystalline penicillin G 3–4 million units intravenously every 4 hours or continuous infusion for 10–14 days
    - b. Alternative regimen
        - i. Procaine penicillin 2.4 million units/day intramuscularly plus probenecid 500 mg 4 times/day for 10–14 days
        - ii. If penicillin allergy: ceftriaxone 2 g/day intramuscularly/intravenously for 10–14 days or patients should be desensitized and given penicillin (see Centers for Disease Control recommendations for skin testing and desensitization)
        - iii. Treatment of sexual partners
    - c. Sexual partners should be presumptively treated if exposed within 90 days preceding the diagnosis in their partner.
    - d. If exposure occurred greater than 90 days, sexual partners should be tested and monitored closely or treated presumptively if serologic test results are not available immediately.

Patient Case

10. M.A. is a 24-year-old woman who presents to the emergency department with severe abdominal pain, fever, dysuria, and a vaginal discharge. She is sexually active with many partners. Her medical history is unremarkable except for recurrent genital herpes (one or two episodes a year). Her medications on admission include BCPs (Ortho Tri-Cyclen) and fluticasone (Flonase) as needed. On physical examination, M.A.'s vital signs include temperature 101.2°F (38°C), pulse rate 92 beats/minute, respiration rate 15 breaths/minute, and BP 117/75 mm Hg. M.A. has adnexal tenderness, cervical motion tenderness, and a vaginal discharge. Which one of the following is the best empiric therapy?
    A. Ampicillin-sulbactam 2 g every 6 hours for 14 days.
    B. Metronidazole 500 mg 3 times/day for 7 days.
    C. Cefotetan 2 g intravenously every 12 hours with doxycycline 100 mg orally every 12 hours for 14 days.
    D. Ceftriaxone 125 mg intramuscularly × 1 with doxycycline 100 mg intravenously 2 times/day for 7 days.

    C. Chlamydial Infection
        1. Can lead to PID, ectopic pregnancy, and infertility
        2. Less dysuria and penile discharge in men compared with gonococcal infection
        3. Treatment
            a. Azithromycin 1 g in a single dose or doxycycline 100 mg 2 times/day for 7 days
            b. Alternatives
                i. Erythromycin base 500 mg 4 times/day for 7 days **or** ofloxacin 300 mg 2 times/day for 7 days **or** levofloxacin 500 mg/day for 7 days **or** erythromycin ethylsuccinate 800 mg 4 times/day for 7 days
            c. Abstain from sexual intercourse for at least 7 days and until sexual partners are adequately treated.

    D. Gonococcal Infection
        1. Penile discharge and dysuria common in men, but women are often asymptomatic (which can lead to PID); symptoms in women include vaginal discharge and dysuria
        2. Treatment
            a. Ceftriaxone 125 mg intramuscularly **or** cefixime 400 mg orally—all as a single dose **PLUS** treatment of chlamydia if not ruled out (fluoroquinolones no longer recommended because of resistance)
            b. Gonococcal infection of the pharynx: ceftriaxone **PLUS** treatment of chlamydia
            c. Alternatives – Spectinomycin 2-g intramuscular single dose or other cephalosporins as a single dose
            d. Abstain from sexual intercourse for at least 7 days and until all sexual partners are adequately treated.

    E. Urethritis
        1. Undiagnosed: treat for both chlamydia and *Gonococcus*
        2. Nongonococcal: treat for chlamydia
        3. Recurrent or persistent: Ensure adherence and no reinfection from infected partner; if these are ensured, treat with [metronidazole or tinidazole] **and** azithromycin for *T. vaginalis*.
        4. All sexual partners within the past 60 days should be assessed and treated.

F. Pelvic Inflammatory Disease
   1. Ascending infection of the female genital tract primarily involving the fallopian tubes
   2. Clinical presentation
      a. Lower abdominal tenderness
      b. Adnexal tenderness
      c. Cervical motion tenderness
      d. Oral temperature greater than 101°F
      e. Abnormal cervical or vaginal discharge
      f. Elevated erythrocyte sedimentation rate
      g. Elevated C-reactive protein
      h. Menorrhagia
      i. Dysuria
      j. Sequelae: abscess in pelvic or fallopian tubes, tubal occlusion, fibrosis, infertility
      k. In general, sexually transmitted and caused by *N. gonorrhoeae*, *C. trachomatis*, anaerobes, gram-negative facultative bacteria, and streptococci
   3. Pelvic inflammatory disease leads to infertility and ectopic pregnancies.
   4. Treatment:
      a. Parenteral treatment
         i. Regimen A: [cefotetan 2 g intravenously every 12 hours or cefoxitin 2 g intravenously every 6 hours] plus doxycycline 100 mg intravenously or orally every 12 hours
            (a) Parenteral therapy can be discontinued 24 hours after clinical improvement and switched to oral therapy for 14 days.
         ii. Regimen B: clindamycin 900 mg intravenously every 8 hours plus gentamicin intravenously/intramuscularly 2-mg/kg loading dose; then 1.5 mg/kg every 8 hours (or once-daily therapy)
            (a) Parenteral therapy can be discontinued 24 hours after clinical improvement and switched to oral for a total of 14 days.
         iii. Alternative regimens
            (a) Ampicillin-sulbactam 3 g intravenously every 6 hours plus doxycycline 100 mg intravenously **or** orally every 12 hours
      b. Oral treatment
         i. Ceftriaxone 250 mg intramuscularly once (other third-generation cephalosporins also acceptable) or cefoxitin 2 g intramuscularly plus probenecid 1 g orally once] plus doxycycline 100 mg 2 times/day for 14 days with or without metronidazole 500 mg orally 2 times/day for 14 days
      c. Sexual partners of patients with PID within the past 60 days should be tested and treated.

Patient Case

11. Which one of the following statements should M.A. tell her sexual partners?
    A. There is no need for concern because PID is not acquired from a sexual partner.
    B. He can resume having sexual intercourse with M.A. as soon as her symptoms improve.
    C. If he had sex with M.A. within the past 60 days, he should be assessed for possible treatment.
    D. He does not need to be tested for human immunodeficiency virus (HIV) because there is no relationship between HIV and other STDs.

G. Bacterial Vaginosis
1. Malodorous vaginal discharge caused by an overgrowth of anaerobic bacteria (circumventing the normal flora of *Lactobacillus*), more than 50% with bacterial vaginosis asymptomatic
2. Infection risk is increased in relation to sexual activity, but it is unknown whether acquired through sexual partner
3. Diagnosis is based on a malodorous vaginal discharge that is high in pH and contains clue cells and whiff test positive (fishy odor after potassium hydroxide 10% added to sample).
4. Bacterial vaginosis can lead to PID and endometritis.
5. Treatment
   a. Nonpregnant women: metronidazole 500 mg 2 times/day for 7 days **or** clindamycin 2% cream, one full applicator at bedtime for 7 days, **or** metronidazole 0.75% gel one full applicator once daily for 5 days
   b. Alternatives: clindamycin ovules 100 mg intravaginally at bedtime for 3 days or clindamycin 300 mg 2 times/day for 7 days
   c. Pregnant women: metronidazole 500 mg 2 times/day for 7 days **or** metronidazole 250 mg 3 times/day for 7 days **or** clindamycin 300 mg 2 times/day for 7 days
   d. Do not use clindamycin cream during pregnancy because of the increased risk of preterm deliveries.
   e. Treatment of sexual partners is not necessary.

H. Trichomoniasis
1. Caused by *T. vaginalis*
2. Men often have no symptoms, but women generally have a malodorous, yellow-green vaginal discharge and vaginal irritation.
3. Treatment
   a. Metronidazole 2 g orally in a single dose or tinidazole 2 g orally in a single dose
   b. Alternative: metronidazole 500 mg orally 2 times/day for 7 days
   c. All sexual partners should be treated.
   d. Metronidazole-allergic patients should be desensitized.

I. Vulvovaginal Candidiasis (VVC)
1. Seventy-five percent of women have at least one episode (40%–45% will have many episodes).
2. Symptoms include pruritus and vaginal discharge.
3. Predisposing factors include OCs, pregnancy, obesity, diabetes mellitus, corticosteroid use, chemotherapy, and antibiotics.
4. Diagnosed by symptoms and potassium hydroxide smear
5. Therapeutic regimens – Note: 1- and 3-day regimens may take up to 7 days for full effect.

Table 21. Therapeutic Regimens for Treatment of Vulvovaginal Candidiasis

Drug	Dose	Length of Therapy
Butoconazole	2% cream: 5 g intravaginally at bedtime (OTC)	3 days
	2% cream: 5 g intravaginally	1 dose
Clotrimazole	1% cream: 5 g intravaginally at bedtime (OTC)	7 days
	100-mg vaginal tablet at bedtime (OTC)	7 days
	Two 100-mg vaginal tablets at bedtime	3 days
Miconazole	2% cream: 5 g intravaginally at bedtime (OTC)	7 days
	100-mg vaginal suppository at bedtime (OTC)	7 days
	200-mg vaginal suppository at bedtime (OTC)	3 days
	1200-mg vaginal suppository × 1 (OTC)	1 dose
Nystatin	100,000-unit vaginal tablet at bedtime	14 days
Terconazole	0.4% cream: 5 g intravaginally at bedtime	7 days
	0.8% cream: 5 g intravaginally at bedtime	3 days
	80-mg vaginal suppository at bedtime	3 days
Tioconazole	6.5% ointment: 5 g intravaginally (OTC)	1 dose
Fluconazole	150-mg oral tablet	1 dose

OTC = over-the-counter.

5. Recurrent VVC (four or more episodes a year) – needs prescription drug treatment, not OTC
    a. Initial treatment for 7–14 days or fluconazole 100-, 150-, or 200-mg dose every third day for three doses
    b. Maintenance: oral fluconazole 100, 150, or 200 mg/week for 6 months
    c. Consider conditions precipitating recurrent VVC: HIV, diabetes mellitus
6. Prophylaxis for VVC while taking antibiotics, recommend OTC 7-day treatment and use a full applicator at bedtime while taking antibiotics

VIII. PROSTATIC INFECTIONS

A. Prostatitis
    1. Symptoms
        a. Urethritis
        b. Asymptomatic
        c. Primarily gram-negative organisms: *C. trachomatis, N. gonorrhoeae, E. coli*
    3. Acute bacterial prostatitis
        a. Therapy duration: 14–28 days
        b. Depends on organism:
            i. Gonorrhea: ceftriaxone 250 mg intramuscularly
            ii. Fluoroquinolones: ciprofloxacin 500 mg 2 times/day, ofloxacin 200 mg 2 times/day
            iii. Cotrimoxazole (trimethoprim-sulfamethoxazole [TMP/SMX]) 960 mg 2 times/day or trimethoprim 200 mg 2 times/day
    4. Chronic bacterial prostatitis (symptoms should have been present for at least 6 months)
        a. Therapy duration: 28 days
        b. Depends on organism:
            i. Fluoroquinolones: ciprofloxacin 500 mg 2 times/day, ofloxacin 200 mg 2 times/day, norfloxacin 400 mg 2 times/day (not for gonorrhea)
            ii. Minocycline 100 mg 2 times/day, doxycycline 100 mg 2 times/day, trimethoprim 200 mg 2 times/day, cotrimoxazole (TMP/SMX) 960 mg 2 times/day

B. Epididymitis
   1. Initial therapy; most likely gonococcal or chlamydial infection
      a. Ceftriaxone 250 mg intramuscularly once plus doxycycline 100 mg 2 times/day for 10 days
   2. Most likely caused by enteric organisms
      a. Ofloxacin 300 mg 2 times/day for 10 days (not for gonorrhea)
      b. Levofloxacin 500 mg/day for 10 days (not for gonorrhea)

IX. MALE SEXUAL DYSFUNCTION

A. Types
   1. Reduced libido from organic or psychological causes
      a. Low serum testosterone concentrations
      b. Increased concentrations of serum prolactin
   2. Ejaculation
      a. Premature
      b. Retarded
      c. Absent
      d. Retrograde
   3. Erectile dysfunction
      a. Persistent (at least 6 months) inability to achieve or maintain an erection of sufficient duration and firmness to complete satisfactory intercourse through vaginal penetration
      b. Psychological
      c. Organic
      d. Mixed
      e. Causes
         i. Vascular because of atherosclerotic plaques, trauma, or irradiation
         ii. Neurologic because of stroke, seizures, or diabetes mellitus
         iii. Hormonal abnormalities because of excess prolactin (hyperprolactinemia) or decreased testosterone concentrations (hypogonadism)
         iv. Medical conditions such as angina, shortness of breath because of asthma or chronic obstructive pulmonary disease
         v. Drugs such as antihypertensives, psychiatric medications (antidepressants and antipsychotics)

B. Treatment of Erectile Dysfunction
   1. Treat organic problems.
      a. Smoking cessation
      b. Control diabetes mellitus.
      c. Control hyperlipidemia.
      d. Control hypertension.
      e. Decrease alcohol intake.
      f. Discontinue illicit drugs.
      g. Lose weight.
      h. Exercise.
      i. Review current medications.

2. Nonpharmacologic treatment
   a. Vacuum pump devices
   b. Venous constriction rings
3. Testosterone replacement
   a. Depot intramuscular injection of testosterone enanthate 200 mg or cypionate 300 mg every 2–3 weeks
   b. Oral testosterone not used because of potential liver toxicity
   c. Scrotal and nonscrotal dermal patches placed daily
      i. Androderm 2.5–10 mg at bedtime on back, abdomen, or arms; rotate sites
   d. One percent testosterone gel 5–10 g every morning
      i. Testim on shoulders, upper arms only
      ii. AndroGel should not be applied to genitals.
   e. Monitor within 1–3 months and at 6- to 12-month intervals.
   f. If no improvement after 3 months, may discontinue treatment
4. Phosphodiesterase inhibitors
   a. Sildenafil (Viagra), tadalafil (Cialis), vardenafil (Levitra)
   b. Inhibits phosphodiesterase type 5 in the penile tissue, preventing the breakdown of cyclic guanosine monophosphate; thus increases smooth muscle relaxation in the corpora cavernosa and enhances penile rigidity
   c. Adverse effects: headache, hot flashes, heartburn, diarrhea, myalgias, hypotension, dizziness, difficulty discriminating blue from green
   d. Contraindications/cautions
      i. Contraindicated with nitrate use
      ii. Caution with cardiovascular disease, hypotension, uncontrolled hypertension, MI/stroke within 6 months, life-threatening arrhythmias, penile deformities, renal/hepatic dysfunction, degenerative retinal disorders
   e. Doses
      i. Sildenafil 50 mg orally × 1; maximal dose 100 mg/day, usually take tablet 1 hour before intercourse
      ii. Tadalafil 10 mg orally × 1; maximal dose 20 mg/day; effects may last up to 36 hours May also use as daily dose without respect to timing of intercourse, tadalafil 2.5–5 mg orally daily
      iii. Vardenafil 10 mg orally × 1; maximal dose 20 mg/day, usually take tablet 1 hour before intercourse
5. Yohimbine
   a. Derivative of African yohimbe tree
   b. α_2-Antagonist
   c. Efficacy controversial, not recommended according to the American Urological Association guidelines
   d. Adverse effects: headaches, dizziness, insomnia, and anxiety
   e. Dose: 5.4 mg orally 3 times/day
6. Alprostadil
   a. Caverject intracavernosal injection 2.5–40 mcg
   b. Muse urethral pellets 125–1000 mcg
   c. Effect may last 30–90 minutes.
   d. Adverse effects: penile pain, cavernosal scarring, priapism
   e. Drug interactions: Do not use with phosphodiesterase inhibitors.

C. Treatment of Premature Ejaculation
   1. Serotonin reuptake inhibitors
      a. Fluoxetine, paroxetine, sertraline, clomipramine
      b. Continuous (daily) or episodic dosing 2–12 hours before intercourse
   2. Topical anesthetics
      a. Lidocaine/prilocaine cream (EMLA) 2.5 g applied 20–30 minutes before intercourse

X. FEMALE SEXUAL DYSFUNCTION

A. Types
   1. Arousal (female sexual arousal disorder) 6%–21%
   2. Orgasm (female orgasmic disorder) 4%–7%
   3. Desire – two types
      a. Hypoactive sexual desire disorder – 10%–46%
      b. Sexual aversion disorder – rare
   4. Pain (dyspareunia, vaginismus, noncoital sexual pain) 3%–18%

B. Treatment
   1. Treat organic problem.
      a. Review medications.
      b. Smoking cessation
      c. Control diabetes mellitus.
      d. Control hyperlipidemia.
      e. Control hypertension.
      f. Decrease alcohol intake.
      g. Discontinue illicit drugs.
      h. Exercise.
   2. Psychotherapy for pain disorders (vaginismus and dyspareunia)
   3. Drugs – off-label uses of medications
      a. Sildenafil 10–50 mg taken 1 hour before sexual intercourse (for female sexual arousal disorder), shown at times to reverse sexual dysfunction caused by selective serotonin reuptake inhibitors
      b. Transdermal testosterone 150–450 mcg, 300 mcg daily – increased sexual satisfaction with sexual activity, increased sexual desire, decreased personal stress in surgically and naturally menopausal women
      c. Testosterone cream 1%, 10 g applied to thigh daily – Used in premenopausal women with decreased testosterone concentrations, improved sexual self-rating scores
      d. Methyltestosterone/estradiol 2.5 mg/1.25 mg daily – Used in surgically menopausal women taking hormone therapy, improved sexual interest or desire
      e. Bupropion 150–300 mg/day – Increased arousal, orgasm in premenopausal women

Patient Case
12. A 65-year-old man presents to his physician complaining of symptoms determined to be erectile dysfunction. He has a history of hyperlipidemia, gastroesophageal reflux disease, and glucose intolerance. His medications include atorvastatin 20 mg orally daily, omeprazole 20 mg orally daily, and aspirin 81 mg as tolerated. He states that he has heard of medications to help with his symptoms but does not want to have to plan his intimate moments. Which of the following drugs might work best for this patient?

   A. Tadalafil.
   B. Vardenafil.
   C. Yohimbine.
   D. Bupropion.

REFERENCES

Osteoporosis/Hormone Replacement Therapy

1. Walsh BW, Kuller LH, Wild RA, et al. Effects of raloxifene on serum lipids and coagulation factors in healthy postmenopausal women. JAMA 1998;279:1445–51.
2. National Osteoporosis Foundation. Physician's guide to prevention and treatment of osteoporosis. Available at *http://www.nof.org/physguide/index.htm*. Accessed December 8, 2009.
3. American College of Obstetricians and Gynecologists. ACOG practice bulletin: clinical management guidelines for obstetricians-gynecologists. Obstet Gynecol 2004;103:203–16.
4. AACE Osteoporosis Task Force. American Association of Clinical Endocrinologists medical guidelines for clinical practice for the prevention and treatment of postmenopausal osteoporosis, 2001 edition, with selected updates for 2003. Endocr Pract 2003;9:545–64.
5. North American Menopause Society. Management of osteoporosis in postmenopausal women: 2006 position statement of the North American Menopause Society. Menopause 2006;13:340–67.
6. North American Menopause Society. Estrogen and progestogen use in postmenopausal women: July 2008 position statement of the North American Menopause Society. Menopause 2008;15:584–602.

Drugs in Pregnancy and Lactation

1. Briggs GG, Freeman RK, Yaffe SJ. Drugs in Pregnancy and Lactation, 7th ed. Philadelphia, PA: Lippincott Williams and Wilkins, 2005.
2. Black RA, Hill DA. Over-the-counter medications in pregnancy. Am Fam Physician 2003;67:2517–24.
3. Koren G, Pastuszak A, Ito S. Drugs in pregnancy. N Engl J Med 1998;338:1128–37.

Complications in Pregnancy

1. Quinlain JD, Hill DA. Nausea and vomiting of pregnancy. Am Fam Physician 2003;68:121–8.
2. Ward RK, Zamorski MA. Benefits and risks of psychiatric medications during pregnancy. Am Fam Physician 2002;66:629–36.
3. Chobanian AV, Bakris GL, Black HR, et al.; National High Blood Pressure Education Program Coordinating Committee. Seventh report of the Joint National Committee on Prevention, Detection, Evaluation, and Treatment of High Blood Pressure. Hypertension 2003;42:1206–52.
4. Gentile S. Clinical utilization of antipsychotics in pregnancy and lactation. Ann Pharmacother 2004;38:1265–71.
5. Zamorski MA, Green LA. NHBPEP report on high blood pressure in pregnancy: a summary for family physicians. Am Fam Physician 2001;64:263–70.
6. Yoder SR, Thornburg LL, Bisognano JD. Hypertension in pregnancy and women of childbearing age. Am J Med 2009;122:890–5.
7. Serlin DC, Lash RW. Diagnosis and management of gestational diabetes mellitus. Am Fam Physician 2009;80:57–62.

Contraception

1. Brown SS, Eisenberg L, eds. The Best Intentions: Unintended Pregnancy and the Well-Being of Children and Families. Washington, DC: National Academy Press, 1995.
2. Hatcher RA Trussell J, Nelson AL, et al. Contraceptive Technology, 19th ed. New York: Ardent Media, 2008.
3. Rosenberg MJ, Waugh MS. Oral contraceptive discontinuation: a prospective evaluation of frequency and reasons. Am J Obstet Gynecol 1998;179(3 Pt 1):577–82.
4. Novák A, de la Loge C, Abetz L, van der Meulen EA. The combined contraceptive vaginal ring, NuvaRing: an international study of user acceptability. Contraception 2003;67:187–94.
5. Oral contraceptives. In: Drug Facts and Comparisons, 4.0. St. Louis, MO: Wolters Kluwer Health, 2009. Available at *http://online.factsandcomparisons.com/*. Accessed December 11, 2009.

Sexually Transmitted Diseases

1. Centers for Disease Control and Prevention. Sexually transmitted diseases treatment guidelines 2006. MMWR 2006;55:1–94. Available at *http://www.cdc.gov/std/treatment/*. Accessed December 7, 2009.

2. Centers for Disease Control and Prevention. Updated recommended treatment regimens for gonococcal infections and associated conditions—United States, April. Available at *http://www.cdc.gov/std/treatment/2006/updated-regimens.htm*. Accessed December 7, 2009.

Prostatic Infections

1. Stern J, Schaeffer A. Chronic prostatitis. Clin Evid 2003;10:994–1002.

2. Wagenlehner FM, Naber KG. Antimicrobial treatment of prostatitis. Expert Rev Anti Infect Ther 2003;1:275–82.

3. Association for Genitourinary Medicine (AGUM), Medical Society for the Study of Venereal Disease (MSSVD). 2002 National Guideline for the Management of Prostatitis. London: Association for Genitourinary Medicine (AGUM), Medical Society for the Study of Venereal Disease (MSSVD), 2002.

4. Prostatitis and chronic pelvic pain syndrome. In: Grabe M, Bishop MC, Bjerklund-Johansen TE, et al. Guidelines on the Management of Urinary and Male Genital Tract Infections. Arnhem, The Netherlands: European Association of Urology (EAU), 2008:79–88.

Sexual Dysfunction (Male and Female)

1. Wespes E, Amar E, Hatzichristou D, et al. Guidelines on erectile dysfunction. Eur Urol 2002;41:1–5.

2. Montague DK, Jarow J, Broderick GA, et al. AUA guideline on the pharmacologic management of premature ejaculation. J Urol 2004;172:290–4.

3. AACE Male Sexual Dysfunction Task Force. American Association of Clinical Endocrinologists medical guidelines for clinical practice for the evaluation and treatment of male sexual dysfunction: a couple's problem—2003 update. Endocr Pract 2003;9:77–95.

4. Montague DK, Jarow J, Broderick GA, et al. Chapter 1. The management of erectile dysfunction: an AUA update. J Urol 2005;174:230–9.

5. Kammerer-Doak D, Rogers RG. Female sexual function and dysfunction. Obstet Gynecol Clin North Am 2008;35:169–83.

ANSWERS AND EXPLANATIONS TO PATIENT CASES

1. Answer: D
Deep vein thrombosis increased with Prempro (conjugated estrogens and medroxyprogesterone acetate). Myocardial infarction and strokes also increased. Fractures actually decreased.

2. Answer: C
Definitions
Normal = BMD within 1 SD of the young adult mean
Osteopenia = BMD between −1 SD and −2.5 SD
Osteoporosis = BMD at least −2.5 SD

3. Answer: B
Start drug therapy:
    a. North American Menopause Society
        i. If BMD T-score is below −2.5 in the absence of risk factors
        ii. If BMD T-score is below −2.0 to −2.5
            (a) With at least one of the following: previous fracture after menopause other than skull, facial bone, angle, finger, and toe; thinness (body weight less than 127 lb or BMI less than 21 kg/m^2); history of hip fracture in a parent (NAMS)
        iii. All postmenopausal women who have had ano steoporotic vertebral fracture
    b. American College of Obstetricians and Gynecologists
        i. If fragility or low-impact fracture
        ii. if BMD T-score is below −2.0 in the absence of risk factors
        iii. If BMD T-score is below −1.5 in the presence of one or more risk factors in section B1
    c. American Association of Clinical Endocrinologists
        i. If low-trauma fracture
        ii. If BMD T-score is below −2.5 with no risk factors
        iii. If BMD T-score is below −1.5 with risk factors in section B1
        iv. Nonpharmacologic preventive measures are ineffective

Bisphosphonates such as alendronate are considered first-line drugs because they inhibit normal and abnormal bone resorption and have been shown to reduce vertebral and non-vertebral fractures by 30%–50%. Nasal Miacalcin is not considered a first-line drug; however, it may be useful for bone pain caused by vertebral compression fractures. Teriparatide (Forteo) is reserved for treating women at high risk of fracture, including those with very low BMD (T-score worse than −3.0) and a previous vertebral fracture. It decreases vertebral fractures by 65% and non-vertebral fractures by 53%.

4. Answer: C
Lisinopril is an ACE inhibitor and is known have some teratogenicity. It is not recommended for women who are trying to conceive or who are pregnant. Methyldopa is the preferred agent for treating hypertension in women who are trying to conceive or pregnant. β-Blockers are not specifically teratogenic but may cause adverse effects in the fetus.

5. Answer: B
An OC with stronger estrogen properties is required because the patient is bleeding through early in the cycle. Ortho-Cept has higher estrogenic properties (intermediate) than Mircette and other options (low). Estrogen deficiency is early or midcycle breakthrough bleeding (days 1–10). Progestin deficiency is late breakthrough bleeding (days 10–28).

6. Answer: C
Micronor is a POP. The patient cannot use Ortho-Evra because she is obese, and she cannot use estrogen products because she has hypertension (YAZ and Ortho-Evra). She also takes an ACE inhibitor, which should not be used with YAZ because of the possibility of hyperkalemia. Mirena is a progestin-only intrauterine system that may used for up to 5 years, which may be appropriate for the patient if she does not want to get pregnant for several years.

7. Answer: C
If dose is 3 hours late, it is considered a missed dose. Patient should take missed dose as soon remembered and use another contraceptive method for the next 48 hours. Missed two or more doses, another contraceptive method until next menses.

8. Answer: B
Treatment of HSV infection substantially decreases the duration of viral shedding, pain, and length of time to complete healing but has no impact on the risk, frequency, latency, or severity of recurrences.

9. Answer: D

Patient-initiated therapy is important for people with occasional recurrences of HSV infection because recurrent infections resolve more rapidly than the initial infection. Antiviral agents should be initiated as soon as possible. Because the patient is experiencing several recurrences (six or more a year), treatment beyond the patient-initiated therapy (valacyclovir 500 mg orally 2 times/day for 5 days when a recurrence is noticed) is insufficient. Therapy beyond 5 days is unnecessary because untreated recurrent infections resolve in 7 days; the choice of acyclovir 500 mg orally 3 times/day for 10 days when a recurrence is noted is therefore incorrect. In addition, suppressive therapy is given 2 times/day or daily—not 3 times/day; therefore, suppressive therapy with famciclovir 250 mg orally 3 times/day is inappropriate. Suppressive therapy with valacyclovir 500 mg/day orally should be offered.

10. Answer: C

Cefotetan 2 g intravenously every 12 hours with doxycycline 100 mg orally or intravenously every 12 hours is an appropriate empiric antibiotic combination for PID. The combination has activity against *N. gonorrhoeae* and *C. trachomatis*, as well as the gram-negative and anaerobic organisms that are often involved. Metronidazole alone would only have activity against anaerobes and would miss the other organisms often involved in PID. Ampicillin-sulbactam has good activity against most organisms in PID; however, it has no activity against atypical organisms (i.e., *C. trachomatis*). Although ceftriaxone and doxycycline are appropriate, the dose of ceftriaxone should be 250 mg, and the duration of doxycycline should be 14 days.

11. Answer: C

Pelvic inflammatory disease is definitely related to sexual activity; therefore, until all partners and the patient have been treated, abstinence from intercourse for at least 7 days is indicated. In addition, although they should be encouraged to be tested for HIV, given the strong relationship between STDs and the risk of HIV, the most appropriate recommendation for a sexually active patient with PID is to have all sexual partners within the past 60 days tested and treated.

12. Answer: A

Tadalafil may be dosed daily without respect to timing of sexual intercourse. Vardenafil should be taken 60 minutes before sexual intercourse. Yohimbine and bupropion are not first line for erectile dysfunction.

ANSWERS AND EXPLANATIONS TO SELF-ASSESSMENT QUESTIONS

1. Answer: C
Definitions
Normal = BMD within 1 SD of the young adult mean
Osteopenia = BMD between −1 SD and −2.5 SD
Osteoporosis = BMD at least −2.5 SD

2. Answer: B
Start drug therapy:
  a. North American Menopause Society
     i. If BMD T-score is below −2.5 in the absence of risk factors
     ii. If BMD T-score is below −2.0 to −2.5
        (a). With at least one of the following: previous fracture after menopause other than skull, facial bone, angle, finger, and toe; thinness (body weight less than 127 lb or BMI less than 21 kg/m2); history of hip fracture in a parent (NAMS)
     iii. All postmenopausal women who have had an osteoporotic vertebral fracture
  b. American College of Obstetricians and Gynecologists
     i. If fragility or low-impact fracture
     ii. If BMD T-score is below −2.0 in the absence of risk factors
     iii. If BMD T-score is below −1.5 in the presence of one or more risk factors in section B1
  c. American Association of Clinical Endocrinologists
     i. If low-trauma fracture
     ii. If BMD T-score is below −2.5 with no risk factors
     iii. If BMD T-score is below −1.5 with risk factors in section B1
     iv. Nonpharmacologic preventive measures are ineffective

Bisphosphonates such as risedronate are considered first-line drugs because they inhibit normal and abnormal bone resorption and have been shown to reduce vertebral and non-vertebral fractures by 30%–50%. Raloxifene is indicated for the prevention of osteoporosis in postmenopausal women. It works as a selective estrogen receptor modulator. Although teriparatide decreases vertebral fractures by 65% and non-vertebral fractures by 54%, it would not be used as first-line therapy because it is administered subcutaneously and is very expensive. Risk factors for osteoporosis include smoking and sedentary lifestyle. Smoking cessation and weight-bearing exercise should be recommended.

3. Answer: C
Warfarin is a category X drug in pregnancy and a known teratogen. If a woman requires anticoagulation and is planning to conceive or is pregnant, she should find an alternative anticoagulant such as a low-molecular-weight heparin (e.g., enoxaparin) or heparin. Warfarin should not be used at any time during pregnancy.

4. Answer: B
Medroxyprogesterone is added to conjugated estrogens to decrease the risk of endometrial cancer. Estrogen alone is not sufficient because the patient has an intact uterus as indicated by her medical history (no surgeries).

5. Answer: B
The efficacy of the OC may be decreased. *(See Answer 5 Table on page 2-258)*

6. Answer: C
The number of patients needed to treat with famciclovir over acyclovir to prevent one recurrent herpes simplex genital infection (1 year of follow-up of study participants on suppressive therapy [acyclovir or famciclovir], with 27% and 24%, respectively, experiencing a recurrent infection) is 33.3 = 1/(0.27 − 0.24). The only information needed is the absolute risk in both groups (which is provided).

7. Answer: C
The patient has a history of DVT, which precludes any estrogen product (Yasmin and Ortho-Evra). Her BP is elevated but not greater than 160/100 mm Hg, which would be a contraindication for estrogen use. She is also obese at 202 lb, so the Ortho-Evra patch is not recommended. Depo-Provera may be an option, but the patient is obese and Depo-Provera is known to cause weight gain. In addition, Depo-Provera has a long return to fertility, and the patient stated she wanted to have children in the near future. Nor-QD is a POP and the best of the choices.

8. Answer: B
A phosphodiesterase inhibitor such as sildenafil may be initiated. Testosterone replacement would not be effective because he has normal testosterone concentrations.

Yohimbine would not be considered first-line therapy because its efficacy is controversial. Serotonin reuptake inhibitors, such as fluoxetine, would be used for the treatment of premature ejaculation.

9. Answer: D

Penicillin G 4 million units every 4 hours intravenously for 14 days after penicillin desensitization is the correct therapy for a patient with neurosyphilis who is allergic to penicillin. Levofloxacin would not cover syphilis. Three doses of benzathine penicillin G are indicated for late latent syphilis, not neurosyphilis. Furthermore, although doxycycline is an alternative for patients who are penicillin allergic, patients with neurosyphilis should be desensitized and given penicillin.

10. Answer: D

Data are continuous and probably normally distributed (given the large population of 350 patients in the study); therefore, a parametric test is indicated. The Student t-test is the appropriate parametric test for comparing two groups. Although ANOVA is a parametric test, it is used to compare more than two groups. A chi-square test is used for nominal data between two groups. The Mann-Whitney U-test is a nonparametric analog to the Student t-test.

Answer 5 Table.

Drugs Interfering with Oral Contraceptive Efficacy		Oral Contraceptives Interfering with the Efficacy of Other Drugs	
Increased	Decreased	Increased	Decreased
Ascorbic acid	Anticonvulsants[a]	Benzodiazepines[b]	Benzodiazepines[c]
Acetaminophen—scheduled	Antibiotics	Theophylline and caffeine	Warfarin
Atorvastatin	Rifampin	Cyclosporine	Thyroid agents
Rosuvastatin	Theophylline	Corticosteroids	Hypoglycemics
NNRTIs[d]	St. John's wort	Alcohol	Methyldopa
Protease inhibitors[e]	NNRTI-nevirapine	β-Blockers	Metformin
	Protease inhibitors[f]	Tricyclic antidepressants	Amprenavir
	Sulfonamides	Ropinirole	
	Griseofulvin	Zolmitriptan	
	Bosentan		
	Tacrolimus		
	Modafinil		

[a]Barbiturates, phenytoin, primidone, carbamazepine, oxcarbazepine, felbamate, topiramate, vigabatrin.
[b]Alprazolam, chlordiazepoxide, diazepam.
[c]Temazepam.
[d]Delavirdine, efavirenz.
[e]Atazanavir, amprenavir, indinavir.
[f]Nelfinavir, ritonavir, lopinavir-ritonavir.
NNRTIs = nonnucleoside reverse transcriptase inhibitors.

    a. Reported antibiotic cases in the literature: tetracycline, minocycline, erythromycin, penicillins, and cephalosporins. Pharmacokinetic studies have not shown decreased OC steroid concentrations with tetracycline, doxycycline, ampicillin, metronidazole, quinolones, or fluconazole.
    b. Proposed mechanisms of drug interactions
        i. Interference of absorption: ethinyl estradiol is conjugated in liver, excreted in bile, hydrolyzed by intestinal bacteria, and reabsorbed as active drug. Non–liver enzyme-inducing antibiotics temporarily decrease colonic bacteria and inhibit enterohepatic circulation of ethinyl estradiol. Gastrointestinal flora have recovered 3 weeks after the introduction of an antibiotic.
        ii. Liver enzyme induction (rifampin and griseofulvin): metabolism of progesterone and estrogen is accelerated
        iii. Use alternative contraception for the length of antibiotic therapy plus 7 days after discontinuing the antibiotic.

PHARMACOKINETICS: A REFRESHER

CURTIS L. SMITH, PHARM.D., BCPS

FERRIS STATE UNIVERSITY

LANSING, MICHIGAN

PHARMACOKINETICS: A REFRESHER

CURTIS L. SMITH, PHARM.D., BCPS

FERRIS STATE UNIVERSITY
LANSING, MICHIGAN

Learning Objectives:

1. Identify and provide examples using basic pharmacokinetic concepts commonly used in clinical practice, including elimination rate constant, volume of distribution (V_d), clearance, and bioavailability.

2. Describe specific pharmacokinetic characteristics of commonly used therapeutic agents.

3. Define important issues as they relate to drug concentration sampling and interpretation.

Self-Assessment Questions:

Answers to these questions may be found at the end of this chapter.

1. J.H., a 65-year-old woman (65 kg), was recently initiated on tobramycin and piperacillin-tazobactam for treatment of hospital-acquired pneumonia. After the first dose of tobramycin 120 mg (infused from noon to 1:00 pm), serum tobramycin concentrations are drawn. They are 4.4 mg/L at 3:00 pm and 1.2 mg/L at 7:00 pm. Which one of the following statements is true about tobramycin?

   A. There are sufficient data to determine the half-life ($t_{1/2}$) but not the V_d.
   B. There are sufficient data to determine both the $t_{1/2}$ and V_d.
   C. There are insufficient data to determine either the $t_{1/2}$ or the V_d.
   D. There are sufficient data to determine the V_d but not the $t_{1/2}$.

2. P.L. is a 60-year-old woman (60 kg) recently initiated on gentamicin and clindamycin. After the first gentamicin dose of 110 mg (infused from 6:00 pm to 6:30 pm), serum gentamicin concentrations are drawn. They are 3.6 mg/L at 7:30 pm and 0.9 mg/L at 11:30 pm. Which one of the following best describes this patient's gentamicin pharmacokinetic parameters?

   A. The $t_{1/2}$ is about 2 hours.
   B. The $t_{1/2}$ is about 3 hours.
   C. The maximum concentration (C_{max}) is about 3.8 mg/L.
   D. The V_d is about 11.6 L.

3. R.O. is a 74-year-old woman initiated on gentamicin 100 mg intravenously every 24 hours for pyelonephritis. On admission, her serum creatinine (SCr) is 1.8 mg/dL. She also has congestive heart failure and is fluid overloaded because of her diminished renal function and nonadherence to her angiotensin-converting enzyme inhibitor and diuretic. A few days into her hospitalization, her SCr is down to 1.1 mg/dL, and she is reinitiated on furosemide and enalapril. Which of the following most likely happened to the gentamicin $t_{1/2}$ in R.O. during her hospitalization?

   A. Her clearance increased, which increased her V_d and decreased her $t_{1/2}$.
   B. Her clearance increased, which increased her elimination rate constant and decreased her $t_{1/2}$.
   C. Her V_d decreased, which increased her clearance and decreased her $t_{1/2}$.
   D. Her V_d decreased, which increased her elimination rate constant and increased her $t_{1/2}$.

4. A patient receives vancomycin 1000 mg intravenously every 24 hours and has a trough concentration, drawn 30 minutes before the next dose, of 6 mg/L. Which one of the following regimens is best for this patient if the goal trough concentration is 10–15 mg/L?

   A. Maintain the dose at 1000 mg intravenously every 24 hours.
   B. Lower the dose to 500 mg, but keep the interval at every 24 hours.
   C. Keep the dose at 1000 mg, but shorten the interval to every 12 hours.
   D. Lower the dose to 500 mg, and shorten the interval to every 12 hours.

5. A 40-year-old, 60-kg woman who smokes presents to the emergency department at 2:00 pm with an acute exacerbation of asthma. She takes theophylline sustained release 300 mg 2 times/day, with the last dose taken at 9:00 that morning. Her theophylline concentration soon after presenting to the emergency department is 7.0 mg/L. She is stabilized and is to be sent home on theophylline sustained release. Which one of the following options is the best regimen for this patient?

   A. Theophylline sustained release 300 mg by mouth every 12 hours.
   B. Theophylline sustained release 600 mg by mouth every 12 hours.
   C. Theophylline sustained release 400 mg by mouth every 8 hours.
   D. Theophylline sustained release 600 mg by mouth every 8 hours.

6. L.R. is a 49-year-old patient with diabetes mellitus and renal failure. He was recently in a car accident and sustained head trauma. He currently receives

phenytoin 100 mg intravenously 3 times/day, and his most recent concentration was 5.6 mcg/mL. You are asked to suggest a new dose to achieve a concentration within the therapeutic range. Laboratory results include sodium 145 mEq/L, potassium 3.9 mEq/L, chloride 101 mEq/L, carbon dioxide 26 mEq/L, blood urea nitrogen (BUN) 95 mg/dL, SCr 5.4 mg/dL, glucose 230 mg/dL, and albumin (Alb) 2.8 g/dL. Which one of the following choices is the best recommendation?

A. Increase the dose to 200 mg intravenously 3 times/day.
B. Increase the dose to 200 mg intravenously 2 times/day.
C. Decrease the dose to 100 mg intravenously 2 times/day.
D. Keep the dose the same.

7. You are asked how the TDx (fluorescence polarization immunoassay) and EMIT (enzyme multiplied immunoassay technique) assays compare with each other. Which one of the following statements is most accurate?

A. Although both are immunoassays, one labels antibody, whereas the other labels antigen.
B. Although both are immunoassays, one uses antibody as a marker, whereas the other uses a radioisotope.
C. Although both are immunoassays, one uses an enzyme label, whereas the other uses a fluorescent label.
D. They are both names for the same assay technique.

8. An elderly patient is seen in the morning medicine clinic for a routine follow-up. Medication history includes digoxin 0.25 mg/day by mouth, furosemide 40 mg/day by mouth, and potassium chloride 10 mEq/day by mouth. All doses were last taken at 8:00 am today at home. The patient has vague complaints of stomach upset, which began 2 days ago, but is otherwise in no apparent distress. A serum digoxin concentration drawn today at 10:00 am is 2.5 mcg/L. Which one of the following statements best describes what should be done next?

A. Admit the patient for administration of digoxin Fab.
B. Tell the patient to skip tomorrow's dose of digoxin and begin 0.125 mg/day by mouth.
C. Administer a dose of activated charcoal.
D. Do nothing today about the digoxin.

9. A research group is analyzing the relationship between various independent patient demographics (e.g., age, height, weight, Alb, creatinine clearance [CrCl]) and phenytoin pharmacokinetics. Which one of the following statistical tests will need to be used to assess the relationship?

A. One-way analysis of variance.
B. Analysis of covariance.
C. Multiple logistic regression.
D. Spearman rank correlation.

10. N.T. is a 24-year-old woman receiving valproic acid for tonic-clonic seizures. Her most recent trough valproic acid concentration was 22 mg/L. Her most recent Alb concentration was 4.1 g/dL. Based on this serum concentration, which one of the following recommendations is best concerning her dose?

A. Continue with the current dose; the concentration is close enough to the therapeutic range.
B. Assess adherence and increase her dose; the concentration is below the therapeutic range.
C. Decrease her dose; the concentration is slightly above the therapeutic range.
D. Assess adherence and then check a free valproic acid concentration and adjust accordingly.

Patient Cases

[handwritten: 24-12 = 1 half life = 3 days]

1. H.R. is receiving vancomycin for a methicillin-resistant *Staphylococcus aureus* bacteremia. H.R. has chronic renal failure. A 1-g intravenous dose of vancomycin is given at noon on March 21. A concentration drawn at 2:00 pm on March 21 is 23.8 mcg/mL. A concentration drawn at 2:00 pm on March 24 is 12.1 mcg/mL. If you were to give a dose at 4:00 pm on March 24 and your goal trough concentration was 10–15 mg/L, when would it be best to give the next dose?
   A. 1 day after the dose on the 24th.
   B. 3 days from the dose on the 24th.
   C. 6 days from the dose on the 24th.
   D. There is not enough information to calculate when to redose.

   [handwritten: $V_d = 42L$, $K = 0.0094$]

2. After the administration of 100 mg of a drug intravenously and 200 mg of the same drug by mouth, the areas under the curves are 50 and 25 mg/L/hour. Which one of the following is the bioavailability of this drug?
   A. 25%.
   B. 37.5%.
   C. 50%.
   D. 100%.

   [handwritten: 100 × 25 / 200 × 50]

3. An infusion of 20 mg/hour of theophylline is initiated. Which one of the following best represents what the serum concentration would be at 48 hours if the $t_{1/2}$ of the drug were 4 hours and the V_d were 0.5 L/kg (your patient weighs 65 kg)?
   A. 3.6 mg/L.
   B. 5.0 mg/L.
   C. 18.2 mg/L.
   D. 30.4 mg/L.

   [handwritten: $V_d = \dfrac{R_0}{K \cdot C_{ss}}$]

I. BASIC PHARMACOKINETIC RELATIONSHIPS

A. Absorption

$$F = \frac{dose_{iv} * AUC_{ev}}{dose_{ev} * AUC_{iv}}$$

[handwritten: extravascular (oral)]

B. Distribution

Rapid intravenous (or oral) bolus:
$$V_d = \frac{F * dose}{Cp_0}$$

Continuous intravenous infusion at steady state:
$$V_d = \frac{R_0}{k * C_{ss}}$$

Continuous intravenous infusion before steady state:
$$V_d = \frac{R_0}{C * k}(1 - e^{-kt}) \text{ and } C = \frac{R_0}{V_d * k}(1 - e^{-kt})$$

Multiple intravenous (or oral) bolus at steady state:
$$V_d = \frac{F * dose}{C_{ss\,max} * (1 - e^{-kt})}$$

Multiple intravenous (or oral) infusion at steady state: $V_d = \dfrac{F * \text{dose}}{k} * \dfrac{1 - e^{-kt'}}{C_{max} - (C_{min} * e^{-kt'})}$

$$C_{ss\,max} = \dfrac{F * \text{dose}}{V_d * (1 - e^{-kt})} \qquad C_{ss\,min} = \dfrac{F * \text{dose}}{V_d * (1 - e^{-kt})} * e^{-kt}$$

C. Clearance

$$\text{Clearance} = \dfrac{\text{dose}}{\text{AUC}} \qquad k = \dfrac{Cl}{V_d} \qquad k = \dfrac{(\ln C_1 - \ln C_2)}{(t_1 - t_2)} \qquad t_{1/2} = \dfrac{0.693}{k}$$

Continuous intravenous infusion at steady state: $\quad \text{clearance} = \dfrac{R_0}{C_{ss}}$

Continuous intravenous infusion before steady state: $\quad \text{clearance} = \dfrac{R_0}{C} * (1 - e^{-kt})$

Multiple intravenous (or oral) bolus at steady state: $\quad \text{clearance} = \dfrac{F * \text{dose}/\tau}{C_{avg}}$

$$\tau = \dfrac{(\ln C_{max} - \ln C_{min})}{k} \qquad C_1 = C_0 * e^{-kt}$$

II. ABSORPTION

A. First-pass Effect
1. Blood perfusing virtually all the gastrointestinal tissues passes through the liver by means of the hepatic portal vein.
    a. Fifty percent of the rectal blood supply bypasses the liver (middle and inferior hemorrhoidal veins).
    b. Drugs absorbed in the buccal cavity bypass the liver.
2. Drugs affected most by the first-pass effect are those with a high hepatic extraction ratio.
3. Example

Amitriptyline	Labetalol	Nitroglycerin
Desipramine	Lidocaine	Pentazocine
Diltiazem	Metoprolol	Propoxyphene
Doxepin	Morphine	Propranolol
Imipramine	Nicardipine	Verapamil
Isosorbide dinitrate	Nifedipine	

B. Enterohepatic Recirculation
    1. Drugs are excreted by the bile into the duodenum, metabolized by the normal flora in the gastrointestinal tract, and reabsorbed into the portal circulation.
    2. Occurs in drugs with 1) biliary (hepatic) elimination and 2) good oral absorption
    3. Drug is concentrated in the gallbladder and expelled on sight, smell, or ingestion of food.

Examples of Compounds Excreted in Bile and Subject to Enterohepatic Cycling

Compound	Entity in Bile
Chloramphenicol	Glucuronide conjugate
Digoxin	Parent
Estrogens	Parent
Imipramine	Parent and desmethyl metabolite
Indomethacin	Parent and glucuronide
Nafcillin	Parent
Rifampin	Parent
Sulindac	Glucuronides of parent and metabolites
Testosterone	Conjugates
Tiagabine	Glucuronide conjugate
Valproic acid	Glucuronide conjugates
Vitamin A	Conjugates

[handwritten: Reason for estrogen-antibiotic interaction]

Patient Case

4. Which one of the following statements best describes P-glycoprotein?
    A. It is a plasma protein that binds basic drugs.
    B. It transfers drugs through the gastrointestinal mucosa, increasing absorption.
    C. It diminishes the effect of cytochrome P450 3A4 (CYP3A4) in the gastrointestinal mucosa.
    D. It is an efflux pump that decreases gastrointestinal mucosal transport.

---

1. P-glycoprotein is an efflux pump (located in the esophagus, stomach, and small and large intestines) that pumps drugs back into the gastrointestinal lumen; it is a more important factor in drug absorption drug interactions than intestinal CYP3A4.
2. CYP3A4 and P-glycoprotein located in small intestinal enterocytes work together to decrease the absorption of xenobiotics.
3. Most CYP3A4 substrates are also P-glycoprotein substrates.
4. Many CYP3A4 inhibitors/inducers also inhibit/induce P-glycoprotein, leading to increases or decreases in bioavailability.
5. Examples of P-glycoprotein absorption drug interactions include quinidine or verapamil and digoxin; rifampin or St. John's wort; and human immunodeficiency virus protease inhibitors.

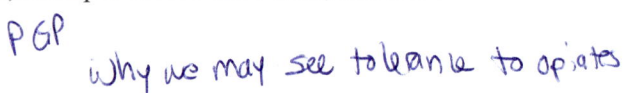

[handwritten: PGP — why we may see tolerance to opiates]

III. DISTRIBUTION

A. Definition: Apparent V_d—proportionality constant that relates the amount of drug in the body to an observed concentration of drug

B. Protein Binding

Protein	Types of Drugs Bound	Molecular Weight	Normal Concentrations (g/L)	(μmol)
Albumin	Acidic	65,000	35–50	500–700
α-1-acid glycoprotein	Basic	44,000	0.4–1.0	9–23
Lipoprotein	Lipophilic and basic	200,000–3,400,000	Variable	Variable

C. P-glycoprotein
1. P-glycoprotein is an efflux pump that mediates blood-brain barrier transport by limiting uptake into or increasing the efflux out of brain epithelial cells.
2. It may be especially important with opioids—induction of P-glycoprotein by chronic use of opioids decreases the opioid effect (tolerance).
3. P-glycoprotein is also found in tumor cells, resulting in the efflux of chemotherapeutic agents out of the cell and, ultimately, multidrug resistance.

IV. CLEARANCE

Enzymes Involved in Drug Metabolism

Oxygenases	Hydrolytic Enzymes
CYP450s	Esterases
Monoamine oxygenases	Amidases
Alcohol dehydrogenases	Epoxide hydrolases
Aldehyde dehydrogenases	Dipeptidases
Xanthine dehydrogenases	
Conjugating Enzymes	
Uridine diphosphate—glucuronyl transferases	
Glutathione *S*-transferase	
Acetyltransferases	
Methyltransferases	

CYP = cytochrome P450.

Patient Case

5. A renal transplant patient receiving cyclosporine receives a diagnosis of community-acquired pneumonia. The patient is admitted to the hospital and initiated on ceftriaxone and a macrolide. Which one of the following macrolides is least likely to interact with cyclosporine?
   A. Erythromycin.
   B. Clarithromycin.
   C. Azithromycin.
   D. All the macrolides inhibit CYP3A4.

1. Introduction
    a. A group of heme-containing enzymes responsible for phase 1 metabolic reactions
    b. Characteristic absorbance of light at 450 nm (thus CYP450)
    c. Primarily located in the membranes of the smooth endoplasmic reticulum in 1) liver, 2) small intestine, and 3) brain, lung, and kidney
    d. Encoded by a supergene family or subfamily; separate genes code for different isoenzymes
    e. Drugs will generally have a high affinity for one particular CYP450, but most drugs also have secondary pathways.
    f. Nomenclature

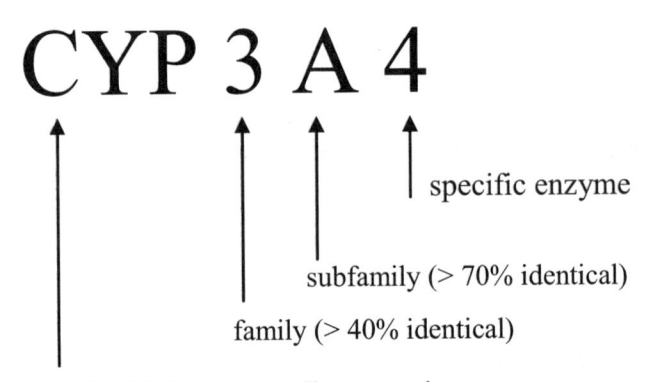

CYP 3 A 4

- specific enzyme
- subfamily (> 70% identical)
- family (> 40% identical)
- GENE for mammalian cytochrome

Figure 1.

2. Distribution of CYP450 isoenzymes in human liver

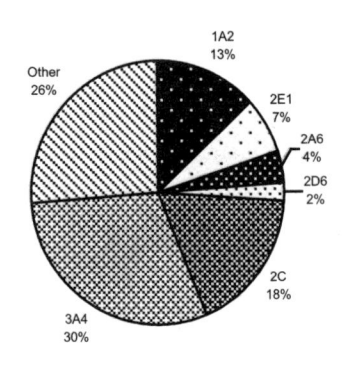

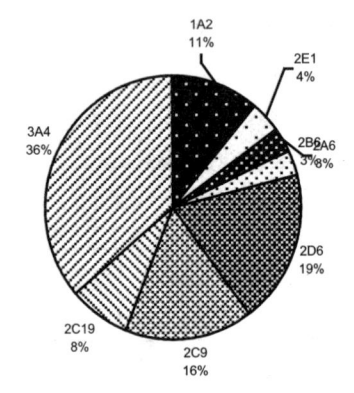

Content (left pie chart):
- Other 26%
- 1A2 13%
- 2E1 7%
- 2A6 4%
- 2D6 2%
- 2C 18%
- 3A4 30%

Role in CYP-mediated Drug Elimination (right pie chart):
- 1A2 11%
- 2E1 4%
- 2B6 3%, 2A6 8%
- 2D6 19%
- 2C9 16%
- 2C19 8%
- 3A4 36%

Figure 2.

3. Distribution of CYP450 isoenzymes in human gastrointestinal tract

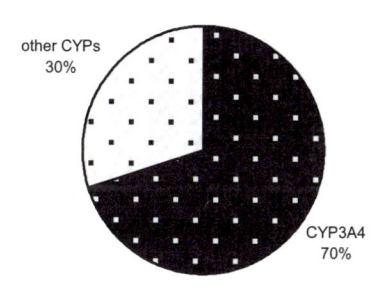

Figure 3.

4. Characteristics of CYP450 metabolism
   a. Inhibition is substrate-independent.
   b. Some substrates are metabolized by more than one CYP450 (e.g., TCAs [tricyclic antidepressants], SSRIs [selective serotonin reuptake inhibitors]).
   c. Enantiomers may be metabolized by a different CYP450 (e.g., warfarin).
   d. Differences in inhibition may exist within the same class of agents (e.g., fluoroquinolones, azole antifungals, macrolides, calcium channel blockers, H2 blockers).
   e. Substrates can also be inhibitors (e.g., erythromycin, verapamil, diltiazem).
   f. Most inducers and some inhibitors can affect more than one isozyme (e.g., cimetidine, ritonavir, fluoxetine, erythromycin).
   g. Inhibitors may affect different isozymes at different doses (e.g., fluconazole).

B. P-glycoprotein
   1. P-glycoprotein is an efflux pump that pumps drugs into the bile; the clinical effect of P-glycoprotein drug interactions in the bile is unknown.
   2. P-glycoprotein pumps drugs from renal tubules into the urine; it also potentially limits the degree of reabsorption.
   3. Examples of drug interactions: quinidine-digoxin, cyclosporine-digoxin, and propafenone-digoxin

C. Pharmacogenetics/Polymorphic Drug Metabolism
   1. Population is divided into poor metabolizers and extensive metabolizers; therefore, metabolism is considered polymorphic.
   2. Definition: coexistence of more than one genetic variant (alleles), which are stable components in the population (more than 1% of population)
   3. Clear antimode results

EM = extensive metabolizer; PM = poor metabolizer; URM = ultrarapid extensive metabolizer.
Figure 4.

4. Phenotype: expression of the trait
    a. Manifestation of the trait clinically
    b. Not necessarily constant
5. Genotype: genetic makeup
    a. Constant: can be tested

Table 1.

Pathway	Substrate	Enzyme	Drug Examples
Oxidation	Debrisoquine, dextromethorphan	CYP2D6	Tertiary amines Fluoxetine Flecainide Propafenone Metoprolol Propranolol Timolol Codeine
Oxidation	Mephenytoin	CYP2C19	Tertiary amines (diazepam) Phenytoin Omeprazole
Acetylation	Isoniazid, caffeine	*N*-acetyltransferase	Clonazepam Dapsone Hydralazine Inamrinone Procainamide Sulfonamides

V. NONLINEAR PHARMACOKINETICS

> **Patient Case**
> 6. C.M. is a 55-year-old man who is initiated on phenytoin after a craniotomy. His current steady-state phenytoin concentration is 6 mg/L at a dose of 200 mg/day by mouth. If his affinity constant (K_m) is calculated to be 5 mg/L, what will happen to his concentration if the dose is doubled (to 400 mg/day by mouth)?
>   A. His concentration will double because phenytoin clearance is linear above the K_m.
>   B. His concentration will more than double because phenytoin clearance is nonlinear above the K_m.
>   C. His concentration will stay the same because phenytoin is an autoinducer, and clearance increases with time.
>   D. His concentration will increase by only 50% because phenytoin absorption decreases significantly with doses greater than 300 mg.

A. Michaelis-Menten Pharmacokinetics

Velocity = Vmax * SKm + S

V_{max} = capacity constant (amount/time)
K_m = affinity constant (amount/volume)
S = substrate concentration (amount/volume)

B. Nonlinear Elimination
   1. Saturation or partial saturation of the elimination pathway

   Rate of elimination = Vmax * CKm + C

   V_{max} = maximum rate of elimination (amount/time)
   K_m = concentration where elimination is ½ V_{max} (affinity constant)
   C = drug concentration

   2. Note: Nonlinearity occurs when concentration is at or above K_m
      a. Example: phenytoin
         i. V_{max} normal = 7 mg/kg/day
         ii. K_m normal = 5.6 mg/L
         iii. 50% variability between individuals

VI. NONCOMPARTMENTAL PHARMACOKINETICS

A. Why Noncompartmental Pharmacokinetics?
   1. Identification of the "correct" model is often impossible.
   2. A compartmental view of the body is unrealistic.
   3. Linear regression is unnecessary—it is easier to automate analysis.
   4. Requires fewer and less stringent assumptions
   5. More general methods and equations
   6. There is no need to match all data sets to the same compartmental model.

B. Definitions
   1. Zero moment—concentration versus time curve
      a. Area under the curve (AUC)

   $$AUC = \sum \frac{(C_n+1 + C_n)}{2} * (t_{n+1} - t_n) ... + \frac{C_{last}}{k}$$

   2. First moment—Concentration * time versus time curve
      a. Area under the first moment curve (AUMC)

   $$AUMC = \sum * (t_{n+1} - t_n) + \frac{C_{last} * t_{last}}{k} + \frac{C_{last}}{k^2}$$

   3. Mean residence time (MRT)

   MRT =

   4. Mean absorption time (MAT)

   $MAT = MRT_{ev} - MRT_{iv}$

C. Pharmacokinetic Parameter Estimation
   1. Clearance

   $$Clearance = \frac{dose}{AUC}$$

2. Volume of distribution at steady state

$$V_{ss} = \frac{dose * AUMC}{AUC^2}$$

3. Elimination rate constant

$k = 1/MRT$

4. Absorption rate constant

$k_a = 1/MAT$

5. Bioavailability

$F = D_{iv} * AUC_{ev} / D_{ev} * AUC_{iv}$

VII. DATA COLLECTION AND ANALYSIS

Patient Case
7. R.K. is a 54-year-old woman with a history of diabetes mellitus and end-stage renal disease. She is receiving gentamicin for *Pseudomonas* pneumonia. A gentamicin concentration is ordered after dialysis. Which one of the following statements is true about obtaining this sample?
   A. The most accurate concentration is obtained immediately after hemodialysis.
   B. Wait a few hours to obtain the concentration because it will decrease significantly within the first few hours after hemodialysis.
   C. Wait a few hours to obtain the concentration because it will increase significantly within the first few hours after hemodialysis.
   D. Wait until the next day so that all the effects of hemodialysis have abated.

A. Timing of Collection
   1. Ensure completion of absorption and distribution phases (especially digoxin and vancomycin, etc.).
   2. Ensure completion of redistribution postdialysis (especially aminoglycosides).

B. Specimen Requirements
   1. Whole blood: Use anticoagulated tube.
   2. Plasma: Use anticoagulated tube and centrifuge; clotting proteins and some blood cells are maintained.
   3. Serum: Use red top, allow to clot, and centrifuge.

Patient Case

8. A drug assay is touted as having high specificity but low sensitivity. Which one of the following statements best describes what this means?
    A. The assay will not be able to distinguish the drug from like products, but it will be able to detect extremely low concentrations.
    B. The assay will not be able to distinguish the drug from like products, and it will not be able to detect extremely low concentrations.
    C. The assay will be able to distinguish the drug from like products and will be able to detect extremely low concentrations.
    D. The assay will be able to distinguish the drug from like products but will not be able to detect extremely low concentrations.

C. Sample Analysis
   1. Assay terminology
      a. Precision (reproducibility): closeness of agreement among the results of repeated analyses performed on the same sample
         i. Standard deviation (SD): average difference of the individual values from the mean
         ii. Coefficient of variation (CV): SD as a percentage of the mean (relative rather than absolute variation)

$$CV = \frac{SD}{mean}$$

   b. Accuracy: closeness with which a measurement reflects the true value of an object
      i. Correlation coefficient—strength of the relationship between two variables
   c. Predictive performance (accuracy)

   Precision: a.k.a. root mean square error (RMSE)

   $$MSE = \frac{1}{N} \sum_{i=1}^{N} pe_i^2 \qquad RMSE = \sqrt{mse}$$

   Bias: a.k.a. mean prediction error (ME)

   $$ME = \frac{1}{N} \sum_{i=1}^{N} pe_i$$

   **Prediction error (pe) is the prediction minus the true value.

   d. Sensitivity: ability of an assay to quantitate low drug concentrations accurately; usually the lowest concentration an assay can differentiate from zero
   e. Specificity (cross-reactivity): ability of an assay to differentiate the drug in question from like substances

D. Assay Methodology
   1. Immunoassays
      a. Radioimmunoassay
         i. Advantages: extremely sensitive (picogram range)
         ii. Disadvantages: Radioimmunoassay kits have limited shelf life because of the short $t_{1/2}$ of labels, nuclear waste, and cross-reactivity.
             **Clinical use for assaying digoxin and cyclosporine

      b. Enzyme immunoassay
         ex. EMIT (enzyme multiplied immunoassay technique)
      c. Fluorescence immunoassay
         TDx (Abbott) (fluorescence polarization immunoassay): most common therapeutic drug monitoring assay
         <u>Advantages</u>: simple, automated, highly sensitive, and stable reagents
         <u>Disadvantages</u>: background interference attributable to endogenous serum fluorescence

   2. High-pressure liquid chromatography
   3. Flame photometry
   4. Bioassay

E. Population Pharmacokinetics in Therapeutic Drug Monitoring
   1. Population pharmacokinetics useful when:
      a. Drug concentrations are obtained during complicated dosing regimens.
      b. Drug concentrations are obtained before steady state.
      c. Only a few drug concentrations are feasibly obtained (limited sampling strategy).

   2. Bayesian pharmacokinetics
      a. Prior population information is combined with patient-specific data to predict the most probable individual parameters.
      b. When patient-specific data are limited, there is greater influence from population parameters; when patient-specific data are extensive, there is less influence.
      c. With small amounts of individual data, Bayesian forecasting generally yields more precise results.

VIII. PHARMACOKINETICS IN RENAL DISEASE

Patient Cases

9. K.M., an 80-year-old white woman (48 kg, 5'4"), is admitted to the hospital for pyelonephritis with sepsis. She has a history of myocardial infarction ×2, congestive heart failure, hypertension, osteoporosis, rheumatoid arthritis, and cerebrovascular accident. On admission, her BUN is 11 mg/dL, her SCr is 0.5 mg/dL, and her Alb is 2.9 g/dL. K.M. is initiated on the following drugs: trimethoprim-sulfamethoxazole intravenously: 240 mg of trimethoprim every 12 hours; lisinopril 10 mg/day by mouth; digoxin 0.125 mg/day by mouth; furosemide 40 mg/day by mouth; cimetidine 400 mg by mouth 2 times/day; acetaminophen 325 mg ii by mouth every 6 hours; calcium carbonate 500 mg by mouth 3 times/day; and carvedilol 6.25 mg by mouth 2 times/day. By the corrected Cockcroft and Gault (C&G) method, which one of the following choices best estimates K.M.'s CrCl?
    A. 64 mL/minute.
    B. 75 mL/minute.
    C. 102 mL/minute.
    D. 120 mL/minute.

10. Which one of K.M.'s drug combinations is most likely to alter her SCr concentrations?
    A. Lisinopril and digoxin.
    B. Trimethoprim-sulfamethoxazole and cimetidine.
    C. Furosemide and calcium carbonate.
    D. Acetaminophen and carvedilol.

A. Estimation of Glomerular Filtration Rate (GFR)/CrCl
   1. Creatinine production and elimination
      a. Creatine is produced in the liver.
      b. Creatinine is the product of creatine metabolism in skeletal muscle.
      c. Creatinine is filtered at the glomerulus, where it undergoes limited secretion.
      d. Creatinine is useful in approximating GFR because
         i. At normal concentrations of creatinine, secretion is low.
         ii. The creatinine assay picks up a noncreatinine chromogen in the blood but not in the urine.
   2. CrCl <u>calculation</u> to estimate GFR
      • CrCl is calculated from a 24-hour urine collection and the following equation:

$$\text{CrCl (mL/minute)} = \frac{\text{volume of urine/1440 minutes} \times [\text{creatinine}]_{\text{urine}}}{[\text{creatinine}]_{\text{plasma}}}$$

      • Normal CrCl
        Healthy young men = 125 mL/minute/1.73 m^2
        Healthy young women = 115 mL/minute/1.73 m^2

      • After age 30, 1% of GFR is lost per year.

3. CrCl estimation to estimate GFR
   a. Factors affecting SCr concentrations:
      i. Gender
      ii. Age
      iii. Weight
      iv. Renal function

      Caveats:
      CrCl estimations worsen as renal function worsens (usually an overestimation).

   b. Jeliffe

      $$\text{CrCl (mL/minute/1.73 m}^2\text{)} = \frac{98 - 0.8(\text{age} - 20)}{\text{SCr}}$$

      - Women: Use 90% of the above equation.

      - Limitations:
        SCr concentration must be stable.
        Adults aged 20–80 years
        Controversy: rounding up SCr in patients with low concentrations (less than 0.7–1 mg/dL)

   c. Cockcroft and Gault (C&G)

      $$\text{CrCl (mL/minute)} = \frac{(140 - \text{age}) * (\text{IBW})}{72 * \text{SCr}}$$

      - Women: Use 85% of the above equation.
        Ideal body weight (IBW) (males) = 50 kg + 2.3 kg for each inch over 5 feet
        IBW (women) = 45.5 kg + 2.3 kg for each inch over 5 feet

      - Limitations:
        SCr concentration must be stable.
        It was developed for adults only.
        Controversy: rounding up SCr in patients with low concentrations (less than 0.7–1 mg/dL)

   d. Corrected versus uncorrected C&G

      - Uncorrected → $\text{CrCl (mL/minute)} = \dfrac{(140 - \text{age}) * (\text{IBW})}{72 * \text{SCr}}$

      $$\text{CrCl (mL/minute/72 kg)} = \frac{(140 - \text{age}) * (\text{IBW})}{72 * \text{SCr}} * \frac{72}{\text{IBW}}$$

      - Corrected → $\text{CrCl (mL/minute/72 kg)} = \dfrac{(140 - \text{age})}{\text{SCr}}$

(a) Corrected C&G equation is normalized to a 72-kg person (similar to most other estimation equations).
(b) Corrected C&G is not influenced by a patient's weight (it is actually influenced by height, because the uncorrected equation uses IBW—a function of height).
(c) Corrected C&G (or weight-adjusted C&G) is better to use for estimating renal function to make dosage adjustments.

e. Modification of diet in renal disease study equation
Full equation:

GFR (mL/minute/1.73 m^2) = 161.5 * (SCr)$^{-0.999}$ * (age in years)$^{-0.176}$ * 1.180 (if patient is African American) * 0.762 (if patient is a woman) * (BUN)$^{-0.170}$ * (Alb)$^{+0.318}$

Simplified four-variable equation:

GFR (mL/minute/1.73 m^2) = 175 * (SCr)$^{-1.154}$ * (age in years)$^{-0.203}$ * 1.212 (if patient is African American) * 0.742 (if patient is a woman)

  (a) These equations actually directly estimate GFR (NOT CrCl).
  (b) These equations are recommended by the American Kidney Foundation and the European Renal Association to estimate renal function (significantly better than C&G).
  (c) Not as accurate when GFR is greater than 60 mL/minute/1.73 m^2
  (d) Controversy: rounding up SCr in patients with low concentrations (less than 0.7–1 mg/dL)

f. Chronic Kidney Disease Epidemiology Collaboration equation

Race and Sex	Serum Creatinine (mg/dL)	Equation
African American		
Female	≤ 0.7	GFR = 166 * (SCr/0.7)$^{-0.329}$ * (0.993)^{Age}
	> 0.7	GFR = 166 * (SCr/0.7)$^{-1.209}$ * (0.993)^{Age}
Male	≤ 0.9	GFR = 163 * (SCr/0.9)$^{-0.411}$ * (0.993)^{Age}
	> 0.9	GFR = 163 * (SCr/0.9)$^{-1.209}$ * (0.993)^{Age}
White or other		
Female	≤ 0.7	GFR = 144 * (SCr/0.7)$^{-0.329}$ * (0.993)^{Age}
	> 0.7	GFR = 144 * (SCr/0.7)$^{-1.209}$ * (0.993)^{Age}
Male	≤ 0.9	GFR = 141 * (SCr/0.9)$^{-0.411}$ * (0.993)^{Age}
	> 0.9	GFR = 141 * (SCr/0.9)$^{-1.209}$ * (0.993)^{Age}

GFR = glomerular filtration rate; SCr = serum creatinine.

  (a) These equations directly estimate GFR (NOT CrCl).
  (b) These equations are more accurate than modification of diet in renal disease at higher GFRs (i.e., greater than 60 mL/minute/1.73 m^2).
  (c) Controversy: rounding up SCr in patients with low concentrations (less than 0.7–1 mg/dL)

g. Pediatric formulas
   DO NOT round up low SCr values in pediatric patients.
   Schwartz

   $$\text{CrCl (mL/minute)} = \frac{K * \text{ht (cm)}}{\text{SCr}}$$

Age	K
Low birth weight ≤ 1 year	0.33
Full term ≤ 1 year	0.45
1 year to adolescence	0.55
Muscular adolescent males	0.7

   Shull

   $$\text{CrCl (mL/minute/1.73 m}^2\text{)} = \frac{(0.035 * \text{age (years)} + 0.236) * 100}{\text{SCr}}$$

   • This is only for those aged 1-18 years.

4. Factors influencing CrCl estimates
   a. Patient characteristics
      i. Age (↓ production of creatinine with age)
      ii. Female sex (↓ production of creatinine)
      iii. Race (production of creatinine in African Americans)
   b. Disease states/clinical conditions
      i. Spinal cord injuries (↓ muscle mass; ↓ creatinine)
      ii. Amputations (↓ muscle mass; ↓ creatinine)
      iii. Cushing syndrome (↓ muscle mass; ↓ creatinine)
      iv. Muscular dystrophy (↓ muscle mass; ↓ creatinine)
      v. Guillain-Barré syndrome (↓ muscle mass; ↓ creatinine)
      vi. Rheumatoid arthritis (↓ muscle mass; ↓ creatinine)
      vii. Liver disease (↓ creatine; ↓ creatinine)
      viii. Glomerulopathic disease (greater amount of creatinine secretion in relation to filtration)
   c. Diet
      i. High-meat protein diets (creatinine ingestion)
      ii. Vegetarians (↓ creatinine ingestion)
      iii. Protein-calorie malnutrition (↓ creatinine ingestion)
   d. Drugs/endogenous substances
      i. Laboratory interaction: alkaline picrate method (NOT kinetic alkaline picrate method, which is more commonly used). Noncreatinine chromogens: in blood but not in urine. Cephalosporins (especially cefoxitin): chromogenic causing false elevations—much greater in urine than in blood. Acetoacetate (increased in fasting individuals, patients with diabetic ketoacidosis): chromogenic causing false elevations
      ii. Pharmacokinetic interaction: drugs compete with creatinine for renal secretion (causing false elevations), trimethoprim, cimetidine, fibric acid derivatives (other than gemfibrozil), dronedarone

B. Drug Dosing in Renal Disease
  1. Loading dose
     a. In general, no alteration is required, but it should be given to hasten achievement of therapeutic drug concentrations.
     b. Alterations in loading dose must occur if the V_d is altered secondary to renal dysfunction.
        i. <u>Example</u>: digoxin
  2. Maintenance dose
     a. Alterations should be made in either the dose or the dosing interval.
        i. Changing the dosing interval:
           (a) Use when the goal is to achieve similar steady-state concentrations.
           (b) Less costly
           (c) Ideal for limited-dosage forms (i.e., oral medications)
        ii. Changing the dose:
           (a) Use when the goal is to maintain a steady therapeutic concentration.
           (b) More costly
        iii. Changing the dose and the dosing interval:
           (a) Often required for substantial dosage adjustment with limited-dosage forms
           (b) Often required for narrow therapeutic index drugs with target concentrations
               (1) If a drug is given more than once daily, then adjust the interval.
               (2) If a drug is given once daily or less often, then adjust the dose.

IX. PHARMACOKINETICS IN HEPATIC DISEASE

Patient Case

11. S.J. is a 55-year-old man with hepatic dysfunction and fungemia caused by *Candida krusei*. He has a small amount of ascites but is not encephalopathic. He is initiated on caspofungin, and the package insert states that doses should be decreased in patients with a Child-Pugh score of 7-9. If he has the following hepatic laboratory values, which one of the following choices is his Child-Pugh score?

    Aspartate transaminase = 85 U/L, alanine transaminase = 56 U/L, alkaline phosphatase = 190 U/L, total bilirubin = 1.8 mg/dL, Alb = 2.9 g/dL, lactic dehydrogenase = 270 U/L, prothrombin time/international normalized ratio = 14.6/1.7, g-glutamyl transferase = 60 U/L

    A. 3.
    B. 5.
    C. 8.
    D. 11.

A. Dosage Adjustment in Hepatic Disease
  1. Clinical response is the most important factor in adjusting doses in hepatic disease.
  2. Low hepatic extraction ratio drugs
     a. Adjustment of maintenance dose is necessary only when hepatic disease alters Cl_{int}.
     b. Alterations in protein binding alone do not require alteration of maintenance dose, even though total drug concentrations decline.

      c. Loading doses may require reduction.
   3. High hepatic extraction ratio drugs
      a. Intravenous administration
         i. Usually necessary to decrease maintenance dose rate
         ii. Consider effect of hepatic disease on protein binding.
      b. Oral administration
         i. Usually necessary to decrease maintenance dose rate

B. Rules for Dosing in Hepatic Disease
   1. Hepatic elimination of high extraction ratio drugs is more consistently affected by liver disease than low extraction ratio drugs.
   2. The clearance of drugs that are exclusively conjugated is not substantially altered in liver disease.

Table 2. Child-Pugh Classification for Liver Disease

	Points 1	Points 2	Points 3
Encephalopathy	0	1 or 2	3 or 4
Ascites	0	+	++
Bilirubin (mg/dL)	< 1.5	1.5–2.3	> 2.3
Alb (g/dL)	> 3.5	2.8–3.5	< 2.8
Prothrombin time (seconds over control)	0–4	4–6	> 6

Pugh score: 5 = normal; 6 or 7 = mild (A); 8 or 9 = moderate (B); > 9 = severe (C).
Alb = albumin.

X. PHARMACODYNAMICS

Patient Case
12. Which one of the following is a reason for a drug to follow clockwise hysteresis?
    A. Formation of an active metabolite.
    B. Delay in equilibrium between the blood and the site of action.
    C. Tolerance.
    D. Increased sensitivity with time.

A. Definition: relationship between drug concentrations and the pharmacologic response

B. Hill equation

$$E = \frac{E_{max} * C^\gamma}{EC_{50}^\gamma + C^\gamma}$$

E = pharmacologic response
E_{max} = maximum drug effect
EC_{50} = concentration producing half of the maximum drug effect
γ = shape factor that accommodates the shape of the curve

Concentration-response Plot

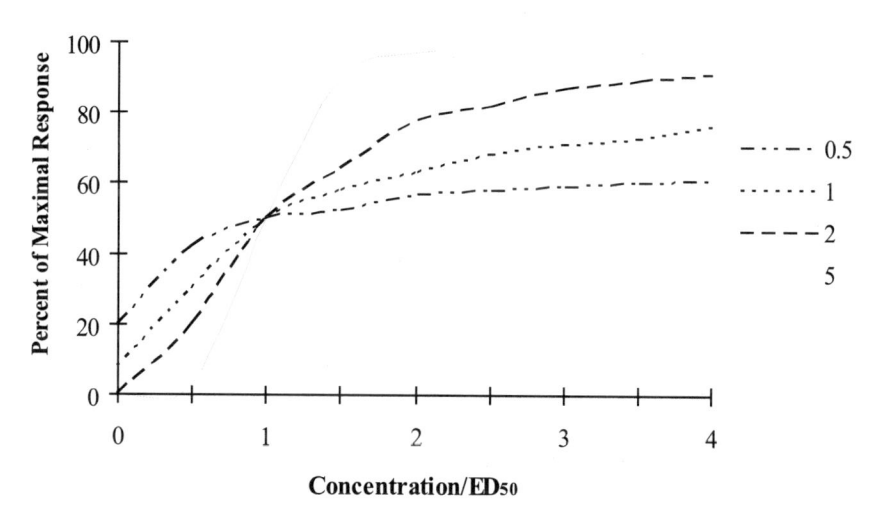

Figure 5.

C. Hysteresis Loops

Definition: Concentrations late after a dose produce an effect different from that produced by the same concentration soon after the dose.

Counterclockwise Hysteresis

Causes:
1. Increased sensitivity
2. Formation of an active metabolite
3. Delay in equilibrium between plasma concentrations and the concentration at the site of action

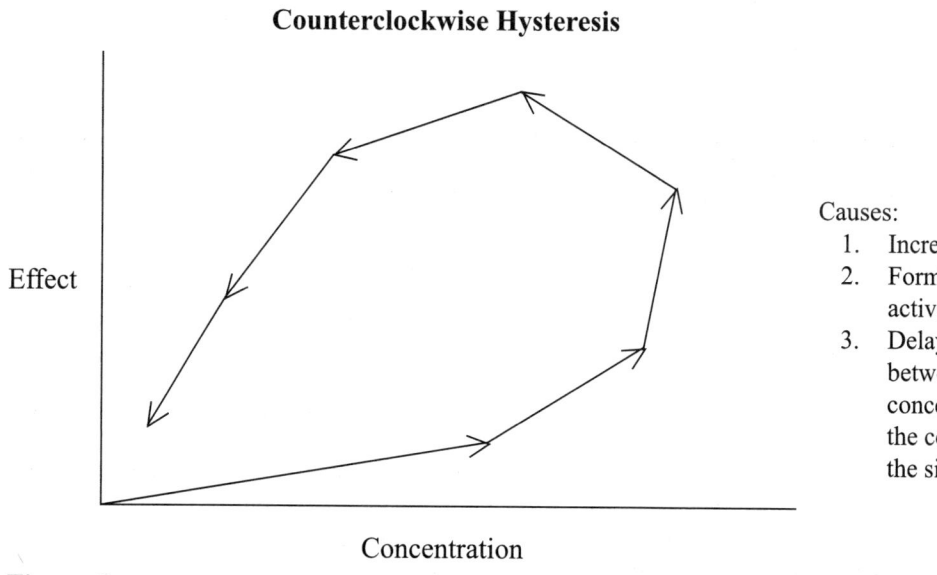

Figure 6.

Clockwise Hysteresis

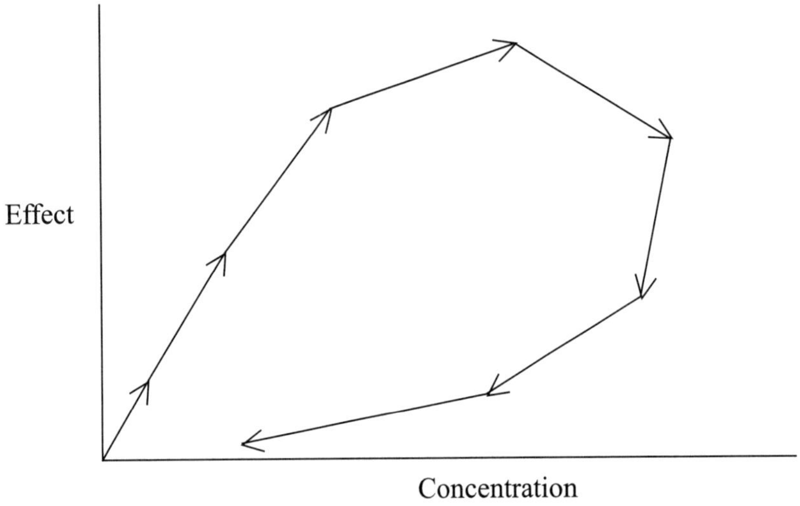

Effect vs Concentration

Causes:
1. Tolerance
2. Formation of an inhibitory metabolite
3. Equilibrium reached faster between arterial blood and site of action vs. venous blood and site of action

Figure 7.

Patient Cases

13. P.L., a 45-year-old man with chronic renal failure, is receiving phenytoin 400 mg/day for a history of tonic-clonic seizures. His phenytoin concentration today is 13.6 mg/L, and his Alb concentration is 4.2 g/dL. Based on his current concentration, which one of the following choices should be recommended with his dose?
    A. Make no changes to his drug regimen.
    B. Keep the total daily dose the same, but change the regimen to 200 mg 2 times/day.
    C. Increase the dose for better seizure control.
    D. Decrease the dose to prevent toxicity.

14. N.R. is a 63-year-old man with renal insufficiency who comes to the emergency department in atrial fibrillation with a ventricular rate of 120 beats/minute. Because of his history of ventricular dysfunction, it is decided to initiate him on digoxin for rate control. Which one of the following is correct regarding dosing in this patient?
    A. The loading dose should remain the same, but the maintenance dose needs to be decreased.
    B. The loading dose needs to be decreased, and the maintenance dose should remain the same.
    C. Neither the loading dose nor the maintenance dose needs to be adjusted.
    D. Both the loading dose and the maintenance dose need to be decreased.

15. P.P. is a 34-year-old man with a history of cerebral palsy and chronic urinary tract infections. He is admitted to the hospital with a *Pseudomonas* urinary tract infection that is resistant to all antibiotics but aminoglycosides. He is initiated on once-daily tobramycin at 400 mg/day intravenously. Which one of the following statements best describes this high-dose, extended-interval aminoglycoside regimen?
    A. It takes advantage of the concentration-dependent killing of aminoglycoside.
    B. It is more efficacious than standard aminoglycoside dosing.
    C. It does not require monitoring of aminoglycoside concentrations.
    D. It will not cause nephrotoxicity.

XI. SPECIFIC DRUG TABLE

Table 3.

Drug	Therapeutic Range	Sampling Issues	Comments
Aminoglycosides	Cp_{max} = 4–10 mg/L Amikacin = 20–30 mg/L Cp_{min} < 2 mg/L Amikacin < 10 mg/L	Duration of infusion, timing of first sample postinfusion (generally should be 0.5–1 hour)	Be familiar with Sawchuk-Zaske method and high-dose, extended-interval dosing
Vancomycin	Cp_{min} = 10–15 mg/L (15–20 mg/L for certain infections including pneumonia, meningitis, and osteomyelitis	Controversial whether to obtain peaks or concentrations altogether	Be familiar with changes in trough concentration recommendations
Phenytoin	10–20 mg/L Free: 1–2 mg/L	In general, obtain trough concentrations	Percent free increases with renal failure and hypoalbuminemia; induces liver enzymes; susceptible to metabolic drug interactions
Carbamazepine	4–12 mg/L		Autoinduction; active metabolite 10,11 epoxide
Phenobarbital	15–40 mg/L		Enzyme inducer
Valproic acid	50–100 mg/L		Saturable protein binding; percent free increases with renal failure and hypoalbuminemia
Digoxin	0.8–2.0 mcg/L	Prolonged distribution period necessitates sampling > 6–12 hours postdose	V_d changes with disease states; susceptible to drug interactions
Cyclosporine	100–250 mcg/L	Whole blood samples	Many drug interactions
Lithium	0.3–1.3 mmol/L	Prolonged distribution necessitates sampling 12 hours postdose	
Theophylline	10–20 mg/L		Treat as continuous infusion with sustained-release dosage forms

Cp = concentration of drug plasma.

Table 4. CYP450 Drug Interactions

Gene Designation	CYP1A2	CYP2C9/10	CYP2C19	CYP2D6	CYP3A4	
Substrates	Acetaminophen Amitriptyline Caffeine Clomipramine Clozapine Estradiol Fluvoxamine Haloperidol Imipramine Mirtazapine Olanzapine Riluzole Ropinirole R-warfarin Tacrine Theophylline Zileuton Zolmitriptan	Amitriptyline Carvedilol (levo) Celecoxib Diclofenac Fluoxetine Fluvastatin Ibuprofen Indomethacin Irbesartan Losartan Phenytoin Piroxicam Rosuvastatin S-warfarin Tamoxifen Tolbutamide Valproic acid Zafirlukast CYP2C8 Rosiglitazone	Amitriptyline Cilostazol Citalopram Clomipramine Diazepam N-desmethyl Diazepam Imipramine Lansoprazole Naproxen Nelfinavir Omeprazole Pantoprazole Phenobarbital Phenytoin Propranolol Rabeprazole (minor) Valproic acid	Amitriptyline Aripiprazole Carvedilol (dextro) Clomipramine Clozapine Codeine Debrisoquine Desipramine Dextromethorphan Donepezil Duloxetine Flecainide Fluoxetine (norfluoxetine) Fluvoxamine Haloperidol Hydrocodone Imipramine Metoprolol Mirtazapine Nortriptyline Oxycodone Paroxetine Propafenone Propranolol Risperidone Thioridazine Timolol Tramadol Trazodone Venlafaxine	Alfentanil Alprazolam Amiodarone Amlodipine Atazanavir Atorvastatin Buspirone Carbamazepine Cilostazol Citalopram Clarithromycin Cyclosporine Dapsone Darunavir Delavirdine Diazepam Diltiazem Donepezil Efavirenz Eplerenone Erlotinib Erythromycin Ethinyl estradiol Felodipine Fentanyl Finasteride Fosamprenavir Gefitinib Gleevec Imatinib Indinavir Irinotecan Itraconazole Ketoconazole Lapatinib Lidocaine Lopinavir Lovastatin Methadone	Midazolam Mirtazapine Nateglinide Nefazodone Nelfinavir Nevirapine Nifedipine Quetiapine Quinidine Rabeprazole Repaglinide Rifabutin Ritonavir R-warfarin Saquinavir Sertraline Sibutramine Sildenafil Simvastatin Sirolimus Tacrolimus Telithromycin Tertiary amines (amitriptyline, clomipramine, imipramine) Tiagabine Tipranavir Trazodone Triazolam Vardenafil Verapamil Voriconazole Zaleplon Zileuton Ziprasidone Zolpidem Zonisamide
Induction	Chargrilled meat Cigarettes Nafcillin Omeprazole Rifampin	Phenobarbital Phenytoin Rifampin Rifapentine	Carbamazepine Phenobarbital Prednisone Rifampin		Carbamazepine Efavirenz Nevirapine Oxcarbazepine Phenobarbital Phenytoin	Pioglitazone Rifabutin Rifampin Rifapentine St. John's wort Topiramate
Inhibition	Amiodarone Cimetidine Ciprofloxacin Diltiazem Erythromycin Fluvoxamine Grepafloxacin Mexiletine Mibefradil Norfloxacin Tacrine Ticlopidine	Amiodarone Fluconazole Fluoxetine Fluvoxamine Isoniazid Leflunomide (metabolism) Omeprazole Sertraline Sulfamethoxazole Trimethoprim Valproic acid Voriconazole Zafirlukast	Cimetidine Felbamate Fluoxetine Fluvoxamine Ketoconazole Lansoprazole Modafinil Omeprazole Oxcarbazepine Pantoprazole Rabeprazole Ticlopidine Topiramate	Amiodarone Bupropion Celecoxib Chlorpheniramine Cimetidine Citalopram Diphenhydramine Escitalopram Fluoxetine Haloperidol Metoclopramide Paroxetine Propafenone Quinidine Ritonavir Sertraline Terbinafine Thioridazine	Amiodarone Aprepitant Atazanavir Cimetidine Clarithromycin Darunavir Delavirdine Diltiazem Erythromycin Fluconazole (large doses) Fluvoxamine Fosamprenavir Grapefruit juice Imatinib	Indinavir Itraconazole Ketoconazole Lopinavir Nefazodone Nelfinavir Norfluoxetine Ritonavir Saquinavir Synercid Telithromycin Tipranavir Verapamil Voriconazole

CYP = cytochrome P450.

REFERENCES

1. Burton ME, Shaw LM, Schentag JJ, eds. Applied Pharmacokinetics & Pharmacodynamics: Principles of Therapeutic Drug Monitoring, 4th ed. Baltimore, MD: Lippincott Williams & Wilkins, 2006.

2. Bauer LA. Clinical pharmacokinetics and pharmacodynamics. In: DiPiro JT, Talbert RL, Yee GC, et al., eds. Pharmacotherapy: A Pathophysiologic Approach, 4th ed. Stamford, CT: Appleton & Lange, 1999:21–43.

3. Winter ME. Basic Clinical Pharmacokinetics, 3rd ed. Vancouver: Applied Therapeutics, 1994.

4. Bauer LA. Applied Clinical Pharmacokinetics. New York: McGraw-Hill Medical, 2001.

5. Matheny CJ, Lamb MW, Brouwer KLR, Pollack GM. Pharmacokinetic and pharmacodynamic implications of P-glycoprotein modulation. Pharmacotherapy 2001;21:778–96.

ANSWERS AND EXPLANATIONS TO PATIENT CASES

1. Answer: C
In 6 days (2 $t_{1/2}$), the concentration will decrease from 35.9 mg/L to about 9 mg/L; now is the time to redose. A 1-g dose given on March 24 will increase the concentration in the blood from 12.1 to 35.9 mg/L (12.1 + 23.8 mg/L). Given that the $t_{1/2}$ is about 3 days, it will take longer than 1 day to reach a concentration of about 10 mg/L. In 3 days (1 $t_{1/2}$), the concentration will decrease from 35.9 mg/L to about 18 mg/L—still too early to redose. Redosing can be figured because plenty of information exists about how to calculate when to redose.

2. Answer: A
F = (100 mg * 25 mg/L/hour)/(200 mg * 50 mg/L/hour).

3. Answer: A
The elimination rate constant equals 0.693/4 hours = 0.17 hour^{-1}. The clearance can be calculated by multiplying the V_d (0.5 L/kg * 65 kg) by the elimination rate constant. Clearance equals 5.5 L/hour. Concentration at steady state will equal the infusion rate divided by clearance. Steady-state concentration = 3.6 mg/L.

4. Answer: D
P-glycoprotein is an efflux pump that pumps drugs back into the gastrointestinal lumen. P-glycoprotein is not a plasma protein, and it does not transfer drugs through the gastrointestinal mucosa but rather pumps drugs back into the gastrointestinal lumen. In addition, P-glycoprotein acts in concert with CYP3A4 to diminish oral absorption.

5. Answer: C
Azithromycin does not inhibit CYP3A4. Erythromycin and clarithromycin are potent inhibitors of CYP3A4 and would be expected to increase cyclosporine concentrations. Cytochrome P450 inhibition is not a drug class effect.

6. Answer: B
By definition, clearance becomes nonlinear once the concentration exceeds the K_m; therefore, the concentrations will more than double. Phenytoin is not a significant autoinducer. Although phenytoin absorption decreases as the dose is increased, it is not clinically significant until a single dose exceeds 400 mg.

7. Answer: C
The correct answer, due to redistribution, is to wait a few hours to obtain the concentration because it will increase significantly within the first few hours after hemodialysis. Waiting a full 24 hours is not necessary.

8. Answer: D
The correct answer is that the assay will be able to distinguish the drug from like products but will not be able to detect extremely low concentrations. High specificity means the assay can distinguish the drug from like products, and low sensitivity means the assay cannot detect extremely low concentrations.

9. Answer: A
The correct answer is 64 mL/minute because a low SCr should be rounded up and because the value must be multiplied by 0.85, given that the patient is a woman. The other answers are incorrect because the SCr is not rounded up and because the value is not multiplied by 0.85.

10. Answer: B
Both trimethoprim-sulfamethoxazole and cimetidine compete with creatinine for secretion in the kidneys, increasing SCr concentrations. Although angiotensin-converting enzyme inhibitors may transiently increase SCr concentrations, digoxin does not affect renal function. Although furosemide may secondarily affect SCr concentrations, calcium does not affect renal function. Acetaminophen and carvedilol generally will not affect SCr concentrations.

11. Answer: C
S.J. has 1 point for not being encephalopathic, 2 points for mild ascites, 2 points for the bilirubin concentration, 2 points for the Alb concentration, and 1 point for the prothrombin time value, for a total of 8 points. Normal patients have a Child-Pugh score of 5, which means no hepatic dysfunction.

12. Answer: C
Tolerance leads to a decrease in effect with time; this is clockwise hysteresis. Formation of an active metabolite, delay in equilibrium between the blood and site of action, and increased sensitivity with time would all lead to an increase in effect with time; this is counterclockwise hysteresis.

13. Answer: D

The dose should be decreased to prevent toxicity. In renal failure, acidic by-products build up in the blood and compete with phenytoin for protein binding. Total concentrations need to be corrected, and this correction leads to a doubling of the concentration. Therefore, the current concentration is too high, and the dose should be decreased. Single doses of 400 mg are fine (doses higher than 400 mg should be divided).

14. Answer: D

Both the loading dose and the maintenance dose need to be decreased. In general, loading doses do not need to be altered in renal dysfunction because they are primarily dependent on the V_d. However, the digoxin V_d is decreased in renal dysfunction. Because digoxin is eliminated renally, the maintenance dose needs to be decreased.

15. Answer: A

Aminoglycosides show concentration-dependent killing, and a high-dose, extended-interval aminoglycoside dose takes advantage of this characteristic. However, it has not proved to be more efficacious than traditional dosing. Aminoglycoside concentrations still need to be monitored with high-dose, extended-interval therapy. In addition, high-dose, extended-interval aminoglycoside dosing can still cause nephrotoxicity (although the incidence is generally diminished).

ANSWERS AND EXPLANATIONS TO SELF-ASSESSMENT QUESTIONS

1. Answer: B
With two concentrations, there are enough data to calculate an elimination rate constant and, therefore, a $t_{1/2}$. In addition, the V_d can be calculated by back extrapolation to the C_{max} and use of appropriate equations (because this was the first dose, and therefore, it is known that the tobramycin concentration was 0 mg/L before the dose was given).

2. Answer: A
The $t_{1/2}$ is about 2 hours. The C_{max} is about 5 mg/L, and the V_d is about 20 L.

3. Answer: B
Her clearance increased because of the improvement in renal function, which increased her elimination rate constant and decreased her $t_{1/2}$. The V_d would not be altered by changes in clearance (they are independent). With the diuresis and angiotensin-converting enzyme inhibitor, her V_d probably decreased, but clearance would not be altered by changes in V_d (they are independent). In addition, if her V_d decreased, her elimination rate constant would decrease, not increase.

4. Answer: C
Because the trough is too low, the interval will have to be shortened to increase the concentration. Changes in dose will have the greatest effect on the peak concentration, and changes in interval will have the greatest effect on the trough concentration.

5. Answer: C
Her dose needs to be increased, and because she is a smoker, the interval should be every 8 hours. Doubling the total daily dose will adequately increase her concentration without causing toxic reactions.

6. Answer: D
Because of the patient's renal failure and low Alb, the total concentration needs to be corrected. The patient's corrected phenytoin concentration is 14.7 mcg/mL. Therefore, no changes need to be made to the dose.

7. Answer: C
Both of these are immunoassays. TDx is a brand name for the Abbott fluorescence polarization immunoassay, which uses a fluorescent label. The term *EMIT* stands for enzyme multiplied immunoassay technique, which is an immunoassay that uses an enzyme label.

8. Answer: D
The digoxin concentration was drawn before the dose taken at 8:00 am had a chance to complete the distribution phase. Once distribution is complete (generally 6-12 hours after the dose), the concentration will be lower and probably within the therapeutic range. Therefore, there is no need for the digoxin antibody, activated charcoal, or lowering of the dose.

9. Answer: C
The correct statistical test is multiple logistic regression. Multiple regression is used to describe the relationship between a dependent variable and two or more independent variables when both the dependent and independent variables are numeric. Analysis of variance is used to describe the relationship between a dependent variable and two or more independent variables when the dependent variable is numeric and the independent variables are nominal. Likewise, analysis of covariance is used to describe the relationship between a dependent variable and two or more independent variables when the dependent variable is numeric and the independent variables are nominal with confounding factors. Spearman rank correlation is a nonparametric test used to describe the relationship between one dependent and one independent variable when the data are ordinal or numeric and not normally distributed.

10. Answer: B
Assessing adherence and increasing her dose, because the concentration is below the therapeutic range, is the correct answer. The valproic acid therapeutic range is 50-100 mg/L, and she is well below this concentration. Although some patients are controlled at lower concentrations, this concentration is most likely too low. She definitely does not need a decrease in dose. Although total valproic acid concentrations are affected by changes in Alb, N.T.'s Alb is normal, and obtaining a free concentration is unnecessary.

ACUTE CARE CARDIOLOGY

JO E. RODGERS, PHARM.D., FCCP, BCPS (AQ CARDIOLOGY)
UNIVERSITY OF NORTH CAROLINA SCHOOL OF PHARMACY
CHAPEL HILL, NORTH CAROLINA

ACUTE CARE CARDIOLOGY

JO E. RODGERS, PHARM.D., FCCP, BCPS (AQ CARDIOLOGY)

UNIVERSITY OF NORTH CAROLINA SCHOOL OF PHARMACY
CHAPEL HILL, NORTH CAROLINA

Acute Care Cardiology

Learning Objectives:

1. Formulate treatment strategies for patients with acute decompensated heart failure and formulate an appropriate pharmacotherapeutic regimen for a given case situation (e.g., warm and wet, cold and dry, other).

2. Create an evidence-based medication regimen for a patient with acute coronary syndrome in a variety of clinical situations (e.g., invasive/ conservative strategy, upstream antiplatelet therapy).

3. Describe an appropriate treatment strategy for atrial and ventricular arrhythmias using evidence-based medicine.

4. Prepare a treatment strategy for a newly diagnosed patient with idiopathic pulmonary arterial hypertension.

5. Select appropriate pharmacologic therapy and develop a monitoring plan for antihypertensive drug therapy for managing hypertensive emergencies.

Self-Assessment Questions:

Answers to these questions may be found at the end of this chapter.

1. A.A. is a 25-year-old woman with a new diagnosis of idiopathic pulmonary arterial hypertension (IPAH). Her home drugs include warfarin 5 mg/day, furosemide 60 mg 2 times/day, and bosentan 62.5 mg 2 times/day. Which one of the following is the best contraceptive strategy for this patient?

    A. Estrogen-progesterone oral contraceptive.
    B. Injectable hormonal contraceptive.
    C. Any hormonal contraceptive and barrier method.
    D. Barrier method only.

2. F.F. is a 64-year-old man with New York Heart Association (NYHA) class III heart failure (HF) admitted for increased shortness of breath, dyspnea on exertion, and decreased exercise tolerance. He admits to dietary nonadherence and has indulged in bacon and eggs, popcorn, and french fries in the past 72 hours. His extremities appear well perfused, but he has 3+ pitting edema in all four extremities. F.F.'s blood pressure (BP) is 115/75 mm Hg. Which one of the following is the best intravenous vasoactive drug to treat this patient if intravenous diuretic therapy fails?

    A. Dobutamine.
    B. Milrinone.
    C. Nesiritide.
    D. Intravenous nitroglycerin.

3. H.E. is a 53-year-old woman admitted to the hospital after the worst headache she has ever experienced. Her medical history includes exertional asthma, poorly controlled hypertension (HTN), and hyperlipidemia (HLD). She is drug nonadherent and has not taken her BP drugs, including clonidine, for 4 days. Vital signs include BP 220/100 mm Hg and heart rate (HR) 65 beats/minute. She receives a diagnosis of a cerebrovascular accident and hypertensive emergency. Which one of the following choices is the best management option for this patient's hypertensive emergency?

    A. Fenoldopam 0.1 mcg/kg/minute.
    B. Nicardipine 5 mg/hour.
    C. Labetalol 0.5 mg/minute.
    D. Enalaprilat 0.625 mg intravenously every 6 hours.

4. W.M., a 69-year-old man, presents to the hospital with 3-mm ST-elevation myocardial infarction (STEMI) within 2 hours of chest pain onset. He is given clopidogrel 300 mg × 1, and he is instructed to chew aspirin (ASA) 81 mg × 4. Abciximab and unfractionated heparin (UFH) are initiated as he is wheeled to the cardiac catheterization laboratory for primary percutaneous coronary intervention (PCI). Four hours after returning to the intensive care unit, a complete blood cell count shows a platelet count of 15×10^3 cells/mm³. Which one of the following is the most likely cause of this patient's thrombocytopenia?

    A. Clopidogrel.
    B. ASA.
    C. UFH.
    D. Abciximab.

5. The Sudden Cardiac Death in Heart Failure trial evaluated the efficacy of amiodarone or implantable cardioverter-defibrillator (ICD) versus placebo in preventing all-cause mortality in ischemic and nonischemic NYHA class II and III patients with HF. There was a 7.2% absolute risk reduction and a 23% relative risk reduction in all-cause mortality at 60 months with an ICD versus placebo. What is the number of patients needed to treat with an ICD to prevent one death versus placebo?

    A. 1.3.
    B. 4.3.
    C. 13.8.
    D. 43.4.

6. A.D. is a 52-year-old woman with a history of witnessed cardiac arrest in a shopping mall; she was resuscitated with an automatic external defibrillator device. On electrophysiologic study, she has inducible ventricular tachycardia (VT). Which one of the following has significantly decreased the incidence of sudden cardiac death over other therapies in a patient population such as this (secondary prevention)?

    A. Propafenone.
    B. Amiodarone.
    C. ICD.
    D. Metoprolol.

7. S.V. is a 75-year-old woman with a history of NYHA class III HF (left ventricular ejection fraction [LVEF] 25%) and many non–ST-elevation MIs (NSTEMIs). She had an episode of sustained VT during hospitalization for pneumonia. Her QTc interval was 380 milliseconds on the telemetry monitor. Which one of the following is the best treatment option for S.V.?

    A. Procainamide.
    B. Metoprolol.
    C. Intravenous magnesium.
    D. Amiodarone.

8. You are working on a review article about newer treatment strategies for antiplatelet and anticoagulant therapy during PCI. You want to ensure that you retrieve all relevant clinical trials and related articles on your subject. Which one of the following comprehensive databases is best to search next to ensure that no key articles were missed?

    A. International Pharmaceutical Abstracts.
    B. Iowa Drug Information Service.
    C. Clin-Alert.
    D. Excerpta Medica.

9. A physician on your team wants you to "do the paperwork" regarding an adverse drug reaction (ADR) that a patient on your team experienced because of nesiritide. The patient had severe hypotension after the initial bolus dose of nesiritide for treatment of decompensated HF, even though his BP was safely in the "normal" range before therapy initiation. The hypotension led to decreased renal perfusion, resulting in oliguric acute renal failure and subsequent hemodialysis initiation. The patient had no known renal insufficiency before developing this complication. Which one of the following statements is correct regarding The Joint Commission requirements for institutional ADR reporting?

    A. A MedWatch form explaining the situation in which the ADR occurred must be completed.
    B. Institutions must create their own definition of "ADR" with which practitioners will be familiar.
    C. Hospital practitioners/staff must use the Naranjo algorithm for assessing the severity of the ADR.
    D. Only severe or life-threatening ADRs need to be reported.

10. Your Pharmacy and Therapeutics Committee wants you to perform a pharmacoeconomic analysis on a new drug available to treat decompensated HF. This drug works through a unique mechanism of action. Unlike other available inotropics (dobutamine, milrinone) that can increase mortality with time, this drug appears to reduce mortality in the long-term setting. However, the price is 10 times higher per day than other available drugs. Your findings will be presented at the next Pharmacy and Therapeutics Committee meeting to make a formulary decision about which medications to stock in your hospital pharmacy. Which of the following types of pharmacoeconomic analysis should be used to determine whether this new drug is a better formulary choice than currently available products?

    A. Cost-minimization analysis.
    B. Cost-effectiveness analysis.
    C. Cost-benefit analysis.
    D. Cost-utility analysis.

I. ACUTE DECOMPENSATED HEART FAILURE

A. Etiology
1. Acute worsening of chronic HF,
2. New cardiac event (e.g., MI, atrial fibrillation [AF]), or
3. Acute massive MI whose initial presentation is severe HF.

B. Hemodynamic Monitoring

Table 1. Hemodynamic Values in Patients with ADHF and Sepsis

Parameter	Normal Value	Typical ADHF Value	Typical Sepsis Value
Mean arterial pressure (MAP) (mm Hg)	80–100	60–80	60–80
Heart rate (HR) (beats/minute)	60–80	70–90	90–100
Cardiac output (CO) (L/minute)	4–7	2–4	5–8
Cardiac index (CI) (L/minute/m^2)	2.8–3.6	1.3–2	3.5–4
Pulmonary capillary wedge pressure (PCWP) (mm Hg)	8–12[a]	18–30	5–8
Systemic vascular resistance (SVR) (dynes/second/cm^{-5})	800–1200	1500–3000	300–800
Central venous pressure (CVP) (mm Hg)	2–6	6–15	2–6

[a]15–18 mm Hg is often desired/optimal in patients with HF to ensure optimal filling pressures.
ADHF = acute decompensated heart failure; CI = CO/BSA (BSA = body surface area); MAP = diastolic blood pressure + [1/3 (systolic blood pressure − diastolic blood pressure)]; SVR = [(MAP − CVP)/CO] × 80.

1. Hemodynamic equations
   a. Blood pressure = CO (cardiac output) × SVR (systemic vascular resistance)
   b. CO = SV × HR, where SV = stroke volume
2. Parameters influencing CO
   a. Heart rate
      i. Also known as chronotropy
      ii. Controlled by autonomic nervous system
   b. Stroke volume
      i. Amount of blood ejected by the heart during systole
      ii. Controlled by four factors
         (a) Inotropy – Ventricular contractility or "squeezing" force
         (b) Afterload – Resistance or pressure that the left ventricle (LV) pumps against to eject blood into the aorta; estimated by the SVR
         (c) Preload – Amount of tension applied to the LV before contraction; equivalent to LV end diastolic volume; estimated by the pulmonary capillary wedge pressure (PCWP)
         (d) Lusitropy – Diastolic relaxation of the ventricle

3. Hemodynamic classification
   a. Subset I – normal
      i. Warm and dry
      ii. Cardiac index greater than 2.2 L/minute, PCWP less than 18 mm Hg
      iii. Goal PCWP 15–18 mm Hg
   b. Subset II – pulmonary congestion
      i. Warm and wet
      ii. Cardiac index greater than 2.2 L/minute, PCWP great than 18 mm Hg
   c. Subset III – hypoperfusion
      i. Cold and dry
      ii. Cardiac index less than 2.2 L/minute, PCWP less than 18 mm Hg
      iii. If PCWP less than 15 mm Hg, remove fluid restriction or administer fluid until PCWP 15–18 mm Hg; then reassess CI
   d. Subset IV – pulmonary congestion and hypoperfusion
      i. Cold and wet
      ii. Cardiac index less than 2.2 L/minute, PCWP greater than 18 mm Hg

C. Clinical Presentation

Table 2. Signs and Symptoms of ADHF

Congestion (elevated PCWP)	Hypoperfusion (reduced CO)
Dyspnea on exertion or at rest	Fatigue
Orthopnea, paroxysmal nocturnal dyspnea	Altered mental status or sleepiness
Peripheral edema	Cold extremities
Rales	Worsening renal function
Early satiety, nausea/vomiting	Narrow pulse pressure
Ascites	Hypotension
Hepatomegaly, splenomegaly	Hyponatremia
Jugular venous distention	
Hepatojugular reflux	

ADHF = acute decompensated heart failure; CO = cardiac output; PCWP = pulmonary capillary wedge pressure.

D. Drug Therapy Overview

Table 3. Overview of ADHF Guideline Recommendations

Diuretic Therapy
i. <u>Recommended</u> as intravenous loop diuretics for patients admitted with fluid overload
ii. When response to diuretics is minimal, the following options <u>should be considered</u>:
(a) Fluid and sodium restriction,
(b) Initiation of increased doses or continuous infusion of loop diuretic,
(c) Addition of a second type of diuretic (metolazone or chlorothiazide), or
(d) Ultrafiltration.
Inotropic Therapy
i. <u>May be considered</u> to relieve symptoms and improve end-organ function in patients with *diminished peripheral perfusion or end-organ dysfunction (low output syndrome)*, particularly if:
(a) Marginal systolic BP (< 90 mm Hg),
(b) Symptomatic hypotension despite adequate filling pressure, or
(c) No response to, or intolerance of, intravenous vasodilators.
ii. <u>May be considered</u> in similar patients with evidence of fluid overload if they respond poorly to intravenous diuretics or manifest diminished or worsening renal function
Vasodilator Therapy
i. <u>May be considered</u> in addition to intravenous loop diuretics to rapidly improve symptoms in patients without symptomatic hypotension
ii. <u>May be considered</u> in patients with persistent symptoms despite maximal loop diuretics and oral drug therapy
iii. **When adjunctive therapy is required in addition to loop diuretics, intravenous vasodilators <u>should be considered</u> over inotropic drugs**
Invasive Hemodynamic Monitoring
i. Routine use of hemodynamic monitoring with invasive intravenous lines (e.g., Swan-Ganz pulmonary artery catheters) <u>is not recommended</u>

ADHF = acute decompensated heart failure; BP = blood pressure.

E. Diuretic Therapy

Table 4. Diuretic Therapy for ADHF

Loop diuretics (ascending limb of loop of Henle)
i. Most widely used and most potent, effective at low CrCl (< 30 mL/minute)
ii. Furosemide (Lasix) most commonly used
Thiazides (distal tubule)
i. Relatively weak diuretics when used alone, not effective at low glomerular filtration rate
ii. Reserved for add-on therapy in patients refractory to loops
Diuretic resistance
i. Increase dose rather than frequency of loop diuretic (Note: Ceiling effect at about 160–200 mg IV furosemide)
ii. Add a second diuretic with a different mechanism of action
(a) Hydrochlorothiazide 12.5–25 mg PO daily, metolazone 2.5–5 mg PO daily
(b) Chlorothiazide 250–500 mg IV daily; consider if gastrointestinal edema
iii. Continuous infusion of loop diuretic – Furosemide 0.1 mg/kg/hour IV doubled every 4–8 hours, max 0.4 mg/kg/hour
Adverse effects: electrolyte depletion (potassium, magnesium), worsening renal function

ADHF = acute decompensated heart failure; CrCl = creatinine clearance; IV = intravenous(ly); PO = orally.

F. Inotropic Therapy

Table 5. Inotropic Therapy for ADHF

	Dobutamine (Dobutrex)	**Milrinone (Primacor)**
Mechanism of action	$β_1$-agonist: Stimulates AC to convert ATP into cAMP to ↑ CO; slight peripheral vasodilation	PDE inhibitor: Inhibits cAMP breakdown in heart to ↑ CO and in vascular smooth muscle to ↓ SVR
Clinical effects	Positive inotropic, chronotropic, lusitropic effects	Positive inotropic and lusitropic effects, no chronotropic effects
Indication	ADHF – Cold and wet or cold and dry exacerbations (if PCWP > 15 mm Hg)	
Dosing	Start 2.5–5 mcg/kg/minute IV, may titrate to maximum 20 mcg/kg/minute	50 mcg/kg IVB, then 0.375 mcg/kg/minute IV; may titrate to maximum 0.75 mcg/kg/minute
Typical dose	5 mcg/kg/minute IV	No bolus, 0.1–0.375 mcg/kg/minute IV
Half-life	2 minutes	1 hour, prolonged to 2–3 hours if CrCl < 50 mL/minute
Elimination	Hepatically metabolized (inactive), renally eliminated	90% renal
Adverse effects	Proarrhythmia, tachycardia, hypokalemia, myocardial ischemia, tachyphylaxis (> 72 hours); possible increased mortality with long-term use	Proarrhythmia, hypotension (avoid bolus), tachycardia, < 1% thrombocytopenia, possible increased mortality with long-term use
Other comments	Recommended if hypotension	Recommended if receiving a β-blocker

AC = adenylate cyclase; ADHF = acute decompensated heart failure; ATP = adenosine triphosphate; cAMP = cyclic adenosine monophosphate; CO = cardiac output; CrCl = creatinine clearance; IV = intravenous(ly); IVB = intravenous bolus; PCWP = pulmonary capillary wedge pressure; PDE = phosphodiesterase; SVR = systemic vascular resistance.

G. Vasodilator Therapy

Table 6. Vasodilator Therapy for ADHF

	Sodium Nitroprusside (Nipride)	Nesiritide (Natrecor)	IV Nitroglycerin
Mechanism of action	Nitric oxide–induced stimulation of GC to convert GTP to cGMP	Recombinant B-type natriuretic peptide binds to natriuretic peptide receptor A to stimulate guanylate cyclase and production of cGMP; natriuretic mechanism unknown	Combines with sulfhydryl groups in vascular endothelium to create S-nitrosothiol compounds, which mimic nitric oxide's stimulation of guanylate cyclase and production of cGMP
Clinical effects	Balanced arterial and venous vasodilator	Hemodynamic effects: ↓ PCWP and SVR, minimal changes in HR or CI Neurohormonal effects: ↓ NE, ET-1, and aldosterone Natriuretic effects: ↑ Urine output and sodium excretion	Preferential venous vasodilator > arterial vasodilator, arterial vasodilation at high doses
Indication	Warm and wet ADHF, alternative to inotropes in cold and wet ADHF, hypertensive crises	Warm and wet ADHF, alternative to inotropes in cold and wet ADHF	Warm and wet ADHF, ACS, or hypertensive crises
Dosing	0.3–0.5 mcg/kg/minute IV, ↑ by 0.5 mcg/kg/minute up to 3 mcg/kg/minute	2 mcg/kg IVB, 0.01 mcg/kg/minute IV, ↑ by 0.005 mcg/kg/minute up to 0.03 mcg/kg/minute	5 mcg/minute IV, ↑ by 5 mcg/minute up to 200 mcg/minute
Typical dose	0.5–1 mcg/kg/minute IV	0.01 mcg/kg/minute IV May omit bolus if low SBP	25–75 mcg/minute IV, titrated to response
Half-life	< 10 minutes	20 minutes	1–4 minutes
Elimination	Cyanide hepatically metabolized, thiocyanate renally excreted	Natriuretic peptide receptor C (no renal/hepatic adjustment)	Inactive metabolites in urine
Adverse effects	Hypotension, cyanide or thiocyanate toxicity	Primarily hypotension (up to 1 hour), tachycardia (less than inotropes)	Hypotension, reflex tachycardia, headache, tachyphylaxis

ACS = acute coronary syndrome; ADHF = acute decompensated heart failure; cGMP = cyclic guanine monophosphate; CI = cardiac index; ET = endothelin; GC = guanylate cyclase; GTP = guanosine triphosphate; HR = heart rate; IV = intravenous(ly); IVB = intravenous bolus; NE = norepinephrine; PAC = pulmonary artery catheter; PCWP = pulmonary capillary wedge pressure; SBP = systolic blood pressure; SVR = systemic vascular resistance.

Patient Cases

1. D.D. is a 72-year-old man admitted to the ward team for HF decompensation. D.D. notes progressively increased dyspnea on exertion (now 10 ft, previously 30 ft) and orthopnea (now four pillows, previously two pillows), increasing bilateral lower extremity swelling (3+), 13.6-kg weight gain in the past 3 weeks, and dietary nonadherence. He has a history of idiopathic dilated cardiomyopathy (LVEF 25%, NYHA class III), paroxysmal AF, and HLD. Pertinent laboratory values are as follows: B-type natriuretic peptide (BNP) 2300 pg/mL (0–50 pg/mL), potassium+ (K+) 4.9 mEq/L, blood urea nitrogen (BUN) 22 mg/dL, SCr 1 mg/dL, aspartate aminotransferase (AST) 40 international units/L, alanine aminotransferase (ALT) 42 international units/L, international normalized ratio (INR) 1.3, partial thromboplastin time (PTT) 42 seconds, BP 108/62 mm Hg, and HR 82 beats/minute. Home drugs include carvedilol 12.5 mg 2 times/day, lisinopril 40 mg/day, furosemide 80 mg 2 times/day, spironolactone 25 mg/day, and digoxin 0.125 mg/day. Which one of the following is best for treating his acute decompensated heart failure (ADHF)?

    A. Carvedilol 25 mg 2 times/day.
    B. Nesiritide 2-mcg/kg bolus, then 0.01 mcg/kg/minute.
    C. Furosemide 120 mg intravenously 2 times/day.
    D. Milrinone 0.5 mcg/kg/minute.

2. After being initiated on intravenous loop diuretics and metolazone 2.5 mg with only minimal urine output and rising creatinine (creatinine clearance [CrCl] now 30 mL/minute), D.D. is transferred to the coronary care unit for further management of diuretic-refractory decompensated HF. His carvedilol dose is now 6.25 mg 2 times/day, and lisinopril and spironolactone are being held. His BP is 110/75 mm Hg, and his HR is 75 beats/minute. Which one of the following best represents other ways in which D.D.'s decompensated HF should be treated?

    A. Nesiritide 2-mcg/kg bolus, then 0.01 mcg/kg/minute.
    B. Sodium nitroprusside 0.3 mg/kg/minute.
    C. Dobutamine 5 mcg/kg/minute.
    D. Milrinone 0.5 mcg/kg/minute.

3. D.D. initially responds with 2 L of urine output overnight, and his weight decreases by 1 kg the next day. However, by day 5, his urine output has diminished again, and his serum creatinine (SCr) has risen to 4.3 mg/dL. He was drowsy and confused this morning during rounds. His extremities are cool and cyanotic, BP is 102/58 mm Hg, and HR is 98 beats/minute. It is believed that he is no longer responding to his current regimen. A Swan-Ganz catheter is placed to determine further management. Hemodynamic values are cardiac index (CI) 1.5 L/minute/m², SVR 2650 dynes/cm⁻⁵, and PCWP 30 mm Hg. Which one of the following is the best drug based on his current symptoms?

    A. Milrinone 0.2 mcg/kg/minute.
    B. Dobutamine 5 mcg/kg/minute.
    C. Nitroglycerin 20 mcg/minute.
    D. Phenylephrine 20 mcg/minute.

II. ARRHYTHMIAS

A. Drug Therapy Overview

Table 7. Antiarrhythmic Drug Classes

Class I Na$^+$ channel blockers	IA – Quinidine, procainamide, disopyramide IB – Lidocaine, mexiletine IC – Propafenone, flecainide, moricizine	Slows depolarization (↑ QT) Slows depolarization Slows depolarization
Class II β-Blockers	Metoprolol, esmolol, atenolol	Slows AV nodal conduction
Class III K$^+$ channel blockers	Amiodarone, sotalol, dofetilide, or ibutilide	Slows repolarization (↑ QT)
Class IV Ca^{2+} channel blockers	Diltiazem, verapamil	Slows AV nodal conduction

AV = atrioventricular; Ca^{2+} = calcium; K$^+$ = potassium; Na$^+$ = sodium.

Table 8. Antiarrhythmic Drug Properties and Dosing (class I and III agents only)

Drug	Adverse Effects, Contraindications, Drug Interactions, Pharmacokinetics	Dosing by Indication
Class IA – Na$^+$ channel blockers		
Quinidine (Quinidex, Quinaglute)	AEs: Nausea/vomiting/diarrhea (30%), "cinchonism"(CNS and GI symptoms, tinnitus), TdP (first 72 hours) DI: Warfarin, digoxin	AF conversion: Avoid use because of GI AEs AF maintenance: Sulfate: 200–400 mg PO every 6 hours Gluconate: 324 mg PO every 8–12 hours
Procainamide (Pronestyl)	AEs: Lupuslike syndrome (30% if > 6 months), hypotension (IV use, 5%), TdP CI: LVEF < 40% PK: Reduce dose in renal and liver dysfunction (active metabolite NAPA)	AF conversion: 1 g IV for 30 minutes, then 2 mg/minute (1-hour efficacy 51%) AF maintenance: No oral agent VT conversion: 20 mg/minute IV until 17 mg/kg, arrhythmia ceases, or QRS widens > 50% VT maintenance: 2–4 mg/minute
Disopyramide (Norpace, Norpace CR, Rythmodan, Rythmodan-LA)	AEs: Anticholinergic effects, TdP, ADHF (negative inotropy) CI: Glaucoma	AF conversion: IR 200 mg (if < 50 kg) or 300 mg (if > 50 kg) PO every 6 hours AF maintenance: 400–800 mg/day in divided doses (Recommended adult dose 600 mg/day given as IR 150 mg PO every 6 hours or as CR 300 mg PO every 12 hours) If < 50 kg, max 400 mg/day If *moderate* renal dysfunction (CrCl > 40 mL/minute) or hepatic dysfunction, max 400 mg/day If *severe* renal dysfunction, 100 mg (IR only, avoid CR) every 8 hours if CrCl 30–40 mL/minute, every 12 hours if CrCl 15–30 mL/minute, or every 24 hours if CrCl < 15 mL/minute

Table 8. Antiarrhythmic Drug Properties and Dosing (class I and III agents only) *(Continued)*

Class IB – Na⁺ channel blockers (inactive)		
Lidocaine (Xylocaine)	AEs: CNS (perioral numbness, seizures, confusion, blurry vision, tinnitus) CI: Third-degree AV heart block PK: Reduce dose in those with HF, liver disease, and renal dysfunction and in the elderly DI: Amiodarone (increased lidocaine levels)	VT/VF conversion: 1–1.5 mg/kg IVB; repeat 0.5–0.75 mg/kg every 3–5 minutes (max 3 mg/kg) (If LVEF < 40%: 0.5–0.75 mg/kg IVP) VT maintenance: 1–2 mg/minute
Mexiletine (Mexitil)	AEs: CNS (tremor, dizziness, ataxia, nystagmus) CI: Third-degree AV heart block	VT maintenance: 200–300 mg every 8 hours
Class IC – Na⁺ channel blockers (Note: Avoid in patients with HF or post-MI)		
Propafenone (Rhythmol)	AEs: Metallic taste, dizziness, ADHF, bronchospasm, bradycardia, heart block (negative inotropy and β-blocking properties) CI: HF (NYHA III–IV), liver disease, valvular disease (TdP) DI: Digoxin ↑ by 70%; warfarin ↑ by 50% as well as drugs that inhibit CYP 2D6, 1A2, 3A4 (increased propafenone concentrations)	AF conversion: 600 mg PO × 1 (efficacy 45% at 3 hours) AF maintenance: 150–300 mg PO every 8–12 hours
Flecainide (Tambocor)	AEs: Dizziness, tremor, ADHF (negative inotropy) CI: HF, CAD, valvular disease, LVH (TdP) DI: Digoxin ↑ by 25%	AF conversion: 300 mg PO × 1 (efficacy 50% at 3 hours) AF maintenance: 50–150 mg PO BID
Class III – K⁺ channel blockers		
Amiodarone (Cordarone)	AEs: Pulmonary fibrosis 3%–17%, hyperthyroidism 3%, hypothyroidism 30%–50%, neurologic toxicity 20%–40%, photosensitivity, corneal deposits, hepatitis, blue-gray skin 15%, TdP < 1%, heart block 14%, hypotension (IV), phlebitis (IV) (Ca²⁺ and β-blocking properties) CI: Iodine hypersensitivity, hyperthyroidism, third-degree AV heart block DI: Warfarin, digoxin, HMG-CoA reductase inhibitors (max simvastatin dose 20 mg/day), phenytoin ↑ ≥ 50%, lidocaine, and others (inhibits CYP3A4/2D6/2C9 and gut *pgp*) *Does **not** increase mortality in patients with HF PK: Half-life 58 days (average)	AF conversion: IV: 5–7 mg/kg IV over 30–60 minutes, then 1.2–1.8 g/day continuous IV or divided oral doses until 10 g total PO: 1.2–1.8 g/day in divided doses until 10 g total
		AF maintenance: 200–400 mg/day PO
		Pulseless VT/VF conversion: 300 mg or 5 mg/kg IVB in 20 mL of D₅W or NS; repeat 150 mg IVB every 3–5 minutes
		Stable VT: 150 mg IVB in 100 mL of D₅W for 10 minutes
		VT/VF maintenance: 1 mg/minute × 6 hours; then 0.5 mg/minute (max 2.2 g/day)
Sotalol	AEs: ADHF, bradycardia, AV block, wheezing, 3%–8% TdP within 3 days of initiation, bronchospasm (β-blocking properties) CI: Baseline QTc > 440 milliseconds or CrCl < 40 mL/minute (AF only) PK: Renally eliminated *Hospitalization **mandatory** for initiation, obtain QTc 2–3 hours after first 5 doses, double-dose every 3 days; NTE QTc > 500 milliseconds	Not effective for AF conversion! AF maintenance (based on CrCl) 80 mg PO BID (> 60 mL/minute) 80 mg PO QD (40–60 mL/minute) Contraindicated < 40 mL/minute VT maintenance (based on CrCl) 80 mg PO BID (> 60 mL/minute) 80 mg PO QD (30–60 mL/minute) 80 mg PO QOD (10–30 mL/minute) 80 mg PO > QOD (< 10 mL/minute)

© 2010 American College of Clinical Pharmacy

Table 8. Antiarrhythmic Drug Properties and Dosing (class I and III agents only) *(Continued)*

Dofetilide (Tikosyn)	AEs: TdP (0.8%; 4% if no renal adjustment), dizziness, diarrhea DI: CYP3A4 inhibitors and drugs secreted by kidney (cimetidine, ketoconazole, verapamil, trimethoprim, prochlorperazine, megestrol), HCTZ CI: Baseline QTc > 440 milliseconds or CrCl < 20 mL/minute PK: Renally eliminated *Hospitalization **mandatory** for initiation, obtain QTc 2–3 hours after first 5 doses, reduce 50% if QTc ↑ > 15%; NTE QTc > 500 milliseconds *Does not increase mortality in patients with HF	AF conversion (based on CrCl) 500 mcg PO BID (> 60 mL/minute) 250 mcg PO BID (40–60 mL/minute) 125 mcg PO BID (20–40 mL/minute) Contraindicated < 20 mL/minute (efficacy 12% at 1 month) AF maintenance: Titrate down based on QTc NTE 500 milliseconds or > 15% ↑ in QTc
Ibutilide (Covert)	AEs: TdP 8%, heart block (β-Blocking properties) DI: CYP3A4 inhibitors or QT-prolonging drugs CI: Baseline QTc > 440 milliseconds, concomitant antiarrhythmic drugs, LVEF < 30% *ECG monitoring during and 4 hours after CV	AF conversion: 1 mg IV (or ≥ 60 kg) 0.01 mg/kg IV (< 60 kg), repeat in 10 minutes if ineffective (efficacy 47% at 90 minutes)
Dronedarone (Multaq)	AEs: Worsening HF, QT prolongation, hypokalemia or hypomagnesemia with potassium-sparing diuretics DI: CYP3A4 inhibitors, QT-prolonging drugs, simvastatin, tacrolimus-sirolimus, and other CYP3A4 substrates with narrow therapeutic range, digoxin and other pgp substrates CI: QTc ≥ 500 milliseconds or PR ≥ 280 milliseconds, NYHA class IV HF or NYHA class II–III HF with recent decompensation, severe hepatic impairment, second- or third-degree AVB or HR < 50 beats/minute PK: Half-life 13–19 hours	AF conversion/AF maintenance: 400 mg PO BID Discontinue if QTc ≥ 500 milliseconds

ADHF = acute decompensated heart failure; AE = adverse effect; AF = atrial fibrillation; AV = atrioventricular; AVB = atrioventricular block; BID = twice daily; CAD = coronary artery disease; CI = contraindication; CNS = central nervous system; CR = controlled release; CrCl = creatinine clearance; CV = cardioversion; CYP = cytochrome P450; D_5W = dextrose 5%; DI = drug interactions; ECG = electrocardiogram; GI = gastrointestinal; HCTZ = hydrochlorothiazide; HF = heart failure; HMG-CoA = 3-hydroxy-3-methylglutaryl coenzyme A; HR = heart rate; IR = immediate release; IV = intravenous; IVB = intravenous bolus; IVP = intravenous push; LVEF = left ventricular ejection fraction; MI = myocardial infarction; MOA = mechanism of action; NS = normal saline; NTE = not to exceed; NYHA = New York Heart Association; pgp = P-glycoprotein; PK = pharmacokinetics; PO = oral; QD = once daily; QOD = once every other day; TdP = torsades de pointes; VF = ventricular fibrillation; VT = ventricular tachycardia.

B. Acute Tachyarrhythmias
 1. Tachycardia with a pulse
    a. Give oxygen; assess airway, breathing, and circulation; and treat reversible causes.
    b. If <u>unstable</u>, administer immediate direct current cardioversion (DCC)
    c. If <u>stable</u>, determine whether QRS complex is narrow or wide
       i. Narrow complex tachycardia (usually **atrial** arrhythmias)
          (a) <u>Regular rhythm</u> – Supraventricular tachycardia (SVT) or sinus tachycardia likely
              (1) Vagal maneuvers and/or adenosine 6-mg intravenous push; then a 12-mg intravenous push (may repeat once) – Use adenosine cautiously in severe coronary artery disease (CAD).

(A) If converts, likely atrial tachycardia (AT), atrioventricular (AV) or AV nodal reciprocating/reentrant tachycardia, or Wolfe-Parkinson White syndrome
(B) If Wolfe-Parkinson White syndrome, avoid verapamil, diltiazem, and digoxin.
(C) If persistent with AV block, likely atrial flutter or AT
   (b) Irregular rhythm – AF or atrial flutter likely
      (1) **Rate control plus anticoagulation** if persistent/permanent AF
      (2) If disabling symptoms, consider adding antiarrhythmic drug therapy or ablation
      (3) If hemodynamically unstable, DCC recommended

Table 9. Atrial Fibrillation – Rate Control and Rhythm Control

Rate Control	
General presentation	β-Blockers or nondihydropyridine calcium channel blockers (diltiazem, verapamil)
If HF and no accessory pathway present	Digoxin[a] or amiodarone
If accessory pathway present	Amiodarone
Rhythm Control	
Unstable, duration less than 48 hours	DCC, IV UFH immediately beforehand
Unstable, duration unknown, or greater than 48 hours	DCC, TEE (rule out thrombus) + IV UFH beforehand
Stable, duration unknown, or more than 48 hours	Before DCC, RC + AC (INR 2–3) 3–4 weeks before and 4 weeks after If AF up to 7 days, either elective DCC or chemical cardioversion[b] • Flecainide, dofetilide, propafenone, ibutilide, or amiodarone • Digoxin and sotalol may be harmful if used for chemical cardioversion of AF; they are not recommended • If AF greater than 7 days, either elective DCC or chemical cardioversion[b] • Dofetilide, amiodarone, or ibutilide

[a]If paroxysmal AF, avoid digoxin.
[b]Quinidine, procainamide, disopyramide, and dofetilide should **NOT** be initiated out of hospital for conversion of AF to sinus rhythm.
AC = anticoagulate; AF = atrial fibrillation; DCC = direct current cardioversion; HF = heart failure; IV = intravenous; RC = rate control; TEE = transesophageal echocardiograph; UFH = unfractionated heparin.

   ii. Wide complex tachycardia (usually **ventricular** arrhythmias)
      (a) Ventricular tachycardia or unknown mechanism
         (1) Intravenous procainamide, sotalol, amiodarone, or lidocaine
         (2) Amiodarone preferred if LV dysfunction or signs of HF
         (3) Prepare for synchronized DCC if drug therapy fails.
      (b) Definite SVT (see narrow complex tachycardia)

2. Premature ventricular contractions
   a. Avoid flecainide, encainide, and moricizine (class IC agents) because of increased mortality in post-MI patients.
   b. β-Blockers are useful for controlling <u>symptomatic</u> premature ventricular contractions.
3. Ventricular tachycardia
   a. Nonsustained VT
      i. If <u>asymptomatic</u> – No therapy required
      ii. If <u>symptomatic</u> – β-Blockers; if unresponsive, then amiodarone or sotalol
   b. Sustained VT (QTc not prolonged)
      i. If <u>unstable</u> – DCC; if refractory to DCC, then amiodarone
      ii. If <u>stable</u> – Procainamide (general presentation); lidocaine (associated with MI); amiodarone, β-blockers, or procainamide (associated with CAD and repetitive idiopathic VT)
   c. Polymorphic VT (prolonged QTc) – Torsades de pointes
      i. Induced primarily when QTc interval is greater than 500 milliseconds
      ii. Withdrawal of any medications that prolong QT and correction of low magnesium ion (Mg^{2+}) or K^+ recommended
         (a) Class I and III antiarrhythmic drugs
         (b) Assess for drug interactions by cytochrome P450 (CYP) 3A4 (e.g., azole antifungals, erythromycin).
         (c) Assess for other QT-prolonging drugs such as pentamidine, haloperidol, ziprasidone, droperidol, sulfamethoxazole-trimethoprim, promethazine, and tricyclic amine antidepressants.
      iii. If <u>unstable</u>, DCC with sedation
      iv. If <u>stable</u>, intravenous Mg^{2+} 1- to 2-g intravenous bolus (maximum 16 g/24 hours)[a]
      v. If associated with MI, lidocaine 1- to 1.5-mg/kg intravenous bolus
   d. Pulseless VT or VF – See advanced cardiac life support (ACLS) algorithm for pulseless VT/VF
4. Pulseless electrical activity or asystole – ACLS algorithm for pulseless electrical activity/asystole

Table 10. Select ACLS Algorithms

Algorithm for Pulseless Ventricular Tachycardia or Fibrillation
CPR/DCC
Epinephrine 1 mg IV/IO every 3–5 minutes
Vasopressin 40 units IV/IO × 1 (replaces first or second epinephrine doses)
Amiodarone 300 mg IV/IO × 1, repeat 150 mg IV/IO × 1 OR Lidocaine 1–1.5 mg/kg IV, repeat 0.5–0.75 mg/kg IV/IO every 5–10 minutes (max 3 mg/kg)
Algorithm for PEA or Asystole
CPR (no DCC)
Epinephrine 1 mg IV/IO every 3–5 minutes
Vasopressin 40 units IV/IO × 1 (replaces first or second epinephrine doses)
If HR < 60 beats/minute for asystole or slow PEA, atropine 1 mg every 3–5 minutes × 3 (total 0.04 mg/kg)

ACLS = advanced cardiac life support; CPR = cardiopulmonary resuscitation; DCC = direct current conversion; HR = heart rate; IO = intraosseous; IV = intravenous; PEA = pulseless electrical activity.

C. Implantable Cardiac Defibrillators (ICDs)
   1. For <u>primary</u> prevention of sudden cardiac death – indicated if nonischemic dilated cardiomyopathy or ischemic heart disease (more than 40 days post-MI), LV ejection fraction (LVEF) 35% or less, NYHA class II or III, receiving optimal chronic medications, and reasonable expectation of survival with a good functional status for more than 1 year
   2. For <u>secondary</u> prevention of sudden cardiac death – indicated if recurrent sustained VT in post-MI patients, normal or near-normal LVEF, receiving optimal chronic medications, and reasonable survival expectation
   3. Contraindications: evolving acute MIs with VT, acute VT after coronary artery bypass grafting (CABG), VF caused by AF, terminal illness, psychiatric disorder, and severe NYHA class IV (non-transplantable) HF

D. Special Patient Populations
   1. Heart failure – Amiodarone and dofetilide (LV dysfunction post-MI) have a neutral effect on mortality.
   2. Acute MI
      a. Encainide, flecainide, moricizine – Increased mortality when used to treat post-MI premature ventricular contractions
      b. Class IA medications – Increased mortality in post-MI survivors
      c. Dofetilide – Neutral effect on mortality in LV dysfunction post-MI

Table 11. Alteration of Defibrillation Threshold

Threshold Alteration	Medications	Comments
Increase threshold	Amiodarone, lidocaine, and mexiletine	Reprogram ICD, increased energy (joules) required
Decrease threshold	Sotalol	May decrease energy needed for DCC

DCC = direct current conversion; ICD = implantable cardiac defibrillator.

Patient Cases

4. C.D. is a 68-year-old man admitted after an episode of syncope with a presyncopal syndrome of seeing black spots and having dizziness before passing out. Telemetry monitor showed sustained VT for 45 seconds. His medical history includes HF NYHA class III, LVEF 30%, MI × 2, HTN × 20 years, LV hypertrophy, diabetes mellitus (DM), and diabetic nephropathy. His drugs include lisinopril 5 mg/day, furosemide 20 mg 2 times/day, metoprolol 25 mg 2 times/day, digoxin 0.125 mg/day, glyburide 5 mg/day, and ASA 325 mg/day. His laboratory tests show BP 120/75 mm Hg, HR 80 beats/minute, BUN 30 mg/dL, and SCr 2.2 mg/dL. Which one of the following is the best therapy to initiate for conversion of his sustained VT?

   A. Amiodarone 150 mg intravenously for 10 minutes, then 1 mg/minute for 6 hours, then 0.5 mg/minute.
   B. Sotalol 80 mg 2 times/day, titrated to QTc about 450 milliseconds.
   C. Dofetilide 500 mcg 2 times/day, titrated to QTc about 450 milliseconds.
   D. Procainamide 20 mg/minute, maximum 17 mg/kg.

5. C.D. presents to the emergency department 3 months after amiodarone maintenance initiation (he refused ICD placement) after a syncopal episode during which he lost consciousness for 30 seconds, according to witnesses. He also complains of rapid HR episodes during which he feels dizzy and light-headed. He feels very warm all the time (he wears shorts, even though it is winter), is unable to sleep, and has experienced a 3-kg weight loss. He received a diagnosis of hyperthyroidism caused by amiodarone therapy. On telemetry, he shows runs of nonsustained VT. With an amiodarone half-life of 50 days, how long do you expect the effects of amiodarone to be provoking tachyarrhythmia episodes in this patient?

   A. Never.
   B. 1 month.
   C. 6 months.
   D. 1 year.

III. ACUTE CORONARY SYNDROMES

A. Definitions and Goals
   1. Definitions

Table 12. UA, NSTEMI, and STEMI Definitions

Unstable angina (UA)	Acute angina at rest, typically prolonged > 20 minutes, ST-segment depression, T-wave inversion, or no ECG changes may occur, but no biomarkers for cardiac necrosis present
Non–ST-elevation MI (NSTEMI)	Same as above, except positive cardiac enzyme biomarkers of necrosis (troponin I or T elevation, CKMB fraction > 5%–10% of total CK)
ST-elevation MI (STEMI)	Same as above, plus ST-elevation of > 1 mm above baseline on ECG

CK = creatine kinase; CKMB = creatine kinase myocardial band; ECG = electrocardiogram; MI = myocardial infarction.

   2. Goals of therapy
      a. Unstable angina (UA)/NSTEMI goals
         i. Prevent total occlusion of the infarct-related artery.
            (a) Glycoprotein (GP) IIb/IIIa inhibitors and anticoagulants
            (b) Percutaneous coronary intervention can be either or both:
               (1) Percutaneous transluminal coronary angiography, (i.e., "balloon")
               (2) Stent implantation
            (c) Thrombolytics have no benefit but have an increased bleeding risk.
         ii. Control chest pain and associated symptoms.
      b. ST-elevation MI goals
         i. Restore patency of the infarct-related artery and minimize infarct size.
            (a) Thrombolytic medications or "door-to-needle" time within 30 minutes
            (b) Percutaneous coronary intervention or "door-to-balloon" time within 90 minutes
               (1) If presenting to a facility without the capability for expert, prompt intervention with primary PCI within 90 minutes, should undergo fibrinolysis unless contraindicated
               (2) Facilitated PCI consists of planned, immediate PCI after an initial pharmacologic regimen such as full- or half-dose fibrinolysis, a GP IIb/IIIa inhibitor, or a combination of such; might be performed as a reperfusion strategy in higher-risk patients when PCI is not immediately available and bleeding risk is low
               (3) Rescue PCI consists of PCI after failed thrombolysis and is indicated in select patients if shock, severe HF, and/or pulmonary edema, hemodynamic or electrical instability, evidence of persistent ischemia
         ii. Prevent complications such as arrhythmias or death.
         iii. Control chest pain and associated symptoms.
B. Invasive or Conservative Treatment Strategy
   1. Calculate thrombolysis in myocardial infarction (TIMI) score (see Table 13) by adding 1 point for each history or presentation finding.
   2. Risk of mortality, new or recurrent MI, or severe recurrent ischemia through 14 days based on TIMI score: score = 0–1, mortality 7%; score = 2, mortality 8%; score = 3, mortality 13%; score = 4, mortality 20%; score = 5, mortality 26%; and score = 6–7, mortality 41%.

Table 13. TIMI Scoring

	TIMI
History	Age
	More than three cardiac risk factors
	– hypertension, diabetes mellitus, hyperlipidemia, smoking, family history
	History of coronary artery disease
Presentation	Severe angina
	ASA within 7 days
	Elevated markers
	ST-segment deviation

ASA = aspirin; TIMI = thrombolysis in myocardial infarction.

Table 14. Selection of Initial Treatment Strategy: Invasive vs. Conservative

Initial Invasive Strategy
Recurrent angina/ischemia at rest with low-level activities despite intensive medical therapy
Elevated cardiac biomarkers (TnT or TnI)
New/presumably new ST-segment depression
Signs/symptoms of HF or new/worsening mitral regurgitation
High-risk findings from noninvasive testing
Hemodynamic instability
Sustained VT
PCI within 6 months
Prior CABG
High-risk score (e.g., TIMI, GRACE)
Reduced left ventricular function (LVEF < 40%)
Initial Conservative Strategy
Low-risk score (e.g., TIMI, GRACE) or patient/physician presence in the absence of high-risk features

CABG = coronary artery bypass grafting; GRACE = Global Registry of Acute Coronary Events; HF = heart failure; LVEF = left ventricular ejection fraction; PCI = percutaneous coronary intervention; TIMI = thrombolysis in myocardial infarction; TnI = troponin I; TnT = troponin T; VT = ventricular tachycardia.

C. Initial Management
   1. "MONA" in UA/NSTEMI, "MONA" plus β-blocker in STEMI

Table 15. "MONA" plus β-Blocker

M = Morphine	• Morphine 1–5 mg IV is reasonable if symptoms are not relieved despite NTG or if symptoms recur
O = Oxygen	• Oxygen if O_2 saturation < 90% or high-risk features for hypoxemia

N = Nitroglycerin	• Nitroglycerin spray or SL tablet 0.4 mg × 3 doses to relieve acute chest pain (if pain is unrelieved after <u>1 dose</u>, call 911)
	• Nitroglycerin IV 5–10 mcg/minute, titrate to chest pain relief or 200 mcg/minute if pain unrelieved by morphine and SL NTG
	  - Hold if MAP < 80 mm Hg
	  - Used in first 48 hours for treatment of persistent chest pain, HF, and HTN
	  - Use should not preclude other mortality-reducing therapies (ACE inhibitor, b-blocker)
	  - No mortality benefits but high placebo crossover rate
	• Contraindication: Sildenafil or vardenafil use within 24 hours or tadalafil use within 48 hours; SBP < 100 mm Hg or ≥ 30 mm Hg below baseline, HR < 50 beats/minute, HR > 100 beats/minute in absence of symptomatic HF or right ventricular infarction

A = Aspirin	• ASA chew and swallow non–enteric-coated 162–325 mg × 1 dose - Clopidogrel – If ASA allergy or considerable gastrointestinal intolerance

β-Blocker	• Oral or intravenous β-blocker (oral route preferred)
	  - Mortality benefit in early phases of acute MI (metoprolol 5.7% vs. placebo 8.9%)
	  - Metoprolol 5 mg IV every 5 minutes × 3 doses, followed by 25–50 mg PO 2 times/day uptitrated as tolerated
	  - IV route reasonable if a tachyarrhythmia or HTN present
	• Contraindications: Hypotension, signs of HF, risk factors for cardiogenic shock, or other relative contraindications (third-degree heart block, active asthma)

Other early hospital therapies	
ACE inhibitors	• Indicated <u>orally</u> within first 24 hours if HF, LVEF < 40%, type 2 diabetes mellitus, or CKD - IV therapy contraindicated because of risk of hypotension • Consider in all patients with CAD • Indicated indefinitely in all patients with LVEF < 40% • ARB indicated if contraindication to ACE inhibitor • Contraindication: Hypotension
CCBs	• Specifically, nondihydropyridine CCBs – verapamil, diltiazem • Recommended if continuing or frequently recurring ischemia and contraindication to β-blocker therapy or recurrent ischemia after β-blockers and nitrates fully used - No real benefit or detriment to mortality; primarily symptom relief effects • Contraindication: Clinically significant LV dysfunction; immediate-release dihydropyridine CCBs should not be administered in the absence of a β-blocker

ACE = angiotensin-converting enzyme; ARB = angiotensin receptor blocker; ASA = aspirin; CAD = coronary artery disease; CCBs = calcium channel blockers; CKD = chronic kidney disease; HF = heart failure; IV = intravenous; LVEF = left ventricular ejection fraction; MAP = mean arterial pressure; N/A = not available; NTG = nitroglycerin; PO = oral; SBP = systolic blood pressure; SL = sublingual.

2. Treatment algorithms for UA/NSTEMI and STEMI (see Tables 16 and 17)

Table 16. UA/NSTEMI Algorithm

Strategy	Early Invasive (PCI ≤12 hours from hospitalization, high-risk patient)	Delayed PCI (PCI > 12 hours from hospitalization)	Early Conservative (no PCI, low-risk patient)
Anticoagulant therapy[a]	Enoxaparin, UFH, fondaparinux (+ UFH added at time of PCI), or bivalirudin	Enoxaparin, UFH, fondaparinux (+ UFH added at time of PCI), or bivalirudin	Enoxaparin or fondaparinux
Antiplatelet therapy	Clopidogrel or prasugrel[b] + abciximab or eptifibatide initiated at time of PCI[c] for patients receiving UFH, enoxaparin, or fondaparinux	Clopidogrel or prasugrel[b] + If high or moderate risk, initiate eptifibatide or tirofiban either before angiography/PCI (if recurrent ischemia) or at time of PCI[c]	Clopidogrel + If positive stress test, abciximab or eptifibatide with UFH or enoxaparin, or bivalirudin at time of PCI

[a]If high risk of bleeding, fondaparinux or bivalirudin preferred. If CABG planned, UFH preferred.
[b]If unlikely to undergo CABG, initiate prasugrel at time of PCI.
[c]After PCI, discontinue NTG and anticoagulation and continue abciximab for 12 hours or eptifibatide for at least 12 hours.
CABG = coronary artery bypass graft; NTG = nitroglycerin; PCI = percutaneous coronary intervention; UFH = unfractionated heparin.

Table 17. STEMI Algorithm[a]

Symptoms ≤ 12 hours	
Clopidogrel or Prasugrel	Clopidogrel
Primary PCI	Fibrinolysis
UFH with abciximab (alternatively eptifibatide or tirofiban) or bivalirudin alone	IV UFH for at least 48 hours or IV and SC enoxaparin for hospitalization, up to 8 days (preferred, selected patients) or IV and SC fondaparinux for hospitalization, up to 8 days

[a]Algorithm for patients with symptoms for 12 hours or less. If symptoms for more than 12 hours, administer clopidogrel with PCI or coronary artery bypass grafting or fibrinolysis for selected patients. If PCI, administer UFH or enoxaparin with abciximab or eptifibatide or bivalirudin alone at time of PCI.
IV = intravenous; PCI = percutaneous coronary intervention; SC = subcutaneous; UFH = unfractionated heparin.

3. Dosing of antiplatelet and anticoagulant therapy (see Tables 18–20)

Table 18. ASA, CLO, PRA Dosing

Aspirin	CLO (Plavix)[a]/PRA (Efficient)[b]
Initial therapy – ASA 162–325 mg nonenteric orally or chewed × 1 Pre-PCI – ASA 75–325 mg before PCI No stent – ASA 75–162 mg/day indefinitely Post-stent – ASA 162–325 mg/day for at least 1 month (*bare metal*), at least 3 months (*sirolimus*), at least 6 months (*paclitaxel*); then 75–162 mg/day indefinitely	Initial therapy – NSTEMI – CLO 300- to 600-mg LD × 1 – STEMI with or without fibrinolytic – CLO 300-mg LD × 1 Pre-PCI – CLO 300- to 600-mg LD or PRA 60-mg LD No stent (STEMI with or without fibrinolytic) – CLO 75 mg/day for at least 14 days and up to 1 year Post-stent – CLO 75 mg/day or PRA 10 mg/day (5 mg/day if < 60 kg) for at least 12 months and up to 15 months (bare metal stent or DES)

[a]Discontinue clopidogrel at least 5 days or PRA at least 7 days before elective CABG. Administer clopidogrel indefinitely if ASA allergy. Avoid LD if patient is 75 years or older.
[b]Initiate PRA in patients with known coronary artery anatomy only to avoid use in patients needing CABG surgery. Avoid PRA if patient is 75 years or older unless patient has DM or history of myocardial infarction.
ASA = aspirin; CABG = coronary artery bypass grafting; CLO = clopidogrel; DES = drug-eluting stent; DM = diabetes mellitus; LD = loading dose; NSTEMI = non–ST-elevation myocardial infarction; PCI = percutaneous coronary intervention; PRA = prasugrel; STEMI = ST-elevation myocardial infarction.

Table 19. GP IIb/IIIa Inhibitor Dosing

	STEMI PCI	UA/NSTEMI with/without PCI	Notes
Abciximab (ReoPro)	0.25-mg/kg IV bolus, then 0.125 mcg/kg/minute (maximum 10 mcg/kg) for 12 hours	Not recommended	Renal adjustment not necessary
Eptifibatide (Integrilin)	180-mcg/kg IV bolus × 2 (10 minutes apart), then 2 mcg/kg/minute for 12–18 hours	180-mcg/kg IV bolus, then 2 mcg/kg/minute for 12–72 hours	If CrCl < 50 mL/minute, reduce infusion 50%; not studied if CrCl >4 mg/dL.
Tirofiban (Aggrastat)	25-mcg/kg IV bolus, then 0.1 mcg/kg/minute for 18 hours	0.4 mcg/kg/minute for 30 minutes (LD infusion), then 0.1 mcg/kg/minute for 18–72 hours	If CrCl < 30 mL/minute, reduce infusion 50%

CrCl = creatinine clearance; GP = glycoprotein; IV = intravenous; LD = loading dose; NSTEMI = non–ST-elevation myocardial infarction; STEMI = ST-elevation myocardial infarction; UA = unstable angina.

Table 20. Anticoagulant Dosing

	Unfractionated Heparin	Enoxaparin (Lovenox)	Fondaparinux (Arixtra)	Bivalirudin (Angiomax)
Classification	—	LMWH	Factor Xa inhibitor	DTI
UA/NSTEMI	60-unit/kg IVB (max 4000 units), 12 units/kg/hour IV (maximum 1000 units/hour) for 48 hours or end of PCI, goal aPTT 1.5–2 × control	1 mg/kg SC BID for 24–48 hours (UA/NSTEMI) or until end of PCI or throughout hospitalization or up to 8 days (STEMI)	2.5 mg SC QD (If STEMI, give initial 2.5 mg IVB)	0.1-mg/kg IVB; then 0.25 mg/kg/hour IV
PCI	Supplemental doses to target ACT[a]	If last dose < 8 hours, none If last dose > 8 hours, 0.3 mg/kg IVB if last dose 8–12 hours prior	UFH 50- to 60-unit/kg IVB throughout hospitalization or up to 8 days	UA/NSTEMI – 0.5-mg/kg IVB, 1.75 mg/kg/hour IV STEMI – 0.75-mg/kg IVB, 1.75 mg/kg/hour IV Discontinue at end of PCI or continue at 0.25 mg/kg/hour if needed (Hold UFH 30 minutes before administration)
STEMI primary PCI[b]	If GP IIb/IIIa, UFH 50–70 units/kg IVB If no GP IIb/IIIa, UFH 70- to 100-unit/kg IVB Supplemental doses to target ACT[a]	—	—	0.75 mg/kg, 1.75 mg/kg/hour IV
Dose adjustments/contraindications	Avoid if history of HIT	If CrCl < 30 mL/minute, 1 mg/kg SC QD Avoid if > 175 kg or CrCl < 15 mL/minute	Avoid if CrCl < 30 mL/minute	Adjust infusion dose in severe renal dysfunction (IVB dose same)

[a]Target ACT 250–300 seconds for primary PCI without GP IIb/IIIa inhibitor and 200–250 seconds in patients given a concomitant GP IIb/IIIa inhibitor.
[b]If STEMI status is post-fibrinolytics, UFH dose – same as UA/NSTEMI and enoxaparin dose – if younger than 75 years, 30 mg IVB, followed immediately by 1 mg/kg subcutaneously 2 times/day (first two doses maximum 100 mg if more than 100 kg), if older than 75 years, no IVB, 0.75 mg/kg subcutaneously 2 times/day (first two doses maximum 75 mg if more than 75 kg).
ACT = activated clotting time; aPTT = activated partial thromboplastin time; BID = twice daily; DTI = direct thrombin inhibitor; HIT = heparin-induced thrombocytopenia; IV = intravenous; IVB = intravenous bolus; LMWH = low-molecular-weight heparin; NSTEMI = non–ST-elevation myocardial infarction; PCI = percutaneous coronary intervention; QD = once daily; SC = subcutaneously; STEMI = ST-elevation myocardial infarction; UA = unstable angina; UFH = unfractionated heparin.

4. Thrombolytic dosing (see Table 21) and adjunctive therapy
   a. Administer within 12 hours of symptom onset (preferably within 6 hours). Ideally, administer within 30 minutes of hospital arrival.
   b. Patients undergoing reperfusion with fibrinolytics should receive anticoagulant therapy for a minimum of 48 hours and preferably for the duration of the index hospitalization, up to 8 days.
   c. Alteplase, reteplase, and tenecteplase require concomitant UFH administration of a 60-unit/kg bolus (maximum 4000 units) and 12 units/kg/hour (maximum 1000 units/hour), with provision for an activated partial prothrombin time of about 50–70 seconds.
   d. Low-molecular-weight heparins can be used in combination with thrombolytics if the patient is younger than 75 years without significant renal dysfunction (SCr is less than 2.5 mg/dL in men and less than 2 mg/dL in women).

Table 21. Thrombolytic Therapy

	Dosing
Alteplase (rt-PA, Activase)	15 mg IV, then 0.75 mg/kg over 30 minutes (max 50 mg), then 0.5 mg/kg (max 35 mg) over 60 minutes
Reteplase (r-PA, Retavase)	10 units IV, repeat 10 units IV in 30 minutes
Tenecteplase (TNK-tPA, TNKase)	< 60 kg, 30 mg IV; 60–69 kg, 35 mg IV; 70–79 kg, 40 mg IV; 80–89 kg, 45 mg IV, > 90 kg, 50 mg IV (about 0.5 mg/kg)
Streptokinase (Streptase)	1.5 million units IV over 60 minutes

IV = intravenously.

Table 22. Contraindications to Thrombolytic Therapy

Relative Contraindications	**Absolute Contraindications**
• BP > 180/110 mm Hg on presentation • History of TIA or CVA < 3 months prior • History of chronic poorly controlled HTN • INR 2–3 on warfarin • Recent trauma, major surgery, CPR, internal bleeding in 2–4 weeks • Streptokinase exposure > 5 days earlier or prior allergic reaction (if given streptokinase again) • Active peptic ulcer • Age > 75 years • Pregnancy • Known intracranial pathology (dementia)	• ANY prior hemorrhagic stroke • Ischemic stroke within 3 months (except in past 3 hours) • Intracranial neoplasm or arteriovenous malformation • Active internal bleeding • Aortic dissection • Considerable facial trauma or closed-head trauma in past 3 months

BP = blood pressure; CPR = cardiopulmonary resuscitation; CVA = cerebrovascular accident; HTN = hypertension; INR = international normalized ratio; TIA = transient ischemic attack.

D. Long-Term Management
1. β-Blockers
   a. Indicated for all patients unless contraindicated
   b. Initiate within a few days of event, if not acute, and continue indefinitely
   c. If moderate or severe LV failure, initiate with gradual titration
2. Angiotensin-converting enzyme (ACE) inhibitors
   a. Indicated for all patients even if no LV dysfunction, HTN, or DM
   b. Give oral ACE inhibitor in low doses to all patients during the first 24 hours of anterior STEMI, HF signs (pulmonary congestion), or LVEF less than 40%, provided no hypotension exists (systolic BP less than 100 mm Hg) or other contraindication, to reduce mortality and remodeling.
   c. Angiotensin receptor blocker if ACE inhibitor intolerant
   d. Avoid intravenous ACE inhibitor post-MI to prevent hypotension.
3. Aldosterone receptor blockers
   a. Indicated if post-MI with LVEF less than 40%, symptomatic HF or DM, and receiving ACE inhibitor; however, contraindicated if CrCl less than 30 mL/minute or K more than 5 mEq/L
4. Warfarin – Indicated either without (INR 2.5–3.5) or with low-dose ASA (75–81 mg/day, INR 2–2.5) if high CAD risk and low bleeding risk if patient does not require, or is intolerant of, clopidogrel
5. Lipid management – Statins indicated with a low-density lipoprotein goal less than 100 mg/dL, with a goal of less than 70 mg/dL reasonable
6. Other goals – Hemoglobin A_{1c} less than 7%, smoking cessation, body mass index 18.5–24.9 kg/m^2, exercise 3 or 4 times/week

Patient Cases

6. J.D. is a 66-year-old, 70-kg woman with a history of MI, HTN, HLD, and DM who presents with sudden-onset diaphoresis, nausea, vomiting, and dyspnea, followed by a bandlike upper chest pain (8/10) radiating to her left arm. She had felt well until 1 month ago, when she noticed her typical angina was occurring with less exertion. Electrocardiography (ECG) showed ST-depressions in leads II, III, and aVF and hyperdynamic T waves. Cardiac enzymes are positive, and she has a diagnosis of NSTEMI. Home medications are ASA 81 mg/day, simvastatin 40 mg every night, metoprolol 50 mg 2 times/day, and metformin 1 g 2 times/day. Which one of the following is the best antiplatelet/anticoagulant strategy for this patient?
    A. ASA 325 mg and clopidogrel 600 mg × 1, then 75 mg/day, UFH titrated to 50–70 seconds immediately plus eptifibatide 180-mcg/kg bolus × 1, then 2 mcg/kg/minute at time of PCI if indicated.
    B. ASA 325 mg and enoxaparin 80 mg subcutaneously 2 times/day plus cardiac catheterization for possible PCI.
    C. Medical management with abciximab 0.25-mg/kg bolus, then 0.125 mg/kg/minute for 12 hours plus enoxaparin 80 mg subcutaneously 2 times/day, ASA 325 mg/day, and clopidogrel 300 mg × 1, then 75 mg/day.
    D. Medical management with ASA 325 mg and clopidogrel 300 mg × 1, then 75 mg/day plus UFH 70-unit/kg bolus; then 15 units/kg/hour.

7. J.D. received a percutaneous transluminal coronary angioplasty and paclitaxel-eluting stent in her right coronary artery. Which one of the following best represents how long clopidogrel therapy should be continued?
    A. 1 month.
    B. 3 months.
    C. 6 months.
    D. At least 12 months.

Patient Cases (continued)

8. Which one of the following is the optimal lifelong ASA dose once dual therapy with clopidogrel after PCI with stent implantation is completed?

    A. 25 mg.
    B. 81 mg.
    C. 325 mg.
    D. 650 mg.

9. R.V., a 52-year-old man with a history of HTN and hypertriglyceridemia, presents to a major university teaching hospital with a cardiac catheterization laboratory. He has 3 hours of crushing 10/10 substernal chest pain radiating to both arms that began while he was eating his lunch (seated), which is accompanied by nausea, diaphoresis, and shortness of breath. He has never before experienced chest pain of this character or intensity. He usually can walk several miles without difficulty and is a 1.5 pack/day smoker. Home medications are lisinopril 2.5 mg/day and gemfibrozil 600 mg 2 times/day. Current vital signs include HR 68 beats/minute and BP 178/94 mm Hg; weight is 100 kg. Electrocardiography shows a 3-mm ST-elevation in leads V_2–V_4, I, and aVL. Serum chemistry values are within normal limits. The first set of cardiac enzymes shows positive myoglobin concentrations, creatine kinase (CK) 175 units/L, myocardial band (MB) 17.4 units/L, and troponin T 0.8 mcg/L (less than 0.1 mcg/L). Which one of the following is best to treat this patient's STEMI?

    A. Cardiac catheterization with primary PCI (stent) of occluded artery, together with abciximab, clopidogrel, ASA, and UFH.
    B. Reteplase 10-unit bolus × 2, 30 minutes apart, plus UFH 60-unit/kg bolus and a 12-unit/kg/hour infusion.
    C. Abciximab 0.25-mg/kg intravenous push and 0.125 mg/kg/minute for 12 hours plus enoxaparin 100 mg subcutaneously 2 times/day plus tenecteplase 25-mg intravenous push × 1.
    D. Tirofiban 0.04 mcg/kg/minute × 30 minutes; then 0.01 mcg/kg/minute plus UFH 60-unit/kg bolus and a 12-unit/kg/hour infusion.

10. W.F. is a 70-year-old male smoker with a history of HTN, benign prostatic hypertrophy, and lower back pain. Three weeks ago, he started experiencing substernal chest pain with exertion (together with dyspnea), which radiated to both arms and was associated with nausea and diaphoresis. Episodes have increased in frequency to 4–5 times/day; they are relieved with rest. He has never had an ECG. Today, he awoke with 7/10 chest pain and came to the emergency department of a rural community hospital 2 hours later. He was acutely dyspneic and had ongoing pain. Home medications are ASA 81 mg/day for 2 months, doxazosin 2 mg/day, and ibuprofen 800 mg 3 times/day. Vital signs include HR 42 beats/minute (bradycardic with complete heart block); BP 104/48 mm Hg; and weight 61 kg. Laboratory results include BUN 45 mg/dL, SCr 1.7 mg/dL, CK 277 units/L, CKMB 35.2 units/L, and troponin T 1.5 mcg/L (less than 0.1 mcg/L). His ECG shows a 3-mm ST-elevation. Aspirin, clopidogrel, and sublingual nitroglycerin were given in the emergency department. Which one of the following best describes how his treatment should be managed?

    A. Alteplase plus enoxaparin.
    B. UFH.
    C. Tenecteplase plus UFH.
    D. Diagnostic cardiac catheterization for possible primary PCI.

IV. PULMONARY ARTERIAL HYPERTENSION

A. Definition, Diagnosis, and Treatment Goals
   1. Pulmonary arterial hypertension (PAH)
      a. Idiopathic pulmonary arterial hypertension (IPAH)
         i. Change in nomenclature during 2003 World Conference on Pulmonary Hypertension; used to be known as primary pulmonary hypertension
         ii. Familial PAH
      b. Secondary causes – Scleroderma (most common), chronic thromboembolic disease, HIV (human immunodeficiency virus), liver disease, connective tissue diseases, medications, toxins, others
   2. Symptoms
      a. Dyspnea with exertion (60% of patients), fatigue, chest pain, syncope, weakness (40%) – Caused by impaired oxygen delivery to tissues and diminished CO
      b. Orthopnea, peripheral edema, liver congestion, abdominal bloating, and other signs of right ventricular hypertrophy and failure occur when disease progresses to involve the heart.
   3. Diagnosis

Table 23. Diagnostic Findings of PAH

Hemodynamic alterations	mPAP > 25 mm Hg, PCWP ≤ 15 mm Hg, and PVR > 3 Wood units on RHC
Electrocardiogram	Signs of RV hypertrophy, right-axis deviation, and anterior ST- and T-wave abnormalities consistent with RV strain pattern
Echocardiography	Estimated RV systolic pressure elevation, enlarged RV, RV dysfunction
Chest radiography	Enlarged pulmonary arteries and diminished peripheral pulmonary vascular markings, RV enlargement
Physical examination	Cool and/or cyanotic extremities, jugular venous distension, pulsatile hepatomegaly, peripheral edema, ascites

mPAP = mean pulmonary artery pressure; PAH = pulmonary arterial hypertension; PCWP = pulmonary capillary wedge pressure; PVR = pulmonary vascular resistance; RHC = right heart catheterization; RV = right ventricle.

   4. World Health Organization functional assessment classification

Table 24. World Health Organization Classification for PAH

Class	Definition
Class I	No symptoms (dyspnea, fatigue, syncope, chest pain) with normal daily activities
Class II	Symptoms with strenuous normal daily activities that slightly limit functional status and activity level
Class III	Symptoms of dyspnea, fatigue, syncope, and chest pain with normal daily activities that severely limit functional status and activity level
Class IV	Symptoms at rest; cannot conduct normal daily activities without symptoms

   5. Treatment goals
      a. Relieve acute dyspnea symptoms.
      b. Improve exercise capacity/quality of life and prevent death.
         i. Acute vasodilator response testing

(a) Use intravenous epoprostenol, inhaled nitric oxide, or intravenous adenosine.
(b) Positive response: Reduction in mean pulmonary artery pressure (mPAP) of at least 10 mm Hg to an absolute mPAP less than 40 mm Hg
(c) Positive response predicts mortality reduction with long-term calcium channel blocker or vasodilator use.

B. Treatment of PAH

Table 25. Initial PAH Treatment Algorithm

Supportive Care
Oxygen to maintain O$_2$ saturation > 90%, diuretic if peripheral edema or ascites
Oral anticoagulation, warfarin (INR 1.5–2.5) if IPAH ± diuretics ± digoxin (Anticoagulation to prevent catheter thrombosis (IV prostaglandin use) and venous thromboembolism)
Immunizations for influenza and pneumococcus
Discuss effective methods of birth control with women of childbearing potential
Positive Response to Acute Vasoreactivity Testing
Initiate oral CCB - If sustained response, continue CCB - If no sustained response, see "Lower Risk" algorithm below
Negative Response to Acute Vasoreactivity Testing

Lower Risk[a]	Higher Risk[b]
First line: ERAs or PDEIs (oral) Alternatives: epoprostenol or treprostinil (IV) Iloprost (inhaled), treprostinil (SC)	Epoprostenol or treprostinil (IV) Iloprost (inhaled) ERAs or PDEIs (oral) Treprostinil (SC)

Reassess: consider combination therapy, investigational protocols, atrial septostomy, lung transplantation

[a]Low risk (good prognosis) if no RV failure, gradual progression of symptoms, WHO class II or III, 6 MW more than 400 m, peak VO$_2$ more than 10.4 mL/kg/minute, minimal RV dysfunction, RAP less than 10 mm Hg, CI more than 2.5 L/minute/m^2, BNP minimally elevated.
[b]High risk (poor prognosis) if RV failure, rapid progression of symptoms, WHO class IV, 6 MW less than 300 m, peak VO$_2$ < 10.4 mL/kg/minute, substantial RV enlargement/dysfunction (or pericardial effusion or right atrial enlargement), RAP greater than 20 mm Hg, CI less than 2 L/minute/m^2, BNP significantly elevated.
BNP = B-type natriuretic peptide; CCB = calcium channel blocker; CI = cardiac index; ERA = endothelin receptor antagonist; INR = international normalized ratio; IPAH = idiopathic pulmonary arterial hypertension; IV = intravenously; MW = minute walk; PDEI = phosphodiesterase inhibitor; RAP = right atrial pressure; RV = right ventricle; SC = subcutaneously; WHO = World Health Organization.

- Reassessment should include functional class determination and 6-minute walk test every 4–6 months, with right heart catheterization less often.
- Satisfactory condition is defined as functional class I or II, ambulated 380 m or greater (or 1250 feet) during 6-minute walk test, with a CI of 2.2 L/minute/m^2 or greater and mean pulmonary arterial pressure less than 12 mm Hg.

Table 26. Overview of PAH Treatment Options if Calcium Channel Blockers Fail

Drug/ Mechanism/ Indication	Dose	Adverse Effects	Considerations

Calcium channel blockers
 	
Class II PAH
	Varies by agent and patient tolerance	Hypotension, headache, dizziness, peripheral edema, cardiac conduction delay (diltiazem)	• Should not be used empirically without positive response to acute vasodilatory response testing!
			• Diltiazem, amlodipine, nifedipine most commonly used
			• Select agent based on HR at baseline
			  - If tachycardic, choose diltiazem
			  - If bradycardic, choose amlodipine, nifedipine

Epoprostenol (Flolan) Prostacyclin analog Class III–IV PAH	1–40 ng/kg/minute IV	Jaw pain, nausea, vomiting, flushing, headache, muscle aches and pain, catheter-related thrombosis, and IV line infections; rebound worsening of symptoms if abruptly discontinued	• Continuous IV infusion by pump • Unstable at acidic pH and room temperature (refrigerate or use ice packs before and during infusion) • Drug requires reconstitution in sterile environment • Medical emergency if infusion interrupted ($t_{1/2}$ – 6 minutes) – Spare drug cassette and infusion pump should be kept available • Costs ≥ $100,000/year
Treprostinil (Remodulin) Prostacyclin analog Class II–IV PAH	1.25- to 40-ng/kg/minute SC infusion	Severe erythema and induration (83%) and injection site pain (85%) limits use; also headache, nausea, diarrhea, rash	• Longer half-life ($t_{1/2}$ – 3 hours) – Longer to seek medical attention than with epoprostenol • Premixed, prefilled syringe easier to administer than epoprostenol • Local treatments (hot and cold packs or topical analgesics) can be used to minimize infusion site discomfort • Moving infusion site every 3 days minimizes irritation
Inhaled iloprost (Ventavis) Prostacyclin analog Class III–IV PAH	2.5 × 1; then 5 mcg/inhalation by nebulizer 6–9 times/day while awake	Mild, transient cough, flushing, headache, syncope	• Requires 6–9 inhalations daily (15 minutes each with jet nebulizer) • Prodose AAD nebulization system required • Inhaled form has less systemic adverse reactions than other prostacyclin analogs • Use no more than every 2 hours
Bosentan (Tracleer) Nonselective endothelin receptor antagonist (ET_A and ET_B) Class III–IV PAH	62.5–125 mg PO twice daily	Peripheral edema 5%–14%, hypotension 7%, increased LFTs 11%, flushing 7%–14%, palpitations 5% Efficacy decreased with CYP2C8/9 and 3A4 inducers, and toxicity increased with 3A4 and CYP2C8/9 inhibitors	• Severe drug interactions with glyburide (increased LFTs) and cyclosporine (decreased efficacy of both cyclosporine and bosentan) • Monitor LFTs monthly • Monitor hemoglobin/hematocrit periodically • Potential teratogen; if childbearing age, use two contraceptive methods (reduced efficacy of hormonal contraceptives); monthly pregnancy test required

Table 26. Overview of PAH Treatment Options if Calcium Channel Blockers Fail *(continued)*

Ambrisentan (Letairis) Selective endothelin receptor antagonist (ET_A only) Class II–III PAH	5–10 mg PO once daily	Peripheral edema 17%, hypotension 0%, increased LFTs 0%–2.8%, flushing 4%, palpitations 5%, fluid retention No CYP drug interactions documented	• Caution with cyclosporine • Monitor LFTs monthly • Potential teratogen (see above comments)
Sitaxsentan (Thelin) (selective endothelin receptor antagonist) ($ET_A \gg ET_B$) Not FDA approved	Not currently FDA approved	Peripheral edema 16%–25%, nausea 18%–23%, increased LFTs 10%, dizziness 10%–14%, headache 45%, nasal congestion, decreased hemoglobin Inhibits CYP2C9 (moderate) as well as 2C19 and 3A4 (weak)	• Contraindicated with cyclosporine (increased sitaxsentan concentrations) • Contraindicated with pregnancy and breastfeeding • Monitor LFTs monthly • Monitor hemoglobin/hematocrit periodically • Drug interaction with warfarin, phenytoin, and tolbutamide (increased concentrations of these medications) because of CYP2C9 inhibition
Sildenafil (Revatio) Phosphodiesterase inhibitor Class II–IV PAH	20 mg PO three times daily	Headache, epistaxis, facial flushing, bluish or blurry vision, light sensitivity, dyspepsia, insomnia	• Half-life 4–5 hours • May augment effects of other vasodilators when used in combination (especially prostacyclin) • Contraindicated in patients receiving nitrates • Avoid combined use with strong CYP3A4 inhibitors (e.g., ritonavir, cimetidine, erythromycin)
Tadalafil (Adcirca) Phosphodiesterase inhibitor Class II–IV PAH	40 mg PO once daily	• Headache, flushing, indigestion, nausea, backache, myalgia, nasopharyngitis, respiratory tract infection	• Half-life 17.5 hours • May augment effects of other vasodilators when used in combination (especially prostacyclin) • Contraindicated in patients receiving nitrates • If CrCl 31–80 mL/minute, initiate 20 mg PO once daily and titrate as tolerated • If CrCl < 30 mL/minute or hemodialysis, avoid use • If Child-Pugh Class A or B, initiate 20 mg PO once daily and titrate as tolerated • If Child-Pugh Class C, avoid use • Avoid combined use with potent CYP3A4 inhibitors as well as CYP3A4 inducers

CCBs = calcium channel blockers; CrCl = creatinine clearance; CYP = cytochrome P450; ET-1 antagonists = endothelin-1 antagonists; FDA = U.S. Food and Drug Administration; PAH = pulmonary arterial hypertension; PO = orally; SC = subcutaneous; IV = intravenous; LFTs = liver function tests.

Patient Case

11. R.W. is a 38-year-old obese woman who presents with increasing symptoms of fatigue and shortness of breath. She could walk only 10–20 feet at baseline and is now short of breath at rest. Her arterial blood gas is pH 7.31/Pco_2 65/Po_2 53/85% O_2 saturation. She has three-pillow orthopnea and 3+ pitting edema in her lower extremities. Medical history is significant only for AF. On computerized tomographic angiography, the pulmonary artery trunk is substantially enlarged, with a mean pressure of 56 mm Hg. Echocardiography shows right atrial and ventricular hypertrophy. Chest radiography detects prominent interstitial markings. Pertinent laboratory test values are BUN 21 mg/dL, SCr 1.2 mg/dL, AST 145 international units/L, ALT 90 international units/L, INR 2.1, and PTT 52 seconds; vital signs include BP 108/62 mm Hg and HR 62 beats/minute. Home medications are warfarin 2.5 mg/day, ipratropium 2 puffs every 6 hours, salmeterol 2 puffs 2 times/day, and diltiazem 480 mg/day. Her diagnosis is IPAH. Based on the options below, which one of the following is the best evidence-based management strategy?

   A. Increase diltiazem to 600 mg/day.
   B. Start sildenafil 20 mg 3 times/day.
   C. Start epoprostenol 2 ng/kg/minute.
   D. Start bosentan 62.5 mg 2 times/day.

V. HYPERTENSIVE CRISES (URGENCY AND EMERGENCY)

A. Definitions
   1. Hypertensive urgency – Acutely elevated BP, particularly diastolic BP greater than 120/130 mm Hg, without evidence of target organ damage
   2. Hypertensive emergency – HTN with evidence of target organ damage to brain, heart, kidneys, eyes (e.g., hypertensive encephalopathy, intracranial hemorrhage, or other acute neurologic deficit, UA or acute MI, acute HF, pulmonary edema [shortness of breath], aortic dissection, retinopathy or papilledema, decreased urine output or acute renal failure, eclampsia)

B. Goals
   1. Hypertensive urgency – Lower mean arterial pressure (MAP) to goal or near goal within 24 hours; oral medications can be used.
   2. Hypertensive emergency – Lower MAP by 25% or diastolic BP to 100/110 mm Hg within 30–60 minutes.

C. Treatment Options

Table 27. Dose, Onset, Duration, and Adverse Effects of Commonly Used Drugs for Hypertensive Emergencies

Drug (onset, duration)	Dose	Adverse Effects
Sodium nitroprusside (Nipride) (immediate, 2–3 minutes after discontinue)	0.25–0.5 mcg/kg/minute, maximum 3 mcg/kg/minute	Cyanide/thiocyanate toxicity, nausea, vomiting, methemoglobinemia CI: renal, hepatic failure Caution: increased ICP
Esmolol (Brevibloc) (1–2 minutes, 10–30 minutes)	500 mcg/kg LD for 1 minute, then 25–50 mcg/kg/minute, maximum 300 mcg/kg/minute	Bronchospasm, HF exacerbation, bradycardia/heart block Caution: acute HF, asthma
Labetalol (Normodyne, Trandate) (5–10 minutes, 3–6 hours)	20–80 mg IV every 15 minutes OR 0.5–2 mg/minute maximum 300 mg/24 hours	Same as esmolol
Nicardipine (Cardene) (1–5 minutes, 15–30 minutes – up to 4 hours if prolonged infusion)	5–15 mg/hour, maximum 15 mg/hour	Reflex tachycardia, nausea, vomiting, headache, flushing Caution: angina/MI, acute HF, increased ICP
Nitroglycerin (2–5 minutes, 5–10 minutes)	5–10 mcg/minute, maximum 100 mcg/minute	Headache, nausea, vomiting, tachyphylaxis, methemoglobinemia Caution: increased ICP
Hydralazine (Apresoline) 10 minutes, 1–4 hours)	5–10 mg IV every 4–6 hours (not to exceed 20 mg/dose)	Reflex tachycardia, headache, flushing Caution: angina/MI, increased ICP, aortic dissection
Enalaprilat (Vasotec) (Within 30 minutes, 12–24 hours)	0.625–1.25 mg IV every 4–6 hours, maximum 5 mg every 6 hours	Renal insufficiency/failure, hyperkalemia CI: pregnancy, renal artery stenosis (Note: long half-life)
Fenoldopam (Corlopam) (< 5 minutes, 30 minutes)	0.1 mcg/kg/minute, maximum 1.6 mcg/kg/minute	Headache, flushing, tachycardia, cerebral ischemia Caution: glaucoma
Clevidipine (Cleviprex) (2–4 minutes, 5–15 minutes)	1–2 mg/hour maximum 16 mg/hour	Renal failure, hepatic failure, and geriatric patients not specifically studied CI: soy/egg product allergy, severe aortic stenosis, defective lipid metabolism Caution: HF, concomitant β-blocker use, reflex tachycardia, rebound hypertension

CI = contraindication; HF = heart failure; ICP = intracranial pressure; IV = intravenous.

Table 28. Dose, Indication, and Adverse Effects of Commonly Used Drugs for Hypertensive Urgencies

Drug	Dose	Adverse Effects
Captopril (Capoten)	6.5–50 mg PO	Renal insufficiency/failure, hyperkalemia CI: pregnancy, renal artery stenosis
Clonidine (Catapres)	0.2 mg PO; then 0.1 mg/hour up to 0.8 mg total	Sedation, dry mouth, dizziness Caution: altered mental status CI: severe carotid artery stenosis
Minoxidil (Loniten)	5–20 mg PO	Tachycardia, edema CI: angina, HF
Nifedipine	10–20 mg PO	Flushing, headache, edema CI: severe aortic stenosis, coronary artery or cerebrovascular disease
Labetalol (Normodyne, Trandate)	200–400 mg PO repeated every 2–3 hours	Bronchospasm, especially in patients with asthma HF exacerbation; bradycardia/heart block Caution: acute HF

CI = contraindication; HF = heart failure; PO = orally.

Table 29. Agents Preferred for Hypertensive Crises Based on Comorbidities

Comorbidity	Preferred Agent(s)
Acute aortic dissection	IV esmolol alone or in combination with nicardipine or nitroprusside (IV β-blocker must precede other agents)
Acute heart failure	IV nitroprusside, IV nitroglycerin, IV nesiritide, or IV ACE inhibitors in combination with IV diuretics If pulmonary edema (Note: Avoid β-blockers)
Acute intracerebral hemorrhage/acute ischemic stroke	IV labetalol, IV nicardipine
Acute myocardial infarction	IV β-blocker in combination with IV nitroglycerin If heart rate < 70 beats/minute, IV nicardipine or IV clevidipine
Acute pulmonary edema	IV nesiritide, IV nitroglycerin, IV nitroprusside
Acute renal failure	IV fenoldopam, IV nicardipine, IV clevidipine
Eclampsia or preeclampsia	IV hydralazine, IV labetalol, IV nicardipine
Hypertensive encephalopathy	IV nitroprusside, IV labetalol, IV fenoldopam, IV nicardipine
Perioperative hypertension	IV clevidipine, IV esmolol, IV nicardipine, IV nitroglycerin, IV nitroprusside
Sympathetic crisis	IV nicardipine, IV fenoldopam, IV clevidipine, IV phentolamine (Note: Avoid unopposed β-blockade)

ACE = angiotensin-converting enzyme; IV = intravenous.

Patient Case
12. A.W., a 68-year-old man with a history of end-stage renal disease on hemodialysis, HTN, CAD post-MI, moderately depressed LVEF, and gastroesophageal reflux disease, presents with acute-onset shortness of breath and chest pain. After his recent dialysis, he had a large barbecue meal with salt and smoked some marijuana laced with cocaine. He was medication nonadherent for 2 days and noticed he had gained 2 kg in 24 hours. His baseline orthopnea worsened to sleeping sitting up in a chair for the past 2 nights before admission. He developed acute-onset chest tightness with diaphoresis and nausea, pain 7/10. He went to the emergency department, where a BP of 250/120 mm Hg was noted. He had crackles halfway up his lungs on examination, and chest radiography detected bilateral fluffy infiltrates with prominent vessel cephalization. His ECG showed sinus tachycardia HR 122 beats/minute and ST depressions in leads 2, 3, and aVF. He was admitted for hypertensive emergency. Laboratory results are as follows: BUN 48 mg/dL, SCr 11.4 mg/dL, BNP 2350 pg/mL, troponin T 1.5 mcg/L (less than 0.1 mcg/L), CK 227 units/L, and MB 22 units/L. Which one of the following medications is best to manage A.W.'s hypertensive emergency?

A. Intravenous nitroglycerin 5 mcg/minute, titrated to 25% reduction in MAP.
B. Labetalol 2 mcg/minute, titrated to 50% reduction in MAP.
C. Sodium nitroprusside 0.25 mcg/kg/minute, titrated to 25% reduction in MAP.
D. Clonidine 0.1 mg orally every 2 hours as needed for 50% reduction in MAP.

REFERENCES

Acute Decompensated Heart Failure

1. Hunt SA, Abraham WT, Chin MH, et al. 2009 focused update incorporated into the ACC/AHA 2005 guidelines for the diagnosis and management of heart failure in adults: a report of the American College of Cardiology Foundation/American Heart Association Task Force on Practice Guidelines developed in collaboration with the International Society for Heart and Lung Transplantation. J Am Coll Cardiol 2009;53:1343–82.
2. Adams KF, Lindenfeld J, Arnold JMO, et al. Executive summary: HFSA 2006 comprehensive heart failure practice guideline. J Card Fail 2006;12:10–38.
3. Nohria A, Lewis E, Warner Stevenson LW. Medical management of advanced heart failure. JAMA 2002;287:628–40.

Acute Coronary Syndromes

1. Antman EM, Hand M, Armstrong PW, et al. 2007 focused update of the ACC/AHA 2004 guidelines for the management of patients with ST-elevation myocardial infarction: a report of the American College of Cardiology/American Heart Association Task Force on Practice Guidelines: developed in collaboration with the Canadian Cardiovascular Society endorsed by the American Academy of Family Physicians. J Am Coll Cardiol 2008;51:210–47.
2. Anderson JL, Adams CD, Antman EM, et al. ACC/AHA 2007 guideline update for the management of patients with unstable angina and non–ST-segment elevation myocardial infarction – executive summary: a report of the American College of Cardiology/American Heart Association Task Force on Practice Guidelines. J Am Coll Cardiol 2007;50:652–726.
3. King SB III, Smith SC Jr., Hirshfeld JW Jr., et al. 2007 focused update of the ACC/AHA/SCAI 2005 guideline update for percutaneous coronary intervention: a report of the American College of Cardiology/American Heart Association Task Force on Practice Guidelines. J Am Coll Cardiol 2008;51:172–209.
4. Kushner FG, Hand M, Smith SC Jr., et al. 2009 focused update of the ACC/AHA guidelines for the management of patients with ST-elevation myocardial infarction (updating the 2004 guideline and 2007 focused update) and ACC/AHA/SCAI guidelines on percutaneous coronary intervention (updating the 2005 guideline and 2007 focused update): a report of the American College of Cardiology/ American Heart Association Task Force on Practice Guidelines. J Am Coll Cardiol 2009;54:2205–41.

Arrhythmias

1. Fuster V, Ryden LE, Cannom DS, et al. ACC/AHA/ESC 2006 guidelines for the management of patients with atrial fibrillation – executive summary: a report of the American College of Cardiology/American Heart Association Task Force on Practice Guidelines and the European Society of Cardiology Committee for Practice Guidelines. J Am Coll Cardiol 2006;48:854–906.
2. Zipes DP, Camm AJ, Borggrefe M, et al. ACC/AHA/ESC 2006 guidelines for the management of patients with ventricular arrhythmias and the prevention of sudden cardiac death – executive summary: a report of the American College of Cardiology/American Heart Association Task Force and the European Society of Cardiology Committee for Practice Guidelines. J Am Coll Cardiol 2006;48:1064–108.
3. Blomström-Lundqvist C, Scheinman MM, Aliot EM, et al. ACC/AHA/ESC 2003 guidelines for the management of patients with supraventricular arrhythmias – executive summary: a report of the American College of Cardiology/American Heart Association Task Force on Practice Guidelines and the European Society of Cardiology Committee for Practice Guidelines. J Am Coll Cardiol 2003;42:1493–531.
4. American Heart Association. 2005 guidelines for cardiopulmonary resuscitation and emergency cardiovascular care. Circulation 2005;112:1–211.

Pulmonary Arterial Hypertension

1. McLaughlin VV, Archer SL, Badesch DB, et al. ACCF/AHA 2009 expert consensus document on pulmonary hypertension. J Am Coll Cardiol 2009;53:1573–619.
2. Badesch DB, Abman SH, Simonneau G, et al. Medical therapy for pulmonary arterial hypertension: updated ACCP evidence-based clinical practice guidelines. Chest 2007;131:1917–28.

3. McLaughlin VV, McGoon MD. Pulmonary arterial hypertension. Circulation 2006;114:1417–31.

Hypertensive Emergency

1. Rhoney D, Peacock WF. Intravenous therapy for hypertensive emergencies, part 1. Am J Health Syst Pharm 2009;66:1343–52.

2. Rhoney D, Peacock WF. Intravenous therapy for hypertensive emergencies, part 2. Am J Health Syst Pharm 2009;66:1448–57.

3. Haas AR, Marik PE. Current diagnosis and management of hypertensive emergency. Semin Dial 2006;19:502–12.

4. Marik PE, Varon J. Hypertensive crises: challenges and management. Chest 2007;131:1949–62.

ANSWERS AND EXPLANATIONS TO PATIENT CASES

1. Answer: C
This patient, who has ADHF, is receiving a b-blocker. Although long-term b-blockers can improve HF symptoms and reduce mortality, b-blockers can worsen symptoms in the short term. It is recommended to keep the maintenance b-blocker therapy at the same or a slightly reduced dose compared with outpatient therapy in patients with ADHF; increasing the dose may acutely worsen symptoms and CO. In patients admitted with volume overload without substantial signs of decreased CO, it is reasonable to try intravenous loop diuretics initially. As gut edema increases, oral loop diuretics (notably furosemide) become less effective because of decreased absorption. Nesiritide is a vasodilatory drug that can be initiated if intravenous loop diuretic therapy fails, but because of its adverse effects and substantial cost, it is not recommended before a trial of intravenous diuretics. Milrinone is an inotropic drug. Because of their adverse effects, inotropes are recommended in cold and wet exacerbations after vasodilatory medications have failed.

2. Answer: A
Nesiritide and sodium nitroprusside are reasonable options if intravenous diuretics fail and the patient needs further diuresis and afterload reduction. Although nesiritide has been linked with the potential for worsening SCr in a meta-analysis, its use is not contraindicated in patients with preexisting renal insufficiency. This patient is showing signs of a warm and wet exacerbation and has experienced treatment failure with intravenous loop diuretics and the addition of the thiazide diuretic metolazone, so nesiritide is the most appropriate option in this patient at this time. Sodium nitroprusside can lead to thiocyanate toxicity in patients with severe renal insufficiency, so it is contraindicated in this case. Dobutamine is typically used in states of low CO decompensation and is counteracted by concomitant b-blocker therapy, making it a poor choice in patients receiving b-blockers. Although milrinone is a more acceptable inotropic agent in a patient receiving b-blockers, the dosing strategy in this case is not appropriate for the degree of renal insufficiency the patient shows. Because of its renal clearance, milrinone must be dose adjusted if CrCl is less than 50 mL/minute.

3. Answer: A
Signs of a decreased CO state in HF, such as increased SCr, decreased mental status, and cool extremities, suggest a cold and wet state, and adjunctive therapy is indicated. Positive inotropic agents, such as milrinone, will increase CO to maintain perfusion to vital organs. Milrinone will also vasodilate the peripheral vessels to unload the heart (↓ SVR). The milrinone dose has been adjusted to accommodate the patient's degree of renal insufficiency. Again, although dobutamine would be a potential choice in this patient, it is not recommended in patients receiving b-blockers. Low-dose nitroglycerin causes venous dilation; however, this patient would benefit from arterial dilation as well. Only higher doses of nitroglycerin will cause arterial dilation. Phenylephrine has no positive beta effects, so it will not augment contractility. In addition, it will cause vasoconstriction through alpha stimulation, which will further increase SVR and likely worsen CO. Vasoconstrictors are reserved for patients in cardiogenic shock. Even though this patient shows signs of significant hypoperfusion, the BP remains preserved.

4. Answer: A
Treatment options for sustained VT are dependent on concomitant disease states, particularly LVEF (40% cutoff). In a patient with LV dysfunction, class I agents such as procainamide are contraindicated. In a patient whose CrCl is less than 60 mL/minute, sotalol requires a considerable dosage reduction to avoid excess torsades de pointes. Sotalol is not an effective cardioversion drug but is more useful for preventing future episodes of arrhythmias (maintaining sinus rhythm) once sinus rhythm is achieved. Dofetilide is indicated only for AF, not for ventricular arrhythmias; similarly, cardioversion rates with dofetilide are low. Amiodarone is first-line therapy for sustained VT in patients with severe renal insufficiency, HF, and structural heart disease.

5. Answer: C
With the prolonged half-life of amiodarone and extensive fat tissue volume of distribution, it would be expected that hyperthyroid adverse effects would last for at least 3–5 half-lives of the drug, which is anywhere from 5 to 8 months. Although therapeutic levels may fall off substantially by then, 1 month is too soon to expect the effects to subside. Even though some iodine and amiodarone molecules will likely remain absorbed in fat stores for years, if not for life, therapeutic levels should not exist for longer than what is predicted by the half-life.

6. Answer: A
In this patient, the presence of ST-depressions on ECG, positive biomarkers for myocardial necrosis, at least three risk factors for CAD, and history of CAD (prior MI), as well as other factors, suggests a high

risk of future events. In such high-risk patients, cardiac catheterization (invasive strategy) is used to determine whether occluded or partially occluded epicardial arteries exist, which can be intervened on, and whether to make an intervention (stent or percutaneous transluminal coronary angiography). Aspirin and clopidogrel or prasugrel is indicated for an early invasive strategy in the management of an NSTEMI. The GP IIb/IIIa inhibitors abciximab or eptifibatide should be initiated at the time of PCI. Unfractionated heparin, enoxaparin, or fondaparinux should be initiated on presentation and would be appropriate to pair with abciximab or eptifibatide. Abciximab was beneficial only in clinical trials of primary PCI or PCI during the abciximab infusion (early invasive strategy). Abciximab was not superior to placebo when used in a conservative medical management strategy without PCI. Unfractionated heparin together with clopidogrel has been studied in medically managed patients not pursuing catheterization (CURE trial) but was studied in a low-risk patient population. Metformin should be held for 24 hours either before or after the catheterization (especially in those with renal dysfunction) to prevent lactic acidosis.

7. Answer: D
Clopidogrel has been studied most commonly for a 30-day poststenting procedure to prevent acute reocclusion of coronary vessels. Because the stent is not endothelialized for a longer period after drug-eluting stent placement compared with traditional stents, a clopidogrel duration of at least 3 months was initially recommended for sirolimus-eluting stent and at least 6 months after paclitaxel drug-eluting stent placement to prevent risk of acute stent thrombosis. However, this recommendation was recently extended to at least 1 year for both of these drug-eluting stents. Although the duration of clopidogrel has changed, that of ASA 162–325 mg/day has remained the same. This dose of ASA should be continued for at least 3 months for sirolimus- and 6 months for paclitaxel drug-eluting stent. After these timeframes, the ASA dose may then be reduced to 75–162 mg/day indefinitely.

8. Answer: B
Doses of ASA lower than 75 mg/day (e.g., 25 mg) have not proved as efficacious as higher doses of ASA after combination therapy with clopidogrel and a PCI procedure. Aspirin 325 mg should be given to all patients after a PCI procedure with stent implantation throughout the recommended duration of clopidogrel therapy (1 month for bare metal stents, 3 months for sirolimus-eluting stents, and 6 months for paclitaxel-eluting stents). Once the recommended duration of dual therapy is completed, patients should receive a reduced dose of 75–162 mg/day to prevent gastrointestinal and bleeding complications, and 81 mg is within this range of doses (Class I, LOE B). There is no evidence that a higher dose of ASA (650 mg) has any benefit over lower doses of ASA, and it has a higher risk of adverse effects; thus, it is not recommended.

9. Answer: A
Although this patient presented within 3 hours of chest pain onset and is a thrombolytic candidate (within less than 6 hours of onset is preferred), up to 95% of patients can achieve normal, brisk TIMI-3 flow rates with primary PCI versus only 50%–60% of patients achieving normal TIMI-3 coronary flow with thrombolytic therapy. Because he is in a hospital that can perform a primary PCI with stent implantation, this is the therapy of choice. Although GP IIb/IIIa inhibitors have been studied in combination with thrombolytics and anticoagulants for STEMI, the slight increase in TIMI-3 blood flow rates was accompanied by a substantially increased risk of bleeding; thus, they are not recommended. Tirofiban and UFH alone are not indicated for treatment of STEMI (recommended for medical management of non-STEMI [NSTEMI] acute coronary syndrome only).

10. Answer: C
Unlike the patient in case 9, this patient presents with a STEMI to a rural community hospital. He presents within the window for thrombolytic therapy consideration (less than 6 hours after chest pain onset). He is experiencing complete heart block and bradycardia, which could indicate an occlusion above the area perfusing his sinoatrial and/or AV nodes. Because he is still having ischemic chest pain and ST-segment elevation, he should benefit from reperfusion therapy. Enoxaparin is a treatment option for medical management, but the patient is at higher risk of bleeding from impaired enoxaparin clearance and requires dosage adjustment. Simply treating this patient conservatively with UFH alone in the setting of ongoing chest pain, shortness of breath, and pulmonary edema is not an optimal choice. Diagnostic catheterization and possible PCI to determine whether an artery can be reperfused are not desirable because of the patient's elevated SCr (CrCl 35 mL/minute). Because of the shorter half-life and ease of administration of tenecteplase, it is preferable to alteplase. Clearance of UFH is not as altered as enoxaparin and would be a more appropriate therapy than enoxaparin in combination with a thrombolytic.

11. Answer: C

This patient is already receiving therapy with calcium channel blockers to control her HR caused by AF. She is taking a considerable dose of diltiazem, and her HR likely will not tolerate further increases in therapy. Sildenafil is indicated for functional class I patients to improve symptoms or for patients whose other therapies have failed. Although bosentan is an attractive oral option to manage her PAH, her liver enzymes are elevated more than 3 times the upper limit of normal. In this setting, administering bosentan is not recommended. If liver transaminases are elevated transiently because of hepatic congestion, bosentan may be reconsidered later. Because this patient is currently in functional class IV with symptoms at rest, epoprostenol is indicated for a survival benefit.

12. Answer: A

Hypertensive emergency should be treated immediately by a 25% reduction in MAP, followed by a slow reduction to goal for 5–7 days. The patient's comorbidities guide the optimal therapy. His dialysis and SCr of 11.4 mg/dL are a contraindication to sodium nitroprusside caused by possible thiocyanate toxicity. Labetalol (β-blockers in general) is controversial in patients who have taken cocaine, but its nonselective nature makes it an option; however, a reduction of 50% initially is too rapid a decrease in BP for safety. Clonidine is not an appropriate drug for hypertensive emergency because its unpredictable oral nature is difficult to titrate and can lead to precipitous drops in BP beyond the goal 25% reduction and possibly stroke or worsening MI. Nitroglycerin is an optimal choice, considering the patient's lack of contraindications to this therapy and his evolving MI.

ANSWERS AND EXPLANATIONS TO SELF-ASSESSMENT QUESTIONS

1. Answer: C
Bosentan is an inducer of CYP3A4 and CYP2C9 isoenzymes. Bosentan decreases the plasma concentrations of all hormonal contraceptive medications, including both estrogen- and progesterone-containing formulations, because of its effects on CYP metabolism. No hormonal contraceptive, including oral, injectable, topical (patch), and implantable formulations, should be used as the only means of contraception because it may not effectively prevent pregnancy in patients taking bosentan. Use of a double-barrier method with a condom and diaphragm plus spermicide is indicated in patients receiving bosentan and hormonal contraceptives. Because bosentan is also a known teratogen, a barrier method alone may not be a sufficient form of contraception.

2. Answer: C
Patients with dietary and/or drug nonadherence most commonly present with warm and wet exacerbation of their HF. Although they are well perfused and their CO has not changed substantially (i.e., their disease has not progressed), their habits have caused them to retain excess fluid. Dobutamine and milrinone primarily increase CO, which is not a considerable problem in warm and wet exacerbations. In addition, the adverse effects of these agents (increased mortality, proarrhythmia) limit their use. Nesiritide is a balanced arterial and venous dilator that decreases afterload and preload, respectively, and is the best choice for this patient without an invasive hemodynamic monitoring catheter in place. Although intravenous nitroglycerin is effective in warm and wet exacerbations, its use requires dosage titration by a Swan-Ganz catheter or central venous catheter, which is not in place in this patient at this time.

3. Answer: B
This patient shows target organ damage from poorly controlled HTN in the form of a cerebrovascular accident. Although fenoldopam is indicated for treating hypertensive emergency, its use is cautioned in patients with stroke symptoms because its dopamine agonist activity can cause cerebral vasodilation and potentially reduced bloodflow to the ischemic areas of the brain. Nicardipine is an appropriate choice in this patient because its calcium channel blocking effects will reduce BP and potentially decrease vasospasm in the cerebral arteries, which may lead to further ischemia or seizure activity. Although labetalol is an effective option for treating H.E.'s hypertensive emergency, she has a history of asthma and a low HR, making labetalol a less-than-ideal option for treating her symptoms. The antihypertensive effects of enalaprilat are dependent on a patient's renin activity, which is not known in this case. Therefore, the BP-reducing effects may be more difficult to control than with a drug having a more consistent effect in individuals. In addition, the bolus nature of the drug is not ideal for tightly controlling BP with a 25% reduction in MAP. Continuous-infusion drugs are preferable for easier titration to effect in a hypertensive emergency.

4. Answer: D
Although several drug classes for treating acute MI are linked with thrombocytopenia, the timeframe in which the thrombocytopenia occurs is a key factor in distinguishing which agent is causative. Although UFH can produce a rapid drop in platelet count on reexposure, the nadir in platelet count is typically around $50 \times 10^3/mm^3$. Adenosine diphosphate inhibitors, particularly ticlopidine, are linked with rare isolated thrombocytopenia. Clopidogrel rarely causes thrombotic thrombocytopenic purpura, which, in turn, causes thrombocytopenia and a constellation of other symptoms (mental status changes, acute renal failure, etc.) usually for longer treatment durations of weeks to months after therapy initiation. Abciximab can cause acute profound thrombocytopenia in about 1.5% of patients treated. The timeframe is almost immediate (usually within 2–24 hours of administration initiation) and causes a nadir of about $20 \times 10^3/mm^3$ platelets.

5. Answer: C
The number needed to treat can be calculated by 1/absolute risk reduction. Because the absolute risk reduction in mortality at 60 months was 7.2% with ICD versus placebo, 1/0.072 would be used to calculate the number of patients needed to treat to prevent one death during this time. About 13.8 patients would need to be treated with ICD to prevent one death in 60 months versus placebo. Other calculations in this fashion, including relative risk reduction and 100% minus the absolute or relative risk reduction, do not provide useful information for interpreting the trial results and yield an incorrect number of patients.

6. Answer: C

The Cardiac Arrest Study Hamburg trial compared ICD implantation with antiarrhythmic therapy in survivors of cardiac arrest for secondary prevention of sudden cardiac death. The propafenone study arm was discontinued early because of a significantly (61%) higher mortality rate compared with ICDs. Although this trial had a small sample size that prevented a statistically significant difference in total mortality from being shown in ICD-treated patients versus patients treated with either amiodarone or metoprolol, the incidence of sudden death was significantly reduced in patients with an ICD implanted (33% vs. 13%, p=0.005). The AVID (Antiarrhythmics Versus Implantable Defibrillators) trial also evaluated ICD implantation versus antiarrhythmic drug therapy (primarily amiodarone) in survivors of sudden cardiac death. Patients implanted with ICDs had a significantly greater rate of survival than those treated with drug therapy (89% vs. 82%, p<0.02).

7. Answer: D

S.V. has a depressed LVEF less than 40%, so her drug therapy options are limited to prevent the development of worsening HF, which could occur if she were administered procainamide for treatment of her arrhythmia. Procainamide is indicated only in secondary prevention of sustained VT in patients with a normal LVEF greater than 40%. Metoprolol is indicated only for the treatment of patients with asymptomatic nonsustained VT and SVT associated with CAD. S.V. had a symptomatic episode of sustained VT. Her QTc interval is not prolonged at 380 milliseconds, so she does not require intravenous magnesium therapy. She qualifies for treatment with either amiodarone or lidocaine. Amiodarone is first-line treatment of patients without contraindications because of its efficacy.

8. Answer: D

International Pharmaceutical Abstracts is a database of primarily pharmaceutical abstracts in more than 750 journals, including foreign and state pharmacy journals, in addition to key U.S. medical and pharmacy journals. Many of the citations are not included on MEDLINE, so a broader search can be performed; however, subject descriptors are not consistently defined in a uniform way, and multiword terms are often cited backward. The Iowa Drug Information Service database offers full-text articles from 1966 to present in about 200 medical and pharmacy journals (primarily based in the United States). It is updated monthly, so newly available articles may take longer to be accessed from this service. The Clin-Alert database contains more than 100 medical and pharmacy journals focused on adverse events, drug interactions, and medical-legal issues. It is used primarily to look up adverse events (especially recent reports) associated with medications. Excerpta Medica is a comprehensive database of more than 7000 journals from 74 countries dating from 1974 to present. Recently published articles appear in the system within 10 days of article publication, and it often contains data not found in a typical MEDLINE search.

9. Answer: B

MedWatch is a post–U.S. Food and Drug Administration (FDA) approval program established by the FDA for health care professionals to report to the FDA the adverse events that occur after a drug is approved. Although it is commonly used only for reporting serious reactions to the FDA, it can be used to report any adverse event. Information recorded on these forms is reported to the manufacturer and is used to determine whether black box warnings are necessary or whether new adverse effects are seen with a drug. The Joint Commission requires that all institutions have a definition of an ADR for the institution that all health care professionals can understand and remember. In addition, The Joint Commission requires that each dose of drug administered be monitored for adverse effects, that each institution have a system for reporting ADRs in place, and that the institution ensure that the reporting mechanism identifies all key ADRs.

10. Answer: B

Because the Pharmacy and Therapeutics Committee wants to discover whether the new drug is worth the extra cost for the added mortality benefits it can provide for patients with decompensated HF compared with available therapies, a cost-effectiveness analysis is the best pharmacoeconomic analysis to perform. Cost-minimization analysis is used to determine whether a therapeutically equivalent drug within a class that provides a therapeutic outcome the same as others available can be used for less cost. Cost-utility analysis is used to determine whether a drug can improve the quality of a patient's life more than other available therapies. Cost-benefit analysis is used to evaluate new programs or services to determine whether they provide enough benefit to be worth the cost of running the program.

OUTPATIENT CARDIOLOGY

**ROBERT L PAGE II, PHARM.D., MSPH, FCCP,
FASHP, FAHA, FASCP, BCPS, CGP**

UNIVERSITY OF COLORADO DENVER
SCHOOLS OF PHARMACY AND MEDICINE
AURORA, COLORADO

OUTPATIENT CARDIOLOGY

ROBERT L PAGE II, PHARM.D., MSPH, FCCP, FASHP, FAHA, FASCP, BCPS, CGP

UNIVERSITY OF COLORADO DENVER
SCHOOLS OF PHARMACY AND MEDICINE
AURORA, COLORADO

Learning Objectives:

1. Recommend patient-specific pharmacologic management of chronic heart failure, with an emphasis on mortality-reducing drugs and their target dosages.

2. Develop an appropriate pharmacologic and monitoring plan for patients with atrial fibrillation.

3. Given a patient with hypertension, outline the optimal pharmacologic management based on practice guidelines and clinical trial evidence.

4. Create an evidence-based drug regimen for a patient with coronary artery disease in both the presence and absence of stable angina.

Self-Assessment Questions:

Answers to these questions may be found at the end of this chapter.

1. R.S., a 58-year-old woman with a history of hypertension, coronary artery disease (CAD) (s/p myocardial infarction [MI] 4 months ago), and dyslipidemia presents to the clinic for follow-up. She is without complaints and specifically has no symptoms of dyspnea or edema. An echocardiogram reveals a left ventricular ejection fraction (LVEF) of 35%. Her drugs include aspirin 325 mg/day, metoprolol succinate 200 mg/day, and simvastatin 20 mg every night. Her vital signs include heart rate (HR) 58 beats/minute and blood pressure (BP) 138/80 mm Hg. Her lungs are clear, and her laboratory results are within the reference range. Which one of the following is the best management of R.S.'s drug therapy?

   A. Continue current therapy.
   B. Initiate digoxin 0.125 mg/day.
   C. Initiate carvedilol 3.125 mg 2 times/day.
   D. Initiate enalapril 5 mg 2 times/day.

2. J.O., a 64-year-old woman with New York Heart Association (NYHA) class III nonischemic dilated cardiomyopathy and an LVEF of 40%, presents to the heart failure (HF) clinic for follow-up. She has no complaints. Her drugs include enalapril 10 mg 2 times/day, furosemide 40 mg 2 times/day, and potassium chloride (KCl) 20 mEq 2 times/day. Her vital signs include BP 130/88 mm Hg and HR 78 beats/minute. Her laboratory results are within normal limits. Which one of the following is the best management of her HF?

   A. Continue current regimen.
   B. Increase enalapril to 20 mg 2 times/day.
   C. Initiate metoprolol extended release 12.5 mg/day.
   D. Initiate digoxin 0.125 mg/day.

3. J.M. is a 65-year-old woman with a history of hypertension and poor drug adherence who presents to her primary care physician with dyspnea and markedly decreased exercise tolerance. An echocardiogram reveals an LVEF of 65% with considerable diastolic dysfunction. J.M.'s drugs include nifedipine extended release 60 mg/day and hydrochlorothiazide 25 mg/day. Her vital signs include HR 98 beats/minute and BP 128/78 mm Hg. Her lung fields are clear to auscultation, and there is no evidence of systemic congestion. Which one of the following is the best pharmacologic management for J.M.?

   A. Discontinue nifedipine and initiate diltiazem 240 mg/day.
   B. Discontinue hydrochlorothiazide and initiate furosemide 40 mg 2 times/day.
   C. Initiate digoxin 0.25 mg/day.
   D. Add enalapril 5 mg 2 times/day.

4. B.W. is a 78-year-old man with a history of hypertension, peripheral arterial disease, reflux disease, and atrial fibrillation (AF). His therapy includes aspirin 325 mg/day, lansoprazole 30 mg every night, atenolol 50 mg/day, lisinopril 10 mg/day, and atorvastatin 20 mg/day. His BP is 132/72 mm Hg, and HR is 68 beats/minute. Which one of the following is the best therapy for B.W. at this time?

   A. Add diltiazem and warfarin.
   B. Add digoxin and increase lisinopril to 20 mg/day.
   C. Discontinue atorvastatin and add warfarin.
   D. Add warfarin and decrease aspirin to 81 mg/day.

5. Z.G. is a 61-year-old man with AF, hypertension, and hypercholesterolemia. His drugs include digoxin 0.25 mg/day, warfarin 5 mg/day, amlodipine 10 mg/day, and pravastatin 20 mg every night. He comes to the clinic today with no complaints except for palpitations and dyspnea when doing yard work. His vital signs include BP 138/80 mm Hg and HR 72 beats/minute. All laboratory results are within normal limits; his international normalized ratio (INR) is 2.4, and his digoxin concentration is 1.1 ng/dL. Which one of the following is the best option to help with Z.G.'s symptoms?

A. Add atenolol 50 mg/day.
B. Increase digoxin to 0.5 mg/day.
C. Continue current regimen; advise Z.G. to avoid activities that cause symptoms.
D. Add verapamil 240 mg/day.

6. R.P. is an 82-year-old African American man with a history of hypertension, a transient ischemic attack, and gout. His drugs include allopurinol 300 mg/day, nifedipine extended release 60 mg/day, and aspirin 81 mg/day. His vital signs include BP 145/85 mm Hg and HR 82 beats/minute. Which one of the following is the best approach to improve R.P.'s BP control?
   A. Add hydrochlorothiazide 50 mg/day.
   B. Add ramipril 2.5 mg/day.
   C. Add atenolol 50 mg/day.
   D. Add diltiazem 240 mg/day.

7. M.L. is a 32-year-old white woman with a history of type 1 diabetes mellitus and hypertension. She takes lisinopril 10 mg/day and uses insulin. During her clinic visit, a pregnancy test is performed to follow up on a positive home pregnancy test the patient performed. The results confirm a pregnancy. Her BP today is 162/105 mm Hg, and HR is 88 beats/minute. Which one of the following is the best therapy for her BP at this time?
   A. Increase lisinopril to 20 mg/day and add hydrochlorothiazide.
   B. Add hydralazine.
   C. Discontinue lisinopril and begin methyldopa.
   D. Discontinue lisinopril and add losartan.

8. You are asked to design a randomized, placebo-controlled, clinical trial to examine the ability of a new ACE inhibitor, Trillionapril, versus enalapril, to reduce coronary events in patients with a Framingham 10-year risk of cardiovascular events of more than 20%. The plan is to include 4500 patients in each group and to monitor them for an average of 4.8 years. Which one of the following statistical tests is best for comparing the proportion of cardiovascular events in patients receiving Trillionapril versus enalapril?
   A. Analysis of variance.
   B. Mann-Whitney U-test.
   C. Student unpaired t-test.
   D. Chi-square analysis.

9. J.T. is a 58-year-old man being discharged from the hospital after undergoing a diagnostic cardiac catheterization when a treadmill test showed some mild abnormalities. His medical history is notable only for hypercholesterolemia. The procedure showed a 70% lesion of the proximal left anterior descending artery, which was stented, in addition to mild luminal irregularities throughout most other arteries. Before admission, his drugs were aspirin 81 mg/day and simvastatin 40 mg every night (past low-density lipoprotein cholesterol [LDL-C] was 120 mg/dL). His BP is 135/75 mm Hg, and his HR is 80 beats/minute. His discharge orders currently include the following drugs: aspirin 81 mg/day, clopidogrel 75 mg/day for 6 months (to ensure stent patency), simvastatin 80 mg every night, and ezetimibe 10 mg/day. Is there anything you would like to do differently regarding his discharge drugs?
   A. Discontinue simvastatin plus ezetimibe and begin atorvastatin 80 mg/day.
   B. Discontinue ezetimibe and add gemfibrozil 600 mg 2 times/day.
   C. Add ramipril 5 mg/day.
   D. Add atenolol 25 mg/day.

10. R.K. is a 67-year-old man with chronic stable angina. He has had worsening chest discomfort with exercise and has been using his "as-needed" nitroglycerin with increasing frequency. His cardiovascular drugs consist of aspirin 325 mg/day, atenolol 100 mg/day, atorvastatin 80 mg/day, and lisinopril 20 mg/day. Today, his BP is 136/80 mm Hg, and HR is 60 beats/minute. During exercise, his HR typically increases to about 85 beats/minute. Which one of the following suggestions to improve his angina symptom control is best?
    A. Add amlodipine 10 mg/day.
    B. Discontinue atenolol and begin extended-release nifedipine 90 mg/day.
    C. Add clopidogrel 75 mg/day.
    D. Add ezetimibe 10 mg/day.

Patient Cases

1. L.S. is a 48-year-old woman with alcohol-induced cardiomyopathy. Her most recent LVEF is 20%; her daily activities are limited by dyspnea and fatigue (NYHA class III). Her medications include lisinopril 20 mg/day, furosemide 40 mg 2 times/day, carvedilol 12.5 mg 2 times/day, spironolactone 25 mg/day, and digoxin 0.125 mg/day. Her most recent laboratory results include the following: sodium (Na) 140 mEq/L, K 4.0 mEq/L, Cl 105 mEq/L, bicarbonate 26 mEq/L, blood urea nitrogen (BUN) 12 mg/dL, serum creatinine (SCr) 0.8 mg/dL, glucose 98 mg/dL, calcium 9.0 mg/dL, phosphorus 2.8 mg/dL, magnesium (Mg) 2.0 mEq/L, and digoxin 0.7 ng/mL. Her vital signs today include BP of 112/70 mm Hg and HR of 68 beats/minute. Which one of the following is the best approach for maximizing the management of her HF?
    A. Increase carvedilol to 25 mg 2 times/day.
    B. Increase lisinopril to 40 mg/day.
    C. Increase spironolactone to 50 mg/day.
    D. Increase digoxin to 0.25 mg/day.

2. J.T. is a 62-year-old man with a history of CAD (MI 3 years ago), hypertension, depression, chronic renal insufficiency (baseline SCr is 2.8 mg/dL), peripheral arterial disease, osteoarthritis, hypothyroidism, and HF with an LVEF of 25%. His medications include aspirin 81 mg/day, simvastatin 40 mg every night, enalapril 5 mg 2 times/day, metoprolol extended release 50 mg/day, furosemide 80 mg 2 times/day, cilostazol 100 mg 2 times/day, acetaminophen 650 mg 4 times/day, sertraline 100 mg/day, and levothyroxine 0.1 mg/day. His vital signs include BP 120/70 mm Hg and HR 72 beats/minute. Laboratory results are within normal limits, except for a SCr of 2.8. Thyroid-stimulating hormone is 2.6 milliunits/L. His HF is stable and considered NYHA class II. Which one of the following is the best approach for maximizing the management of his HF?
    A. Discontinue metoprolol and begin carvedilol 12.5 mg 2 times/day.
    B. Increase enalapril to 10 mg 2 times/day.
    C. Add spironolactone 25 mg/day.
    D. Add digoxin 0.125 mg/day.

I. HEART FAILURE

A. Background: HF is a complex clinical syndrome that can result from any structural or functional cardiac disorder that impairs the ability of the ventricle to fill with or eject blood.
   1. Systolic dysfunction (decreased EF less than 40%)
      a. Impaired wall motion
      b. Dilated ventricle
      c. Two-thirds attributable to CAD
      d. One-third attributable to nonischemic cardiomyopathy
         i. Hypertension
         ii. Thyroid disease
         iii. Valvular disease
         iv. Cardiotoxins
             (A) Alcohol
             (B) Chemotherapeutic agents
                 (1) Anthracyclines
                 (2) Cyclophosphamide
                 (3) 5-Fluorouracil
                 (4) Trastuzumab
         v. Myocarditis
         vi. Idiopathic

2. Diastolic dysfunction (preserved/normal EF)
   a. Accounts for about 30% of patients with HF
   b. Impaired ventricular relaxation and filling
   c. Normal wall motion
   d. Most are caused by hypertension and age-related decreases in the elastic properties of the cardiovascular system.
   e. Some are caused by various cardiomyopathies (e.g., restrictive, infiltrative, hypertrophic).
3. Primary symptoms
   a. Dyspnea
   b. Fatigue
   c. Edema
   d. Exercise intolerance
4. Stages of HF

Table 1.

Stage	Description	Patient Population
A	At high risk of HF but without structural heart disease or symptoms of HF	Patients with hypertension, atherosclerotic disease, diabetes mellitus, obesity, or metabolic syndrome OR patients using cardiotoxins or having a family history of cardiomyopathy
B	Structural heart disease but without signs or symptoms of HF	Patients with a previous MI, left ventricular remodeling, or asymptomatic valvular disease
C	Structural heart disease with prior or current symptoms of HF	Patients with known structural heart disease and shortness of breath, fatigue, and/or reduced exercise tolerance
D	Refractory HF requiring specialized interventions	Patients who have marked symptoms at rest despite maximal medical therapy (e.g., those who are recurrently hospitalized or cannot be safely discharged from the hospital without specialized interventions)

HF = heart failure; MI = myocardial infarction.

5. New York Heart Association classification of HF

Table 2.

NYHA Functional Class	Description
I	No limitations in physical activity because of HF symptoms
II	Symptoms of HF with normal level of activity
III	Marked limitations in physical activity because of HF symptoms
IV	Symptoms of HF at rest

HF = heart failure; NYHA = New York Heart Association.

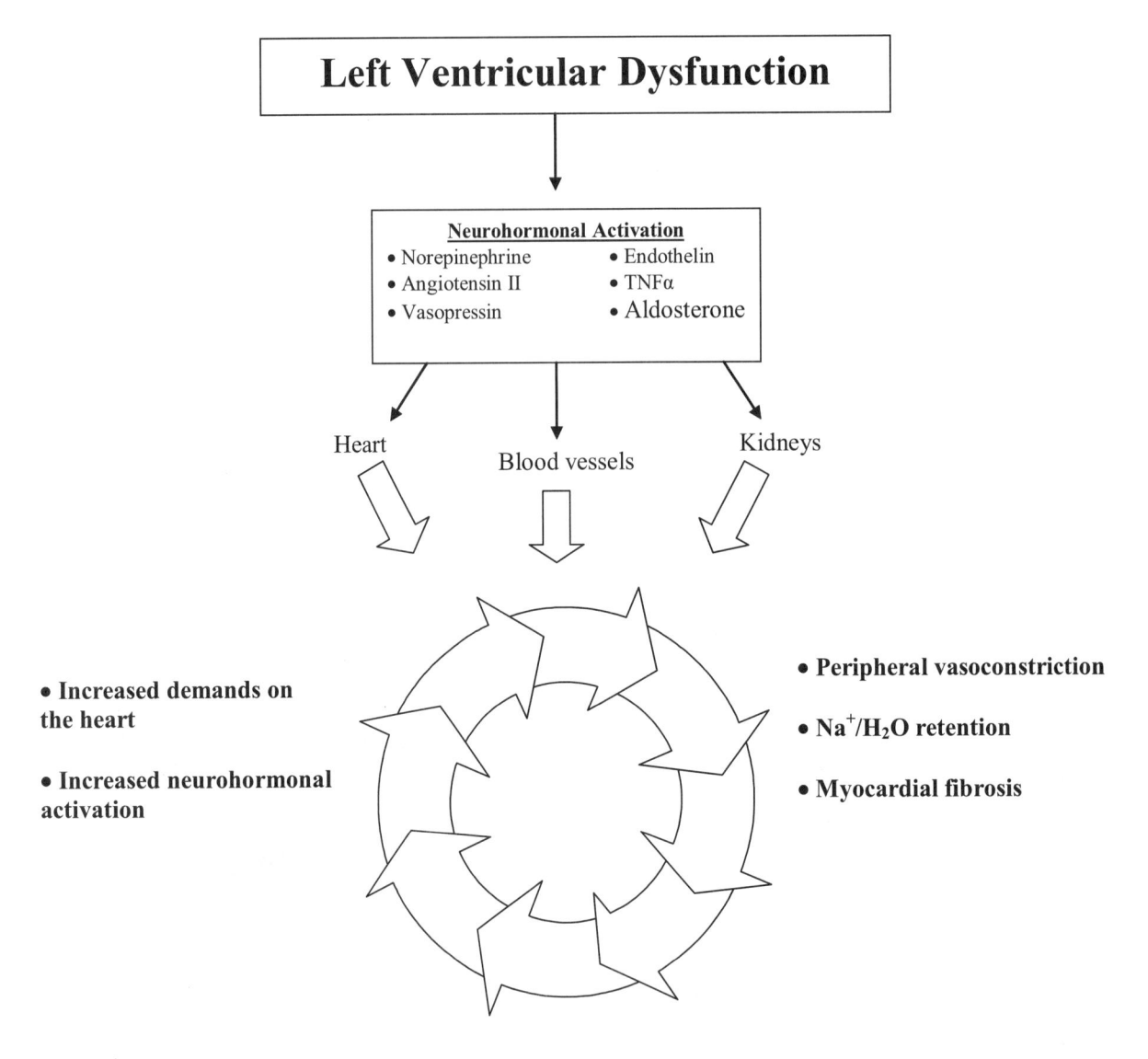

Left Ventricular Dysfunction

Neurohormonal Activation
- Norepinephrine
- Angiotensin II
- Vasopressin
- Endothelin
- TNFα
- Aldosterone

Heart → Increased demands on the heart; Increased neurohormonal activation

Blood vessels

Kidneys → Peripheral vasoconstriction; Na^+/H_2O retention; Myocardial fibrosis

Figure 1.
H_2O = water; Na = sodium; TNFα = tumor necrosis factor alpha.

- B. Pharmacologic Therapy for Systolic HF
    1. Principles of therapy
        a. Block the compensatory neurohormonal activation caused by decreased cardiac output that promotes further cardiac deterioration and damage.
        b. Prevent/minimize Na and water retention.
        c. Eliminate or minimize symptoms of HF (increase quality of life).
        d. Slow the progression of cardiac dysfunction.
        e. Decrease mortality.
    2. Management of fluid overload with diuretics
        a. Short-term benefits (days)
            i. Decreased jugular venous distension
            ii. Decreased pulmonary congestion
            iii. Decreased peripheral edema

  b. Intermediate-term benefits (weeks to months)
    i. Decreased daily symptoms
    ii. Improved cardiac function
    iii. Increased exercise tolerance
  c. Long-term benefits (months to years): no benefit on mortality
  d. Diuretic caveats
    i. Never use as the only therapy for HF because they have no effect on disease progression or mortality
    ii. If a patient has fluid overload, initiate and adjust therapy to result in 1–2 lb of weight loss per day (may be more aggressive in the inpatient setting).
    iii. Chronic therapy should be adjusted to maintain a euvolemic state.
    iv. Monitor and replace K and Mg as needed, especially with loop diuretics (goal with cardiovascular disease is K of 4.0 mEq/L or higher and Mg of 2.0 mEq/L or higher to minimize arrhythmias).
    v. Loop diuretics are recommended because of greater diuretic capabilities.
     a. Loop diuretics retain efficacy with decreased renal function.
    vi. May combine loop diuretic with another class (e.g., thiazide diuretic) for synergy if needed

Table 3.

Diuretic Class	Examples	Increase in Sodium Excretion (%)
Loop	Furosemide, bumetanide, torsemide	25–30
Thiazide	Hydrochlorothiazide, metolazone, chlorthalidone	5–8
Potassium sparing	Amiloride, triamterene, spironolactone	2–3

3. Neurohormonal blockade
  a. Angiotensin-converting enzyme (ACE) inhibitors
    i. Benefits of ACE inhibitor
     (A) Decreased mortality (about 25% relative risk reduction vs. placebo)
     (B) Decreased hospitalizations (about 30% relative risk reduction vs. placebo)
     (C) Symptom improvement
     (D) Improved clinical status
     (E) Improved sense of well-being
    ii. Mechanism of action
     (A) Blocks production of angiotensin II
      (1) Decreases sympathetic stimulation
      (2) Decreases production of aldosterone and vasopressin
      (3) Decreases vasoconstriction (afterload)
     (B) Increases bradykinins (decreases their metabolism)
      (1) Increases vasodilatory prostaglandins
    iii. Place in therapy
     (A) Should be used in all patients with LV dysfunction (even if asymptomatic)
    iv. Dosing considerations
     (A) Start low and increase dose every 1–4 weeks to goal.
     (B) Benefits of high versus low doses

(C) Patient may notice improvement in several weeks.

Table 4.

Drug	Starting Dosage	Target Dosage	Maximal Dosage
Captopril	6.25 mg TID	50 mg TID	50 mg TID
Enalapril	2.5 mg BID	10 mg BID	20 mg BID
Lisinopril	2.5–5 mg/day	20 mg/day	40 mg/day
Perindopril	2 mg/day	8 mg/day	16 mg/day
Ramipril	1.25–2.5 mg/day	5 mg BID	10 mg/day
Trandolapril	1 mg/day	4 mg/day	4 mg/day

Note: Fosinopril and quinapril may be used; however, they do not have the same magnitude of mortality-reducing data as the above-listed ACE inhibitor.
BID = 2 times/day; TID = 3 times/day.

v. Monitoring
  (A) Serum creatinine, BP, and K in 1–2 weeks after starting or increasing the dose, especially in high-risk individuals (e.g., those with systolic BP less than 90 mm Hg, with serum Na concentrations less than 130 mmol/L, or receiving high loses of loop diuretics)
    (1) Serum creatinine may rise (up to a 0.5-mg/dL increase is acceptable) because of renal efferent artery dilation (results in a slightly decreased glomerular filtration rate).
      (a) Rarely, acute renal failure occurs, especially if the patient is intravascularly depleted (be careful to avoid overdiuresis).
      (b) Use cautiously in patients with a baseline SCr more than 3.0 mg/dL (NOT a contraindication; they should still be used, just with smaller dosage changes and increased monitoring).
    (2) Monitor BP and symptoms of hypotension (e.g., dizzy, light-headed).
      (a) Blood pressure may be low to begin with because of low cardiac output. BP = CO × SVR
      (CO = cardiac output, SVR = systemic vascular resistance).
      (b) In HF, as cardiac output increases because of decreased systemic vascular resistance, BP may decrease slightly or remain about the same.
      (c) Symptoms of hypotension are often not present with small dose increases. Remember to treat the patient, not the number.
    (3) Potassium may rise because of decreased glomerular filtration rate and decreased aldosterone.
      (a) Use cautiously in those with a baseline K greater than 5.0 mEq/L.
  (B) Ninety percent of people tolerate ACE inhibitors.
    (1) Angioedema (less than 1%) – could switch to angiotensin II receptor blockers (ARBs; cross-reactivity is 2.5%)
    (2) Cough (5%–10%) – could switch to ARBs (less than 1%)
b. β-Blockers
  i. Benefits of β-blockade (when added to an ACE inhibitor)
    (A) Decreased mortality (about 35% relative risk reduction vs. placebo)
    (B) Decreased hospitalizations (about 25% relative risk reduction vs. placebo)
    (C) Symptom improvement
    (D) Improved clinical status

(E) Improved sense of well-being
ii. Mechanism of action
(A) Blocks the effect of norepinephrine and other sympathetic neurotransmitters on the heart and vascular system
(1) Decreases ventricular arrhythmias (sudden death)
(2) Decreases cardiac hypertrophy and cardiac cell death
(3) Decreases vasoconstriction and HR
(B) Carvedilol also provides β-blockade.
(1) Further decreases systemic vascular resistance (afterload)
iii. Place in therapy
(A) Should be used in all stable patients (e.g., those not receiving intravenous inotropic or diuretic therapy, those without peripheral and pulmonary congestion) with LV dysfunction (even if asymptomatic)
iv. Dosing considerations
(A) Added to existing ACE inhibitor therapy (at least at a low dose) when HF symptoms are stable and patients are euvolemic
(B) Start low and increase (double) the dose every 2–4 weeks (or slowly, if needed) to goal.
(C) Avoid abrupt discontinuation; can precipitate clinical deterioration
(D) Patient may notice improvement in several months.
(E) Benefits of high versus low doses

Table 5.

Agent	Starting Dosage	Target Dosage
Bisoprolol	1.25 mg/day	10 mg/day
Carvedilol	3.125 mg BID	25 mg BID[a]
Metoprolol succinate extended release[b] (metoprolol CR/XL)	12.5–25 mg/day	200 mg/day

[a]Fifty milligrams 2 times/day if weight is more than 85 kg.
[b]Few or no data exist with metoprolol tartrate.
BID = 2 times/day; CR = controlled release; XL = extended release.

v. Monitoring
(A) Blood pressure, HR, and hypotension, dizziness (monitor in 1–2 weeks)
(1) Significant hypotension, bradycardia, or dizziness occurs in about 1% of patients on β-blocker therapy when titrated slowly. If these appear, lower the dose by 50%. Discontinue the drug only if patient has heart block or is in cardiogenic shock.
(2) With carvedilol, dizziness and hypotension are more common, usually occurring within 24–48 hours of a dosage increase.
(3) The net decrease in HR at goal doses of β-blocker is only 10–15 beats/minute from baseline.
(B) Increased edema/fluid retention (monitor in 1–2 weeks)
(1) From 1% to 2% more common than placebo (in euvolemic, stable patients)
(2) Responds to diuretic increase
(C) Fatigue or weakness
(1) From 1% to 2% more common than placebo

(2) Usually resolves spontaneously in several weeks
(3) May require dosage decrease or discontinuation
- c. Aldosterone blockade
    - i. Patient population
        - (A) Class III and IV HF
        - (B) Left ventricular dysfunction immediately after MI
    - ii. Benefits of spironolactone in class III and IV HF
        - (A) Decreased mortality (30% relative risk reduction vs. placebo)
        - (B) Decreased hospitalizations for HF (35% relative risk reduction vs. placebo)
        - (C) Improved symptoms
    - iii. Benefits of eplerenone (a selective aldosterone blocker) with LV dysfunction after MI
        - (A) Decreased mortality (13% relative risk reduction vs. placebo)
    - iv. Mechanism of action
        - (A) Blocks effects of aldosterone in the kidneys, heart, and vasculature
            - (1) Decreases K and Mg loss
                - (a) Decreases ventricular arrhythmias
            - (2) Decreases Na retention
                - (a) Decreases fluid retention
            - (3) Eliminates catecholamine potentiation
                - (a) Decreases BP
            - (4) Blocks direct fibrotic actions on the myocardium
    - v. Place in therapy
        - (A) Should be considered in all patients with class III and IV HF who are receiving background therapy with an ACE inhibitor, diuretic, and β-blocker or after an MI with LV dysfunction
        - (B) Avoid use in combination with both ACE inhibitor and ARB; the effects of all three agents on K have not been adequately characterized.
    - vi. Dosing considerations
        - (A) Dosing
            - (1) Spironolactone 12.5–25 mg/day
            - (2) Eplerenone 25–50 mg/day
        - (B) Avoid use if SCr is greater than 2.5 mg/dL or serum K is greater than 5.0 mEq/L.
    - vii. Monitoring
        - (A) Potassium within 1 week of starting therapy
            - (1) Hyperkalemia was reported in only 2% of patients in the trial; however, in practice, it occurs in about 10% of patients.
            - (2) Decrease dose by 50% or discontinue if K is greater than 5.5 mEq/L.
        - (B) Gynecomastia
            - (1) For spironolactone, gynecomastia was reported at a rate of 10% in clinical trials.
            - (2) Eplerenone: A selective aldosterone blocker, it has only been studied in a very narrow subset of the HF population (post-MI with decreased EF); may be considered in class III and IV patients with painful gynecomastia
4. Digoxin
    - a. Benefits of digoxin
        - i. Improves symptoms
        - ii. Improves exercise tolerance

- iii. Small decrease in hospitalizations
- iv. No effect on mortality
  - b. Mechanism of action (in HF) by Na-K adenosine triphosphatase inhibition
    - i. Decreases central sympathetic outflow by sensitizing cardiac baroreceptors
    - ii. Decreases renal reabsorption of Na
    - iii. Minimal increase in cardiac contractility because of the inhibition of Na-K adenosine triphosphatase. This is not thought to cause beneficial effects in HF.
  - c. Place in therapy
    - i. Should be considered in patients with symptomatic LV dysfunction despite optimal ACE inhibitor (or ARB), β-blocker, spironolactone (if appropriate), and diuretic therapy
  - d. Dosing considerations and monitoring
    - i. Serum concentrations of 0.5–0.8 ng/dL are effective in HF.
      - (A) Minimizes the risk of adverse effects and ventricular arrhythmias associated with increased concentrations
      - (B) Risk of toxicity increased with age and renal dysfunction
      - (C) Risk of toxicity increased in the presence of hypokalemia or hypomagnesemia
    - ii. For most patients, 0.125 mg/day is adequate to achieve the desired serum concentration. Loading doses are not recommended in the population.
    - iii. Useful initial agent for patient with concomitant AF
    - iv. Drug interactions. Digoxin concentrations are increased with concomitant:
      - (A) Clarithromycin-erythromycin
      - (B) Amiodarone, dronedarone
      - (C) Itraconazole, posaconazole, voriconazole
      - (D) Cyclosporine
      - (E) Verapamil
5. Hydralazine-isosorbide dinitrate
   a. Benefits
      - i. Decreases mortality 39% versus placebo
      - ii. Decreases hospitalizations 33% versus placebo
   b. Mechanism of action
      - i. Hydralazine
        - (A) Vasodilator
        - (B) Enhances effect of nitrates
      - ii. Isosorbide dinitrate
        - (A) Stimulates nitric acid signaling in the endothelium
   c. Place in therapy
      - i. African Americans with NYHA class II–IV HF, already receiving an ACE inhibitor (or ARB), β-blocker, and diuretic therapy
      - ii. Decreases mortality versus placebo; however, ACE inhibitors have shown a 28% relative risk reduction in death compared with hydralazine-isosorbide dinitrate.
      - iii. A reasonable alternative in patients unable to take an ACE inhibitor or ARB because of severe renal insufficiency, hyperkalemia, or angioedema
   d. Dosing consideration
      - i. Hydralazine (25–75 mg orally 3 or 4 times/day); isosorbide dinitrate (10–40 mg orally 3 times/day). Titrate on the basis of BP.

ii. Fixed-dose BiDil (hydralazine 37.5 mg plus isosorbide dinitrate 20 mg) with a goal dose of 2 tablets 3 times/day
     e. Monitoring
        i. Headache
        ii. Hypotension
        iii. Drug-induced lupus with hydralazine
6. Angiotensin II receptor blockers
   a. Have never been proved superior to ACE inhibitors at target HF dosages
   b. Current role is as an ACE inhibitor substitute for patients unable to take an ACE inhibitor because of cough.
   c. The best ARB to use on the basis of available data is candesartan 32 mg/day or valsartan 160 mg 2 times/day (target doses).

Patient Case

3. Which one of J.T.'s (from case 2) drugs may be adversely affecting his cardiac prognosis?
   A. Acetaminophen.
   B. Sertraline.
   C. Cilostazol.
   D. Levothyroxine.

C. Nonpharmacologic Therapy
   1. Prevent further cardiac injury.
      a. Discontinue smoking.
      b. Reduce weight if obese.
      c. Control hypertension.
      d. Control diabetes mellitus.
      e. Minimize alcohol to two or fewer drinks per day for men, one or fewer drinks per day for women
      f. Eliminate alcohol if cardiomyopathy is alcohol induced.
   2. Limit Na to 2 g/day.
   3. Restrict fluid intake to 2 L/day if serum Na is less than 130 mmol/L or if there is fluid retention despite aggressive diuresis and dietary Na restriction.
   4. Modest exercise program
      a. Benefits of therapy
         i. Possible modest effects on all-cause hospitalization and all-cause mortality
         ii. Safe for patients with HF
   5. Annual influenza vaccine and pneumococcal vaccine every 5 years
   6. Monitor and appropriately replace electrolytes (minimize risk of arrhythmias).
   7. Monitor for thyroid disease.
      a. Hypothyroidism may be masked by HF symptoms.
      b. Hyperthyroidism will worsen systolic dysfunction.
   8. Screen for and treat depression.

D. Drugs to Avoid or Use with Caution
 1. Nonsteroidal anti-inflammatory drugs (NSAIDs; including selective cyclooxygenase-2 inhibitors)
    a. Promote Na and water retention
    b. Blunt diuretic response
 2. Corticosteroids
    a. Promote Na and water retention
 3. Class I and III antiarrhythmic agents (*except* amiodarone and dofetilide)
    a. Negative inotropic activity
    b. Proarrhythmic effects
    c. Amiodarone and dofetilide have been proven safe in patients with HF.
    d. Avoid with dronedarone.
 4. Calcium channel blocking agents (*except* amlodipine and felodipine)
    a. Negative inotropic activity
    b. Neurohormonal activation
    c. Amlodipine and felodipine have been proven safe in patients with HF.
 5. Minoxidil
    a. Fluid retention
    b. Stimulation of the renin-angiotensin-aldosterone system
 6. Thiazolidinediones
    a. Fluid retention
 7. Metformin
    a. Increased risk of lactic acidosis (black box warning)
 8. Anagrelide
    a. Positive inotropic activity
    b. Tachycardia
 9. Amphetamines
    a. α- and β-agonist activity, tachycardia
    b. Atrial and ventricular arrhythmias
 10. Cilostazol
    a. Inhibition of phosphodiesterase III, causing increased ventricular arrhythmias
 11. Itraconazole
    a. Negative inotropic activity
 12. Pregabalin
    a. Lower extremity edema, HF exacerbation
    b. Inhibition of calcium channels

In contrast to the large number of trials and the patients with systolic dysfunction who have been studied, there is a lack of objective data to guide therapy for patients with diastolic dysfunction. The following recommendations are based primarily on the consensus opinion of cardiovascular experts.

E. General Treatment Goals of Diastolic Dysfunction
 1. Control hypertension according to published guidelines.
    a. Hypertension impairs myocardial relaxation.
    b. Hypertension promotes cardiac hypertrophy.
 2. Control tachycardia.
    a. Tachycardia decreases the time for the ventricular and coronary arteries to fill with blood.
    b. Control of HR improves symptoms of HF.

c. Can use β-blockers, dihydropyridine calcium channel blockers, and/or digoxin
3. Reduce preload (but not too much!).
    a. Ventricular filling pressure is primarily determined by central blood volume.
    b. Symptoms of breathlessness can be relieved by the use of diuretics or nitrates.
    c. Patients with diastolic dysfunction are more preload-dependent for ventricular filling. Decreasing the preload too much may cause unexpected hypotension.
4. Aggressively investigate, repair, and treat myocardial ischemia.
    a. Myocardial ischemia impairs ventricular relaxation.
    b. Any ischemia possibly contributing to diastolic dysfunction warrants aggressive therapy.

F. Pharmacologic Therapy for Diastolic Dysfunction
    1. Angiotensin-converting enzyme inhibitors
        a. Benefits of therapy
            i. Reduction in unplanned hospitalizations
            ii. Improvement in NYHA class
            iii. Improvement in exercise tolerance
    2. Angiotensin II receptor blockers
        a. Benefits of therapy
            i. The addition does not improve outcomes in patients with maximized background therapy and well-controlled BP.
    3. Digoxin
        a. Benefits of therapy
            i. No effect on all-cause mortality or on all-cause or cardiovascular hospitalizations
            ii. Possible increase in unstable angina admissions
    4. β-Blockers, verapamil, diltiazem
        a. Benefits of therapy
            i. Targeted symptom relief

II. ATRIAL FIBRILLATION

Patient Case
4. P.M. is a 52-year-old man with a history of hypertension and a transient ischemic attack 2 years ago. He visits his primary care doctor with the chief complaint of several weeks of a "fluttering" feeling in his chest on occasion. He thinks it is nothing; however, his wife insists he have it checked. For his hypertension, he takes verapamil 240 mg/day and aspirin 81 mg/day. His laboratory data from his past visit were all within normal limits. His vital signs today include BP 130/78 mm Hg and HR 76 beats/minute. An electrocardiogram reveals an irregularly irregular rhythm, with no p-waves, and a ventricular rate of 74 beats/minute. A diagnosis of AF is made. Which one of the following is the best approach for managing his AF?

   A. Begin digoxin 0.25 mg/day.
   B. Begin atenolol 50 mg/day.
   C. Begin amiodarone 400 mg 2 times/day, tapering to goal dose of 200 mg/day for the next 6 weeks.
   D. Begin warfarin 7.5 mg/day; adjust to a goal INR of 2.5.

A. Background
   1. Prevalence
      a. Most common arrhythmia: 2.2 million Americans
      b. Prevalence increases with age.
      c. Common comorbidity in patient with valvular heart disease or HF
   2. Symptoms
      a. Some patients have no symptoms.
      b. At worst, an embolic event or symptoms of HF may be present.
      c. Most patients have some degree of:
         i. Palpitations
         ii. Chest pain
         iii. Dyspnea
         iv. Fatigue
         v. Light-headedness
         vi. Syncope
      d. Symptoms vary with ventricular rate, underlying functional status, AF duration, and individual patient perceptions.
   3. Classification (more than one of these may exist in a given patient):
      a. Paroxysmal—spontaneous self-termination within 7 days of onset
      b. Persistent—lasting more than 7 days
      c. Permanent—a commonly used but arbitrary classification
      d. Recurrent—two or more episodes

B. Pathophysiology
   1. Cardiac conduction

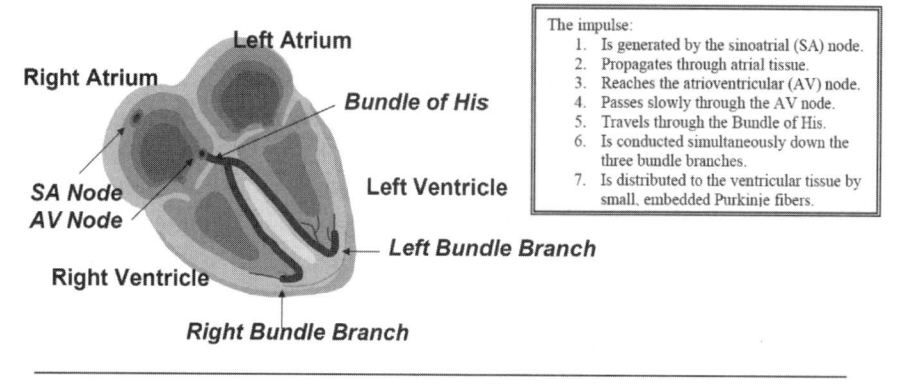

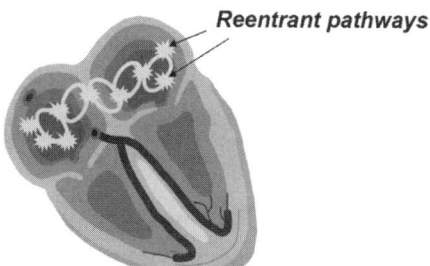

Figure 2.

2. Electrocardiogram findings
   a. No p-waves
   b. Irregularly, irregular rhythm
   c. Rate may be fast or slow (depending on the rate of atrioventricular node conduction).

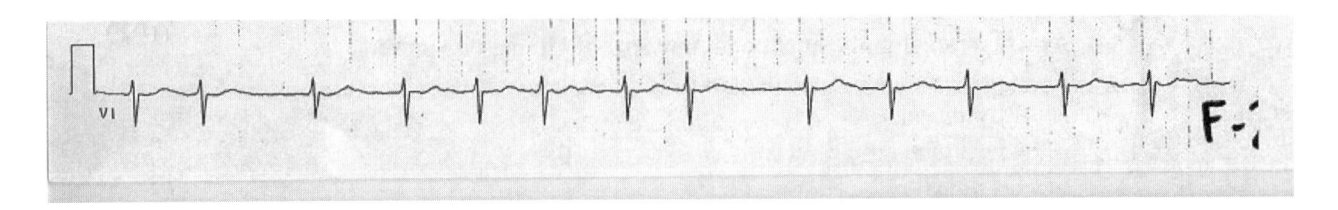

Figure 3.

3. Why do these abnormal impulses develop?

Table 6.

Atrial Distension	High Adrenergic Tone
Chronic hypertension	Alcohol withdrawal
Mitral valve disease	Thyrotoxicosis
Cardiomyopathy	Sepsis
Congenital defects	Binge drinking
Pulmonary hypertension	Cocaine
Acute pulmonary embolus	Amphetamines
	Excessive theophylline, caffeine
	Sympathomimetics
	Surgery

C. Pharmacologic Therapy
   1. Ventricular rate control
      a. If patients have a rapid ventricular rate, atrioventricular node blockade is required.
      b. The goal HR is 60–80 beats/minute at rest and 90–115 beats/minute during exercise.
      c. Select the best agent based on individual clinical response and concomitant disease states that may increase or decrease the desirability of one of the three approaches.
      d. These therapies have no effect on cardioversion:
         i. β-Blockade
            (A) Any agent with β-blockade can be used and dosed to the goal HR.
            (B) Selective $β_1$-antagonists, such as atenolol, may be preferred.
            (C) Labetalol or carvedilol if additional β-blockade is desirable (e.g., hypertension or cocaine exposure).
            (D) Sotalol or propafenone (class III antiarrhythmic) if rhythm control necessary
            (E) Effective for controlling exercise-associated HR increases
         ii. Calcium channel blockade
            (A) Verapamil or diltiazem
               (1) Avoid use if there is concomitant systolic dysfunction.
               (2) May be preferred over β-blocker in patients with asthma/severe chronic obstructive pulmonary disease
               (3) Also effective for controlling exercise-associated HR increases
         iii. Digoxin

(A) Often ineffective alone for controlling ventricular rate in AF, especially during exercise or movement (because of minimal effectiveness with sympathetic stimulation)
(B) Should be included in regimen if patient has systolic HF
(C) May also be effective if additional HR control is needed when a patient is receiving a β-blocker, diltiazem, or verapamil

2. Anticoagulation
3. The average annual stroke rate is 5% per year without anticoagulation.
    a. A patient's individual risk may vary from about 1% to 20% per year based on his or her risk factors. (This risk is INDEPENDENT of current cardiac status [i.e., normal sinus rhythm or AF].)
    b. Risk stratification and treatment determination

Table 7.

Step 1. Based on the patients past medical history, determine the patients risk factors for stroke.

High Risk Factors	Moderate Risk Factors	Weak Risk Factors
Prior stroke, transient ischemic attack, or embolus Mitral valve disease Prosthetic heart valve[a]	Hypertension HF LV dysfunction (EF < 35%) Older than 75 years Diabetes mellitus	Aged 65–74 years Woman CAD Thyrotoxicosis

[a] If mechanical prosthetic valve, INR is determined by valve specifics (minimum INR = 2.5).
CAD = coronary artery disease; EF = ejection fraction; HF = heart failure; LV = left ventricular.

Step 2. Based on number and specific risk factors, determine antithrombotic therapy.

Warfarin[A]: Goal INR = 2.5 (2–3)	Warfarin[A]: Goal INR = 2.5 (2–3) or Aspirin 81–325 mg/day	Aspirin 81–325 mg/day
• Any high-risk factor • Two or more moderate risk factors	• One moderate-risk factor • Any weak risk factors	• No risk factors (< 65 years old and no cardiovascular disease or diabetes mellitus)

[A] With warfarin treatment, the average annual risk of stroke decreases to about 1%.
INR = international normalized ratio.

Adapted with permission from Lippincott, Williams & Wilkins. Fuster V, Ryden LE, Cannom DS, et al.; American College of Cardiology/American Heart Association Task Force on Practice Guidelines; European Society of Cardiology Committee for Practice Guidelines; European Heart Rhythm Association; Heart Rhythm Society. ACC/AHA/ESC 2006 guidelines for the management of patients with atrial fibrillation: a report of the American College of Cardiology/American Heart Association Task Force on Practice Guidelines and the European Society of Cardiology Committee for Practice Guidelines (Writing Committee to Revise the 2001 Guidelines for the Management of Patients with Atrial Fibrillation): developed in collaboration with the European Heart Rhythm Association and the Heart Rhythm Society. Circulation 2006;114:e257–e354.

Table 8.

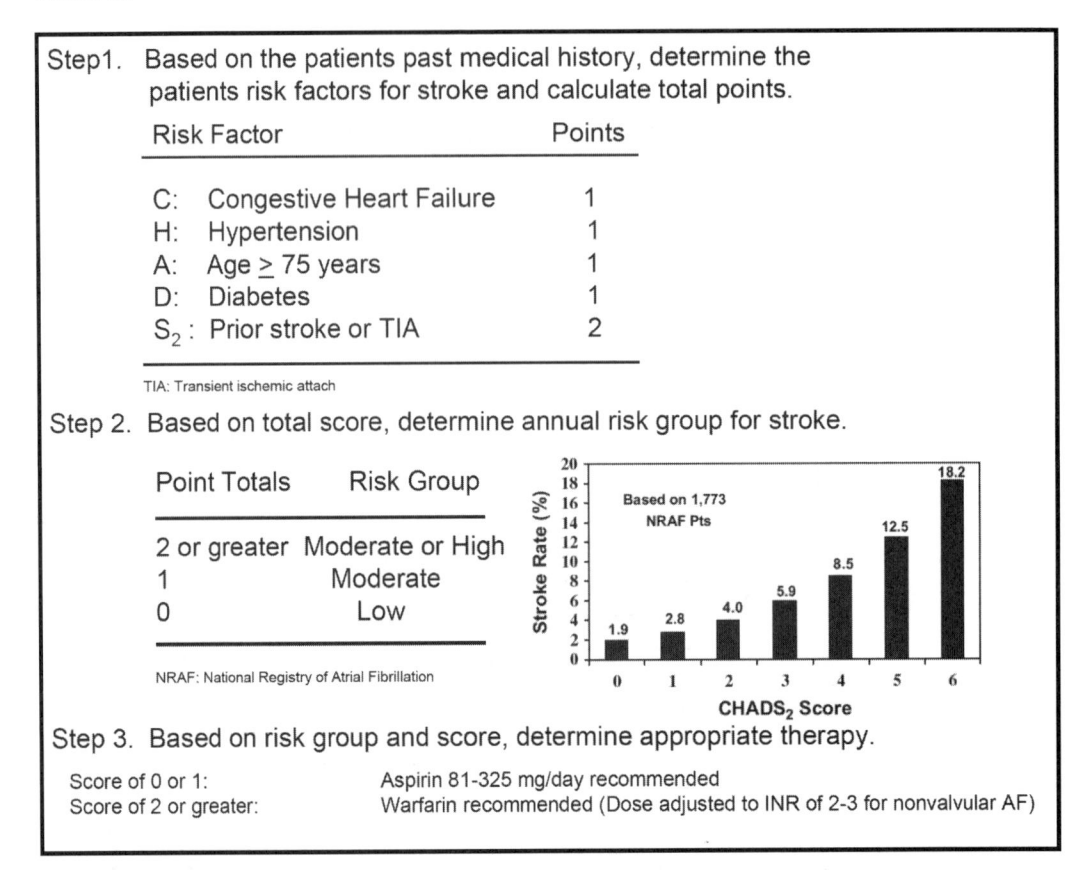

Step 1.	Based on the patients past medical history, determine the patients risk factors for stroke and calculate total points.

Risk Factor	Points
C: Congestive Heart Failure	1
H: Hypertension	1
A: Age ≥ 75 years	1
D: Diabetes	1
S_2: Prior stroke or TIA	2

TIA: Transient ischemic attach

Step 2. Based on total score, determine annual risk group for stroke.

Point Totals	Risk Group
2 or greater	Moderate or High
1	Moderate
0	Low

Stroke rates by CHADS₂ Score (Based on 1,773 NRAF Pts): 0 → 1.9, 1 → 2.8, 2 → 4.0, 3 → 5.9, 4 → 8.5, 5 → 12.5, 6 → 18.2

NRAF: National Registry of Atrial Fibrillation

Step 3. Based on risk group and score, determine appropriate therapy.

Score of 0 or 1: Aspirin 81-325 mg/day recommended
Score of 2 or greater: Warfarin recommended (Dose adjusted to INR of 2-3 for nonvalvular AF)

Adapted from Gage BF, Waterman AD, Shannon W, Boechler M, Rich MW, Radford MJ. Validation of clinical classification schemes for predicting stroke: results from the National Registry of Atrial Fibrillation. JAMA 2001;285:2864–70.
Reprinted with permission from the American Medical Association.

- e. Role of clopidogrel
    - i. ACTIVE A (New Engl J Med 2009;360:2066–78): Compared with aspirin alone, patients with AF receiving 75 mg/day of clopidogrel and aspirin who had an increased risk of stroke and for whom warfarin was unsuitable had a significant reduction in major vascular events but an increased risk of bleeding.
    - ii. ACTIVE W (Lancet 2006;367:1903–12): Compared with clopidogrel and aspirin, warfarin had a significantly lower rate of vascular events in patients with AF plus one or more risk factors for stroke. No difference existed in bleeding between groups.
- f. Bleeding
    - i. Minor hemorrhage increased with therapeutic warfarin therapy
    - ii. Major hemorrhage not increased with warfarin therapy with INR 2–3
    - iii. Risk of intracranial hemorrhage increased with INR greater than 4

Outpatient Cardiology

> **Patient Case**
> 5. H.D. is a 67-year-old man with a history of hypertension, moderate mitral valve insufficiency, and AF for 4 years. His drugs include ramipril 5 mg 2 times/week, sotalol 120 mg 2 times/week, digoxin 0.125 mg/day, and warfarin 5 mg/day. He visits his primary care physician today with increased fatigue on exertion and palpitations with no lower or upper extremity edema. His vital signs today include BP 115/70 mm Hg and HR 88 beats/minute; all laboratory results are within normal limits, except for an INR of 2.8. His electrocardiogram shows AF. An echocardiogram shows an LVEF of 35%–40%. Which one of the following is the best approach for managing his AF?
> A. Discontinue sotalol and begin metoprolol succinate 12.5 mg/day.
> B. Add aspirin 325 mg/day.
> C. Discontinue sotalol and begin amiodarone 400 mg 2 times/day, tapering to goal dose of 200 mg/day for the next 6 weeks.
> D. Add metoprolol 25 mg 2 times/day.

4. Rhythm control: Since the publication of the Atrial Fibrillation Follow-up Investigation of Rhythm Management (AFFIRM) trial (N Engl J Med 2002;34:1825–33), it has been known that maintaining normal sinus rhythm offers no advantage over controlling the ventricular rate (in the typical elderly patient with AF). In fact, the rhythm control group had a higher incidence of hospitalizations, gastrointestinal adverse effects, and symptoms of HF. However, in specific patients with intractable and intolerable symptoms, despite adequate rate control (dyspnea and palpitations), restoration and maintenance of normal sinus rhythm may be desirable.

Table 9.

	Pros	Cons
Rate control strategy	Easy to achieve and maintain	Electrical and structural remodeling because of continued atrial fibrillation makes future attainment of NSR virtually impossible
Rhythm control strategy	If patient is symptomatic with fatigue and exercise intolerance, these may improve if NSR is attained (especially in the patient with HF)	Adverse effects of medications, cost of medications and monitoring, likelihood of atrial fibrillation recurrence

HF = heart failure; NSR = normal sinus rhythm.

    a. If cardioversion is attempted (electric or pharmacologic), the absence of atrial thrombi must be ensured.
        i. Thrombi present plus cardioversion = 91% stroke rate
        ii. Without anticoagulation (caused by decreased or stagnant bloodflow in the atria)
            (A) Atrial fibrillation for greater than 48 hours = 15% rate of atrial thrombus
            (B) Atrial fibrillation for greater than 72 hours = 30% rate of atrial thrombus
    b. Ensure safe cardioversion by either:
        i. Transesophageal echocardiogram to visualize the atria OR
        ii. Three or more weeks of therapeutic anticoagulation (INR greater than 2.0)
    c. Oral pharmacologic agents to induce/maintain normal sinus rhythm
        i. Class I antiarrhythmics: contraindicated in patients with HF
            (A) Often third line because of frequent dosing requirements and adverse effect profiles; some patients require hospitalization for initiation because of proarrhythmic effects; only about 50% efficacy at 1 year

(1) Quinidine
(2) Disopyramide
(3) Propafenone
(4) Flecainide

(B) However, flecainide and propafenone may be considered <u>first-line</u> therapies for patients without structural heart disease (see figure below).

ii. Class III antiarrhythmics

(A) Amiodarone: 85%–95% efficacy
(1) In addition, has electrophysiologic properties of classes I–IV
(2) Oral loading dose required (400 mg/day 2 or 3 times/day × 2 weeks and then 400 mg/day for 4 weeks, followed by a 200-mg/day maintenance dose). Achieving a loading dose of 10 g is desirable. Many different regimens exist.
(3) Long half-life of about 60 days
(4) In addition, has atrioventricular nodal blocking properties; may help control HR if AF recurs
(5) Hepatically metabolized inhibitor of cytochrome P450 (CYP) enzymes CYP3A4, CYP1A2, CYP2C9, CYP2D6, and P-glycoprotein
(6) Minimal incidence of ventricular arrhythmias
(7) Drug interactions (many)
   (a) Digoxin – Increased digoxin exposure. Lower initial digoxin dose by 50%
   (b) Warfarin – Increased warfarin exposure. Lower warfarin dose by 25%
   (c) Simvastatin – Increased simvastatin exposure. Do not exceed dose of 20 mg/day.
   (d) β-Blockers (particularly carvedilol) –Additive bradycardia, increased β-blocker exposure
(8) Extensive monitoring for noncardiac adverse effects
   (a) Liver function tests: baseline and every 6 months
   (b) Thyroid function tests: baseline and every 6 months
   (c) Chest radiography: baseline and annually
   (d) Pulmonary function tests (including D_LCO_2 [carbon dioxide diffusion in the lungs]): baseline and for unexplained dyspnea or chest radiographic abnormalities
   (e) Ophthalmologic examination: for symptoms of visual impairment

iii. Class I–IV agents

(A) Dronedarone: 21%–25% efficacy
(1) Amiodarone analog that specifically lacks the iodine moiety that contributes to the pulmonary, thyroid, hepatic, and ocular toxicity of amiodarone
(2) Has complex antiarrhythmic properties that span all classes of the Vaughan-Williams classification
(3) Dose: 400 mg twice daily with morning and evening meal
(4) Hepatically metabolized CYP3A4 substrate and a moderate CYP3A4, CYP2D6, and P-glycoprotein inhibitor
(5) Half-life only 24 hours
(6) Can increase SCr within 7 days (by 0.1 mg/dL – not clinically important)
(7) Contraindicated in NYHA class II or III HF with recent decompensation requiring hospitalization, severe liver impairment, NYHA class IV HF, HR less than 50 beats/minute, and strong CYP3A4 inhibitors

(8) Compared with placebo in the ATHENA trial (N Engl J Med 2009;360:668–78), high-risk patients with a history of paroxysmal or persistent AF or atrial flutter within the past 6 months receiving dronedarone had a lower incidence of hospitalization for cardiovascular causes or death from any cause; risk of cardiovascular death, death from arrhythmias, and incidence of stroke.

(9) Based on Andromeda study (N Engl J Med 2008;358:2678–87), dronedarone compared with placebo showed an increased mortality in patients with HF (LVEF less than 35% and NYHA classes II–IV).

(10) One meta-analysis (J Am Coll Cardiol 2009;54:1089–95) found dronedarone less effective than amiodarone for the maintenance of sinus rhythm, but with fewer adverse effects.

(11) Drug interactions
   (a) Digoxin: increased digoxin exposure, so lower dose of digoxin by 50%
   (b) Diltiazem, verapamil, β-blockers: excessive bradycardia and increased exposure of these agents, so initiate these drugs at lowest dose. Diltiazem and verapamil can increase dronedarone exposure, so monitor electrocardiogram.
   (c) Statins with CYP3A metabolism: Increased statin exposure. Follow statin package labeling for CYP3A4 inhibitors.
   (d) CYP3A4 inhibitors: AVOID
   (e) Cyclosporine, tacrolimus, sirolimus: Increased exposure of these agents, monitor serum concentrations closely

(12) U.S. Food and Drug Administration Risk Evaluation and Mitigation Strategy
   (a) See the following Web site: *www.fda.gov/downloads/Drugs/DrugSafety/PostmarketDrugSafetyInformationforPatientsandProviders/UCM187494.pdf*

(B) Sotalol: 50%–60% efficacy
   (1) Renal excretion; hence, dose adjustment and vigilant QTc (corrected noninvasive cardiac output) monitoring necessary in renal impairment
   (2) May be initiated in outpatient setting in patients with little or no heart disease, normal baseline QTc, normal serum electrolytes, and normal renal function
   (3) Contraindicated in patients with HF and CrCl less than 40 mL/minute

(C) Dofetilide: 50%–60% efficacy
   (1) Must be initiated in the hospital (2- to 3-day stay). Dose titrated on the basis of renal function and QTc response
   (2) Hepatically metabolized by CYP3A
   (3) Renal elimination through renal cationic secretion; check QTc if renal function acutely declines
   (4) Safe to use in patients with HF
   (5) Drug interactions:
      (a) Cimetidine, verapamil, ketoconazole, hydrochlorothiazide, and trimethoprim alone or in combination with sulfamethoxazole: AVOID
      (b) CYP3A4 inhibitors: increased dofetilide exposure, so use with caution
      (c) Triamterene, metformin, amiloride: increased dofetilide exposure, so use with caution

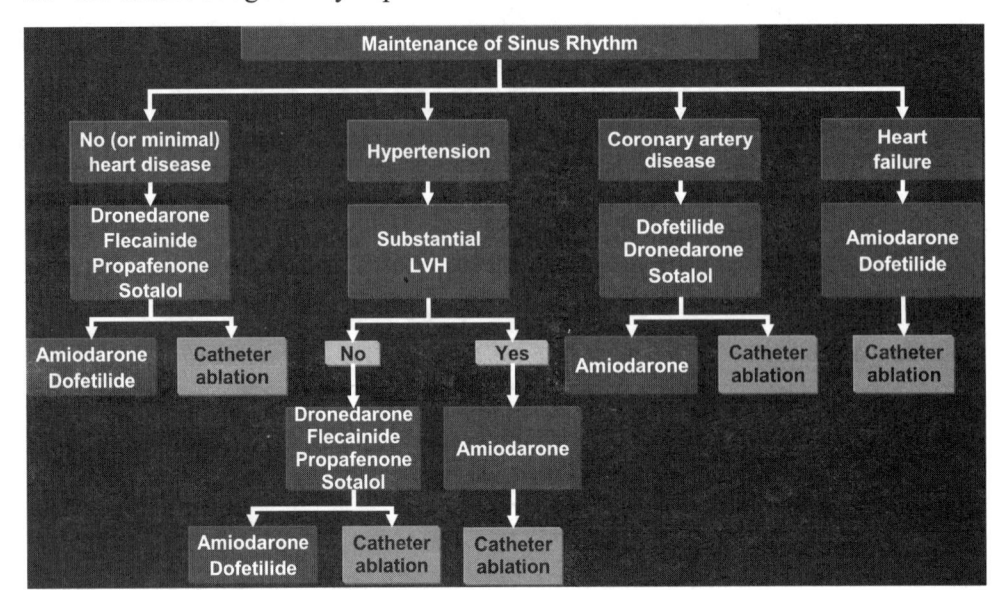

iii. The choice of agent may depend on comorbidities.

Figure 4.

CAD = coronary artery disease; LVH = left ventricular hypertrophy.

Adapted with permission from Lippincott, Williams & Wilkins. Fuster V, Ryden LE, Cannom DS, et al.; American College of Cardiology/American Heart Association Task Force on Practice Guidelines; European Society of Cardiology Committee for Practice Guidelines; European Heart Rhythm Association; Heart Rhythm Society. ACC/AHA/ESC 2006 guidelines for the management of patients with atrial fibrillation: a report of the American College of Cardiology/American Heart Association Task Force on Practice Guidelines and the European Society of Cardiology Committee for Practice Guidelines (Writing Committee to Revise the 2001 Guidelines for the Management of Patients with Atrial Fibrillation): developed in collaboration with the European Heart Rhythm Association and the Heart Rhythm Society. Circulation 2006;114:e257–e354.

5. Nonpharmacologic therapies
    a. Electrical cardioversion (low-energy cardioversion, sedation highly desirable, can be used in an emergency if patient is hemodynamically unstable)
    b. Atrioventricular nodal ablation: Ablate atrioventricular node and chronically pace the ventricles.
    c. Pulmonary vein ablation: This relatively new therapy ablates the origin of the abnormal atrial foci, which is often near the pulmonary vein–atrial tissue intersection.

III. HYPERTENSION

Definition: Hypertension is considered a BP of 140/90 mm Hg or higher or antihypertensive drug therapy.

   A. Background
      1. Statistics
         a. Most common chronic disease in the United States
         b. Affects 50 million Americans

c. Normotensive 50-year-old lifetime risk of developing hypertension is 90%.
d. For each 20-mm increase in systolic BP and 10-mm increase in diastolic BP, there is a 2-fold increased risk of cardiovascular disease (e.g., stroke, MI).
e. Only 31% of patients with hypertension have it under adequate control.
2. Etiology
   a. Essential hypertension: 90% (no identifiable cause)
      i. Contributed to by obesity and Na intake
   b. Secondary hypertension
      i. Primary aldosteronism
      ii. Renal parenchymal disease
      iii. Thyroid or parathyroid disease
      iv. Medications (e.g., cyclosporine, NSAIDs, sympathomimetics)
3. Diagnosis
   a. Periodic screening for all individuals older than 21 years
   b. Patient seated quietly in chair for at least 5 minutes
   c. Use appropriate cuff size (bladder length at least 80% the circumference of the arm).
   d. Take BP at least 2 times, separated by at least 2 minutes.
   e. The average BP on two separate visits is required to diagnose hypertension accurately.
4. Benefits of lowering BP
   a. Forty percent decrease in stroke
   b. Twenty-five percent decrease in MI
   c. Fifty percent decrease in HF
5. Effects of lifestyle modifications on BP

Table 10.

Modification	Recommendation	Approximate Systolic BP Reduction
Weight reduction (if more than 25 kg/m^2)	Attain/maintain BMI less than 25 kg/m^2	5–20 mm Hg per 10-kg weight loss
Adopt DASH eating plan (includes substantial potassium intake)	Consume a diet rich in fruits, vegetables, and low-fat dairy products with a reduced content of saturated and total fat	8–14 mm Hg
Dietary sodium restriction	Reduce dietary sodium intake to no more than 2.4 g of sodium	2–8 mm Hg
Physical activity	Engage in regular aerobic physical activity such as brisk walking (at least 30 minutes/day, most days of the week)	4–9 mm Hg
Moderation of alcohol consumption	Limit consumption to: Men: 2 drinks/day Women: 1 drink/day	2–4 mm Hg

BMI = body mass index; BP = blood pressure; DASH = Dietary Approaches to Stop Hypertension.

Patient Cases

6. D.W. is a 50-year-old African American man being discharged from the hospital after an acute MI. His medical history is significant for hypertension. He was taking hydrochlorothiazide 25 mg/day before hospitalization. An echocardiogram before discharge shows an LVEF of more than 60%. His vital signs include BP 150/94 mm Hg and HR 80 beats/minute. Which one of the following is the best approach for managing his hypertension?
   A. Discontinue hydrochlorothiazide and add diltiazem.
   B. Continue hydrochlorothiazide and add metoprolol.
   C. Discontinue hydrochlorothiazide and add losartan.
   D. Continue hydrochlorothiazide and add losartan.

7. T.J. is a 45-year-old white woman with a history of type 2 diabetes mellitus treated with glyburide 5 mg/day. She presents to the clinic for a routine follow-up of her diabetes. Her BP today (average of two readings) is 138/88 mm Hg, HR is 70 beats/minute, and laboratory results are Na 140 mEq/L, K 4.0 mEq/L, Cl 102 mEq/L, bicarbonate 28 mEq/L, BUN 14 mg/dL, and SCr 1.8 mg/dL. Of note, at her last visit, her BP was 136/85 mm Hg. Which one of the following is best for managing her hypertension at this time?
   A. Begin lifestyle modifications.
   B. Begin lifestyle modifications and add losartan 50 mg/day.
   C. Begin lifestyle modifications and add lisinopril 2.5 mg/day.
   D. Begin lifestyle modifications and add atenolol 25 mg/day.

B. Therapeutic Management
   1. Patient classification and management in adults
      a. Primary classification based on systolic BP

Table 11.

BP Classification	Systolic BP (mm Hg)	Diastolic BP (mm Hg)	Lifestyle Modification
Normal	< 120 AND	< 80	Encourage
Prehypertension	120–139 OR	80–89	Yes
Stage 1 hypertension	140–159 OR	90–99	Yes
Stage 2 hypertension	≥ 160 OR	≥ 100	Yes

BP = blood pressure.

   2. Select treatment goal.

Table 12.

Goal BP values recommended by the AHA (2007)	
Most Patients for General Prevention (Primary Prevention Patients)	< 140/90 mm Hg
Patients with: • Diabetes, • Significant chronic kidney disease**, • Known coronary artery disease (myocardial infarction, stable angina, unstable angina), • Non-coronary atherosclerotic vascular disease (ischemic stroke, transient ischemic attack, peripheral arterial disease, abdominal aortic aneurism) or • Framingham risk score ≥ 10%	< 130/80 mm Hg
Patients with left ventricular dysfunction (systolic heart failure)	120/80 mm Hg
**Significant chronic kidney disease is considered to be moderate-to-severe chronic kidney disease, defined as: estimated GFR < 60 ml/min/1.73 m2 (correlating to a serum creatinine > 1.3 mg/dL in women or > 1.5 in men); or albuminuria (> 300 mg/day or > 200 mg/g creatinine). Framingham risk score calculated using the risk calculator available at: http://www.nhlbi.nih.gov/guidelines/cholesterol/risk_tbl.htm	

Disclaimer: The JNC7 (2003) recommends a goal BP of less than 140/90 mm Hg for all patients, except for diabetes and chronic kidney disease, in which they recommend less than 130/80 mm Hg. Therefore, the AHA 2007 guidelines are more recent, include more updated evidence, and are more aggressive. Follow the AHA recommendations for now until the JNC8 guidelines are published (in 2010). The JNC8 will then be the primary guidelines to follow.

Adapted with permission from Lippincott, Williams & Wilkins. Rosendorff C, Black HR, Cannon CP, et al.; American College of Cardiology/American Heart Association Council for High Blood Pressure Research and the Councils on Clinical Cardiology and Epidemiology and Prevention. Treatment of hypertension in the prevention and management of ischemic heart disease. A scientific statement from the AHA Council for High Blood Pressure Research and the Councils on Clinical Cardiology and Epidemiology and Prevention. Circulation 2007;115:2761–88.

3. Select appropriate therapy.

Figure 5.

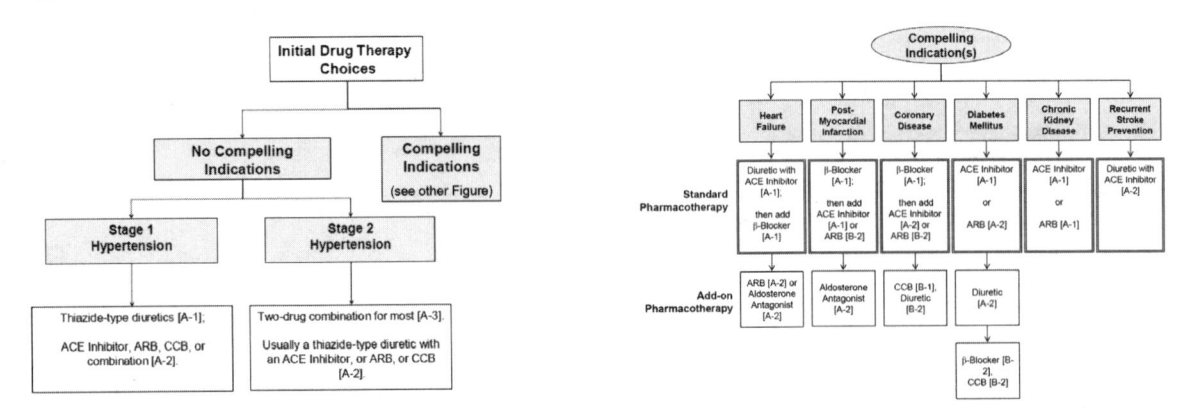

NOTE: Strength of recommendation [A, B, and C = good, moderate, and poor evidence to support recommendation] and quality of evidence [1 = Evidence from more than 1 properly randomized, controlled trial. 2 = Evidence from at least 1 well-designed clinical trial with randomization, from cohort or case-controlled analytic studies; or dramatic results from uncontrolled experiments or subgroup analyses. 3 = Evidence from opinions of respected authorities, based on clinical experience, descriptive studies, or reports of expert communities] are in brackets.

ACE = angiotensin-converting enzyme; ARB = angiotensin receptor blocker; CCB = calcium channel blocker.

Modified from Saseen JJ, MacLaughlin EJ. Hypertension. In: DiPiro JT, Talbert RL, Yee GC, Matzke GR, Wells BG, Posey LM, eds. Pharmacotherapy: A Pathophysiological Approach, 7th ed. New York: McGraw-Hill, 2008:Chapter 15.

4. Considerations with specific antihypertensive agents
   a. β-Blockers
      i. Caution with asthma, severe chronic obstructive pulmonary disease (especially higher doses) because of pulmonary β-blockade
      ii. Increased risk of developing diabetes compared with ACE inhibitor, ARB, and calcium channel blocker; use caution in patients at high risk of diabetes mellitus (e.g., family history, obese)
      iii. May mask some signs of hypoglycemia in patients with diabetes mellitus
      iv. May cause depression
   b. Thiazides
      i. May worsen gout by increasing serum uric acid
      ii. Increased risk of developing diabetes compared with ACE inhibitor, ARBs, and calcium channel blocker; use caution in patients at high risk of diabetes mellitus (e.g., family history, obese)
      iii. May assist in the management of osteoporosis by preventing urine calcium loss
   c. Angiotensin-converting enzyme inhibitors and ARBs
      i. Contraindicated in pregnancy
      ii. Contraindicated with bilateral renal artery stenosis
      iii. Monitor K closely, especially if renal insufficiency exists or another K-sparing drug is in use.
      iv. Presence of diabetic nephropathy should influence choice of ACE inhibitor versus ARB

Table 13.

Nephropathy		Agent
Type 1	Any level of proteinuria	ACEI
Type 2	Microalbuminuria	ACEI or ARB
Type 2	Macroalbuminuria and renal insufficiency (i.e., elevated serum creatinine)	ARB

ACEI = angiotensin-converting enzyme inhibitor; ARB = angiotensin II receptor blocker.

4. Considerations within specific patient populations
   a. Patients with ischemic heart disease: Potent vasodilators may cause reflex tachycardia, thereby increasing myocardial oxygen demand (hydralazine, minoxidil, and dihydropyridine calcium channel blocker) (can attenuate this by also using an atrioventricular nodal depressant (non-dihydropyridine calcium channel blocker or β-blocker)
   b. Elderly patients:
      i. Caution with antihypertensive agents and orthostatic hypotension
      ii. Initiate with low dose and titrate slowly.
   c. African American patients: β-Blockers and ACE inhibitors are generally less effective as monotherapy than in white patients; however, combination therapy with thiazides improves effectiveness and should still be used if comorbid conditions dictate.
   d. Pregnant women
      i. Methyldopa and hydralazine are recommended if a new therapy is initiated. Most antihypertensives (except for ACE inhibitors and ARBs) can be safely continued in pregnancy.
5. Monitoring
   a. Have the patient return in 4 weeks to assess efficacy.
   b. May have patient follow-up sooner if BP particularly worrisome
   c. If there is an inadequate response from the first agent (and adherence verified) and no compelling indication exists, initiate therapy with a drug from a different class.

IV. CHRONIC CAD AND CHRONIC STABLE ANGINA

Coronary artery disease is a general term that does not discriminate between the various phases the individual may cycle between for several decades. These phases include asymptomatic disease, stable angina, progressive angina, unstable angina, non–ST-segment elevation MI, and ST-segment elevation MI.

Based on the manifestations a patient is experiencing, some therapies may be added or modified. However, several basic treatment rules apply to all individuals with CAD, regardless of the symptoms they may experience.

The following mnemonic, developed for patients with chronic stable angina, can be applied to all patients with CAD.
A = Aspirin and Antianginal Therapy
B = β-Blocker and BP
C = Cigarette Smoking and Cholesterol
D = Diet and Diabetes
E = Education and Exercise
Obviously, not all patients with CAD have diabetes or smoke cigarettes, but it is a way to remember the primary areas that should be addressed, as applicable, in all patients with CAD.

A few important recommendations:
Weight reduction/maintenance to 18.5–24.9 kg/m^2;
Physical activity for 30–60 minutes/day 7 days/week (minimum of 5 days/week);
Low-density lipoprotein cholesterol less than 100 mg/dL;
Blood pressure less than 130/80 mm Hg;
No smoking and no environmental exposure to smoke;
Reduce intake of saturated fats (to less than 7% of total calories), *trans*-fatty acids, and cholesterol (to less than 200 mg/day);
If diabetic, glycosylated hemoglobin less than 7%; and
Influenza vaccine each year

Patient Cases

8. L.J., a 58-year-old white man, is discharged from the hospital after a non–ST-segment elevation MI. His medical history is significant for hypertension. He was taking hydrochlorothiazide 12.5 mg/day before hospitalization. An echocardiogram shows an LVEF of more than 60%. His vital signs include BP 130/65 and HR 64 beats/minute, and he states that he feels great. His drug regimen consists of aspirin 81 mg/day, atenolol 50 mg/day, hydrochlorothiazide 25 mg/day, atorvastatin 80 mg/day, and sublingual nitroglycerin 0.4 mg as needed for chest pain. Which of the following represents the best action to take in response to this discharge regimen?
    A. Discontinue hydrochlorothiazide; add diltiazem extended release 240 mg/day.
    B. Continue hydrochlorothiazide; add amlodipine 5 mg/day.
    C. Discontinue hydrochlorothiazide; add ramipril 5 mg/day.
    D. Continue hydrochlorothiazide; add vitamin E.

9. L.W. is a 64-year-old woman with a significant coronary disease history, having had two MIs and three stent placements in the past 10 years. Her LVEF is more than 60%. She has developed shortness of breath and chest heaviness with activity for the past several months, despite being adherent to her medications. She says she is requiring up to three doses of her sublingual nitroglycerin per day; however, she has severely curtailed her activity to avoid the discomfort. She takes aspirin 325 mg/day, simvastatin 40 mg every night, enalapril 10 mg 2 times/day, and metoprolol titrate 50 mg 2 times/day. Her BP is 132/80 mm Hg, and her HR is 72 beats/minute. Which one of the following regimens is best to improve her stable angina symptoms and increase her activity level?
    A. Discontinue metoprolol tartrate and begin diltiazem extended release 240 mg/day.
    B. Have her take a sublingual nitroglycerin before exertion.
    C. Add isosorbide mononitrate 60 mg every morning.
    D. Increase metoprolol tartrate to 100 mg 2 times/day and add isosorbide mononitrate 60 mg every morning.

A. Therapeutic Management
   1. Antiplatelet therapy
      a. Aspirin
         i. Inhibits synthesis of thromboxane A_2
         ii. Indicated in all patients with CAD, unless contraindicated
         iii. Dose at 75–162 mg/day.
         iv. Decreases cardiovascular events by about one-third
      b. Clopidogrel
         i. Prevents adenosine diphosphate–mediated platelet activation
         ii. A dose of 75 mg/day if aspirin absolutely contraindicated
         iii. Magnitude of benefit not clear; however, appears to be about that of aspirin
      c. Dipyridamole: should be avoided in symptomatic CAD
         i. Increases exercise-induced myocardial ischemia
         ii. No benefit over aspirin in the absence of symptomatic CAD
   2. Lipid-lowering therapy (see Ambulatory Care—Disorders of Lipid Metabolism)
      a. Low-density lipoprotein cholesterol should be less than 100 mg/dL.
      b. Reduction in LDL-C to less than 70 mg/dL or use of a high-dose statin is reasonable.
      c. In high- or moderately high-risk patients, the intensity of lipid-lowering therapy should be sufficient to achieve a 30%–40% reduction in LDL-C.
      d. If triglycerides are 200–499 mg/dL, non–high-density lipoprotein concentrations should be less than 130 mg/dL; however, less than 100 mg/dL is also reasonable if triglycerides are 200–499 mg/dL or higher.
      e. Can consider the addition of plant stanols/sterols (2 g/day) or viscous fiber (greater than 10 g/day) to lower LDL-C
      f. For risk reduction, encourage omega-3 fatty acids in the form of fish or capsule (1 g/day) in all patients.
   3. Angiotensin-converting enzyme inhibitors
      a. Angiotensin-converting enzyme inhibitors (specifically ramipril 10 mg/day) have been shown to greatly decrease cardiovascular events in patients with CAD (and no LV dysfunction) at high risk of subsequent cardiovascular events.
      b. An ACE inhibitor should be considered in patients with an LVEF of 40% or less and in patients with hypertension and established CAD, diabetes mellitus, and/or chronic kidney disease.
      c. Consider using in lower-risk patients with a mildly reduced or normal LVEF in whom cardiovascular risk factors are well controlled and revascularization has been performed.
      d. Postulated mechanisms: plaque stabilization
   4. Angiotensin II receptor blockers
      a. Recommended for those with hypertension, those with indications for and intolerance of ACE inhibitors, those with HF, or those who have had an MI with an EF of 40% or less

Additional Therapies for Chronic Stable Angina

Definition: predictable angina symptoms with exertion
Goal: Reduce symptoms of ischemia, increase physical function, and improve quality of life.
    In general, achieved by either:
        Decreasing myocardial oxygen demand OR
        Increasing myocardial oxygen supply

5. β-Blockers
    a. Pharmacologic effects: decreased inotropy and HR (decreased oxygen demand)
    b. Goal resting HR 55–60 beats/minute (less than 50 beats/minute if angina symptoms continue)
    c. Goal exercise HR of no more than 75% HR associated with angina symptoms
    d. Contraindications: severe bradycardia (HR less than 50 beats/minute), high-degree atrioventricular block (without pacemaker), sick sinus syndrome (without pacemaker)
6. Calcium channel blockers
    a. Pharmacologic effects
        i. Decrease coronary vascular resistance and increase coronary bloodflow (increase oxygen supply)
        ii. Negative inotropy, to varying degrees; nifedipine much greater than amlodipine and felodipine (decrease oxygen demand)
        iii. Decrease HR (verapamil and diltiazem only)
    b. Place in therapy
        i. Added to β-blocker therapy to achieve HR goals
        ii. Instead of β-blocker therapy when unacceptable adverse effects emerge
        iii. Short-acting calcium antagonists (nifedipine, nisoldipine) have been associated with increased cardiovascular events and should be avoided (except in slow-release formulations).
    c. Contraindications for non-dihydropyridines : systolic HF, severe bradycardia, high-degree atrioventricular block (without pacemaker), and sick sinus syndrome (without pacemaker)
    d. Contraindications for dihydropyridines: LV dysfunction (except amlodipine and felodipine)
7. Nitrates
    a. Pharmacologic effects:
        i. Endothelium-dependent vasodilation, dilates epicardial arteries and collateral vessels (increased oxygen supply)
        ii. Decreased LV volume because of decreased preload mediated by venodilation (decreased oxygen demand)
    b. Place in therapy
        i. A scheduled nitrate is useful in conjunction with β-blockade or non-dihydropyridine calcium channel blocker (which blunts the reflex sympathetic tone with nitrate therapy).
        ii. As-needed sublingual or spray nitrate is necessary to relieve effort or rest angina.
        iii. In addition, as-needed nitrates can be used before exercise to avoid ischemic episodes.

c. Contraindications: hypertrophic obstructive cardiomyopathy, inferior wall MI, severe aortic valve stenosis, sildenafil and vardenafil within 24 hours, tadalafil within 48 hours
8. Aldosterone receptor blockers
   a. Place in therapy
      i. Can be used in patients post-MI without significant renal dysfunction (SCr should be less than 2.5 mg/dL for men and 2.0 mg/dL for women) or hyperkalemia (K should be less than 5.0 mEq/L) who are receiving a β-blocker and ACE inhibitor (or ARB), have an EF of 40% or less, and have either HF or diabetes mellitus
9. Ranolazine
   a. Pharmacologic effects
      i. Inhibits myocardial fatty acid oxidation, causing increased glucose oxidation (a less oxygen-consuming process)
      ii. Increases "oxygen efficiency"
   b. Place in therapy
      i. Ideal role is not clear. Currently, either as monotherapy or as an add-on to maximally tolerated conventional therapy (β-blocker plus calcium channel blocker plus nitrate) with continued symptoms
      ii. Important points
         (A) Heart rate or BP effects are not present; thus, bradycardia and hypotension are not a concern.
         (B) Dose-related QT prolongation
         (C) Metabolized by CYP3A
            (1) Avoid in hepatic dysfunction or disease.
            (2) Avoid use with strong 3A inhibitors including ketoconazole, itraconazole, clarithromycin, nefazodone, nelfinavir, ritonavir, indinavir, and saquinavir.
            (3) Avoid use with 3A inducers such as rifampin, rifabutin, rifapentine, phenobarbital, phenytoin, carbamazepine, and St. John's wort.
            (4) Limit the dose to 500 mg 2 times/day in patients receiving including diltiazem, verapamil, aprepitant, erythromycin, fluconazole, and grapefruit juice.

REFERENCES

Heart Failure

1. Hunt SA, Abraham WT, Chin MH, et al. 2009 focused update incorporated into the ACC/AHA 2005 guidelines for the diagnosis and management of heart failure in adults. A report of the American College of Cardiology Foundation/American Heart Association Task Force on Practice Guidelines developed in collaboration with the International Society for Heart and Lung Transplantation. J Am Coll Cardiol 2009;53:e1–e90.
2. Jackevicius CA, Page RL, Chow S, et al. High impact articles related to the management of heart failure: 2008 update. Pharmacotherapy 2009;29:82–120.
3. Amabile CM, Spencer AP. Keep your heart failure patient safe: a review of potentially dangerous medications. Arch Intern Med 2004;164:709–20.
4. Adams KF, Lindenfeld J, Arnold JMO, et al. HFSA 2006 comprehensive heart failure practice guideline. J Card Fail 2006;12:e1–e122.

Atrial Fibrillation

1. Fuster V, Rydén LE, Cannom DS, et al. ACC/AHA/ESC 2006 guidelines for the management of patients with atrial fibrillation: a report of the American College of Cardiology/American Heart Association Task Force on Practice Guidelines and the European Society of Cardiology Committee for Practice Guidelines (Writing Committee to Revise the 2001 Guidelines for the Management of Patients with Atrial Fibrillation). Circulation 2006;114:e257–e354.
2. Singer DE, Albers GW, Dalen JE, et al. Antithrombotic therapy in atrial fibrillation. Chest 2008;133:546S–592S.
3. The Atrial Fibrillation Follow-up Investigation of Rhythm Management (AFFIRM) Investigators. A comparison of rate control and rhythm control in patients with atrial fibrillation. N Engl J Med 2002;347:1825–33.

Hypertension

1. Chobanian AV, Bakris GL, Black HR, et al. The Seventh Report of the Joint National Committee on Prevention, Detection, Evaluation, and Treatment of High Blood Pressure: the JNC 7 report. JAMA 2003;289:2560–72.
2. Rosendorff C, Black HR, Cannon CP, et al. Treatment of hypertension in the prevention and management of ischemic heart disease: a scientific statement from the American Heart Association Council for High Blood Pressure Research and the Councils on Clinical Cardiology and Epidemiology and Prevention. Circulation 2007;115:2761–88.
3. Appel LJ, Brands MW, Daniels SR, et al. Dietary approaches to prevent and treat hypertension: a scientific statement from the American Heart Association. Hypertension 2006;47:296–308.

CAD and Chronic Stable Angina

1. Gibbons RJ, Abrams J, Chatterjee K, et al. ACC/AHA 2002 guideline update for the management of chronic stable angina: a report of the American College of Cardiology/American Heart Association Task Force on Practice Guidelines (Committee to Update the 1999 Guidelines for the Management of Patients with Chronic Stable Angina). Circulation 2006;114:e257–e354.
2. Gibbons RJ, Abrams J, Chatterjee K, et al. 2007 chronic angina focused update of the ACC/AHA 2002 guidelines for the management of patients with chronic stable angina. A report of the American College of Cardiology/American Heart Association Task Force on Practice Guidelines Writing Group to develop the focused update of the 2002 guidelines for the management of patients with chronic stable angina. Circulation 2007;116:2762–72.
3. Smith SC, Allen J, Blair SN, et al. ACC/AHA guidelines for the secondary prevention for patients with coronary and other atherosclerotic vascular disease: 2006 update. Circulation 2006;13:2363–72.

ANSWERS AND EXPLANATIONS TO PATIENT CASES

1. Answer: A
At this time, the best option is to increase L.S.'s carvedilol to the goal dose of 25 mg 2 times/day. Despite her HR of 68 beats/minute, it is safe to increase the β-blocker. Appropriate monitoring would include signs and symptoms of hypotension and bradycardia. Her ACE inhibitor is already at the target dose; hence, it should be increased to the maximal dose only if there is another indication to do so (hypertension or proteinuria). Spironolactone 25 mg is the recommended dose for HF; increasing to 50 mg/day is not warranted. Her digoxin concentration of 0.7 ng/dL is within the desired range of 0.6–1.0 ng/dL, so no dosage increase is warranted because this would not improve efficacy and would only increase the risk of toxicity/arrhythmia.

2. Answer: B
Increasing the ACE inhibitor to target doses should be achieved in all patients, if possible. J.T.'s BP of 120/72 mm Hg safely permits increasing the enalapril from 5 mg to 10 mg 2 times/day. There is no consensus that carvedilol is preferred over extended-release metoprolol for patients with HF. Spironolactone is not appropriate to initiate because J.T.'s HF is not NYHA class III or IV, and his baseline SCr concentration is greater than 2.5 mg/dL. Digoxin should be added only in patients who continue to have symptoms or hospitalizations despite optimal therapy with an ACE inhibitor, β-blocker, and diuretic. J.T. has minimal symptoms, and his therapy has opportunities for optimization.

3. Answer: C
Cilostazol, a phosphodiesterase III inhibitor, is associated with an increased risk of ventricular arrhythmias and death in patients with HF. Acetaminophen is the drug of choice for mild to moderate pain in patients with HF because NSAIDs can lead to water retention and worsening HF symptoms. The selective serotonin reuptake inhibitors have no contraindications to use. Properly dosed thyroid replacement therapy, as evidenced by his therapeutic thyroid-stimulating hormone concentration, is also beneficial because both hypothyroidism and hyperthyroidism have negative consequences in patients with HF.

4. Answer: D
The patient is experiencing minimal symptoms with his AF; thus, an antiarrhythmic should not be considered. Even if he had significant symptoms with his AF, the noncardiac adverse effects of amiodarone would make it an unattractive antiarrhythmic in a healthy 52-year-old man. His ventricular rate is well controlled with his verapamil therapy; hence, no additional atrioventricular node blockade is warranted with either a β-blocker or digoxin. If additional atrioventricular node blockade were desired, digoxin would not be ideal because of a significant drug interaction with his verapamil therapy. P.M. has a significant risk factor for stroke with AF and a prior transient ischemic attack, as well as hypertension. Furthermore, this patient has a $CHADS_2$ score (congestive HF, hypertension, age older than 75 years, diabetes, and prior stroke of transient ischemic attack) of 3, so anticoagulation with warfarin to a goal INR of 2.5 is indicated.

5. Answer: A
With the new diagnosis of HF, H.D. can no longer receive sotalol. Discontinuing this drug is very important so that his risk of arrhythmic death is not increased. Adding metoprolol is a reasonable approach at this time to decrease his HR to less than 80 beats/minute, and β-blockade with bisoprolol, metoprolol, or carvedilol is indicated with the new diagnosis of HF. There is no indication for aspirin therapy in this patient, and his anticoagulation is adequately managed with his INR of 2.8 on warfarin therapy. If rhythm control is desired, amiodarone and dofetilide are the only two drugs that have been proven safe and effective in patients with decreased EFs. However, amiodarone is not an attractive option at this time because it is not clear whether his AF symptoms are bothersome enough to warrant this agent, which has several long-term adverse effects. The drug interactions between amiodarone and digoxin and warfarin would have to be addressed before initiating amiodarone.

6. Answer: B
With his history of MI, D.W. has a compelling reason to have a β-blocker as part of his antihypertensive regimen. In general, African Americans do not respond as well as whites to the antihypertensive effects of β-blockade; however, it should still be used. The maintenance of hydrochlorothiazide in his regimen increases the likelihood of adequate BP control because African Americans typically respond well to diuretic therapy, bearing in mind that most individuals require two or more drugs to attain adequate BP control. The regimens without a β-blocker are not appropriate because of D.W.'s medical history. Therapy consisting of losartan or diltiazem is inferior to β-blockade in this patient population.

7. Answer: C

The BP goal in individuals with diabetes mellitus or chronic renal dysfunction is less than 130/80 mm Hg. Despite the categorization of prehypertension, the presence of diabetes warrants immediate therapy to attain a more aggressive goal BP of less than 130/80 mm Hg than in the nondiabetic population. The presence of diabetes presents a compelling reason to include an ACE inhibitor in the absence of any contraindication. Lisinopril initiated at a low dose of 2.5 mg/day is appropriate given her level of renal dysfunction and mildly elevated BP. Angiotensin-converting enzyme inhibitors are superior to ARBs in patients with diabetes, so losartan is not an ideal agent to initiate at this time. Likewise, no compelling indication is present for using a β-blocker in this patient; therefore, an atenolol-based regimen is less desirable than the ACE inhibitor regimen. In all situations, lifestyle modifications should be emphasized to this patient.

8. Answer: C

Because the patient is post-MI, his BP goal is less than 130/80 mm Hg, which he has achieved. Therefore, no decision must be made based on improved BP control. Because he is post-MI, he has a compelling indication for β-blocker therapy, which he is already receiving. He has not provided any information to indicate the need for additional antianginal therapies, so the addition of a calcium channel blocker is not necessary. He is taking appropriate antiplatelet and cholesterol-lowering drugs according to the requirements for individuals with CAD. An ACE inhibitor is indicated in all patients with CAD unless a contraindication exists. Ramipril is reasonable to add to this patient's regimen, and discontinuing hydrochlorothiazide may be desirable to minimize the occurrence of hypotension. However, hydrochlorothiazide could also be continued if the likelihood of hypotension was thought to be low. Vitamin E therapy is not recommended in patients with CAD because of the lack of benefit in this patient population.

9. Answer: D

Both β-blockers and calcium antagonists can be used to achieve HR goals in patients with stable angina. However, this patient has a compelling indication for β-blockade over calcium antagonism (status post-MI), and the dose has room to be increased. Therefore, replacing the β-blocker with a non-dihydropyridine calcium antagonist is not ideal. Although nitroglycerin as needed can be used before exertion to minimize the occurrence of angina, it should be used only after other goals have been achieved, such as a resting HR of 65–60 beats/minute. The only available option that incorporates increased HR control with β-blockade is Answer D, which also incorporates standing nitrate therapy. Adding a nitrate by itself is not advisable because of the potential for reflex tachycardia in an individual who already has a higher than desired HR. The addition of a nitrate (increased oxygen supply) and increased β-blockade (decreased oxygen demand) is the best option for this patient.

ANSWERS AND EXPLANATIONS TO SELF-ASSESSMENT QUESTIONS

1. Answer: D
R.S. has LV systolic dysfunction, probably secondary to her MI 4 months ago. Angiotensin-converting enzyme inhibitors are considered the cornerstone of therapy for LV systolic dysfunction based on evidence that they slow the progression of HF and reduce symptoms, hospitalizations, and mortality in this patient population. Angiotensin-converting enzyme inhibitors should be initiated in all patients with systolic dysfunction. This patient does not have any contraindications for using an ACE inhibitor. Digoxin is not indicated unless a patient is symptomatic on optimal HF therapy. R.S. is neither symptomatic nor on optimal therapy. β-Blockers are recommended, and R.S. is already taking a β-blocker at the target dose. Thus, no rationale exists for adding carvedilol.

2. Answer: C
J.O. is taking the target dose of enalapril, and further increases in the enalapril dose are not necessary unless the patient remains hypertensive once target doses of all agents shown to reduce morbidity and mortality in HF are reached. The addition of β-blocker therapy, initially at a low dose, together with ACE inhibitor therapy, is recommended for further reductions in morbidity and mortality and for slowing the progression of HF. Digoxin is indicated only in symptomatic patients, despite optimal therapy.

3. Answer: A
J.M. has diastolic dysfunction, which is a problem with ventricular relaxation. The preferred therapy is either a β-blocker or a non-dihydropyridine calcium channel blocker, both of which slow the HR and permit greater time for the ventricle to fill with blood. Nifedipine can cause reflex tachycardia, which potentiates diastolic dysfunction by reducing ventricular filling time. Diuretics should be used cautiously because patients with diastolic dysfunction are often fluid-dependent (preload) for maximal ventricular filling. In addition, J.M. has no symptoms of systemic congestion, suggesting a need for increased diuresis. Digoxin does not have a role in managing diastolic dysfunction, and although ACE inhibitors are first-line therapy for systolic dysfunction, they can be considered in diastolic dysfunction if further antihypertensive therapies are needed after the HR is decreased.

4. Answer: D
B.W. has two moderate risk factors (hypertension and age older than 75) as well as a $CHADS_2$ score of 2, making him a candidate for warfarin therapy because of his AF. This will greatly decrease his risk of stroke from about 5% per year to about 1% per year. Because his HR is much less than 80 beats/minute with the atenolol therapy, there is no reason to discontinue this, nor is there a reason to add an additional rate control drug, such as digoxin or diltiazem. With his peripheral vascular disease, atorvastatin therapy is necessary, and his BP is well controlled; therefore, increasing the lisinopril dose is not warranted. To derive the beneficial antiplatelet effects for cardiovascular event prevention, 81 mg of aspirin is adequate. Aspirin 325 mg is also effective but has a greater risk of bleeding with concomitant warfarin.

5. Answer: A
Z.G. is experiencing a rapid ventricular response with exercise/strenuous activity, causing the sensation of palpitations and dyspnea. Digoxin alone exhibits poor control of the ventricular rate during times of high sympathetic influence (e.g., exercise). It is common to require additional therapy to control the ventricular rate adequately. A β-blocker such as atenolol is a good choice to maintain HR during activity. Better agents than verapamil exist because of verapamil's drug interaction with digoxin. The subsequent digoxin concentration may cause symptoms of toxicity. Similarly, doubling the digoxin dose would about double the current serum concentration to 2.2 ng/dL, which should be avoided. Instructing the patient to avoid activity is not desirable because physical activity should be encouraged and supported in all patients, especially in those with risk factors for cardiovascular disease.

6. Answer: B
R.P.'s BP goal is less than 130/80 mm Hg. His therapy with nifedipine is likely highly effective; however, additional therapy is necessary to achieve his goal BP. Ideally, a low-dose diuretic could be added. However, his history of gout makes hydrochlorothiazide a less attractive option, especially at such a large dose (50 mg). Angiotensin-converting enzyme inhibitors are the drug of choice for patients with a history of stroke, and ramipril is a reasonable selection in this patient, whose history includes a transient ischemic attack. An initial dose of 2.5 mg is reasonable in this elderly man. No

indications are present in R.P. to suggest the need for a β-blocker or a non-dihydropyridine calcium channel blocker.

7. Answer: C
During pregnancy, ACE inhibitors and ARBs are contraindicated because of associations with fetal growth restriction, neonatal renal failure, skeletal abnormalities, and fetal death. Methyldopa is preferred as first-line therapy for hypertension in pregnancy based on reports of stable uteroplacental bloodflow and fetal hemodynamics during methyldopa therapy, and there is no evidence of long-term adverse effects on child development. In addition, hydralazine is considered safe in pregnancy; however, the ACE inhibitor should be discontinued for this option to be a reasonable alternative.

8. Answer: D
The proportion of patients receiving Trillionapril who have an event will be compared with the proportion of patients receiving enalapril who have an event. The best statistical test for comparing two proportions (count data) is chi-square analysis. Chi-square analysis is appropriate to analyze nominal or categorical data. An analysis of variance is appropriate when there are more than two treatment groups. The Student unpaired t-test is for continuous data. The Mann-Whitney U-test is appropriate for continuous data that are not normally distributed.

9. Answer: C
This patient has newly diagnosed CAD. All patients with CAD should be taking at least aspirin, lipid-lowering therapy to a goal of less than 100 mg/dL, and an ACE inhibitor. This patient is already receiving appropriate antiplatelet therapy, and the proposed modifications to his lipid-lowering regimen appear reasonable to reach an LDL-C concentration of less than 100 mg/dL. The other lipid-lowering regimens offered are not obviously better at reaching the stated goal. An ACE inhibitor is missing from this patient's discharge regimen, so the addition of ramipril is warranted. A β-blocker is not required because no myocardial damage (infarction) has occurred. However, if additional BP lowering is required, a β-blocker is a reasonable choice because the patient is at high risk of future cardiovascular events.

10. Answer: A
R.K. appears to have sufficient HR control, both at rest and with exercise, so it is desirable to continue his β-blocker therapy. Discontinuing his atenolol and adding nifedipine, which is devoid of HR effects, would not be ideal and might even worsen his angina symptoms because of a relative tachycardia, despite the increased myocardial oxygen supply. Adding amlodipine to the existing HR control therapy is the best choice because it optimizes the oxygen supply, which has not yet been pharmacologically addressed. Adding antiplatelet therapy with clopidogrel or increasing therapy for dyslipidemia will not affect his acute angina symptoms.

TYPES OF ECONOMIC AND HUMANISTIC OUTCOMES ASSESSMENTS

KATHLEEN M. BUNGAY, PHARM.D., FCCP
THE HEALTH INSTITUTE, NEW ENGLAND MEDICAL CENTER
BOSTON, MASSACHUSETTS

LISA A. SANCHEZ, PHARM.D.
PE APPLICATIONS
HIGHLANDS RANCH, COLORADO

TYPES OF ECONOMIC AND HUMANISTIC OUTCOMES ASSESSMENTS

Kathleen M. Bungay, Pharm.D.;
and Lisa A. Sanchez, Pharm.D.

Outline

Frequent misuse and misunderstandings exist regarding what pharmacoeconomics is and what it encompasses. This chapter will assist readers in clarifying their understanding of pharmacoeconomics and lead to an increased understanding of its principles, methods, and applications.

I. Definitions
   A. Pharmacoeconomics—typically defined as the description and analysis of the costs and consequences of pharmaceuticals and pharmaceutical services and its effects on individuals, health care systems, and society. These costs and consequences typically include both economic and humanistic assessments.
      1. A division of outcomes research. However, not all outcomes research is pharmacoeconomic research.
   B. Outcomes research—more broadly defined as studies that attempt to identify, measure, and evaluate the end results of health care services in general; includes not only clinical effects, but also economic and humanistic outcomes such as functional status, well-being, and satisfaction with care. Proponents of outcomes research believe that all three types of outcomes should be measured. (Reference: Figure 1. Components of Contemporary Clinical Decision Making; Reference: Table 1. Some Economic and Humanistic Pharmacoeconomic Evaluations)

II. A proposed model for outcomes evaluations
   A. Proposed that evaluation of drug therapy and related services should always include assessments of economic, clinical, and humanistic outcomes.
   B. The economic, clinical, and humanistic outcome (ECHO) model organizes outcomes of medical care along three general dimensions: clinical, economic, and humanistic.
      1. Economic outcomes—direct, indirect, and intangible costs compared with the consequences of medical treatment alternatives.
      2. Clinical outcomes—medical events that occur as a result of disease or treatment (outside the scope of this program).
      3. Humanistic outcomes—consequences of disease or treatment on patient functional status, or quality of life, measured along several dimensions, e.g., physical functioning, social functioning, general health perceptions and well-being. (Reference: Figure 2. The Conceptual Model: Economic, Clinical, and Humanistic Outcome [ECHO] Model)
   C. The ECHO model recognizes intermediary outcomes
      1. Economic outcomes have intermediaries introduced from the clinical and humanistic side of the model.
         a. From the clinical side are direct costs of medical care associated with each treatment, not just the direct cost of the pharmaceutical products; laboratory testing, emergency department visits, inpatient hospitalizations, and costs of retreatment from product failure also included.
         b. From humanistic side are the indirect, or productivity costs associated with the time lost from work.

c. Direct nonmedical costs for transportation to the hospital, or physicians office for treatment also included.
2. Humanistic outcomes have intermediaries that affect the individual's subjective evaluation of outcomes.
   a. Examples of the intermediaries are listed here and in Figure 3: side effects; efficacy/effectiveness; patient's willingness or ability to pay; adherence to drug regimen (compliance); patient's knowledge; drug dosing schedules. (Reference: Figure 3. Alternative conceptualizations of the relationship between therapeutic interventions and outcomes)

III. Economic outcomes assessment
   A. Costs
      1. Costs—the resources consumed by a program or treatment alternative. Costs must be identified, relevant to the perspective(s) chosen, prior to measurement and comparison.
         a. Direct medical costs—costs incurred for medical products and services used for the prevention, detection, and treatment of a disease.
            i. Examples: hospitalization, drugs, laboratory testing, supplies
               a) Fixed costs represent overhead costs
               b) Variable costs—vary as a function of volume
         b. Direct nonmedical costs—costs for nonmedical services that are the result of illness or disease, but do not involve purchasing medical services.
            i. Examples: special food, transportation for health care, family care
         c. Indirect costs—costs of morbidity and mortality resulting from illness or disease.
            i. Examples: lost productivity, premature death
               a) Human capital method
               b) Willingness to pay
         d. Intangible costs—costs of pain, suffering, grief, and other nonfinancial outcomes of disease and medical care.
         e. Incremental costs—additional costs incurred to obtain an additional unit of benefit from an alternative strategy.
         f. Opportunity costs—money spent on one resource that cannot be spent for other purposes; the value of the next best use that is forgone.
   B. Consequences
      1. Positive versus negative
         a. Full evaluations must measure both desirable and undesirable outcomes.
      2. Intermediate versus final
         a. Intermediate outcomes are commonly used to demonstrate clinical efficacy because their usage reduces the costs and time required to conduct a clinical trial.
      3. Balancing costs and consequences is the essence of pharmacoeconomic evaluation.
   C. Perspectives: The pharmacoeconomic question being asked usually determines the appropriate perspective or viewpoint to be used. (Reference: Figure 4. Potential Perspectives for Pharmacoeconomic Evaluations)
      1. Patient—the ultimate consumer of health care services. Costs, from patients' perspective, are essentially what they pay for a product or service (the portion not covered by insurance).
      2. Provider—the health care professional or care organization; costs from this perspective are the actual costs of providing a product or service, regardless of the charge.
      3. Payer—insurers, government, or employers; the cost to the payer are the charges for health care products and services allowed (reimbursed) by the payer.
      4. Society—costs include patient morbidity and mortality costs, and the overall costs of giving and receiving medical care.
      5. Controversy in choosing perspective
         a. Many researchers assert that society is the best perspective for all economic evaluations.
   D. Misuse of pharmacoeconomic terms: Many have demonstrated that pharmacoeconomic terminologies are commonly misused.
   E. Economic Assessments: The basic task of economic evaluations is to identify, measure, value, and compare the costs and consequences of the alternatives being considered.
      1. Partial economic evaluation include a simple descriptive tabulation of outcomes or resources consumed.
      2. Full economic evaluation helps to assess the economic benefit of a program, service, or treatment.
         a. Requires two distinguishing features of economic evaluation.
            i. Comparison of two or more treatment alternatives.
            ii. Both costs and consequences of the alternatives are examined.
         b. Limitations of full economic analyses. (Reference: Table 2. Common Economic Evaluation Methodologies)
      3. Cost of illness (COI)

a. Definition—involves identifying all the direct and indirect costs of a particular disease or illness within a health care system.
b. Yields a total cost of a disease that can be compared to the cost of implementing a prevention or treatment strategy.
4. Cost-minimization analysis (CMA)
   a. Definition—compares the costs of two or more treatment alternatives that have a demonstrated equivalence in therapeutic outcome (i.e., therapeutically equivalent alternatives).
   b. Results expressed as a total cost per treatment alternative; allows for separate examination of the relevant cost components.
   c. Used to determine the least costly alternative.
5. Cost-benefit analysis (CBA)
   a. Definition—method to compare the costs and benefits of treatment alternatives or programs; costs and benefits expressed in monetary terms.
   b. Results are expressed as either a cost-to-benefit ratio, or as the net cost or benefit.
   c. Example: if cost for treatment is $100 and value of outcome of treatment is $1000, cost-benefit ratio is: benefit ÷ cost = $1000 ÷ $100 = 10/1 benefit of $1 million and cost of $100,000 also yields cost-benefit ratio of 10/1
   d. Used to compare treatment alternatives or programs, particularly when deciding how to allocate scarce resources.
6. Cost-effectiveness analysis (CEA)
   a. Definition—method to compare treatment alternatives, or programs where cost is measured in monetary terms and consequences in units of effectiveness or natural units.
      i. May be less expensive, and at least as effective as the comparator.
      ii. May be more expensive while providing an additional benefit worth the additional cost.
      iii. May be less expensive and less effective when the extra benefit is not worth the extra cost.
   b. Results are expressed as average cost-effectiveness ratios, or as the incremental cost of using one alternative over another.
   c. For example: drug A has 90 percent cure rate, drug B has 95 percent cure rate; drug A costs $50,000 to treat 100 patients, drug B costs $100,000 to treat 100 patients
   d. Calculation of cost-effectiveness ratios:
      drug A costs $50,000/100 patients ÷ 90 cures/100 patients = $555/cure
      drug B costs $100,000/100 patients ÷ 95 cures/100 patients = $1053/cure
   e. Calculation of incremental cost-effectiveness ratio:
      $100,000 - $50,000
      95 cures - 90 cures
      = $10,000/additional cure with drug B
   f. Used to compare competing programs or treatment alternatives that differ in therapeutic outcome
7. Cost-utility analysis (CUA)
   a. Definition—method to compare treatment alternatives or programs where costs are measured in monetary terms and outcome is expressed in terms of patient preferences or quality of life.
   b. Results are expressed as dollars per quality-adjusted life-year (QALY) gained, or some other patient-weighted utility measure.
   c. Used to compare treatments or programs using terms of patient preference, or quality of health care, or when outcomes cannot be expressed in monetary terms.

IV. Techniques for analysis
   A. Discounting
      1. Definition—an analysis that adjusts (reduces) future costs and consequences to reflect present fiscal value.
      2. Discounting costs—based on the time value of money; because the value of money decreases over time, future costs must be adjusted (discounted) to present time values.
      3. Discount rate—discount rate of 3–8 percent should be used (often reflective of current interest rates used by banking institutions).
   B. Sensitivity analysis
      1. Definition—an analysis that tests robustness of study conclusions; sensitive variables (or assumptions) are varied over a range of plausible results and the impact on study results is observed.
      2. Variables include percent efficacy (or effectiveness), incidence of specific adverse drug reactions, and dominant costs.
   C. Decision analysis
      1. Definition—an explicit, quantitative, and prescriptive approach to choosing between competing treatment alternatives or programs.

2. Tool used in decision analysis is a decision tree; allows for the graphic presentation of treatment alternatives, outcomes, and probabilities. (Reference: Figure 5. Decision Tree)
   D. Incremental cost analysis
      1. Definition—an analysis that examines the extra cost of one program or treatment alternative relative to the additional effect provided by that alternative.
      2. formula: $\dfrac{\text{Cost B} - \text{Cost A}}{\text{Effect B} - \text{Effect A}}$

V. Applied Pharmacoeconomics
   A. Definition—putting pharmacoeconomic principles, methods and theories into practice to assess the value of pharmaceutical products and services used in "real-world" practice settings.
   B. Primary application—to inform local decision making.
      1. Specific applications of economic assessments
         a. Formulary management
         b. Clinical guidelines
         c. Drug use policies
         d. Service or program evaluation
         e. Individual patient treatment decisions

VI. Humanistic Outcomes Assessment
   A. Background
      1. Measurement of health
         a. Case study
   B. Evolution of today's health status outcome measures
      1. During the 1940s, physicians first began to measure patient functioning;
         a. Karnofsky Functional Status for Patients with Cancer
         b. New York Heart Association Classification
      2. When social science methods and clinical expertise came together in the 1970s, the first modern health-status questionnaires emerged.
         a. Quality of Well-Being Scale,
         b. Sickness Impact Profile,
         c. Health Perceptions Questionnaire,
         d. Older Americans Resources and Services (OARS) questionnaire
      3. The next generation developed in the 1980s and 90s
         a. Health Insurance Experiment (HIE) health surveys
         b. Duke-UNC Health Profiles
         c. Nottingham Health Profile
         d. Medical Outcomes Study health surveys, including the SF-36 Health Survey
      4. Variations in medical care in small areas
         a. Typically traced to the work of John Wennberg, who uncovered a phenomenon known as small-area variation.
         b. Wennberg and colleagues noticed large disparities in the rates of various medical procedures in different geographic areas.
      5. The Rand HIE
         a. In 1990, health expenditures accounted for 12.4 percent of GNP, whereas that proportion was 4 percent in 1980, and the rate of growth was exceeding the rate of inflation, questions surfaced.
         b. This quandary prompted the federal government to support a large-scale controlled trial, now known as HIE.
            i. One purpose of the HIE was to learn whether the direct cost of medical care, when borne by consumers, affects their health.
            ii. Presented one of the first major challenges for measuring health status.
            iii. A consequence of this challenge resulted in one of the most extensive applications of psychometric theory and methods (long used in educational testing), to the development and refinement of health status surveys.
            iv. The measurement goal in the HIE was to construct the best possible scales for measuring a broad array of functioning and well-being concepts.
            v. HIE demonstrated the potential of scales, constructed from self-administered surveys, as reliable and valid tools for assessing changes in health status.
            vi. It left two questions unanswered:
               a) Can methods of data collection and scale construction work in sicker and older populations?
               b) Could scales that are more efficient be constructed?

                    vii. The answer to these questions was the challenge accepted by the Medical Outcomes Study (MOS) investigators.
            6. Medical Outcomes Study
                a. Two-year observational study designed to help understand how specific components of the health care system affected the outcomes of care.
                b. Original purpose was to develop more practical tools for monitoring patient outcomes, and their determinants, in routine practice using state-of-the-art psychometric techniques.
            7. Agency for Health Care Policy and Research (AHCPR)/Agency for Healthcare Research and Quality (AHRQ)
                a. To enhance the quality, appropriateness, and effectiveness of health care services and access to services, the federal government established AHCPR (Omnibus Budget Reconciliation Act of 1989).
                    i. The act, sometimes referred to as the Patient Outcomes Research Act, called for the establishment of a broad-based, patient-centered outcomes research program.
                b. In 1999, the agency was reauthorized as AHRQ.
    C. Evaluating the Quality of Care
        1. Structure denotes the attributes of the settings in which care occurs. Evaluations of structure address the relatively stable characteristics of the providers of care, of the tools and resources they have at their disposal, and of the physical and organizational settings in which they work.
        2. Process of care denotes what is actually done in giving and receiving care. It includes the patient's activities in seeking care and carrying it out, as well as the practitioner's activities in making a diagnosis and recommending, or implementing, treatment.
        3. Outcomes of care denote the effects of care on the health status of patients and populations. Improvements in patients' knowledge and salutary changes in patients' behaviors are included under a broad definition of health status, and so is the degree of each patient's satisfaction with care.
    D. Definitions
        1. Quality of Life
            a. Quality of life refers to an evaluation of all aspects of our lives, including where and how we live, how we play, and how we work.
        2. Health
            a. Health is one of 12 domains of life to be considered when researching and evaluating overall quality of life.
            b. The other 11 domains are listed in Table 3 and include: community; education; family life; friendships; housing; marriage; nation; neighborhood; self; standard of living; and work.
        3. Health-related quality of life
            a. Encompasses only those aspects of life that are dominated, or significantly influenced by personal health or activities performed to maintain, or improve health.
            b. Is a specifically focused area of investigation within the larger field of health services and quality-of-life research. Standardized questionnaires are used to capture health-related quality-of-life data.
            c. The term health-related quality of life was adopted by researchers to set their research apart from the more global concept of quality of life, and to more accurately reflect the scope of their research.
    E. Measurement
        1. Measurement is a set of numbers or rules used to quantify a physical attribute. Examples of measurement devices are rulers, thermometers, and scales.
        2. Health has distinct components that must be measured and interpreted individually to fully understand health at a given time, as well as changes over time.
            a. Clues about the components are found in the definitions of health offered by the World Health Organization, as well as in dictionaries.
                i. The World Health Organization has defined health as a state of complete physical, social, and mental well-being, not merely the absence of disease or infirmity.
                ii. Dictionary definitions also identify both physical and mental dimensions of health. The former pertains to the body and bodily needs, the latter to the mind and, particularly, to the emotional and intellectual status of the individual.
                iii. Health connotes completeness, where nothing is missing from the person; it also connotes proper function, where all is working efficiently. The dictionary also suggests well-being, soundness, and vitality as important components of health.
            b. Both World Health Organization and dictionary definitions provide precedents for the dimensionality of health and, specifically, for the distinction between physical and mental health.
            c. Two features of these definitions are crucial
                i. The dimensionality of health.
                ii. The existence of a full range of health states, ranging from disease to well-being.
        3. Range of measurement

            a. Many measurement scales artificially restrict the range of individual differences enumerated. Consistent with a disease orientation, most disease-specific measures emphasize the negative end of the health continuum.
            b. Figure 7 illustrates how both the positive and negative ends of the range might be considered when evaluating mental health status.
    F. Measurement strategy
        1. To provide an assessment of health-related quality of life, one of three approaches is usually taken.
            a. Focus on general health status
            b. Disease-specific-focused on specific aspects of the disease under study.
            c. Both generic and disease specific.
        2. Though measurement strategies may be slightly different, there are some commonly agreed upon and frequently measured general health concepts.
            a. Physical functioning
            b. Mental functioning
            c. Social and role functioning
            d. General health perceptions
    G. General health status measures
        1. Not disease or disorder specific.
        2. Relevant to all ages, races, sexes, and socioeconomic backgrounds.
        3. Permit examination of treatment benefits in comparable units.
        4. Advantages
            a. Used for monitoring patients with more than one condition.
            b. Can compare patients with different conditions by providing a common yardstick.
            c. Used to assess the relative benefits of different treatments.
            d. The same measures can be appropriately applied to both general (well) and patient (sick) populations; can be used with people of any age, gender, or race.
        5. Disadvantages
            a. Do not cover areas of health status that are important to particular groups of patients who may experience specific improvements or disabilities in functioning due to their disease state.
            b. Need to use additional questionnaires for disease- or condition-specific set of questions.
            c. Not specific to any particular disease state; not able to capture symptoms or domains specifically related to one disease state (e.g., dexterity with arthritis). (Reference: Table 5 lists these key health concepts and indicates how they might be assessed)

VII. Components Common to Many General Health Status Measures
    A. Physical functioning
        1. Physical functioning as it relates to health-related quality-of-life assessment typically refers to the limitations, or disability, experienced by the patient over a defined period.
        2. Questions focus on observable and important physical limitations easily noticed and evaluated by the patient or observer.
    B. Social and Role Functioning
        1. Social functioning
            a. Social functioning is defined as the ability to develop, maintain, and nurture mature social relationships.
                i. Frequency of social contacts.
                ii. Nature of those contacts within the social network or community.
        2. Role functioning
            a. Concerned with the impact health has on a person's ability to meet the demands of that person's normal life role. Work for pay, homemaking duties, and schoolwork are all covered by questions asking about this concept.
            b. Identify everyday role situations or activities that can be directly affected or limited by disease, illness, or treatment.
            c. Whereas most role limitations are due to physical health problems, role limitations are observed both in the presence, and in the absence of, physical limitations.
    C. Mental Health
        1. Disease often affects behavioral, as well as physical aspects of a person's life. General health status assessments, therefore, usually include questions covering aspects of psychological health.
    D. General Health Perceptions
        1. General health perceptions address the person's overall beliefs and evaluations about his or her health.

VIII. Disease-Specific Health Status Instruments
    A. Some limitations or problems with patients' health are unique to their specific disease state.

B. Batteries of questions were designed for use with specific patient populations, and are used to supplement a general health status instrument.
C. These more narrowly focused disease-specific measures request detailed information about the impact a specific disease, and its treatment, have on the patient, from the patient's perspective.
D. In addition, using disease-specific measures allows inclusion of questions of specific interest.
E. Among some specific areas previously investigated with disease-specific questionnaires are sexual functioning, nausea and vomiting, pain, cancer, arthritis, epilepsy, HIV infection, anxiety and depression, asthma, and rhinitis.

IX. Psychometric Theory
A. The underlying theory that supports the design of health surveys, consisting of scales measuring attributes of a person or a population's health.
B. Same theories that support the creation of educational measurements (e.g., Standardized Achievement Tests).
C. A person who studies these theories and conducts research or measurement of such attributes as intelligence, pain, mental well-being, or functioning is usually a doctorate level research psychologist and can be known as a psychometrician.
D. In recent years has produced, in the health sciences literature devoted to measuring health status, a daunting array of already available scales.
E. Perhaps the most common error committed by clinical researchers is to dismiss the existing scales too lightly, and embark on the development of a new instrument with an unjustifiably optimistic and naïve expectation that they can do better.
F. A comprehensive set of standards, widely used in the assessment of psychology and education, is the manual called Standards for Educational and Psychological Tests, published by the American Psychological Association (1974).

X. Psychometric Considerations
A. Psychometrics is the science of testing questionnaires to measure attributes of individuals.
B. It is used in the field of health assessment to translate people's behavior, feelings, and personal evaluations into quantifiable data.
C. These data, once captured, must be both relevant and correct if they are to provide useful insights into health-related quality of life.
   1. Reliability—the relationship between true variation and random error. Evaluations assess the consistency and repeatability of measurement.
   2. Validity—refers to the extent to which differences in scale scores reflect the true differences in the individuals studied.
   3. Useful scales must be sensitive to change, and be accepted by the investigators and respondents.

XI. Use of Patient-Reported Health Status
A. Monitoring the health of populations.
B. Evaluating health care policy.
C. Conducting clinical trials of alternative treatment.
D. Designing systems for monitoring and improving health care outcomes.
E. Individual Patient Care Decisions
   1. Controversies in using health status assessments.
   2. Contributions of technology and modern test theory to the use of health status instruments.
   3. Advances in using health status assessments for individual patient care decisions.
      a. Standardized measures capturing patient perspectives are likely to become more acceptable as a piece of evidence of which providers and their patients can make decisions about treatment and a treatment's efficacy.
      b. Mature theoretical models, sophisticated measurement techniques, and enhanced technology for use in measurement, make the routine use of individual patient results in their own care more promising than ever before.
   4. Two practical concerns of the critics of use of health-related quality-of-life assessments in individual patient care are:
      a. Respondent burden and;
      b. Reliability of scores obtained from shorter questionnaires.
   5. Modern test theory offers the potential for individualized, comparable assessments for the careful examination and application of different health status measures.
      a. One such theory is Item Response Theory (IRT). Researchers report that IRT has a number of potential advantages over the currently used Classical Test Theory in assessing self-reported health outcomes.
      b. Applications of the IRT models are ideally suited for implementing computer adaptive testing. IRT methods are also reported to be helpful in developing better health outcome measures, and in assessing change over time.

6. Patients increasingly have more access to computer technology. It is becoming more practical to use assessments using a computer.
    a. Patients answering questions about a health status concept using dynamic assessment technology are requested only to complete the number of questions needed (minimizes response burden) to establish a reliable estimate.
    b. The resulting scores for an individual are estimated to meet the clinical measures of precision.

XII. Case Study Continued

XIII. Patient Satisfaction
   A. Another outcome suggested by a popular quality-of-care model for how to evaluate the quality of health care is that of patient satisfaction.
   B. Empirical studies show that patients' expressions of dissatisfaction are potent predictors of disenrollment from a physician or a health plan.
   C. A consumer's evaluation of the care received, known as consumer evaluation or patient satisfaction, is both similar and different from a patient's assessment of health status.
      1. The same psychometric techniques are used to obtain information, and to evaluate the accuracy of the information.
      2. The science of obtaining the information is similar.
      3. The information is unique and different from what is asked about health status.
      4. Both reports and ratings are used in patient satisfaction surveys.
         a. Reports are descriptions.
         b. Ratings are evaluations that require a judgment by the evaluator (patient).
   D. There are many different patient satisfaction surveys available.
      1. Attributes that are commonly evaluated, regardless of the care setting include:
         a. The clinician's scientific knowledge and skill;
         b. The quality of clinician-patient communications;
         c. The provision of humane interpersonal treatment;
         d. And the degree of the patient's trust in the care provider.
   E. One setting in which patient satisfaction surveys are becoming increasingly important is that of primary care.
      1. Four distinguishing and shared multiple characteristics are considered essential and unique to this area of health care and provide attributes that can be evaluated by patients. These characteristics include:
         a. Accessibility to care;
         b. Continuity of care;
         c. The comprehensiveness of care and;
         d. How well a patient's care is integrated into a coherent and continuing whole.

XIV Other Measures of Outcomes
   A. The concept of work functioning must be included as an outcome to meet the evaluation needs of employers, who have become a significant form in health care.
   B. The ability to quantify the constituent parts of the losses in work productivity is growing in importance, and will undoubtedly be an important measured health domain.

XV. Conclusion

Learning Objectives

1. Identify and define the terminology and basic components of health economics, outcomes research, and pharmacoeconomics.
2. Differentiate between full and partial economic evaluations.
3. Define direct, indirect, intangible, incremental, and opportunity costs, and classify them based on the perspective taken.
4. Discuss the controversies related to the perspective taken for an economic analysis.
5. Discuss the controversies related to discounting costs and benefits.
6. Differentiate between the application of outcomes research results to system decisions and individualization of patient therapy.
7. Discuss the identification and measurement of appropriate outcomes in health economics research.
8. Understand the evolution and scientific basis for the use of patient self-reported health status assessments.
9. Characterize contemporary developments in content, measurement, and uses of personal health measures.
10. Distinguish between population-based and individual level measures of health.
11. Understand the basic concepts underlying the measurement of health-related quality of life.
12. Differentiate between generic and disease-specific health-related quality-of-life instruments.
13. Discuss uses of health status assessments with other health care professionals.
14. Understand the technological improvements going on in the field of health status measurement.

Abbreviations in This Chapter

ACER	Average cost-effectiveness ratio
AHCPR	Agency for Health Care Policy and Research
AHRQ	Agency for Healthcare Research and Quality
CBA	Cost-benefit analysis
CEA	Cost-effectiveness analysis
COI	Cost of illness
CMA	Cost-minimization analysis
CUA	Cost-utility analysis
ECHO	Economic, clinical, humanistic outcomes
HIE	Health Insurance Experiment
HRQOL	Health-related quality of life
IRT	Item Response Theory
MOS	Medical Outcomes Study
MOS SF-36	Medical Outcomes Study, short form, 36 items
OARS	Older Americans Resources and Services
QALY	Quality-adjusted life-year

Introduction

Frequent misuse of pharmacoeconomic terms abounds. Misconceptions, such as pharmacoeconomics equals cost-containment, and pharmacoeconomics compromises clinical decision making, have lead to apprehension by many health care professionals as they evaluate the economic and humanistic outcomes of health care products and services. Pharmacoeconomics is not about determining the cheapest health care alternatives, but is about determining those alternatives that provide the best health care outcome per dollar spent. This chapter should assist in clarifying many of these misconceptions, leading to an increased understanding of pharmacoeconomic principles, methods, and its application to health care today.

Definitions

Pharmacoeconomics typically is defined as the description and analysis of the costs and consequences of pharmaceuticals and pharmaceutical services, and its impact on individuals, health care systems, and society. Pharmacoeconomics is a division of outcomes research and, typically, addresses both economic and humanistic outcomes. However, not all outcomes research is pharmacoeconomic research.

Outcomes research is more broadly defined as studies that attempt to identify, measure, and evaluate the end results of health care services. As depicted in Figure 1, not only clinical effects, but also economic and humanistic outcomes are included. Thus, proponents of outcomes research believe in measuring, not only the clinical and cost impacts of health care, but also the outcomes that take the patient's perspective into account. Some of the economic and humanistic outcomes to be addressed are listed in Table 1.

Economic, Clinical, and Humanistic Outcomes Model

It has been proposed that the evaluation of drug therapy and related services should include an assessment of economic, clinical, and humanistic outcomes (ECHO) model

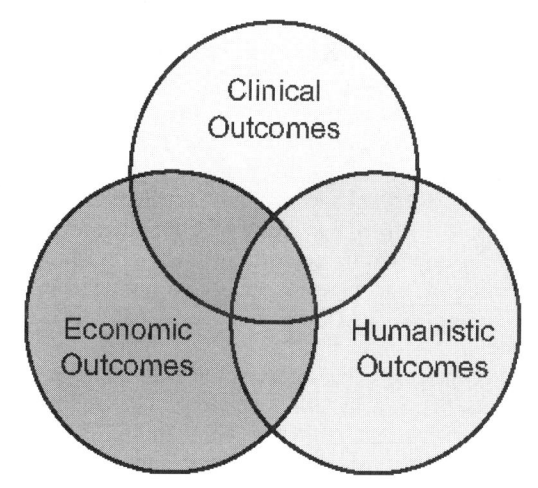

Figure 1. Components of Contemporary Clinical Decision-Making

Table 1. Some Economic and Humanistic Pharmacoeconomic Evaluations

Economic Evaluations	Humanistic Evaluations
Cost-of-illness	Quality of Life
Cost-minimization analysis	Patient preferences
Cost-benefit analysis	Patient Satisfaction
Cost-effectiveness analysis	Willingness-to-pay
Cost-utility analysis	

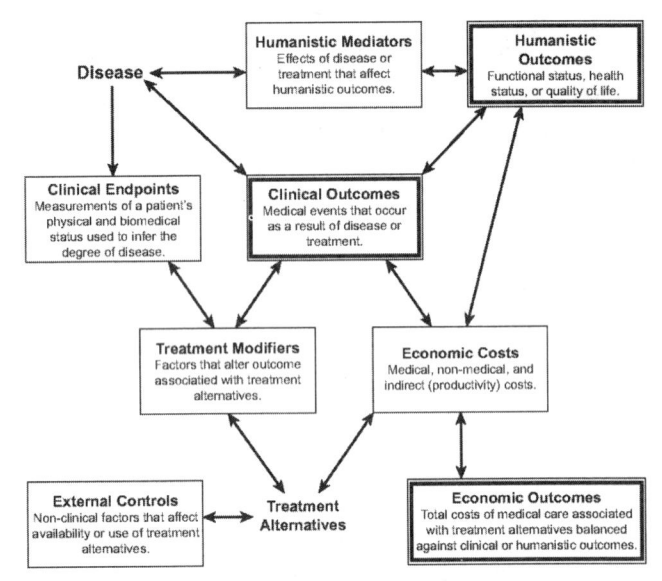

Figure 2. The Conceptual Model: Economic, Clinical, and Humanistic Outcomes (ECHO) Model.
Reprinted with permission from Kozma CM, Reeder CE, Shulz RM. Economic, clinical, and humanistic outcomes: a planning model for pharmacoeconomic research. Clin Ther 1993;15:1121–32.

(see Reference 13). In their proposed model, the ECHO model, depicted in Figure 2, it is assumed that the outcomes of medical care can be classified along these three dimension. Clinical outcomes are defined as medical events that occur as a result of disease or treatment. Economic outcomes are defined as direct, indirect, and intangible costs, compared with the consequences of medical treatment alternatives. Humanistic outcomes are defined as the consequences of disease or treatment on patient functional status, or quality of life. Multiple variables important for understanding the value of alternatives exist within each type of outcome. The authors propose that all three of these outcomes need to be balanced simultaneously to assess value.

Some of the many variables that need to be balanced are intermediate outcomes, or intermediaries. The ECHO model proposes some examples of intermediaries. The economic outcomes have intermediaries introduced from the clinical and humanistic side of the model. The clinical outcomes have intermediaries introduced from the direct costs of medical care associated with each treatment. These intermediaries include the costs of laboratory testing, emergency department visits and inpatient hospitalizations, and costs of retreatment from product failures. As you can see, these costs are more than just the direct costs of pharmaceutical products. Direct nonmedical costs for transportation to the hospital or physician's office for treatment also must be included. Humanistic outcomes have intermediaries, including indirect costs such as time lost from work, that must be added.

Additional humanistic intermediaries are proposed. Examples of these intermediaries include adverse reactions, efficacy or effectiveness of a drug, the patients' willingness or ability to pay, patient compliance, patient knowledge, and dosing requirements such as frequency of administration. Figure 3 depicts a suggested framework for the relationship between the choice of a therapeutic agent and humanistic outcome. Before improvements in health status and patient satisfaction were widely recognized as goals of therapy, the decision about the success of an intervention was based on a favorable balance between the effectiveness and the safety from the clinician's point of view. In this model, effectiveness and safety are no longer the only factors considered to evaluate success. The effects of symptom relief and adverse events, from the patient's perspective, become the main measure of success. For example, even though selective serotonin-reuptake inhibitors are shown to be very effective in the treatment of depression, some patients report insomnia and nightmares. On a depression rating scale, the patient may achieve a score that indicates relief from the symptoms of depression. Patients may simultaneously report in a self-administered health-related quality-of-life (HRQOL) questionnaire they have low vitality and low scores in role-functioning, both indicating poor functioning from the patient's viewpoint. When the patient is questioned about the low scores, it could be discovered that she is a single parent who needs to maintain a job to support her children. Her job requires concentration and alertness during the day, and the drug, although effective and seemingly safe, interferes with her daily functioning, and what is important to her.

Another intermediate factor is the patient's ability, or willingness, to pay for the prescribed therapy. The patient's perception of the effectiveness, or experience, of side effects on health status, as well as financial constraints, can influence willingness to continue to purchase the drug. Nonadherence to therapy, a significant problem with drugs effectiveness, can actually have a positive effect on functional health status as perceived by the patient. The relationship of compliance to outcomes is of growing importance as the study of health status and patient satisfaction matures. It is impossible to establish a relationship between a therapeutic intervention, and its outcome, without the assurance that the patient has taken the prescribed therapy. In addition to willingness to pay and compling, patients' knowledge of their therapy and the dosing schedule influence the humanistic outcomes and each other. Even though many of these relationships are

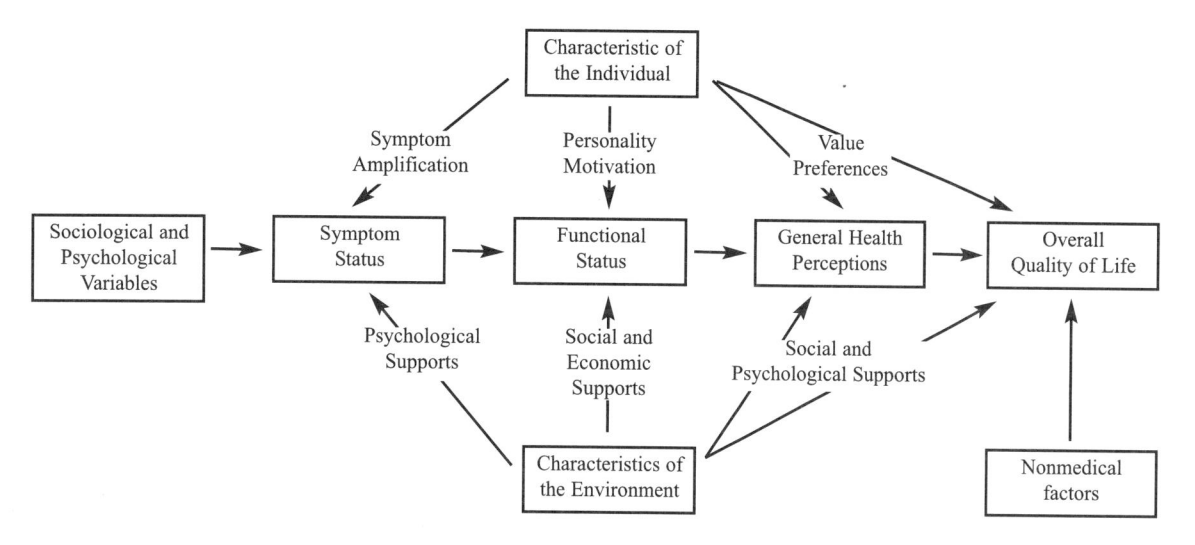

Figure 3. Relationships among measures of patient outcome in a HRQOL conceptual model.
Wilson IB, Cleary PD. Linking clinical variables with health-related quality of life. A conceptual model of patient outcomes. JAMA 1995;273(1):59–65. Reprinted with permission.

studied, there is much room for advancement in understanding the relationships of each of these intermediate variables to humanistic outcomes.

The methods of pharmacoeconomic evaluation strive to assess the value of pharmaceutical products and services, and incorporate several types of outcomes, including those of a clinical, economic, and humanistic nature, in assessing this value to the health care system. This series focuses on the assessment of economic and humanistic outcomes and its applications to patient care. The assessment of clinical outcomes is beyond the scope of the series, and will be addressed in global terms only.

Costs

Traditional cost-containment measures are not always synonymous with improved patient care. Thus, attention has turned toward demonstrating the value of health care. It is critical that the health care products and services used in today's institutions and organizations achieve the highest possible benefit from the dollars spent. Quantification of the value of health care products and services, especially pharmaceuticals, is critical today.

Before a full discussion of the methods of economic evaluation can take place, it is important to examine closely the various categories of costs and consequences that can be included in an economic evaluation. A full evaluation of the relevant costs and consequences differentiates pharmacoeconomics from traditional cost-containment strategies and drug use evaluations. Costs are defined as the value of the resources consumed by a program or treatment alternative. Consequences are defined as the effects, outputs, and outcomes of the program or treatment alternative. This section focuses on identifying, measuring, and comparing the costs, or economic outcomes of health care interventions.

A comparison of two or more treatment alternatives should extend beyond a simple comparison of drug acquisition costs. Cost categories that need to be considered include direct, indirect, and intangible costs. Other costs often discussed in pharmacoeconomic evaluations include opportunity and incremental costs. Including these various cost categories, when appropriate, will provide a more accurate estimate of the total economic impact of a health care program, or treatment alternative, on a specific population, organization, or patient. Each of these types of cost categories are discussed in greater detail.

Direct Costs

Direct costs are the resources consumed in the prevention, detection, or treatment of a disease or illness. These costs can be divided into direct medical and direct nonmedical costs. Direct medical costs quantify the fundamental transactions associated with medical care, and are the costs that contribute to the portion of gross national product spent on health care. An example of costs associated directly with health care interventions include hospitalizations, drugs, medical supplies and equipment, laboratory and diagnostic testing, and physician visits.

Direct medical costs can be further subdivided into fixed and variable costs. Fixed costs represent the overhead costs that are relatively constant and not readily influenced at the treatment level. Thus, they are typically not included in most pharmacoeconomic evaluations. Some examples of fixed costs are those incurred for heat, rent, and lighting. Variable costs, on the other hand, vary as a function of volume and include drugs, fees for a professional service, and supplies. Thus, as a greater number of services are used, more funding must be consumed to provide these services. Shifts in variable costs are particularly important as a means of assessing the cost-effectiveness of a treatment alternative.

Some controversy exists as to whether personnel costs should be considered as fixed or variable costs. For example, in a hospital setting, one might ask whether switching from a treatment that requires administration 4 times daily to one administered once daily truly saves time for pharmacy technicians, pharmacists, and nurses. Some argue that staffing of these personnel is relatively constant, regardless of the number of patients or number of doses, and that such a change would not cause the hospital to lay off personnel. Others feel that an intervention, such as the one described, frees time for these personnel to perform other activities that provide value and, thus, should be treated as a variable cost. Certainly in this time of "downsizing" or "rightsizing," personnel are often viewed as variable costs by administrators.

Direct nonmedical costs also contribute a significant portion to the total direct cost of a treatment alternative. These are the costs for nonmedical services that are the result of illness or disease, but do not involve the purchase of medical services. Thus, these costs are consumed to purchase services other than medical care, and include resource expenditures borne by patients in seeking care. For example, direct nonmedical costs may include transportation to and from health care facilities, extra trips to the emergency department, attendant child or family care expenses, special diets or clothes, and various other out-of-pocket expenses.

Indirect Costs

Indirect costs are also necessary to consider in the full economic evaluation of a program or treatment alternative. Indirect costs are a less obvious, but no less important source of resource consumption, especially from the perspective of the patients. Indirect costs are those costs that result from morbidity and mortality. These costs are related to changes in production capacity that result from disease or health care interventions. Morbidity costs are costs incurred from missing work, that is, lost productivity. Mortality costs are the costs incurred due to premature death.

To estimate indirect costs, two techniques typically used are the human capital method, and the willingness-to-pay method. Each method attempts to estimate different types of costs. The human capital approach attempts to value morbidity and mortality losses based on an individual's earning capacity. Thus, the value of a life is directly related to income. To estimate the earnings foregone or gained as a result of the illness, the human capital approach uses standard labor wage rates. Because all segments of the population do not have the same level of earnings, using this approach raises an ethical dilemma. Some individual groups such as the elderly, children, and the homeless earn virtually nothing at all. Thus, valuing "imputed" wages of some segments of the population may be an acceptable means of more fairly assigning a value to indirect costs.

In the willingness-to-pay approach, patients are explicitly asked how much money they would be willing to spend to reduce the likelihood of illness. The values obtained through this method are often unreliable because there may be up to 200-fold differences in valuations of life due to pay estimates that are not realistic relative to ones ability. It should be noted that while the willingness-to-pay approach incorporates indirect and intangible costs, the human capital approach considers only changes in work loss and productivity due to morbidity and mortality.

Intangible Costs

Intangible costs are probably the most difficult costs to measure. Intangible costs are those costs incurred that represent nonfinancial outcomes of disease and medical care, and which are not properly expressed in monetary terms. Examples of intangible costs include pain, suffering, inconvenience and grief. Typically, these types of costs are identified in an economic analysis, but often not formally quantified. These costs can either be presented as a caveat in the discussion of the results of an economic evaluation or converted into a common unit of outcome measurement such as a quality-adjusted life-year (QALY).

Incremental Costs

As medical interventions become increasingly intense, costs typically increase. However, due to the economic principle of decreasing incremental returns, the additional outcome gained per additional dollar spent typically decreases. At some point of increasing expenditures, there may be no additional benefits, or even a reduction in outcome. Thus, incremental costs may be another way to assess the economic impact of a program or treatment alternative on a population. Incremental costs represent the additional cost that a program or treatment alternative imposes over another, compared to the additional effect, benefit, or outcome it provides. In other words, incremental costs are the extra costs required to purchase an additional unit of effect.

Opportunity Costs

If a resource is used to purchase a program or treatment alternative, then the opportunity to use it for another purpose is lost. This is referred to as an opportunity cost. This cost represents what could have been produced or purchased with the same resources if the treatment alternative in question was not purchased. In other words, opportunity cost is the value of the alternative that was forgone.

Consequences

Full pharmacoeconomic analyses provide an assessment of the efficiency, and are determined according to the amount of output per unit of input, of one alternative versus another. Compared to the costs of the inputs, the outcomes, or consequences of a disease and its treatment, comprises an equally important component of this research. Although the assessment of costs is relatively similar across the various methods, the manner in which consequences are assessed represents the key distinction among these techniques. Regardless of the method used, good assessments of relative consequences of competing alternatives allows researchers to balance the costs of a program or treatment with their consequences or benefits.

Positive versus Negative Consequences

Most often, benefits of drug therapy are characterized in terms of beneficial effects to the patient. However, a comprehensive assessment of benefits will address both positive and negative effects of competing alternatives. Positive consequences may translate into life-years gained, cases cured, disability days avoided, and improved functional status and well-being. Conversely, because drug products are not devoid of adverse effects, negative consequences also may result. Negative consequences can include harmful side effects, exacerbation of disease, drug toxicity, treatment failure, or even death. Thus, the balancing of positive and negative consequences is critical. For example, the consequences component of an analysis of an aminoglycoside would reflect not only the positive consequences associated with curing an infection, but the potential negative consequences associated with drug toxicities, such as nephrotoxicity.

Intermediate versus Final Consequences

Intermediate consequences are commonly used in clinical trials to demonstrate clinical efficacy because their use reduces the cost and time required to conduct a clinical trial. For example, achieving a decrease in low-density lipoprotein cholesterol levels achieved with a lipid-lowering agent is an intermediate consequence. This intermediate outcome serves as a proxy for more relevant final outcomes, or consequences, expressed as a decrease in myocardial infarction rate and an increase in lives saved. Intermediate consequences are used often in cost-effectiveness analyses as proxies predictive of final consequences of interest. The challenge lies in finding intermediate outcome indicators that can reliably predict long-term effects.

Balancing Costs and Consequences

Balancing costs and consequences is the essence of pharmacoeconomic evaluation. Regardless of the method of economic evaluation used, the objective of pharmacoeconomic research is to provide information regarding the relative value of treatment alternatives through an explicit attempt to balance the costs and consequences of each alternative. Typically, results of this approach will be reported in terms of a cost per unit of effect. The primary distinction among the various methods of economic evaluation rests in the valuation of the consequence side of the equation. This chapter summarizes specific methodological approaches of balancing costs and consequences. Subsequent chapters describe each method in greater detail.

Perspectives

Many perspectives are possible in the economic and humanistic evaluation of medical care. Perspective refers to the point of view from which the economic analysis is performed. These perspectives, or viewpoints, will influence the costs and consequences identified, measured, and compared for a program or treatment alternative. An economic evaluation can be conducted from a single perspective, or multiple perspectives. Common perspectives include those of the patient, provider, payer, and society. The value of a treatment alternative will be heavily dependent on the point of view taken. A variety of perspectives are shown in Figure 4.

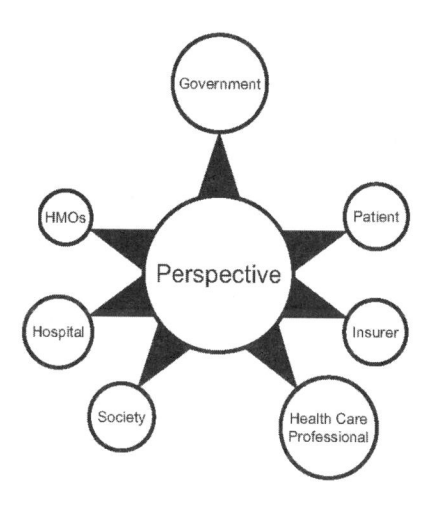

Figure 4. Potential Perspectives for Pharmacoeconoic Evaluations

Patient Perspective

Patients are the ultimate consumers of health care services. Costs from the perspective of patients are essentially what they pay for a product or service, that is, the portion not covered by insurance. Other costs incurred due to illness or treatment, including morbidity and mortality costs, may be captured using this perspective. Consequences from a patient's perspective are the clinical effects of a program or treatment alternative. Costs from a patient's perspective might include insurance co-payments and out-of-pocket drug costs. Also, indirect costs, in terms of health-related work and living limitations are also important from the patient perspective. Additionally, patients are concerned with the positive and negative consequences of a given treatment. The patient's perspective should be considered when assessing the impact of drug therapy on quality of life, or if a patient will pay out-of-pocket expenses for a health care service.

Provider Perspective

Costs from the provider's perspective are the true expense of providing a product or service, regardless of the charge. Few providers are prepared to identify and measure their true economic costs. Charge data may be more readily available, but are usually not reflective of the true costs of health care. Providers can be hospitals, managed care organizations, or private practice physicians. The primary costs from a provider's perspective are of a direct nature. For example, drugs, hospitalization, laboratory tests, supplies, and salaries of health care professionals may be appropriately identified and measured from a provider's perspective. Indirect costs, on the other hand, may be less important from the provider perspective since these expenses are not realized by the provider. When making formulary management, or drug use policy decisions, the viewpoint of the health care organization should dominate. The exception would be when making decisions for a Medicaid or Medicare formulary where the government, or societal perspectives, should dominate.

Payer Perspective

Payers include insurance companies, the government, or employers. Medicare, Blue Cross/Blue Shield, and Motorola are all examples of payers. The costs to the payer are those charges for health care products and services allowed, or reimbursed, by the payer. Again, the primary cost from a payer's perspective are direct costs. However, indirect costs, such as lost workdays and decreased productivity also may contribute to the total cost of health care to the payer. For example, if a patient has peptic ulcer disease, his or her employer may lose the patient's services for 30 days out of the work year. This represents an indirect cost to the employer, who incurs the loss of 30 productive days for this employee. The payer's perspective should be used when insurance companies and employers are contracting with managed care organizations, or selecting employee health care benefits.

Societal Perspective

Society is another potential perspective for pharmacoeconomic evaluations. This perspective is the broadest of all perspectives because it is the only one that considers the benefit to society as a whole. Many researchers assert that society is the best perspective for all economic evaluations. In general, all direct and indirect costs are included in an economic evaluation performed from a societal perspective. Costs from a societal perspective include patient morbidity and mortality costs, and the overall costs of giving and receiving medical care. Also, the perspective that dominates in the health economic literature is that of society. From a societal perspective, all of the important costs and consequences an individual member of society could experience may be included in a complete evaluation of a health care program or treatment alternative. In countries with nationalized medical systems, society is the predominant perspective.

Controversy in Choosing a Perspective

There is some controversy surrounding the issue of a study perspective. Many researchers assert that society is the only relevant, as well as the best perspective from which to conduct an economic analyses from. However, in the United States these studies can be very resource intensive, in terms of time and money. Further, in the real world, organizations may need to focus solely on a single perspective to obtain the data necessary to inform timely decision-making on a local level. Regardless of the perspective chosen, perspective is fundamental because all costs and consequences identified, measured and compared will depend on it.

Misuse of Pharmacoeconomic Terms

No phenomenon has contributed more to the confusion surrounding pharmacoeconomic terminology than the indiscriminate use of these terms in the health care literature. Several studies were conducted in recent years documenting this misuse of economic terminology. Undoubtedly, the most commonly misused term is "cost-effective." The issue was first raised when in 1986 when various misinterpretations of the term cost-effective were reported in the New England Journal of Medicine (see Reference 6). Once common misinterpretation equates cost-effectiveness with "cost-savings." A second misinterpretation equates cost-effectiveness with being "most effective." Both of these interpretations are incorrect, as each considers only one-half of the cost versus consequences.

Economic Assessments

The fundamental task of economic evaluations is to identify, measure, value, and compare the costs and consequences of the alternatives being considered. The two distinguishing features of economic evaluations are that there is a comparison of two or more treatment alternatives, and that both costs and consequences of the alternatives are examined. Pharmacoeconomic evaluations may consist of either partial or full economic evaluations. In general, a full economic evaluation encompasses both of these important features, whereas a partial economic evaluation addresses only one of these features.

Full Evaluations

Full economic evaluations are necessary to comprehensively assess the economic costs and benefits of program and treatment alternatives. Full economic evaluations include cost-minimization analysis (CMA), cost-benefit analysis (CBA), cost-effectiveness (CEA), and cost-utility analysis (CUA). Although each of these methods vary in several important ways, they can all provide a comprehensive analysis of both the costs and consequences of evaluated alternatives. Full economic evaluations are necessary for evaluating an intervention as part of a resource allocation decision. They are also useful for determining what drugs to include, or exclude, to or from a formulary list, or as part of a disease management program.

Limitations of Full Economic Analyses

Full economic evaluations do have some limitations. Each method for comparing costs and consequences has its own distinct limitations and assumptions associated with it, thus, practitioners must be aware of these. Further, although the quality and usefulness of the information is much greater with a full economic evaluation, the amount of time and effort necessary to conduct the evaluation is also much greater.

Various methods of economic evaluation are listed in Table 2 and include cost-of-illness (COI) evaluation, CMA, CBA, CEA, and CUA. Each method, except COI, is used to compare competing programs or treatment alternatives. Also, they are similar in that they measure cost in dollars, but differ in their measurements of outcomes and applications. The purpose of this section is to introduce

Table 2. Common Economic Evaluation Methodologies

Methodology	Cost Unit	Outcome Unit
Cost-of-illness	Dollars	Not assessed
Cost-minimization	Dollars	Assumed to be equivalent in comparative groups
Cost-benefit	Dollars	Dollars
Cost-effectiveness	Dollars	Natural units or units of effect
Cost-utility	Dollars	Quality-adjusted life years or other utility

these methods to readers. A more complete in-depth discussion of each of these methodologies is presented in upcoming chapters.

Partial Evaluations

Partial economic evaluations examine only a portion of the costs versus the consequences question. They may include only a simple descriptive tabulation of outcomes or resources consumed. If only consequences or costs of a program's service or treatment are described, then the evaluation illustrates a simple outcome or cost description and is not considered a full evaluation (which evaluates both costs and consequences and compares them to other treatment options). For example, a study in which the costs and consequences are described, but not compared to alternative options, is referred to as a cost-outcome analysis. Other examples of partial evaluations include efficacy evaluations and cost analyses. A cost analysis compares the costs of two or more alternatives without regard to outcome.

Cost of Illness

A COI evaluation identifies and estimates the overall cost of a particular disease in a defined population. This method, often referred to as burden of illness, measures the direct and indirect costs associated with a specific disease or illness. The costs of many diseases in the United States are estimated, including diabetes mellitus, peptic ulcer disease, and cancer.

By identifying the direct and indirect costs of an illness, one can determine the relative value of a treatment or prevention strategy. For example, by determining the cost of a particular disease to society, the costs of a prevention strategy could be subtracted to yield the cost-benefit of implementing this strategy nationwide. Cost-of-illness is not used to compare competing treatment alternatives, but to provide an estimation of the financial burden of a disease. Thus, the value of prevention and treatment strategies can be measured against this illness cost. This economic evaluation methodology is further examined and described in Chapter 6.

Cost-minimization Analysis

Cost-minimization analysis is a tool used to compare two or more treatment alternatives that are equal in efficacy. Cost-minimization analysis compares the costs of treatment alternatives in dollars. Outcomes are not compared because of the underlying assumption that the treatment alternatives are therapeutically equivalent. Thus, the primary focus of this analysis is to determine the least costly alternative.

Cost-minimization analysis is a relatively straightforward and simple method for comparing competing programs or treatment alternatives. However, if no evidence exists to support the therapeutic equivalence of the alternatives being compared, another method should be used. It should be noted that CMA only shows a cost-savings of one treatment or program over another. An example of the appropriate use of CMA would be to compare a brand-name product to a generic equivalent. Because the outcomes associated with the two drugs are equivalent, costs alone can be compared. Cost-minimization analysis also may be useful when comparing therapeutic agents in the same therapeutic class, assuming that they have demonstrated equivalency in safety and efficacy. The costs of these agents would be identified, measured, and compared. However, the costs must extend beyond those for drug acquisition, and should include all relevant costs incurred for preparing, administering, and monitoring the drugs. This economic evaluation methodology is further examined and discussed in Chapter 7.

Cost-benefit Analysis

Costs and outcomes, or benefits, are both valued in monetary units when performing a CBA. In a CBA, the benefits accrued from a program or intervention, and all of the costs of providing a program or intervention, are identified and converted into equivalent dollars in the year they will occur.

Results of these analyses are typically expressed as either a cost-benefit ratio, or a net cost or benefit. For example, if the cost associated with a treatment is $100, and the outcome resulting from the treatment is valued at $1000, then the cost-benefit ratio, would be expressed as the benefit ($1000) divided by the cost ($100) or as 10:1. This ratio could be interpreted as a treatment alternative that produces $10 of benefit for every $1 spent. Alternatively, by subtracting the costs, $100, from the benefits, $1000, these results could be expressed as a $900 net benefit. Thus, when comparing two treatment alternatives, the alternative with the greatest cost-benefit ratio, or net benefit, would be considered the most efficient use of resources. It should be noted that the results of a CBA are most commonly expressed as a net cost or benefit, because it is sometimes misleading to simply compare ratios. A program that costs $100,000 and results in a benefit of $1,000,000 also yields a cost-benefit ratio of 10:1. However, the relative magnitude of these costs and benefits are dramatically different from others that yields 10:1.

The appropriate time to use CBA is when comparing treatment alternatives or programs where outcome can be expressed in monetary terms. Using CBA, treatment alternatives with different outcomes also can be compared because they are converted into the common denominator of dollars. Cost-benefit analysis may be an appropriate method to use when justifying and documenting the value of an existing pharmacy service, or the potential worth of a new one. Cost-benefit analysis may be particularly useful when allocating scarce funds to competing programs. This economic evaluation methodology is further examined and discussed in Chapter 8.

Cost-effectiveness Analysis

When treatment alternatives are not therapeutically equivalent, or when it is not desirable to express outcomes in monetary units, CEA may provide a more comprehensive evaluation method. Cost is measured in monetary units and outcomes are expressed in terms of obtaining a specific therapeutic objective. These outcomes are expressed in physical, natural, or nondollar units such as cases cured, lives saved, or mm Hg drop in blood pressure. Cost-effectiveness analysis allows researchers to summarize the health benefits and resources used by competing programs so that policy-makers can choose among them. The difference between a cost-effective alternative and one with cost-savings is that cost-savings refers to a competing alternative that is less expensive. However, a cost-effective alternative does not always mean the comparator is less expensive. In fact, a product or service may be considered cost-effective compared to competing alternatives if one of the following three conditions are met. First, a cost-effective alternative may be less expensive, and at least as effective as its comparator. Second, a cost-effective alternative may be more expensive while providing an additional benefit that is worth the additional cost. Third, a cost-effective alternative may be less expensive and less effective in those cases where the extra benefit is not worth the extra cost.

Cost-effectiveness analysis attempts to reveal the optimal alternative, which may not always be the least costly alternative, for accomplishing a desired objective. In this regard, cost-effectiveness need not be cost reduction, but instead should be considered as cost optimization. Cost-effectiveness analysis provides the means to determine and promote the most efficient drug therapy. Another way to say this is that CEA seeks to identify the alternatives that yield the best health care outcome per dollar spent.

The results of a CEA can be expressed either as the average cost-effectiveness ratio (ACER), or as the incremental cost-effectiveness ratio. Average cost-effectiveness ratios represent the average cost of obtaining a specific therapeutic outcome, spread over a large population. An incremental cost-effectiveness ratio represents the additional cost, and additional benefit, when one option is compared to the next most expensive or intensive option.

The decision to use average versus incremental cost-effectiveness ratios is controversial. An ACER reflects the cost per benefit of a new strategy independent of other alternatives, whereas an incremental cost-effectiveness ratio reveals the cost per unit of benefit of switching from one treatment strategy that may already be in operation to another treatment strategy.

Making a formulary management decision regarding whether to add drug A or drug B to the formulary can best illustrate this concept. Imagine drug A is an antibiotic with a 90 percent efficacy, or cure rate, with a total treatment cost for 100 patients of $50,000. The ACER of drug A is calculated by dividing the cost, $50,000, by the outcome, 90 cures, to yield an ACER of $555 per cure. Drug B has a 95 percent cure rate and costs $100,000 to treat 100 patients, yielding an ACER of $1053 per cure.

To determine the incremental cost-effectiveness ratio, or additional cost required to obtain additional cures with drug B, the cost of drug A, $50,000, is subtracted from the cost of drug B, $100,000, and this is then divided by the cures from drug A, 90, subtracted from the cures resulting from drug B, 95. Thus, the incremental cost for each additional cure with drug B is $50,000 divided by five cures or $10,000 per cure.

($100,000 - $50,000)
(95 - 90 cures)
= $10,000 per cure

Using the ACER, it appears that the additional benefit gained by using drug B costs $498 per cure, which is the difference between the ACERs of drug B and drug A. However, this cost represents the difference per patient, spread over the 100 patients that were treated. Only the incremental cost-effectiveness ratio allows you to pose the question of whether one additional cure is worth spending $10,000 when a cure with drug A can be achieved for $555. The decision to use drug A or B is often dependent on the severity of the infection. A cost of $10,000 to cure one case of otitis media may be deemed excessive by a pharmacy and therapeutics committee, but it may be acceptable to use drug B in cases of life-threatening sepsis.

Cost-effectiveness analysis is useful when comparing competing programs or treatment alternatives that differ in therapeutic or clinical outcome. By calculating a summary measurement of efficiency, alternatives with different costs, efficacy rates, and safety rates can be fairly compared along a level playing field. This economic evaluation methodology is further examined and discussed in the Cost-Effectiveness Analysis chapter.

Cost-utility Analysis

At times, it is desirable to include a measure of patient preference, or quality of life, when comparing competing treatment alternatives. Using CUA, the costs of a treatment alternative are expressed in monetary terms and outcomes or consequences are expressed in terms of patient preference or quality-adjusted life-years. Cost-utility analyses can compare cost, quality, and the quantity of patient years. This method is useful when evaluating programs or alternatives that are life-extending, yet with significant side effects, such as cancer chemotherapy, and those that produce reductions in morbidity, rather than mortality, such as occurs with the treatment or arthritis.

The results of a CUA are most often expressed as a cost per QALY gained, or some other health state utility measurement. Quality-adjusted life-years represent the number of full years at full health that are valued equivalently to the number of years as experienced. For example, a full year of health in a disease-free patient would equal 1.0 QALY, while a year spent receiving dialysis might be valued significantly lower, perhaps as a 0.5 QALY.

Because QALYs and other utility measures are highly subjective measurements, there is a lack of agreement on which scales should be used to measure utility. Also, quantifying patient preferences or quality of health care outcomes is complex; thus, CUA may be limited in scope of application from a managed care or institutional perspective. However, when quality of life is the most important health outcome being examined, CUA is a method one may consider to use. This economic evaluation methodology is further examined and described in Chapter 10.

Techniques for Analysis

Discounting

Discounting, or adjusting for differential timing, should be performed if the costs and consequences of program and treatment alternatives accrue during different periods of at least 1 year in duration. To be fair and for accurate comparison, the costs and consequences of various alternatives should be evaluated at the same point in time. Discounting will assist in ensuring a fair and complete comparison is possible.

When costs, or consequences of a program or treatment alternative, will occur in the future, these costs and consequences should be reduced or discounted to be more reflective of current fiscal values. Many investigators will repeat the analyses, varying the discount rates, to examine the effects on costs and consequences. Although, there is no standard discount rate specifically recommended for pharmacoeconomic evaluations, current banking interest rates are often viewed as a benchmark. Many investigators recommend that net costs should be discounted to their present value using a rate of 3–8 percent per annum. However, the modal rates used in economic evaluation of health care products and services appear to be about 5 percent.

Sensitivity Analysis

A standard approach for managing uncertainty in an economic evaluation is to perform a sensitivity analysis. Because of the methodological controversies and the almost universal need to make assumptions when conducting economic evaluations, sensitivity analysis is an essential component of any pharmacoeconomic evaluation. Sensitivity analysis is a tool that tests the robustness of economic evaluation results and conclusions. Underlying assumptions or sensitive variables are varied over a range of plausible results. Holding other evaluation parameters constant, the study results are then recalculated. If changing the values of specific variables does not substantially alter the results, one has more confidence in the original findings. Thus, sensitivity analysis provides a measure of robustness, which also may enhance extrapolation of the results.

Variables include those that are clinically relevant. For example, a drug's rate of efficacy, incidence of adverse drug reactions, and dominant cost values may be varied. A sensitivity analysis may reveal at what point one drug gains or loses a cost-effective advantage and due to what variables.

Also, the threshold value for changing a drug-use decision may be revealed through sensitivity analysis.

Decision Analysis

Decision analysis is a technique often used in pharmacoeconomic evaluations to structure the logical and chronological order of the analysis. This technique represents an explicit, quantitative, and prescriptive approach to choosing among treatment alternatives. Decision analysis is a systematic, quantitative method of describing clinical problems, identifying possible courses of action, assessing the probability and value of outcomes, and finally making a calculation to select the optimum course of action. Because making drug therapy decisions usually involves these steps, a decision analysis approach often provides a valuable way of structuring many pharmacoeconomic evaluations, especially CEAs.

The tool used in decision analysis is a decision table or decision tree. A decision tree, shown in Figure 5, allows investigators to graphically display all treatment alternatives being compared, the relevant outcomes associated with these alternatives, and the probabilities of these outcomes occurring in a patient population. This tree can allow for the algebraic conversion of all of these variables into one summary measurement, often a cost-effectiveness ratio, to allow for a meaningful comparison of two or more treatment alternatives.

Incremental Cost Analysis

Although the results of economic evaluations are often expressed as averages, it is often more instructive and informative to assess the incremental costs. Incremental cost analysis assesses the additional cost that one treatment, service, or program imposes over another compared with the additional benefits or successes it provides. Thus, incremental analysis focus on the additional costs and additional clinical outcomes of alternative strategies. Incremental cost analysis should be considered for any

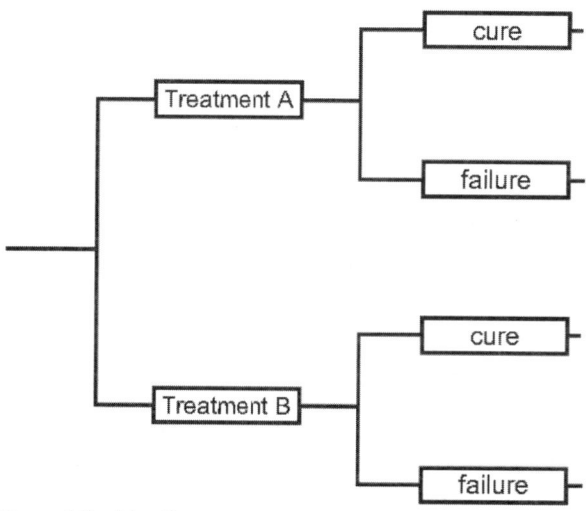

Figure 5. Decision Tree

economic assessment method as a further means of evaluating the data.

Incremental cost analysis is useful when prioritizing health care programs or services for policy decision making. This analysis also may be more useful than average summary measures of efficiency when assessing the value of an alternative that is more expensive but has a greater effect. Thus, incremental cost analysis can be used to answer the question "Is the extra effect worth the extra cost?"

Applied Pharmacoeconomics

Much of the focus of pharmacoeconomics to date is on defining terminology and refining methods and techniques of analyses. Unfortunately, not as much effort is placed on how to apply these methods in the real world to assist pharmacy practitioners and administrators to inform decisions at a local level. Applied pharmacoeconomics is defined as putting pharmacoeconomic principles, methods, and theories into practice to quantify the "value" of pharmacy products and pharmaceutical care services used in "real-world" environments.

There are many benefits that can be realized by applying pharmacoeconomic principles and methods to pharmacy and medical practices. Economic assessments can assist in balancing cost and outcome when determining the most efficient use of health care products and services. When assessing the value of an existing health care service, or the potential worth of implementing a new one, these methods are useful. In general, the application of pharmacoeconomic principles is viewed as a tool to assist health care decision-makers to make better health care decisions. The appropriate application of pharmacoeconomic principles and methods facilitates systematic quantification of the value of health care products and services.

Primary Application of Pharmacoeconomics

The primary application of economic assessments is for contemporary clinical decision making. Common drug use decisions, including formulary management, practice guidelines, drug policy, individual patient treatment, and resource allocation, can be supported using pharmacoeconomic techniques. Economic outcomes data can be powerful tools in determining and promoting the most efficient use of drugs in institutions and organizations. The use of pharmacoeconomics to support each of these decision types is discussed further.

Specific Applications of Economic Evaluations
Formulary Management

Although a formulary is often viewed as a cost-containment tool, it does not always represent a list of the least expensive alternatives. In fact, the purpose of many formularies today is to optimize therapeutic outcomes while controlling costs. Therefore, formulary management decisions should extend beyond evaluating only safety and efficacy, or drug acquisition costs, and include an assessment of the value of health care products and services.

Pharmacoeconomics can assist in determining and supporting various formulary management decisions by providing data regarding which agents are the most efficient for a particular hospital or managed care organization. These data can influence the following formulary decision options:

- Inclusion of newly marketed or other target drugs;
- Exclusion of newly marketed or other target drugs;
- Inclusion, with restriction, of newly marketed or other agents;
- Deletion of drugs from the formulary;
- Curtailing the use of nonformulary items;
- Influencing physician prescribing patterns.

Economic outcomes data can provide critical support for these various formulary decision options.

Practice/Clinical Guidelines

In our current cost-conscious health care environment, it may not be sufficient to determine the treatment alternatives that are the best value, or the most cost-effective. It is also important to determine the best way to use these treatment alternatives in hospitals and managed care organizations. Development of drug use guidelines, policies, or protocols can assist in influencing prescribing and promoting the most cost-effective and desirable use of drugs.

The recent expansion of the outcomes movement fostered by the Agency for Health Care Policy and Research (AHCPR) has sought to standardize the parameters of medical care nationally though decreasing procedural variance, improving therapeutic outcomes, and increasing the appropriateness of medical services paid for by third-party insurers. Although there are many diseases and conditions that have no guideline initiatives, many hospitals and managed care organizations are working to develop guidelines specific to their setting. Pharmacoeconomic principles and methods can be used to determine the treatment alternatives and dosing regimens that are the best value for patients, hospitals, organizations, and payers. A drug use guideline based on a rigorous pharmacoeconomic evaluation may have increased acceptance by other health care practitioners.

Drug Use Policy

At an institution, organization, or government level, policies regarding the appropriate use of health care products and services are made. These policies may be implemented to promote the most efficient use of health care products and services, especially pharmaceuticals. Successful policies can have a significant impact on influencing physician prescribing patterns and the provision of high-quality patient care for the resources available.

A successful drug policy should use the results of pharmacoeconomic evaluations for its development. The health care professionals who may be affected by this policy should be consulted in the policy development phase. Adequate time and resources must be spent on the strategic implementation of the policy. Furthermore, educational strategies should be used, including verbal, written, and on-line communication. However, a policy will only be as successful as the pharmacoeconomic data, implementation, and educational strategies chosen.

Service or Program Resource Evaluation

The principles and methods of pharmacoeconomics can be useful in determining the value of an existing pharmacy or medical service, or estimating the potential worth of implementing a new service. With fewer health care resources available at most hospitals and managed care organizations, competition for these resources has increased. The determination of economic outcomes can provide the means to demonstrate that a specific pharmacy service maximizes the resources allocated to it by hospital administration.

Through the use of pharmacoeconomic methods like CBA, the return on investment, or other benefits produced by one service, can be compared to another service. Practitioners and administrators can use these data to make more informed resource allocation decisions.

Individual Patient Treatment

When applying the principles and methods of economic outcomes assessment to practice, the most important, but also the most difficult application, is the decision about an individual patient's therapy. Most pharmacoeconomic studies, by design, evaluate different patient groups. Thus, it can be difficult to translate the results to an individual who may not exactly parallel the study group's characteristics. Traditionally, clinical decisions have included assessments of the safety and efficacy, or the clinical outcomes, of drug therapy. Today's decisions also should consider economic and humanistic outcomes of drug therapy.

As our awareness expands from considering just safety, efficacy, and cost in clinical decision making, we also should begin to account for the human consequences. Many researchers, pharmaceutical manufacturers, insurers, employer groups, government agencies, physician groups, and clinicians are now taking an active interest in using pharmacoeconomic principles to measure and monitor humanistic outcomes of health care.

Humanistic Outcome Assessments

In the past decade or so, the situation in clinical research has become more complex. The effects of new drugs or surgical procedures on quantity of life are likely to be marginal. Conversely, there is an increased awareness of the impact of health care on the quality of human life. Therapeutic efforts in many disciplines of medicine, especially those increasing numbers who care for patients with chronic, long-term disease states, are directed equally, if not primarily, to improvement of the quality life, not the quantity of life.

With therapeutic efforts focusing more on improving patient function and well-being, the need increases to understand the relationships between traditional clinical and HRQOL, especially since it is increasingly used as an outcome in clinical trials, effectiveness research, and research on the quality of care. Factors that have facilitated this increased usage include the accumulating evidence that measures of health status are valid and reliable. In an effort to promote a better understanding of linking clinical variables to HRQOL, a valuable distinction between basic clinical medicine and social science approaches to patients' health has been published (see Reference 31). Their model linking clinical variables with HRQOL, includes five levels or subdivisions: biological and physiological factors; symptoms; functioning; general health perceptions; and overall quality of life.

Case Study

A 72-year-old white male with a history of diabetes mellitus, coronary artery disease, hypertension, and emphysema is seen in a general medicine clinic with complaints of increasing shortness of breath and chest pressure. He was seen 8 weeks previously for similar complaints, at which time verapamil 80 mg/3 times/day was prescribed. The patient stated that he took the verapamil for about 10 days, but discontinued therapy because "it was not working." Since then, he noted a gradual decline in his exercise tolerance. He had previously been able to walk one city block without symptoms, but he now becomes short of breath and feels "chest heaviness" when walking across the room. The patient denies palpitations and orthopnea, but does state that he has not been sleeping well lately. His social history is that of a widower who lives with his daughter and one grandson. He denies alcohol use and he quit smoking 5 years ago. Physical examination reveals an elderly, pale, thin male sitting comfortably in a chair. His blood pressure is 135/90 mm Hg, his heart rate is 80 beats per minute, and his respiratory rate is 16 breaths per minute. His lungs are clear and his cardiac examination is normal. There is no evidence of ascites or pedal edema.

Take a few minutes to think about what is missing from the case that would improve your understanding of this patient and his health.

Common to all of health status assessment tools is a theoretical framework that views the measurement of biologic functioning as an essential, but inadequate component for comprehensively evaluating health. Beyond the documentation of organ system function lies the need to assess general well-being and behavioral functioning. This broader assessment of health is seen as necessary because basic biologic abnormalities can extend into a person's behavioral functioning and sense of well-being, disrupting the person's HRQOL. The impact a disease can have on a person's life can be likened to a rock dropped into the center of a still pond as depicted in Figure 6. Ripples are sent out over the entire surface of the water or the entirety of life, extending far beyond central organ dysfunction. All of the outer circles are eventually affected and need to be addressed in a HRQOL assessment to have a comprehensive understanding of a patient's condition.

Missing from the case, as presented, is information about this patient's functioning, how he is doing, how he gets around, how he feels, what his social situation and support system consists of, and level of functioning to which he expects to return.

Evolution of Today's Health Status Outcome Measures

During the 1940s, physicians first began to measure patient functioning; the Karnofsky Functional Status for Patients with Cancer and the New York Heart Association Classification were among the instruments developed during that period. The first health-status measures distinguished among functional states and included symptoms, anatomic findings, occupational status, and daily living activities. Studies began in the 1950s when clinicians examined the functional status of patients with severe disabilities. When social science methods and clinical expertise came together in the 1970s, the first modern health-status questionnaires emerged. The early tools were quite long, but the data they captured were valid, reproducible, and relevant. The focus was multidimensional, providing assessments of physical, psychological, and social health. The development, refinement, and use of the early instruments helped to establish the foundation for today's studies. Typical measures of this period include the Quality of Well-Being Scale, the Sickness Impact Profile, the Health Perceptions Questionnaire, and the Older Americans Resources and Services (OARS) questionnaire; they were used in health services and clinical research as outcome measures. The next generation developed in the 1980s and 90s were the Rand Health Insurance Experiment (HIE) health surveys, the Duke-UNC Health Profiles, the Nottingham Health Profile, and the Medical Outcomes Study (MOS) health surveys, including the SF-36 Health Survey. For a more detailed discussion of the history and development of health status assessment, see the *Proceedings of the Advances in Health Assessment Conference:* Palm Springs, California. For a more exhaustive list of questionnaires, readers are directed to Spilker.

Variations in Medical Care in Small Areas

The impetus for research on rationality of processes in health care delivery, an issue that the field of outcomes research and guidelines development are meant to address, typically is traced to the work of John Wennberg, who uncovered a phenomenon known as small-area variation. In brief, Wennberg and colleagues noticed large disparities in the rates of various medical procedures in different geographic areas. The differences could not be attributed to differences in the populations, but instead appeared to indicate differences in physician cultures of different regions, where certain treatment strategies became the norm. For example, a 10-fold difference in rates of tonsillectomy was observed just within the six New England states.

The Rand HIE

When it became apparent in the United States, in 1990, that health expenditures accounted for 12.4 percent of the GNP, whereas that proportion was 4 percent, in 1980, and that the rate of growth of health care expenditures was exceeding the rate of inflation, as well as growth in our economy, questions surfaced. Does spending more buy better health? In individual cases, the answer may be an obvious yes or no, but in the population as a whole as of 1983, the point of diminishing (or absent) returns was difficult to identify. This quandary prompted the federal government to support a large-scale controlled trial, now known as the HIE.

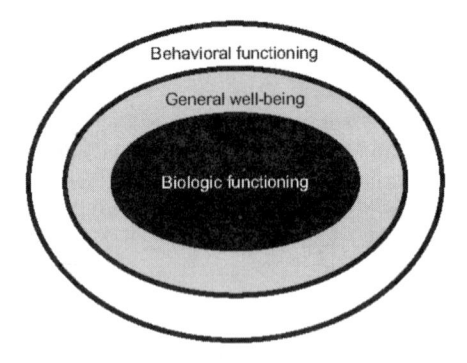

Figure 6. Health Status Concepts
Reprinted with permission from Ware JE.
Conceptualizing and measuring generic health outcomes. Cancer 1991;67(suppl 3):774–9.

One purpose of the HIE was to learn whether the direct cost of medical care, when borne by consumers, affects their health. The researchers found that the more people had to pay for medical care, the less of it they used. Free care had no effect on major health habits that are associated with cardiovascular disease and some types of cancer. Secondly, the study detected no effects of free care for the average enrollee on any of the five general self-assessed health measures.

In addition to these remarkable findings, the HIE presented one of the first major challenges for measuring health status. A consequence of this challenge resulted in one of the most extensive applications of psychometric theory and methods (long used in educational testing), to the development and refinement of health status surveys. Researchers developed or adapted measures to evaluate the effect of cost sharing on health status. At that time, the comprehensive set included four distinct categories—general health, health habits, physiological health, and the risk of dying from any cause related to risk factors. General health was operationally defined as—physical functioning, role functioning, mental health, social contacts, and health perceptions.

The measurement goal in the HIE was to construct the best possible scales for measuring a broad array of functioning and well-being concepts; it demonstrated the potential of scales, constructed from self-administered surveys, as reliable and valid tools for assessing changes in health status. However, it left two questions unanswered: Can methods of data collection and scale construction work in sicker and older populations? In addition, could scales that are more efficient be constructed? The answer to these questions was the challenge accepted by the MOS investigators.

Medical Outcomes Study

The MOS was a 2-year observational study designed to help understand how specific components of the health care system affected the outcomes of care. One of the two original purposes of the MOS was to develop more practical tools for monitoring patient outcomes, and their determinants, in routine practice using state-of-the-art psychometric techniques. The study, and its many implications and conclusions, are mentioned here for completeness, but any of the multiple publications resulting from this study should be consulted for further details.

Agency for Health Care Policy and Research Agency for Healthcare Research and Quality

To enhance the quality, appropriateness, and effectiveness of health care services and access to these services the federal government in Public Law 101-239 (Omnibus Budget Reconciliation Act of 1989) established the Agency for Health Care Policy and Research (AHCPR). The act, sometimes referred to as the Patient Outcome Research Act, called for the establishment of a broad based, patient-centered outcomes research program. In addition to the traditional measures of survival, clinical endpoints and disease–and treatment-specific symptoms and problems, the law mandated measures of "functional status and well-being and patient satisfaction." In 1999, then President Clinton signed the Health Care Research and Quality Act, reauthorizing AHCPR as the Agency for Healthcare Research and Quality (AHRQ) until the end of fiscal year 2005. Presently, its mission is to improve the outcomes and quality of health care, reduce its costs, address patient safety and medical errors, and broaden access to effective services and improve the quality of health care services.

However, there is a difference between quality-of-life assessment and quality of care assessment. Evaluating and improving the quality of health care services includes improving a patient's health status, but the two are not synonymous. Quality health status outcomes are one facet of defining quality health care, though arguably an ultimate outcome.

Evaluating the Quality of Care

The best measure of quality is not how well or how frequently a medical service is given, but how closely the result approaches the fundamental objectives of prolonging life, relieving distress, restoring functioning, and preventing disability. Lembeche PA. Am J Public Health 1952;42:276–86.

Before attempting to assess the quality of care, either in general, or in any particular situation, it is necessary to come to an agreement on what constitutes quality. To measure quality without a firm foundation of prior agreement on how to define it is to court disaster. The author of a well-established conceptual model suggests measuring quality by observing the performance of other health professionals (see Reference 5). The health professional's management of a clearly definable episode of illness in a given patient is defined as the simplest unit of care. It is possible to divide this management into two domains: the technical and the interpersonal. Technical care is the application of the science and technology of medicine and other health sciences, to the management of a personal health problem. Its accompaniment is the management of the social and psychological interactions between the client and the practitioner. Technical care has been called "the science of medicine" and its counterpart, interpersonal care, is often referred to as "the art of medicine." Assessment of the quality of health care has been classified into three categories. They are structure, process, and outcome. The following section will describe what each of these categories represents, who is involved in the evaluation, and what methods are used to monitor each. Each will be illustrated using an example from a pharmacy practice setting.

Structure of Care

Structure denotes the attributes of the settings in which care occurs. Evaluations of structure address the relatively stable characteristics of the providers of care, of the tools and resources they have at their disposal, and of the physical and organizational settings in which they work. This includes the attributes of material resources, such as facilities, equipment, and money; of human resources such as the number and qualifications of personnel; and of organizational structure such as medical staff organization, methods of peer review, and methods of reimbursement. The concept of structure includes the human, physical, and financial resources that are needed to provide medical care. The term embraces the number, distribution, and qualifications of professional personnel, and so too the number, size, equipment, and geographic disposition of hospitals and other facilities. But the concept also goes beyond the factors of production to include the ways in which the financing and delivery of health services are organized, both formally and informally. The presence of health insurance is an aspect of structure. Structure includes the organization of the medical staff in a hospital, and the presence or absence of a quality review effort. To summarize, the basic characteristics of structure are that it is relatively stable, that it functions to produce care, or is a feature of the environment of care, and that it influences the kind of care provided. Inspectors, engineers, architects, national licensing boards, and medical boards complete evaluation of the quality of the structure of a health system. The measurement of structure has many different units. For example, the number of licensed physicians, assurance that all practicing physicians are licensed, and that the building conforms to fire and safety codes are all measures of structure. Researchers have proposed examples of structure criteria by which to evaluate the quality of pharmaceutical care (see Reference 9). These criteria are numerous and include a variety of characteristics, some of which are the presence of appropriate drug information references, having sufficient inventory and record-keeping capabilities, having adequate physical space, availability of trained technicians, and financial stability.

Process of Care

The *process* of care denotes what is actually done in giving and receiving care. It includes the patient's activities in seeking care and carrying it out, as well as the practitioner's activities in making a diagnosis and recommending or implementing treatment. The primary objective of evaluation is to examine a set of activities that go on within and between practitioners and patients. Quality of the process of care is viewed as normative behavior. The norms are derived either from the science of medicine, or the ethics and values of society. Measurements of process are determined by previous scientific research and discoveries and through published literature that defines accepted standards. Most evaluations of the process of care have roots in peer review. One example of how the system monitors processes through the use of Peer Review Standard Organizations for physician peer review. In this system, peers have developed, discovered, or otherwise set precedents for practice standards that become accepted by the medical community. The evaluation of process is then conducted by applying those accepted practice standards to the applicable health care professionals. A judgment concerning the quality of the process is made either by direct observation or by review of recorded information. Dispensing drugs to a patient is one measure of the process of pharmaceutical care. In one proposed strategy, there are both technical and interpersonal aspects to this process of care (see Reference 5). The technical responsibilities of the pharmacist include gathering prescription information, entering the prescription into a computer, reviewing the patient's profile, obtaining the drug from stock, labeling the drug container, assessing if the correct drug and dosage is prescribed, checking for drug allergies and drug interactions, monitoring for adverse events, and assessing if the patient is adherent to their regimen. In this example, the interpersonal skills of listening, being empathetic to the patient, being friendly, and showing concern and consideration are equally important elements of the process of dispensing a drug.

Outcomes of Care

The *outcomes* of care denote the effects of care on the health status of patients and populations. Improvements in patients' knowledge and salutary changes in patients' behaviors are included under a broad definition of health status, and so is the degree of each patient's satisfaction with care. Although most health professionals agree that quality outcomes are a goal of care, little emphasis is placed on their evaluation, and even less on documenting achievement of success. Because patient knowledge, behaviors, and satisfaction are the outcomes of interest, patients are the best sources of information for evaluating these outcomes. These patient-based evaluations are accomplished by using surveys that are scientifically designed and tested for reliability and validity. Surveys also may be interviewer administered or take place by telephone. The use of patients' assessments of their care and their health has received increased attention over the past few decades. Currently, patient self-administered questionnaires are used for making health care policy decisions as well as in clinical practice. However, the methods used to create these questionnaires predate the current awareness in the health care community.

Definitions

Quality of Life refers to an evaluation of all aspects of our lives, including such things as where we live, how we live, how we play, and how we work. Health-related quality of life encompasses only those aspects of life that are dominated or significantly influenced by personal health or activities performed to maintain or improve health.

Health-related quality of life1 is a specifically focused area of investigation within the larger field of health services and quality of life research. Standardized questionnaires are used to capture health-related quality of life data in a variety of research settings. These standardized questionnaires may be self-administered, or completed via telephone or personal interview, by observation, or by postal survey. More recently, computers and Internet technology have become a mode of administration. Health is just one of 12 domains of life that are considered when researching and evaluating a person's overall quality of life. The other 11 domains are listed in Table 3 and include community, education, family life, friendships, housing, marriage, nation, neighborhood, self, standard of living, and work. The term HRQOL was adopted by researchers to set their research apart from the more global concept of quality of life and to more accurately reflect the scope of their research.

Measurement

Now that we have defined HRQOL, and know what it is that we want to measure, we need to discuss a mechanism for achieving this goal. *Measurement* is a set of numbers or rules used to quantify a physical attribute. Examples of measurement devices are rulers, thermometers, and scales. Think for a moment how you might go about measuring a table. To measure a table, you need to measure the attributes of that table so you can describe it to someone who has never seen it. You would say that it has four legs, that each leg is 10 inches high, and that the table is 4 feet long and 3 feet wide. Width, length, and height are all attributes of the table. In the same way, physical functioning and mental health are attributes of health. One cannot just expect to be able to measure health—you need to measure the attributes of health. An important feature of health is its dimensionality.

Health has distinct components that must be measured and interpreted individually to fully understand health at a given point in time, as well as changes over time. Clues about the components can be found in the definitions of health offered by the World Health Organization as well as in dictionaries. The World Health Organization has defined *health* as a state of complete physical, social, and mental well-being, not merely the absence of disease or infirmity. Dictionary definitions also identify both physical and mental dimensions of health. The former pertains to the body and bodily needs, the latter to the mind, and particularly, to the emotional and intellectual status of the individual. Health connotes completeness, where nothing is missing from the

Table 3. Twelve Domains of Life

Community	Marriage
Education	Nation
Family Life	Neighborhood
Friendships	Self
Health	Standard of Living
Housing	Work

person; it also connotes proper function, where all is working efficiently. The dictionary also suggests well-being, soundness, and vitality as important components of health. Thus, both the World Health Organization and dictionary definitions provide clear precedents for the dimensionality of health and, specifically, for the distinction between physical and mental health. Empiric evidence in support of this distinction is also quite convincing. To summarize, two features of these definitions are crucial; namely, the dimensionality of health and the existence of a full range of health states ranging from disease to well-being.

Many measurement scales artificially restrict the range of individual differences enumerated. Consistent with a disease orientation, most disease specific measures emphasize the negative end of the health continuum. The result is a substantial loss of information. The situation is analogous to a scale for measuring weight that ends at 100 pounds. All objects weighing more are assigned the same score. This would be satisfactory in a world where nothing weighed more than 100 pounds or where differences greater than 100 pounds were irrelevant. Figure 7 illustrates how both the positive and negative ends of the range might be considered when evaluating mental health status. In measuring health, just as in measuring the table, it is important to be able to express each attribute in relationship to the others. To do this, a complete strategy is needed.

Measurement Strategy

To provide an assessment of HRQOL, one of three approaches is usually taken. Researchers can either select tools that focus on general health status, or they can chose tools that are more narrowly focused on specific aspects of the disease under study. For a comprehensive picture of patients' HRQOL, it is often desirable to include both types of assessment tools in research projects having a HRQOL objective. As mentioned, it is important to remember that health is a multidimensional concept that extends over a wide range of a continuum. For example, measurement of mental health necessitates inclusion of both negative and positive ends of the spectrum. Measurement of physical health should include elucidation of vigorous activities as well as basic functions such as bathing and dressing oneself.

Though measurement strategies for different health status instruments may be slightly different, there are some commonly agreed upon and frequently measured general health concepts that can be identified and discussed. These concepts are 1) physical functioning; 2) mental functioning; 3) social and role functioning; and 4) general health perceptions. By denoting a measure as a general health status measure, it is understood that the questions are not disease or disorder specific, and they cover a range of health states from a life-threatening condition to an overall sense of well-being. General measures evaluate aspects of health relevant to all ages, races, sexes, and socioeconomic backgrounds and permit examination of treatment benefits in comparable units.

Medical outcomes study researchers compared and reported the functional status and well-being of patients with chronic conditions using general health measures (see Reference 27). The authors reported the usefulness of generic (nondisease specific) health measures for monitoring progress and for use as outcomes in studies of patients with chronic conditions. The authors maintain that there are several advantages of general measures of functional status and well-being over disease specific measures. Among these, they note, first, they are useful for monitoring patients with more than one condition, and secondly, for comparing patients with different conditions by providing a common yardstick. Lastly, the same measures can be appropriately applied to both general (well) and patient (sick) populations with the advantage of comparing patient groups (sicker) against the healthy standard of a general population.

Commonly Measured Domains of Health in General Health Status Assessment

General health status instruments evaluate aspects of health relevant to all ages, races, sexes, and socioeconomic backgrounds. Questions in a general health status questionnaire are not defined by the disease or disorder under study. These questions have historically covered the full range of the state of disease or illness, and have therefore emphasized the negative end of the health continuum. Increasingly, this limitation in older general health status instruments is being recognized and outcomes researchers are now constructing general health status tools that extend measurements into the well-being end of the health spectrum. General health status tools are, by definition, multidimensional and evaluate at least four key health concepts, which include physical functioning, social and role functioning, mental health, and general health perceptions. Table 4 lists these key health concepts and indicates how they might be assessed.

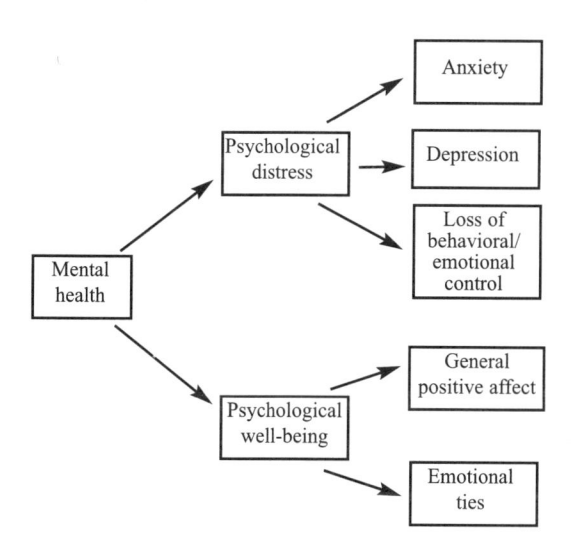

Figure 7. Positive and negative ends of mental health status

Physical Functioning

Physical functioning, as it relates to HRQOL assessment, typically refers to the limitations, or disability, experienced by the patient over a defined period. The questions focus on observable and important physical limitations easily noticed and evaluated by the patient or observer. Among such limitations are difficulties in walking, eating, or dressing. In the past, questions concentrated on the negative end of the physical functioning continuum and provided no insight into the well range of physical functioning where activities such as playing sports and running might be noted. Measures of physical functioning should not be confined only to limitations and disabilities. Rather, these measures also should include questions regarding activities of daily living, energy level, satisfaction with physical condition, and ability to perform all levels of activities ranging from the most basic to the most vigorous. Without questions covering the entire continuum of this domain, only those people with physical limitations or disabilities will be identified, evaluated, and segmented for research purposes; any differences among respondents without significant physical limitations or disabilities will be lost by assessments that do not include the well end of the range. In addition to physical limitations, specific concepts often included in general health status questions about physical abilities, days in bed, bodily pain, and more recently, physical well-being. Table 5 delineates these components of the physical domain, and how they are incorporated into a variety of general health assessment instruments.

Social and Role Functioning

Although social and role functioning are often thought of as a single entity and used interchangeably, they are distinct concepts in terms of HRQOL. Social functioning questions address the extent to which a person participates in social interactions, and also the satisfaction derived from these interactions and from the social network that person has established. Role functioning questions are concerned with those duties and responsibilities that are limited by an individual's health.

Social Functioning

Social functioning is defined as the ability to develop, maintain, and nurture mature social relationships. Social well-being is separated into two areas that include the frequency of social contacts and the nature of those contacts within the social network or community. Both of these areas must be considered together. Evaluating only the frequency of contacts in isolation from the nature of those contacts may offer no insight or the wrong insight into the person's state of social functioning; therefore, including a person's assessment of the adequacy of his or her social network is essential when evaluating social functioning in the context of HRQOL. It is known that belonging to a community, family, or neighborhood provides a strong sense of being wanted, loved, and valued, and has significant influence on assessments of mental health, as well as on social health.

Role Functioning

Role functioning as a component of health is concerned with the impact health has on a person's ability to meet the demands of that person's normal life role. Work for pay, homemaking duties, and schoolwork are all covered by questions asking about this concept. A role function assessment should identify everyday role situations or activities that can be directly affected or limited by disease, illness, or treatment. Whereas most role limitations are due to physical health problems, it has been noted that role limitations are observed both in the presence and in the absence of physical limitations.

Mental Health

Disease often affects the behavior, as well as the physical aspects of a person's life. General health status assessments, therefore, usually include questions covering aspects of psychological health. These questions typically focus on the frequency and intensity of symptoms of psychological distress. Anxiety and depression are common themes in mental health components of general health status instruments, but scales focusing only on these two concepts do not adequately cover the full mental health continuum. Perceptions of psychological well-being, life satisfaction, and cognitive functioning are also needed if a comprehensive assessment of the mental health domain by a health-related quality of life instrument is to be achieved. Although general health status questionnaires covering the mental health domain are not intended for use as diagnostic tools, some questions are used as screens for certain disorders such as depression.

General Health Perceptions

General health perceptions address the person's overall beliefs and evaluations about his or her health. Questions covered in this area focus on each person's health preferences, values needs, and attitudes. Assessments of general health perceptions are necessary because they allow consideration of individual differences in reactions to pain, perceptions of difficulty, the level of effort required, or the degree of worry or concern about health. Unlike questions that focus on measures of limitations, pain, and dysfunction to assess other health domains of interest, questions covering general health perceptions address positive feelings. These questions can be positively framed, thereby allowing the full spectrum of HRQOL to be evaluated.

Advantages of generic health status measures are that they can be used to assess the relative burden of different conditions, and to assess the relative benefits of different treatments. The questionnaires can be used with people of any age, gender, or race. For example, elderly patients with arthritis and young patients with hypertension can be asked the same questions without suspicion that their age or disease state differences will confound their answers. In a general health status instrument, patients may be asked if they believe their health is excellent, very good, good, fair, or poor. A general questionnaire would not ask about nausea related to cancer chemotherapy treatment, but may ask if the patient is less energetic, or more calm and peaceful.

Disadvantages of generic instruments are that, by design, they do not cover areas of health status that are important to

Table 4. Summary of Information About Widely Used General Health Surveys

	QWB	SIP	HIE	NHP	QLI	COOP	EURO-QOL	DUKE	MOS FWBP	MOS SF-36
CONCEPTS										
Physical functioning	•	•	•	•	•	•	•	•	•	•
Social functioning	•	•	•	•	•	•	•	•	•	•
Role functioning	•	•	•	•	•	•	•	•	•	•
Psychological distress		•	•	•	•	•	•	•	•	•
Health perceptions (general)			•	•	•	•	•	•	•	•
Pain (bodily)		•	•	•		•	•	•	•	•
Energy/fatigue	•		•	•				•	•	•
Psychological well-being		•						•	•	•
Sleep		•		•				•	•	
Cognitive functioning		•						•	•	
Quality of Life						•			•	
Reported health transition						•			•	
CHARACTERISTICS										
Administration method (S = self, I = interviewer, P = proxy)	I, P	S, I, P	S, P	S, I	S, P	S, I	S	S, I	S, I	S, I, P
Scaling method (L = Likert, R = Rasch, T = Thurstone, U = utility)	U	T	I	T	L	L	U	L	L	L, P
Number of questions	107	136	86	38	5	9	9	17	149	36
Scoring options (p = profile, SS = summary scores, SI = single index)	SI	P,SS,SI	P	P	SI	P	SI	P, SI	P	P, SS

QWB = Quality of Well-Being Scale (1973)
SIP = Sickness Impact Profile (1976)
HIE = Health Insurance Experiment surveys (1979)
NHP = Nottingham Health Profile (1980) (1992)
QLI = Quality of Life Index (1981) (1992)
COOP = Dartmouth Function Charts (1987)
EUROQOL = European Quality of Life Index (1990)
DUKE = Duke Health Profile (1990)
MOS FWBP = MOS Functioning and Well Being Profile
MOS SF-36 = MOS 36-Item Short-Form Health Survey

Reprinted with permission from Ware JE. The status of health assessment 1994. Annu Rev Public Health 1995;16:327–54.

specific groups of patients who may experience specific improvements, or disabilities, in functioning due to their disease state. For instance, general health status questionnaires do not include self-esteem, a concept that is very important to patients with cystic fibrosis. For this reason, additional types of questionnaires that consider a disease- or condition-specific set of questions were designed for many disease states.

Disease-specific Health Status Instruments

Some limitations or problems with patients' health are unique to their specific disease state. For this reason, batteries of questions were designed for use with specific patient populations, and are used to supplement a general health status instrument. These more narrowly focused disease-specific measures request detailed information about the impact of a specific disease and the effect of treatment on the patient, from the patient's perspective. While items in both general health status measures and in disease-specific measures may appear to ask the same question, those in a disease-specific tool are phrased to direct patients to think about their disease, its symptoms, or its treatment, rather than the disease or limitations in general. In addition, using disease-specific measures allows inclusion of questions of specific interest. Among some specific areas previously investigated with disease-specific questionnaires are: sexual functioning; nausea and vomiting; pain; cancer; arthritis; epilepsy; HIV infection; anxiety and depression; asthma, and rhinitis.

Psychometric Theory

The design of health surveys, consisting of scales measuring the attributes of a person or a population's health, are supported by an underlying theory known as psychometric theory. Health status scales development also can be viewed as a unique application of the design and theory that support the creation of educational measurements for instance, Standardized Achievement Tests. A person who studies these theories and conducts research or measurement of such attributes as intelligence, pain, mental well-being, or functioning, is usually a doctorate level research psychologist and can be known as a *psychometrician*.

One readily apparent feature of health sciences literature devoted to measuring health status is the daunting array of already available scales. Paradoxically, if you proceed a little further to find an instrument for your intended purpose, you may conclude that none of the existing scales is quite right. Many researchers tend to magnify the deficiencies of existing measures and underestimate the effort required to develop an adequate new measure. Perhaps the most common error committed by clinical researchers is to dismiss the existing scales too lightly, and embark on the development of a new instrument with an unjustifiably optimistic and naïve expectation that they can do better. The development of scales requires considerable investment of both mental and fiscal resources. A comprehensive set of standards, widely used in the assessment of psychology and education, is the manual called Standards for Educational and Psychological Tests, published by the American Psychological Association (1974). In addition to these standards, there are a number of compendia of measuring scales.

Psychometric Considerations

The literature is ever expanding with reports of general health and disease-specific, HRQOL research. As with any field of research, the studies reported in the literature meet various levels of scientific rigor. Readers of these reports must have a basic understanding of psychometrics to draw proper conclusions from HRQOL findings.

Psychometrics is the science of testing questionnaires to measure attributes of individuals. It is used in the field of health assessment to translate people's behavior, feelings, and personal evaluations into quantifiable data. These data, once captured, must be both relevant and correct if they are to provide useful insights into HRQOL. Two psychometric properties that any measurement scale or instrument must possess include reliability and validity. In addition, useful scales must be sensitive to change and be accepted by the investigators and respondents. When measuring reliability, the scientist is concerned with the relationship between true variation and random error. Evaluations assess the consistency and repeatability of measurement. Validity refers to the extent to which differences in scale scores reflect the true differences in the individuals studied. Whereas the goal is to elicit observed differences that are indeed true differences among respondents, factors such as how the measure is administered, who administers the form, where it is administered, and when it is administered, can affect responses across groups of study participants, and, therefore, can add a degree of uncertainty to the findings of a HRQOL assessment.

Use of Patient-reported Health Status

Applications of general health surveys are numerous, and include monitoring the health of general populations, evaluating health care policy, conducting clinical trials of alternative treatments, designing systems for monitoring and improving health care outcomes, and making clinical decisions in medical practice. Standardized health surveys have the potential to become new laboratory tests in medical practice. Without these tests, patient functioning, and well-being affected by disease and treatment, are unlikely to be discussed during a typical medical visit. Two-thirds to three-fourths of adults in the United States have reported that physicians rarely, or never, ask about the extent of their limitations in performing everyday activities, even in the presence of chronic conditions. As a result, clinicians may not be well-informed about their patient's functional status, well-being, or changes over time. Scientists have proposed that one solution might be to standardize functional and well-being assessments for every medical practice. Such routine assessments could be useful for a number of reasons. They would ensure that all important dimensions of functional status and well-being are considered consistently. They would detect, explain, and track changes in functional capacity over time. Third, their use would make it possible to better consider the patient's total functioning when choosing among therapies. They would guide the efficient use of community resources and social services, and fifth, they could more accurately predict the course of chronic disease. Such data would make it possible for clinicians to better inform patients about the tradeoffs involved in alternative treatments. A great potential exists for standardized measures of functional status and well-being administered routinely and incorporated into existing clinical databases. Meyer and associates published an example of experiences with the use of a short-form general health status measure in a dialysis unit. The clinicians involved in this project related that patients' scores enhance, rather than simply summarize, the collective understanding of a conscientious dialysis team.

In the dialysis unit, health status surveillance revealed new information that was qualitatively different from other assessments made in the care of these patients. The authors suggested that patient-based health status assessment can

Table 5. Items Measuring Generic Health Concepts

Concepts	Definition	Abbreviated items*
Physical		
Physical limitations	Limitations in performance of self-care, mobility, and physical activities	Needs help with bathing, dressing, in bed chair, couch, for most of day Does not walk at all
Physical abilities	Ability to perform everyday activities	Able to walk uphill, up stairs Able to participate in sports, strenuous activities
Days in bed	Confinement to bed due to health problems	During past 30 days, number of days health keeps one in bed all day or most of day
Bodily pain	Ratings of the intensity, duration frequency of bodily pain and limitations in usual activities due to pain	During the past 3 months, how much pain one has had How much pain interfered with thing
Physical well-being	Personal evaluation of physical condition	Ratings of physical shape or condition
Mental		
Anxiety/depression	Feelings of anxiety, nervousness, tenseness, depression, moodiness, downheartedness	Depressed or very unhappy Bothered by nervousness, or nerves
Psychological well-being	Frequency and intensity of general positive affect	Happy, pleased, satisfied with life Wakes up expecting an interesting day Feels cheerful, lighthearted
Behavioral/emotional control	Control of behavior, thoughts, and feelings during specified period	Feels emotionally stable Loses control of behavior, thoughts, feelings Laughs or cries suddenly
Cognitive functioning	Orientation to time and place, memory, attention span, and alertness	Feels confused, forgets a lot, makes more mistakes than usual
Social and role		
Interpersonal contacts	Frequency of visits with friends and relatives Frequency of telephone contacts with close friends or relatives during specific periods of time	Number of friends visited Going out less often to visit people How often on telephone with close friends/relatives in past month
Social resources	Quantity and quality of social ties, network	Number of close friends, people to talk with
Role functioning	Freedom from limitations in performance of usual role activies (e.g., work, housework, school) due to poor health	Limited in kind or amount of major role activity Working shorter hours Health causes problems at work Unable to work because of health
General health perceptions		
Current health	Self-rating of health at present	In general, is health excellent, good, fair or poor?
Health outlook	Expectations regarding health in the future	I expect to have a very healthy life

Adapted with permission of Ware JE. The Health Institute, New England Medical Center, Boston, MA.

improve the management of individual patients, and can contribute to the epidemiology of treatment of endstage renal disease. Health status assessment offers a language in which to phrase experiences that the individual patient may find difficult to express, or may not even think to formulate, or remember, unless prompted. It provides a thread along which to reconstruct experiences. By objectifying the patient's subjective experiences, health status assessment makes the experience more accessible to the staff who shares responsibility for care. It puts the patient's experience on their agenda for discussion, even when the technical aspects of care do not compete for attention.

Advantage of Health Status Assessment Information

Self-administered surveys allow patients a voice in their care. It permits the patient to communicate to those caring for them, about what matters most. This may be information that one needs to know, but does not have time to elicit. Analogously to providing a common language for patients and health professionals, the general HRQOL information also can provide a standard, or a common language, for different disciplines of health professionals. For example, a Nephrologist and a Psychiatrist can use a common metric to discuss a dialysis patient's emotional health. A standardized method of asking patients about their functioning and well-being can be efficiently used in treatment decisions, and as a monitoring parameter for efficacy and toxicity. The information also may be a tool, or indicator, for compliance assessments.

Health-related quality of life can be used to add important information to the evaluation of the effectiveness of an intervention. For example, does the 34-year-old otherwise healthy woman, diagnosed with depression, who just started an antidepressant feel better or worse? One could just simply ask her that question when you see her 4 weeks after the start of her therapy. As pharmacists, we commonly ask, "Are you having any side effects?" If the patient tells you she has diarrhea, you may form an impression of that diarrhea, which seems like a mild side effect. However, having her answer survey questions about her functioning can reveal how trivial or nontrivial the impact of her diarrhea is to her everyday activities. What would happen if her diarrhea limits her ability to function as the checkout person in the grocery store? She cannot leave her post frequently to go to the bathroom, and if she does, she could be fired and not be able to provide for her two young children that she is raising alone. The patient sees the limitation imposed by diarrhea as considerable, and knowing a little more about her functioning conveys a bit of a different message to us than just knowing she is having diarrhea. A discussion using information from a patient self-administered health status survey also could lead to the patient revealing that she has decided to stop taking her drugs. She did not think it was working, and the diarrhea was not worth the hassle.

Advances in Health Status Assessments for Individual Patient Care Decisions

Standardized measures capturing patient perspectives on their physical functioning, social and role functioning, mental health, and general health perceptions are likely to become more acceptable as an additional piece of evidence on which providers, and their patients, can make decisions about treatment and the treatment's efficacy. Mature theoretical models, sophisticated measurement techniques, and enhanced technology for use in measurement, make the routine use of individual patients results in their own care more promising than ever before.

Two practical concerns of the critics of use of HRQOL assessments in individual patient care are: 1) respondent burden; and 2) reliability of scores obtained from shorter questionnaires. Current researchers struggle with the competing demands invoked by the everyday use requiring shorter forms and the reliability of a result obtained from fewer questions. Specifically, concerns are raised about the reliability of the result, and the interpretation, since with popular outcomes measures the standard error around a single person estimate is large and not satisfying enough to ensure stable conclusions.

Modern test theory offers the potential for individualized, comparable assessments for the careful examination and application of different health status measures. One such theory is Item Response Theory (IRT). Researchers report that IRT has a number of potential advantages over the currently used Classical Test Theory in assessing self-reported health outcomes. Applications of the IRT models are ideally suited for implementing computer adaptive testing. IRT methods are also reported to be helpful in developing better health outcome measures, and in assessing change over time.

Patients increasingly have more access to computer technology. It is becoming more practical to use assessments using a computer. Patients answering questions about a health status concept, using dynamic assessment technology, are requested only to complete the number of questions needed (minimizes response burden) to establish a reliable estimate. The resulting scores for an individual are estimated to meet the clinical measures of precision.

In summary, the study of HRQOL requires a multidimensional approach. Assessments should include components that evaluate, at a minimum, the health concepts of physical, social and role functioning, mental health, and perception of general health. Additionally, the full continuum of these concepts should be included, from the most limited, to the healthiest. Approaches to capture HRQOL data include the self-administered questionnaire (paper and pencil, or computer), personal and telephone interviews, observation, and a postal survey. The assessment instruments must possess acceptable reliability, validity, and sensitivity, and the investigators, as well as the participants, must accept them. Psychometrics is an essential part of HRQOL research, especially in today's research environment that requires shorter, more focused measures.

Existing health outcomes measures, drawn from classic test theory and emerging approaches based on item response theory, offer exciting opportunities for appreciably expanded applications in biomedical and health services research, clinical practice, decision making, and policy development. The research agenda of measurement scientists includes challenges to: 1) refine and expand measurement techniques that rely on IRT; 2) improve measurement tools to make them more culturally appropriate for diverse populations, and more conceptually and psychometrically equivalent across such groups; 3) address long standing issues in preference- and utility-based approaches, particularly in the elicitation of preference responses and scoring instruments; and 4) enhance the ways in which data from outcomes measurement tools are calibrated against commonly understood clinical and lay metrics, are interpreted, and are made useable for different decision-makers.

With the advances in measurement that promise to continue, knowledgeable clinicians will become the transportation for these measures to include in patient care. It is suggested interpretation is, in part, an issue of familiarity, and repeated applications of measures can lead to a better understanding. Ideally, a better understanding of what patients tell their providers about their health status can be used for decision making, which require the patients to more actively and routinely participate in their own care.

Case Study Continued

Now back to the case of Mr. A to consider the following questions. You have stumbled on the results of a questionnaire filed in the outpatient chart. Apparently, the patient filled one out at his last visit in the clinic, about 8 weeks ago, dated Oct. 1, 1995. There was another questionnaire filled out earlier today, Dec. 7, 1995, in the clinic. The results of these questionnaires are listed at the end of this section, as Appendices A and B. Please look at the scores for each of the scales and the changes in the scores. There is a brief interpretation guide attached as Appendix C. For another point of comparison of this patient's scores, you also can use the normative values supplied in Appendix D. There are three sets of values listed. The first set is for the general United States population, the second is for the population in Mr. A's age range, and the third is for patients with similar medical conditions. Take some time now to interpret the results of these questionnaires. What other questions do you have for this patient? Think of at least four additional questions. Reflect on the differences between your questions earlier in this section and those you are asking now.

After questioning Mr. A, you find that this month is the second anniversary of his wife's death. He is very sad about this, and is feeling that he wants to give up now. How does this information change your original plan and problem list? Appendix E gives Mr. A's scores 1 year after this clinic visit, dated December 5, 1996, for comparison.

Patient Satisfaction

Another outcome suggested by a well-accepted model for how to evaluate the quality of health care, is that of patient satisfaction (see Reference 5). During the last decade, organization-wide quality improvement efforts in both service and manufacturing sectors of the United States have embraced consumer evaluations of goods and services as a way to monitor product quality. In the health care setting, consumer satisfaction surveys have evolved, from marketing tools, to measures of quality of the product or service delivered. Empirical studies show that patients' expressions of dissatisfaction are potent predictors of disenrollment from a physician or a health plan. Studies of satisfaction with physicians have documented the importance of access, communication, technical quality, and interpersonal quality of care. The concept of assessing patient satisfaction is introduced here and explored further in Chapter 16.

A consumer's evaluation of the care received, known as *consumer evaluation*, or *patient satisfaction*, is both similar and different from a patient's assessment of health status. The same psychometric techniques are used to obtain information, and to evaluate the accuracy of the information. The science of obtaining the information is similar. However, the information that is requested of the patients, that is, the consumers, is unique and very different from what is asked about health status. Both reports and ratings are used in patient satisfaction surveys. Reports are descriptions, whereas ratings are evaluations that require a judgment by the evaluator. For instance, a patient may be asked how long the wait was before being seen by the physician, which is a report; the patient also may be asked if the wait was too long, requiring a judgment.

There are many different patient satisfaction surveys available. Attributes that are commonly evaluated, regardless of the care setting, include the clinician's scientific knowledge and skill, the quality of clinician-patient communications, the provision of humane interpersonal treatment, and the degree of the patient's trust in the care provider. One setting in which patient satisfaction surveys are becoming increasingly important is that of primary care. Four distinguishing and shared multiple characteristics are considered essential and unique to this area of health care, and provide attributes that can be evaluated by patients. These characteristics include accessibility to care, continuity of care, the comprehensiveness of care, and how well a patient's care is integrated into a coherent and continuing whole. As competition in the health care market has increased, many health care delivery organizations have come to view patient satisfaction as an important consumer supplied indicator of quality and a potential benchmarking device when studied over time.

Other Measures of Outcomes

Those seeking to evaluate the impact of the health care system on the health of an individual or population are forced to include multiple outcomes to accommodate both external and internal needs. So far this chapter has focused on economic outcomes and humanistic outcomes. Within the humanistic outcomes category, the basic concepts included in assessments of health status and patient satisfaction were identified. However, as noted, the identification of perspective is important. In the restructuring of health care, the perspective of the employer has become a significant force. To meet the evaluation needs of employers, the concept of work functioning must be included as an outcome. For example, in 1990, the cost of depression to society was estimated to be $44 billion. Of this, $11.7 billion was attributed to reductions in productive capacity, due to excess absenteeism. The ability to quantify the constituent parts of the losses in work productivity is developmental. However, it is growing in importance, and will undoubtedly be an important measured health domain.

Traditionally, simple measures that ask the patient about lost days from work and days in bed were used to measure work functioning. Many popular health status measures include questions on limitations in daily work activities. However, these concepts are still in need of further development. A conceptual basis for measuring the ability to function in work roles may be found in the recent disability literature. Within this literature, disability encompasses the total inability to work, as well as the less severe limitations in work-role functioning. The Institute of Medicine and the World Health Organization, in the development of terminology and classification systems for disability and functional limitations, have established a fundamental instrument development guideline. They suggest that a person's ability to function in work roles will result from two sets of variables: 1) the characteristics of that person's illness or impairment; 2) the requirements of the work situation. Both of these areas are presently under study.

Conclusion

The methods of pharmacoeconomic evaluation strive to assess the value of health care in terms of outcomes of a clinical, economic, and humanistic nature. This chapter has provided several key definitions and concepts that will be built on in later chapters of this book. Further discussion of how to actually perform and apply the results of economic methodologies will be presented in detail as well. Detailed information regarding the conduct and application of humanistic outcomes assessments will be presented in Chapters 14 and 18.

Because "quality-of-life" represents the broadest range of human experiences, use of this general term in the health field has led to considerable confusion, particularly because of the overlap with the more specific concept, health status. To make the meaning more specific and retain the important aspects of life quality, the term "health-related "quality-of-life" is both useful and important.

Annotated Bibliography

1. Barr JT, Schumacher GE. Applying decision analysis to pharmacy management and practice decisions. Top Hosp Pharm Manage 1994;13:60–71.

    In this paper, decision analysis is presented and applied to a typical management situation. Decision analysis is an explicit, quantitative, and prescriptive approach for choosing among alternative outcomes. Literature examples of using pharmacy-related decision analysis are provided, including its use in formulary additions, cost-effectiveness analysis, drug therapy evaluation, therapeutic drug monitoring, and health policy issues.

2. Bootman JL, Townsend RJ, McGhan WF. Principles of pharmacoeconomics, 2nd ed. Cincinnati: Harvey Whitney Books Company, 1996.

    Designed principally for the student as an introduction to pharmacoeconomics, the authors present various techniques, tools, and strategies used to evaluate the economic contribution of specific drug therapies at a policy level and for individual patients. Chapters 6 and 7 will be of particular interest to readers seeking information on outcomes measurement, as overviews of cost-utility analysis and health-related quality of life (HRQOL) measurement, respectively, are presented. The bibliographies in these chapters include many of the key theoretical and empiric citations for these two approaches to measurement. This book is a good starting point for those who wish to read further.

3. Crane VS. Economic aspects of clinical decision-making: applications of clinical decision analysis. Am J Hosp Pharm 1988;45:548–53.

    Clinical decision analysis as a basic tool for decision making is described, and potential applications of decision analysis in six areas of clinical practice are identified in this paper. Applications of clinical decision analysis in the areas of diagnostic testing, patient management, product and program selection, research and education, patient preferences, and health care-policy evaluation are described. Decision analysis offers health professionals a tool for making quantifiable, cost-effective clinical decisions, especially in terms of clinical outcomes.

4. Detsky AS, Nagiie IG. A clinician's guide to cost-effectiveness analysis. Ann Intern Med 1990;113:147–54.

    The authors describe how cost-effectiveness analysis can be used to help set priorities for funding health care programs. For each intervention, the costs and clinical outcomes associated with that strategy must be compared with an alternate strategy for treating the same patients. This paper also discusses the distinction between cost-effectiveness analysis and incremental cost-effectiveness analysis. If an intervention results in improved outcomes, but also costs more, the incremental cost per incremental unit of clinical outcome should be calculated and the incremental cost-effectiveness ratios ranked to set funding priorities. By using this list, the authors maintain the person responsible for allocating resources can maximize the net health benefit for a target population derived from a fixed budget. Because clinicians should participate in policy-making, they must understand the role of this technique in setting funding priorities and allocating health care resources.

5. Donnabedian A. The quality of care: how can it be assessed? JAMA 1988;260:1743–8.

    The author states that although much is known about assessing quality, much remains to be known. Before assessment can begin, one must decide how quality is to be defined. It is further asserted that quality depends on a number of factors: 1) whether one assesses only the performance of practitioners or also the contributions of patients and of the health care system; 2) how broadly health and responsibility for health are defined; 3) whether the maximally effective or optimally effective care is sought; and 4) whether individual or social preferences define the optimum. The need for more detailed information about the causal linkages among structural attributes of health care settings, the processes of care, and the outcomes of care is discussed. The author states the components or outcomes of care to be sampled must be specified, appropriate criteria and standards formulated, and the necessary information obtained to assess quality. Definitions of structure, process, and outcomes are given.

6. Doubilet P. The use and misuse of the term "cost-effective" in medicine. N Engl J Med 1986;314:253–6.

   This paper describes the inconsistencies in the definitions and interpretations of the term cost-effectiveness by authors in medical literature sources. Cost-effectiveness criteria vary considerably and the following interpretations are discussed: 1) cost-effectiveness is equivalent to "cost-savings;" 2) the more effective therapy is also the most cost-effective therapy; 3) cost-effectiveness is the option that is cost-saving while providing equal or better health; 4) cost-effective therapy is that having an outcome worth its corresponding cost relative to competing alternatives. The first two interpretations are incorrect because they only examine one side of the cost-effectiveness equation. The third and fourth interpretations can both be considered correct interpretations of the term. The authors stress it is imperative to standardize terms, such as cost-effectiveness to enhance its usefulness and application to health care policy and clinical decision-making.

7. Drummond MF, Stoddart GL, Torrance GW. Methods for the economic evaluation of health care programmes, 2nd Ed. Oxford: Oxford University Press, 1997.

   This second edition of a landmark textbook, originally published in 1986, discusses in detail the methodological principles of economic evaluation in health care and has been used in courses teaching economic evaluation. The text is not structured like a standard textbook, with detailed discussion of theoretical concepts, but rather concentrates on practical methodological issues that evaluators need to resolve in undertaking an economic evaluation.

8. Eisenberg JM. Clinical economics: a guide to the economic analysis of clinical practices. JAMA 1989;262:2879–86.

   This paper discusses the tools of economics that can be applied to the analysis of medical practice. The focus of the analysis is to improve physicians' choices of ways to use social and individual resources for clinical interventions in the hope of improved health. Types of economic evaluations including cost-identification, cost-effectiveness, cost-benefit, and cost-utility analyses are presented. In addition, useful discussions on study perspectives and determination of health care costs are provided.

9. Farris KB, Kirking DM. Assessing the quality of pharmaceutical care II: applications of concepts of quality assessment from medical care. Ann Pharmacother 1993;27:215-23. Bungay KM, Wagner AK. Comment: assessing the quality of pharmaceutical care. Ann Pharmacother 1993;27:1542.

   The authors propose a framework to facilitate quality assessment of pharmaceutical care. The structure-process-outcome paradigm is presented as a framework for quality assessment of pharmaceutical care. It is recommended that structure be assessed at periodic intervals because it identifies the potential for the provision of quality care. The process of care should be documented, and it is recommended that these variables be linked to outcomes before either structure or process is used to make inferences about the quality of pharmaceutical care. Outcomes assessment will require an interdisciplinary approach. Examples of structure and process criteria are provided for use as a model to integrate pharmaceutical care into a health care system. The editorial comments discuss possible additions to the author's published choices of health outcomes variables.

10. Freund DA, Dittus RS. Principles of pharmacoeconomic analysis of drug therapy. PharmacoEconomics 1992;1:20–32.

    This paper outlines some of the basic principles of pharmacoeconomic analysis. The authors recommend that every analysis should have an explicitly stated perspective, which, unless otherwise justified, should be a societal perspective. Various methods of economic evaluations are reviewed. A discussion of modeling frameworks, such as influence diagrams and decision trees, is also included.

11. Hatoum HT, Freeman RA. The use of pharmacoeconomic data in formulary selection. Top Hosp Pharm Manage 1994;13:47–53.

    This paper encourages pharmacists to improve their knowledge and use of pharmacoeconomic data in formulary selection. Changes in the formulary selection process, particularly concerning use of cost-containment strategies, are described. An overview is presented of the origin, as well as the potential impact of pharmacoeconomic data upon formulary management. The need to balance the economic benefit with the clinical advantages for any proposed new drug for formulary inclusion remains the most critical decision to be made by pharmacists.

12. Katz DA, Welch HG. Discounting in cost-effectiveness analysis of healthcare programmes. PharmacoEconomics 1993; 3:276–85.

    This paper discusses the application of discounting to economic evaluations. Discounting is described as a technique used to make fair comparisons of programs whose costs and outcomes occur at different times. The agreements and disagreements among health economists regarding the need for discounting, and the procedures for discounting costs and benefits are presented. The authors also describe the method of constant rate discounting, which uses the same rate to discount costs and benefits.

13. Kozma CM, Reeder CE, Shulz RM. Economic, clinical, and humanistic outcomes: a planning model for pharmacoeconomic research. Clin Ther 1993;15:1121–32.

    This paper describes a theoretical framework for identifying, collecting, and using outcomes data to assess the value of pharmaceutical treatment alternatives. The Economic, Clinical, and Humanistic Outcomes model depicts the value of a pharmaceutical product or service as a combination of traditional clinical-based outcomes with more contemporary measures of economic efficiency and quality. The model should assist health services researchers in planning, conducting, and evaluating pharmaceutical products and services from a multidimensional perspective. This framework represents a comprehensive framework for medical decision-making.

14. Lee JT, Sanchez LA. Interpretation of "cost-effective" and soundness of economic evaluations in pharmacy literature. Am J Hosp Pharm 1992;48:2622–7.

    Interpretations of the term "cost-effective" in the pharmacy literature are discussed. Sixty-five studies evaluating cost issues were identified in the pharmacy literature. The adequacy of these studies was evaluated according to ten methodologic criteria. In 36 (55 percent) articles, "cost-savings" was incorrectly equated to "cost-effectiveness." Of the 10 criteria, only 50 percent or more of the studies evaluated satisfied three. Criteria least often satisfied dealt with the identification of relevant costs and consequences of each strategy, discounting, incremental analysis, and sensitivity analysis. The authors conclude that many pharmacoeconomic studies incorrectly used the term cost-effective and inadequately addressed basic methodologic components.

15. Meyer KM, Espindle DM, DeGiacomo JM, Jenuleson CS, Kurtin PS, Davies AR. Monitoring dialysis patients' health status. Am J Kidney Dis 1994;24:267–79.

    The authors report 3 years experience with quarterly assessments of self-reported health of dialysis outpatients using the Medical Outcomes Study, short form, 36 items (MOS SF-36). Program logistics and results are described, including reliability coefficients, standard deviations, and standard errors of measurement for the MOS SF-36 in this patient population. Two case reports compare information obtained from the MOS SF-36 with the dialysis team's assessments of the patient, as recorded in the medical record. The comments of two patients on reviewing their MOS SF-36 results are also summarized. Patient reactions to the health status assessment program are explored, and potential benefits and areas for further work are outlined. The authors report that serial measurement of dialysis patients' health status allowed for recognition of clear patterns in individual patient's responses. Patterns sometimes suggested that the patient was either substantially more or less impaired than the dialysis team had thought. Changes in these patterns, both transient and protracted, frequently exceeded 95 percent confidence intervals for patient-level scores.

16. Pathak DS, MacKegian LD. Assessment of quality of life and health status selected observations. J Res Pharm Econ 1992;9:31–52.

    This paper focuses on conceptual and methodological issues involved in the definition and measurement of the construct of HRQOL. Conceptual issues discussed include quality of life versus HRQOL, defining HRQOL, need for a comprehensive framework to investigate the construct HRQOL, and demographic characteristics as determinants of HRQOL. Methodological issues discussed are new psychometric terms versus traditional terms, multi-attribute utility measurement and external validation, measurement of value versus utility, and time-related phenomena and the assessment of temporary and cyclical health states. Because these conceptual and methodological issues remain unresolved, caution is recommended in applying current assessment methods to set health care priorities. It is proposed that the true value of HRQOL assessments resides not in the final values obtained through such assessments, but in the explication of the process used in the valuation of subjective outcomes that cannot be adequately captured by objective measure.

17. Sanchez LA. Pharmacoeconomics and formulary decision-making. Pharmaco-Economics 1996;8(Suppl 2):S16–25.

    This paper describes how pharmacoeconomic data can be used to support various formulary management decisions. For example, these data can support the inclusion or exclusion of a drug on, or from, the formulary and support practice guidelines that promote the most cost-effective, or optimal use, of pharmaceutical products. Various strategies, including using published pharmacoeconomic studies, using economic modeling techniques, and conducting local pharmacoeconomic research, can be used to incorporate pharmacoeconomics into formulary decision making. Criteria for evaluating the pharmacoeconomic literature, suggestions for using economic models and suggested guidelines for conducting pharmacoeconomic projects are discussed. Furthermore, the process for formulary action and the influence of pharmacoeconomics on formulary management in a United States hospital are presented in this paper.

18. Sanchez LA. Expanding the role of pharmacists in pharmacoeconomics: how and why? PharmacoEconomics 1994; 5:367–75.

    The purpose of this paper is to illustrate the value of pharmacoeconomics in modern, pharmacy-practice settings, motivate pharmacists to expand their current roles to include pharmacoeconomics, and provide strategies for incorporating pharmacoeconomics into traditional pharmacy roles. Strategies, including use of published pharmacoeconomic literature, economic modeling and local pharmacoeconomic research, are presented.

19. Sanchez LA, Lee JT. Use and misuse of pharmacoeconomic terms: a definitions primer. Top Hosp Pharm Manage 1994;13:11–22.

    Given the current cost-conscious health care environment, pharmacists must now be able to assess the effect of an agent from safety, efficacy, and value considerations. This article describes the various methodologies that may be used in performing pharmacoeconomic analyses and highlights the use and misuse of pharmacoeconomic terminology. Case studies relating the use of these methods to the pharmacy practice setting are presented. The technical nuances of the various methods are explained to promote a better understanding of the appropriate use of these techniques and the terminology used to describe them.

20. Schrogie JJ, Nash DB. Relationship between practice guidelines, formulary management, and pharmacoeconomic studies. Top Hosp Pharm Manage 1994;13:38–46.

    This paper describes how pharmacy and therapeutics committees can use pharmaco-economic and outcomes studies as tools to evaluate and implement clinical guidelines for patient care. Ways in which the results of studies can help optimize the clinical effects and control the costs of drug therapy are discussed. The use of these data to assist in positioning products in competitive environments is described. A four-part classification of research studies is offered as an aid to strategic research planning.

21. Spilker B, ed. Quality of life and Pharmacoeconomics in Clinical Trials 2nd ed. Philadelphia, PA: Lippincott Williams & Wilkins Publishers, 1996. Revised edition of Quality of Life Assessment in Clinical Trials (1990).

    A comprehensive reference for clinical investigators who conduct quality of life assessments. The volume is divided into 11 sections: introduction to the field; standard scales, tests, and approaches; specific scales, tests, and measures; choosing and administering tests and treatments; analyzing, interpreting, and presenting data; special perspectives on quality of life issues; cross-cultural and cross-national issues; health policy issues; special populations to assess quality of life; specific problems and diseases; and pharmacoeconomics. Expanded to four times its predecessor's size and scope, the Second Edition reflects the rapid progress made worldwide in quality of life assessment and the growing importance of quality of life issues and pharmacoeconomics in health care decision-making. The editor has assembled more than 200 experts from diverse clinical, research, and social science disciplines to provide a comprehensive reference on the methodology, interpretation, and use of quality of life and pharmacoeconomic studies. The Second Edition features all-new sections on pharmacoeconomics and on crucial health policy issues such as outcomes research. The greatly expanded coverage of quality of life assessment includes a new section on cross-cultural and cross-national issues, more detailed information on specific tests, scales, and measures, and more comprehensive guidelines on choosing and administering tests and treatments and analyzing, interpreting, and presenting data.

22. Streiner DL, Norman GR. Health measurement scales: a practical guide to their development and use. 2nd ed. New York: Oxford University Press, 1999.

This is the second edition initiated in recognition of significant developments in the field of measurement since its first printing. This book is organized in chronological sequence according to the order that someone faced with the problem of developing a new instrument might encounter topics. Chapter 2 provides an overview of the criteria that the authors recommend be used to assess any measurement instrument. By reviewing this section, the reader should be able to peruse the literature to see if any available instrument is suitable. In the remaining chapters, the authors assume an unsuccessful search, and provide detailed information regarding the steps involved in developing a new scale. Finally, the appendices provide additional resources for locating further information about health status measurement, including an annotated bibliography of references for existing scales.

23. Udvarhelyi S, Colditz GA, Rai A, et al. Cost-effectiveness and cost-benefit analyses in the medical literature. Ann Intern Med 1992;116:238–44.

The objective of this paper was to determine whether published cost-effectiveness and cost-benefit analyses have adhered to basic analytic principles. Seventy-seven articles published either from 1978-1980 or 1985-1987 in general medical, surgical, and medical subspecialty journals were reviewed based on six fundamental principles of economic evaluations. The study results revealed that only three of the 77 articles reviewed met all six principles. Articles in general medical journals were more likely to use analytic methods appropriately. The authors concluded that greater attention should be devoted to ensuring the appropriate use of analytic methods for economic analyses, and readers should make note of the methods used when interpreting the results of economic analyses.

24. Katz S, Akpom CA, Papsidero JA, Weiss ST. Measuring the health status of populations. In: Berg RL, ed. Health status indexes: proceedings of a conference conducted by Health Services Research. Chicago: Hospital Research and Educational Trust, 1972:39.

In this article, the history of population and individual-level health measurement is reviewed. Key issues facing the field in the early 1970s are examined.

25. McDowell I, Newell C. Measuring health: a guide to rating scales and questionnaires, 2nd ed. New York: Oxford University Press, 1996.

An update of the 1987 edition, this text provides an overview of the field of health status assessment, including the history, techniques, and future directions of measurement. The authors review 88 rating scales and questionnaires that measure physical disability, social health, psychological well-being, depression, mental status, pain, general health status, and quality of life. The description of each scale or questionnaire includes its purpose, conceptual basis, reliability, validity, and a copy of the measure.

26. Patrick DL, Erickson P. Health status and health policy: allocating resources to health care. New York: Oxford University Press, 1993.

Patrick and Erickson propose and explicate the Health Resource Allocation Strategy as a process for comparing costs and outcomes of alternative options when selecting medical and health care interventions with the greatest benefit in relation to cost. They provide a guide to the development and application of health status and quality of life measures, emphasizing those based on utility theory, and they examine contemporary uses of such measures, including preventing disease and promoting health, assessing the cost-benefit of technology, and improving access to care. A compilation of disease-specific measures appears in Chapter 5; the appendix illustrates four utility-based indexes: Disability/Distress Index; Health Utilities Index; Quality of Well-Being Scale; and the EuroQol instrument. The glossary defines key terms.

27. Stewart AL, Ware JE Jr., eds. Measuring functioning and well-being: the Medical Outcomes Study approach. Durham, NC: Duke University Press, 1992.

In this book, the authors provide a comprehensive account of a broad range of self-reported measures of functioning and well-being developed for the Medical Outcomes Study, a large-scale investigation of how patients fare with health care in the United States. Many of these measures were derived from those used in earlier health policy research, including the Health Insurance Experiment (HIE). The authors address conceptual and methodologic issues involved in measuring physical, social, and role functioning; psychological distress and well-being; general health perceptions; energy and fatigue; sleep; and pain. Information is also presented on the construction, reliability, and validity of each measure, along with administration, scoring, and interpretation guidelines. The appendix includes copies of each measure; a glossary defines key terms; and the bibliography offers citations for most of the articles and books in health status assessment and related measurement methods for the past 50 years.

28. Testa MA, Simonson DC. Assessment of quality-of-life outcomes. N Engl J Med 1996;334:835–40.

Quality of life assessments and a conceptual scheme of quality of life are reviewed in this article. The article also addresses properties of measurement scales, selecting an assessment instrument, and interpreting quality of life effects.

29. Manning WG, Leibowitz A, Goldberg G, et al. A controlled trial of the effect of a prepaid group practice on use of services. N Engl J Med 1984; 310:1505–10.

This is an important paper, reporting results of the Rand HIE. The HIE was the first, and still the largest, randomized health services research study ever conducted. Patients were randomly assigned to fee-for-service or health maintenance organization plans to study differences in service use and health outcomes associated with these systems. The article reports the findings with respect to use. Overall expenditures on services were lower in the health maintenance organizations, attributable primarily to differences in rates of hospitalization. The study found that health maintenance organization patients were hospitalized 40 percent less than equivalent fee-for-service patients. Ambulatory care use was similar in the two systems. Subsequent research has validated these findings, both the magnitude and nature of the use differences.

30. Ware JE, Rogers WH, Davies AR, et al. Comparison of health outcomes at a health maintenance organization with those of fee-for service care. Lancet 1986;1:1017–22.

   This landmark article from the Rand HIE shows that the health outcomes associated with managed care differ for patients at different levels of illness and socioeconomic status. In particular, the authors report that outcomes in managed care were worse for patients who were poor and sick at the outset of the study. For nonpoor and/or well patients, managed care had beneficial health effect.

31. Wilson IB, Cleary PD. Linking clinical variables with health-related quality of life. A conceptual model of patient outcomes. JAMA 1995; 273(1):59–65.

   This article provides the clinician with an introduction to health services research concepts. In this article, the authors present a conceptual model, a taxonomy of patients outcomes that categorizes measures of patient outcome according to the underlying health concepts they represent and porpoises specific causal relationships between different health concepts, thereby integrating the two models of health described. This article is valuable to clinicians in practice, and in research settings since it discusses the conceptual intersection of those two worlds.

32. Wennberg J, Gittelson A. Variations in medical care among small areas. Sci Am 1982;246:120–34.

   This is a valuable paper in which the phenomenon of small-area variation associated with six surgical procedures are described. It is one of the first empiric studies of small-area variation in the United States. The authors studied the rates of selected procedures in the six New England states. The results provide powerful evidence that area norms, rather than universally shared scientific criteria, determine medical treatments provided to patients. This field of work led to the call for research, including clinical practice guideline development, health outcomes research, and cost-effectiveness analysis of medical interventions, to try to bring greater rationality to medical care.

Conferences

A variety of conferences have been convened since the early 1970s to address issues of health status measurement—theoretical, conceptual, empiric, and historical. The published proceedings from these conferences include many of the now-classic articles in the health measurement field, and their citation lists contain many others. The following publications direct the interested reader to these sources.

1. Berg RL, ed. Health status indexes: proceedings of a conference conducted by health services research. Chicago: Hospital Research and Educational Trust, 1973.
2. Fowler FJ, ed. The proceedings of the Conference of Measuring the Effects of Medical Treatment. Med Care 1995;33(4): supplement.
3. Health status indexes: work in progress. Health Services Res 1976; 11(4): special issue.
4. Katz S, ed. The Portugal conference: measuring quality of life and functional status in clinical and epidemiological research. J Chronic Dis 1987;40(6): special issue.
5. Lohr KN, ed. Advances in health status assessment: conference proceedings. Med Care 1989;27(3): supplement.
6. Lohr KN, ed. Advances in health status assessment: fostering the application of health status measures in clinical settings—proceedings of a conference. Med Care 1992;30(5): supplement.
7. Lohr KN, Ware Jr JE, eds. Proceedings of the advances in health assessment conference. J Chronic Dis 1987;40: supplement 1.
8. Patrick DL, Chiang YP, eds. Health Outcomes Methodology: Symposium Proceedings. Med Care 2000;38(9): supplement II.

Self-Assessment Questions

1. Proponents of outcomes research believe that which one of the following is true?
   A. Outcomes research is synonymous with pharmacoeconomics.
   B We should measure not only the clinical and cost impacts of health care, but also the outcomes that take the patients perspective into account.
   C. Only clinical effects, and not functional status or well-being, should be included as outcomes.
   D. All outcomes research is pharmacoeconomic research.

2. The economic, clinical, and humanistic outcomes (ECHO) model recognizes the existence of intermediate outcomes. Which one of the following is an example of an intermediate outcome?
   A. A patient's physical functioning or mental well-being.
   B. A specific laboratory value.
   C. The total cost of hospitalization.
   D. Adherence to a drug regimen.

3. Which one of the following statements best describes economic outcomes?
   A. The direct, indirect, and intangible costs compared with the consequences of medical treatment alternatives.
   B. The medical events that occur as a result of a disease or treatment.
   C. The consequences of a disease or treatment on a patient's functional status or quality of life.
   D. The cost-savings associated with a disease or treatment alternative.

4. Which one of the following best represents a direct medical cost?
   A. Pain.
   B. Transportation.
   C. Mortality.
   D. Medical professional time.

5. Lost productivity is an example of which one of the following cost categories?
   A. Direct medical cost.
   B. Direct nonmedical cost.
   C. Indirect cost.
   D. Intangible cost.

6. Which one of the following statements regarding the perspective of economic evaluations is true?
   A. Economic evaluations are valid only if conducted from a single perspective.
   B. Economic evaluations can be conducted from multiple perspectives.
   C. Economic evaluations should only be conducted from the perspective of the patient.
   D. Society is the only valid perspective for economic evaluations.

7. From the perspective of a provider, which one of the following is a direct cost of health care?
   A. The amount paid out-of-pocket by patients directly to their physicians for a clinic visit.
   B. The patient charge for a visit to an emergency department.
   C. The prescription cost of insulin at the community pharmacy.
   D. The salary of the clinical pharmacist who monitors a patient's therapy.

8. From the perspective of an employer, indirect costs are best described by which one of the following?
   A. Hospitalization costs borne by the patient.
   B. Drug effects on patient functioning.
   C. Loss of patient income associated with missed workdays.
   D. Family caregiving costs.

9. The costs and consequences of health care can be different depending on the perspective of the evaluation. Costs from a patient's perspective are best described as which one of the following?
   A. Essentially, what patients are charged for a product or service.
   B. Essentially, the true cost of providing a product or service, regardless of the charge.
   C. Essentially, the charges allowed for a health care product or service.
   D. Essentially, the cost of giving and receiving medical care, including patient morbidity and mortality.

10. Which one of the following constitutes a full economic evaluation?
    A. Two antibiotics are compared and relative cure rates are determined.
    B. The costs for treatment of hypertension by general practice physicians, versus pharmacists, are considered in light of the blood pressure control achieved.
    C. The costs and efficiency of treatment of hypercholesterolemia with a new HMG-CoA reductase inhibitor are determined.
    D. The acquisition costs of two therapeutically equivalent antihypertensive agents are compared.

11. Which one of the following is an example of a partial economic evaluation?
    A. A comparison of the costs and consequences of two alternatives.
    B. A cost-utility analysis.
    C. A comparison of the costs of two equally effective alternatives.
    D. A quality of life comparison of multiple treatment alternatives.

12. Which one of the following is true of partial economic evaluations?
    A. Partial evaluations should be performed as components of full economic evaluations.
    B. Partial evaluations assess all important components necessary for a complete economic analysis.
    C. Partial evaluations may provide a description of the costs, or consequences, of competing alternatives.
    D. Partial evaluations compare the costs and consequences of two treatments.

13. Which one of the following statements is *not* true about cost-minimization analysis?
    A. Cost-minimization analysis is a tool used to compare the costs of two or more treatment alternatives.
    B. Cost-minimization analysis shows only a cost-savings of one treatment alternative over another.
    C. Cost-minimization analysis measures costs of treatment alternatives in dollars and a assumes comparable efficacy.
    D. Cost-minimization analysis is a method to be used when no evidence exists to support the therapeutic equivalence of two or more treatment alternatives.

14. When conducting a cost-benefit analysis (CBA), the results are best expressed as which one of the following?
    A. Cost-benefit ratio.
    B. Average cost per utility.
    C. cost-savings.
    D. Incremental cost ratio.

15. When quantifying the value of a clinical pharmacy service, which one of the following economic evaluation methods is the best to use?
    A. Cost-benefit analysis.
    B. Cost-effectiveness analysis.
    C. Cost-minimization analysis.
    D. Cost-utility analysis.

16. Which one of the following statements does not describe a cost-effective treatment alternative?

A. Less expensive and less effective, where the lost benefit was worth the extra cost.
B. Less expensive and at least as effective.
C. More expensive with an additional benefit worth the additional cost.
D. Less expensive and less effective, where the extra benefit is not worth the extra cost.

17. A cost-effectiveness analysis would be best applied to which one of the following situations?
    A. When comparing two or more treatment alternatives that differ in clinical outcome.
    B. When comparing two or more treatment alternatives that are equal in clinical outcome.
    C. When comparing two or more treatment alternatives that differ in humanistic outcome.
    D. When comparing two or more treatment alternatives that differ in cost.

18. Which one of the following statements best describes an incremental cost-effectiveness ratio?
    A. A summary measurement of efficiency.
    B. The cost per benefit of a new strategy, independent of other treatment alternatives.
    C. The cost to obtain an extra benefit realized when switching from one strategy to another.
    D. The cost per quality-adjusted life-year (QALY) gained.

19. When comparing treatment alternatives, which one of the following is the most correct application for cost-utility analysis?
    A. Alternatives that are life-extending with serious side effects.
    B. Alternatives that differ in cost.
    C. Alternatives that differ in efficacy and safety.
    D. Alternatives that are similar in clinical and humanistic outcomes.

20. Which one of the following statements about discounting is not true?
    A. When costs and consequences of a treatment alternative occur in the future, they should be reduced to reflect current fiscal value.
    B. Discounting is the process of adjusting for differential timing.
    C. There is one standard discount rate that should be used in pharmacoeconomic analyses.
    D. Comparisons of programs or treatment alternatives should be made at the same time.

21. Which one of the following statements regarding discounting is true?
    A. Researchers should always use a 5 percent discount rate.
    B. Costs incurred today to initiate a new program should be discounted.
    C. Discounting can be useful when comparing acute and long-term treatment strategies.
    D. Benefits should not be discounted.

22. The primary reason to perform a sensitivity analysis is to accomplish which one of the following?
    A. Test the robustness of the economic evaluation conclusions.
    B. Reveal sensitive variables of the economic evaluation.
    C. Uncover the range of plausible values.
    D. Allow for a meaningful comparison of treatment alternatives.

23. Which one of the following statements is *not* true regarding the application of pharmacoeconomics to pharmacy practice?
    A. Pharmacoeconomics can be a powerful tool for determining the most efficient use of drugs.
    B. Pharmacoeconomics can assist pharmacy and therapeutics committees in incorporating clinical, economic, and humanistic outcomes of drug therapy into formulary management decisions.
    C. Pharmacoeconomics can provide data to support individual patient treatment and resource allocation decisions.
    D. Use of pharmacoeconomic data ensures that organizational drug-use policies will influence physician prescribing patterns.

24. Which one of the following formulary decision options would be *least* influenced by the inclusion of pharmacoeconomic data?
    A. Inclusion or exclusion of newly marketed agents.
    B. Inclusion with restriction of newly marketed agents.
    C. Deletion of drugs from the formulary.
    D. Determination of the least expensive to purchase alternative.

25. Which one of the following is true regarding health and quality of life?
    A. Quality of life is encompassed by a person's lifestyle, including work and economic status.
    B. Health or HRQOL refers only to those aspects of life dominated, or significantly influenced, by personal health or activities performed to maintain health.
    C. Quality of life is divided into physical and mental dimensions of functioning and well-being.
    D. The concept of health includes marital status, education, and religious beliefs.

26. Which one of the following activities is a dimension of general health status measurement?
    A. Carrying a bag of groceries.
    B. Physical functioning.
    C. Playing sports.
    D. Bathing or dressing.

27. Which one of the following pairs illustrates two opposite extremes of mental well-being? These two attributes can be used to describe the range of a mental health continuum.
    A. Psychological distress and physical distress.
    B. Physical distress and psychological well-being.

C. Psychological well-being and psychological distress.
D. High physical energy and physical weariness.

28. Which one of the following features could be described as one of the most striking differences between traditional clinical measures of a patient's health and measures of health status?

    A. The source of the data is patient self-administered questionnaires.
    B. The collection of data from patients is a new phenomenon, whereas collection of laboratory data dates back many years.
    C. Clinicians can use the clinical data, but not health status data, in decision-making.
    D. Clinical data are "hard data", whereas, health status data are not as scientifically rigorous in their standards of measurement.

29. The following are characteristics of a good scale for measuring health status. Which one of the following is true of generic/general health status measures, but *not* true of disease specific measures?

    A. The concepts can be measured in patients of all ages, races, and socio-demographic characteristics.
    B. The concepts being measured include all possible dimensions of health for a patient population.
    C. The measurement framework extends across the entire range of a dimension, from disease to well-being.
    D. The measurement must be sensitive to change over time to be used in clinical practice.

30. The categorization of structure, process, and outcome published in the early 1960s (see Reference 5) was designed to evaluate which one of the following?

    A. Patients satisfaction with care.
    B. The quality of health care.
    C. Health policy changes.
    D A patients self-assessment of the health care system.

31. Which one of the following best describes a difference between patient satisfaction and health status?

    A. Patient satisfaction results are required for accreditation by JCAHO; health status results are not.
    B. Health status measurements of functioning and well-being are required by law for drug approval; patient satisfaction results are not.
    C. Patient satisfaction is measured with a combination of reports and ratings; health status doesn't use ratings.
    D. Health status is measured using psychometric techniques; patient satisfaction is not.

32. It has been proposed that one solution to increase clinicians' information about the functional status, well-being, and changes over time of their patients might be to standardize these assessments in everyday medical practice. Such routine assessments could be useful for all except which one of the following purposes?

    A. To replace the need for referral to specialists in assessment of functional or emotional problems.
    B. To detect, explain, and track changes in functional capacity over time.
    C. To make it possible to better consider the patients total functioning when choosing among therapies.
    D. As guidance for efficient use of community resources and social services.

33. Which one of the following are *not* characteristics of the measurement and use of individual level patient self-reported health status information?

    A. Standardized method of asking patients about their functioning and well being can be efficiently used in treatment decisions and as a monitoring parameter for efficacy and toxicity of treatment.
    B. Concerns have been raised about the reliability and interpretation of the results from individual, patient-level, health status information.
    C. Modern psychometric test theory, such as Item Response Theory, offers potential for individual patient-level, health status assessment, and use in clinical care.
    D. Existing health outcome assessments drawn from classic test theory can no longer be used.

Appendix A

MOS SF-36™ HEALTH SURVEY

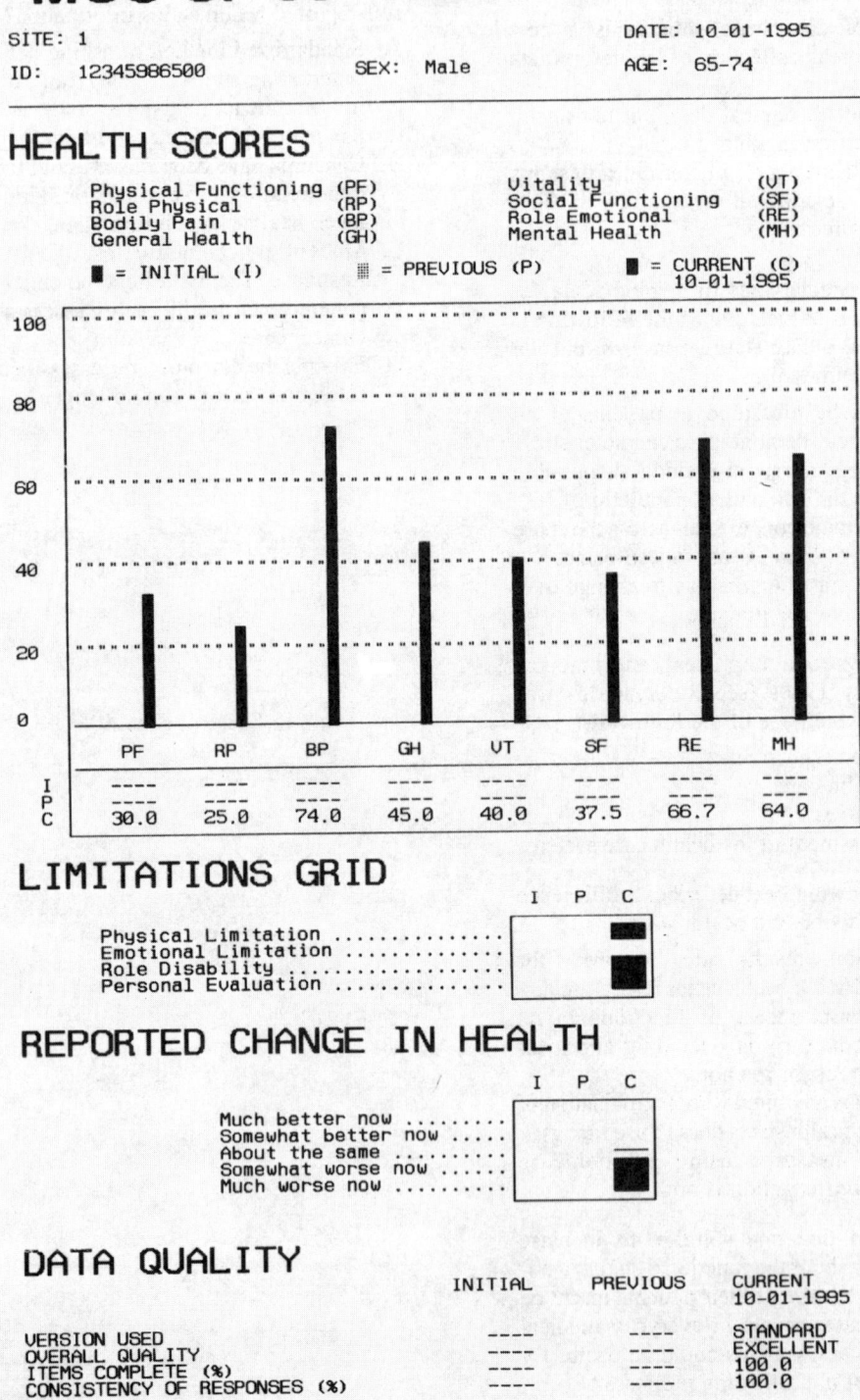

SITE: 1　　　　　　　　　　　　　　　　　　　　DATE: 10-01-1995
ID: 12345986500　　　　　　SEX: Male　　　　　AGE: 65-74

HEALTH SCORES

Physical Functioning (PF)　　　Vitality (VT)
Role Physical (RP)　　　　　　Social Functioning (SF)
Bodily Pain (BP)　　　　　　　Role Emotional (RE)
General Health (GH)　　　　　Mental Health (MH)

■ = INITIAL (I)　　　▦ = PREVIOUS (P)　　　■ = CURRENT (C) 10-01-1995

	PF	RP	BP	GH	VT	SF	RE	MH
I	----	----	----	----	----	----	----	----
P	----	----	----	----	----	----	----	----
C	30.0	25.0	74.0	45.0	40.0	37.5	66.7	64.0

LIMITATIONS GRID

　　　　　　　　　　　　　　　　　　　I　P　C
Physical Limitation
Emotional Limitation
Role Disability
Personal Evaluation

REPORTED CHANGE IN HEALTH

　　　　　　　　　　　　　　　　　　　I　P　C
Much better now
Somewhat better now
About the same
Somewhat worse now
Much worse now

DATA QUALITY

	INITIAL	PREVIOUS	CURRENT 10-01-1995
VERSION USED	----	----	STANDARD
OVERALL QUALITY	----	----	EXCELLENT
ITEMS COMPLETE (%)	----	----	100.0
CONSISTENCY OF RESPONSES (%)	----	----	100.0

Copyright(C) 1993, 2000 by John E. Ware, Jr., Ph.D.
SF-36(R) is a registered trademark of Medical Outcomes Trust
Ware, J.E., Snow, K.K., Kosinski, M. SF-36(R) Health Survey: Manual and Interpretation Guide. Lincoln, RI: QualityMetric Incorporated, 1993, 2000.

Appendix B

MOS SF-36™ HEALTH SURVEY

SITE: 1 DATE: 12-07-1995
ID: 12345986500 SEX: Male AGE: 65-74

HEALTH SCORES

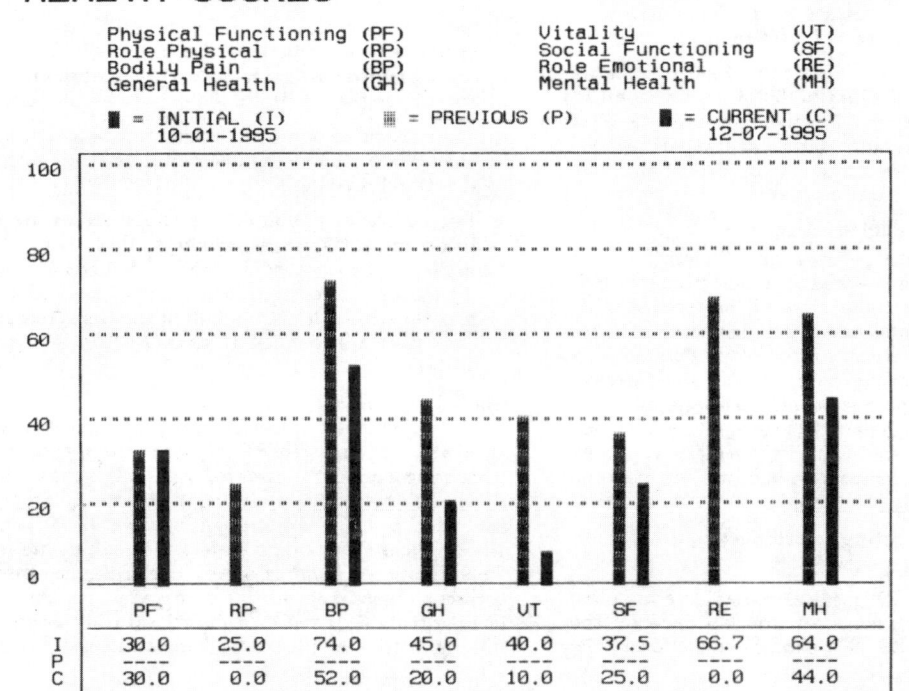

Physical Functioning (PF) Vitality (VT)
Role Physical (RP) Social Functioning (SF)
Bodily Pain (BP) Role Emotional (RE)
General Health (GH) Mental Health (MH)

■ = INITIAL (I) ▓ = PREVIOUS (P) ■ = CURRENT (C)
10-01-1995 12-07-1995

	PF	RP	BP	GH	VT	SF	RE	MH
I	30.0	25.0	74.0	45.0	40.0	37.5	66.7	64.0
P	----	----	----	----	----	----	----	----
C	30.0	0.0	52.0	20.0	10.0	25.0	0.0	44.0

LIMITATIONS GRID

Physical Limitation
Emotional Limitation
Role Disability
Personal Evaluation

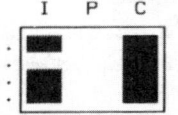

REPORTED CHANGE IN HEALTH

Much better now
Somewhat better now
About the same
Somewhat worse now
Much worse now

DATA QUALITY

	INITIAL 10-01-1995	PREVIOUS	CURRENT 12-07-1995
VERSION USED	STANDARD	----	STANDARD
OVERALL QUALITY	EXCELLENT	----	SATISFACT
ITEMS COMPLETE (%)	100.0	----	100.0
CONSISTENCY OF RESPONSES (%)	100.0	----	93.3

Copyright(C) 1993, 2000 by John E. Ware, Jr., Ph.D.
SF-36(R) is a registered trademark of Medical Outcomes Trust
Ware, J.E., Snow, K.K., Kosinski, M. SF-36(R) Health Survey: Manual and Interpretation Guide. Lincoln, RI: QualityMetric Incorporated, 1993, 2000.

Appendix C

SF-36 HEALTH STATUS SURVEY RESULTS:
INTERPRETATION GUIDE FOR INDIVIDUAL PATIENT REPORTS (RT Version 1.0)

About the SF-36

The SF-36 (Short-Form, 36 Item) Health Survey is a patient-based, generic health status assessment survey that obtains patients' assessments of their functioning and well-being (how they feel), and perceptions of their health in general. The SF-36 has been used to assess the health status of both general and chronic disease populations. Its reliability in these populations has been documented, and its validity in relation to such clinical indicators as presence or absence of disease, severity within disease category, and changes in disease-related symptoms over time has been demonstrated by investigators.

The information about a patient's functional status and well-being obtained with the SF-36 can be useful in assessing and obtaining a better understanding of a patient's overall health status. Data obtained with the SF-36 should be interpreted within the context of all other information available about the patient.

SF-36 Scoring

The SF-36 measures eight different health concepts, each of which is scored on a scale from 0 to 100. Points in between are percentages of the total possible score. All scales are scored so that a higher score indicates better health. For instance, on the Bodily Pain scale, a higher score indicates <u>less</u> pain, and on the Physical Functioning scale, a higher score indicates <u>better</u> physical functioning. Each item in the SF-36 belongs to, and is used in the scoring of, only one of the eight scales. The table below lists each health concept and indicates the meaning of low and high scores for each concept.

Interpreting the Report

Background

The patient's ID (medical record or encounter) number, gender and age range, and the date on which the patient completed the SF-36, are indicated just below the report title *(MOS SF-36 Health Survey)*.

Health Scores

This section reports the patient's scores on each of the eight health concepts (commonly referred to as the eight SF-36 *scales*). Scale scores for each of three possible time points are displayed. A histogram format is used to indicate the eight scale scores at each point in time.

- The scale names (and their corresponding abbreviations in parentheses) are indicated above the graph. Scale abbreviations are used to indicate the corresponding bar in the histogram.

- Initial (I), previous (P), and current (C) dates of survey completion are shown underneath the time point legend. Previous date indicates the most recent date of survey completion before the current administration.

- The vertical axis ranges from 0 to 100 (the range for each SF-36 scale). The horizontal axis lists each scale (by its abbreviation).

- Initial, previous, and current scale scores are listed below the bar(s) corresponding to that scale. "NA" is indicated if a score could not be calculated for a scale on a particular date (scale scores cannot be calculated for a given scale if less than half of the items comprising that scale are completed). **NOTE:** "0.0" is a possible scale score.

Confidence Intervals

Confidence intervals are particularly useful in evaluating changes in SF-36 scores over time and in comparing a patient's scores to benchmark scores. The size of the 90 percent confidence interval (CI) around an individual patient's score ranges between +/- 10 points for the Physical Functioning scale and +/- 23 points for the Role Emotional scale. For any one scale, one would be correct 90 percent of the time or more in concluding that a change truly occurred or a difference truly exists if the difference between the scores being compared exceeds the 90 percent CI for that scale.

Health Concept (Scale Name Bolded)	Lowest Possible Score (0)	Highest Possible Score (100)	Confidence Interval*
Physical Functioning	Limited a lot in performing all physical activities including bathing or dressing	Performs all types of physical activities including the most vigorous without limitations due to health	+/- 10
Role limitations due to physical problems	Problem with work or other daily activities as a result of physical health	No problems with work or other daily activities as a result of physical health	+/- 19
Bodily Pain	Very severe and extremely limiting pain	No pain or limitations due to pain	+/- 12
General Health	Believes personal health is poor and likely to get worse	Believes personal health is excellent	+/- 15
Vitality	Feels tired and worn out all of the time	Feels full of pep and energy all of the time	+/- 13
Social Functioning	Extreme and frequent interference with normal social activities due to physical and emotional problems	Performs normal social activities without interference due to physical or emotional problems	+/- 21
Role limitations due to Emotional problems	Problems with work or other daily activities as a result of emotional problems	No problems with work or other daily activities as a result of emotional problems	+/- 23
General Mental Health	Feelings of nervousness and depression all of the time	Feels peaceful, happy, and calm all of the time	+/- 12

Copyright(C) 1993, 2000 by John E. Ware, Jr., Ph.D.
SF-36(R) is a registered trademark of Medical Outcomes Trust
Ware, J.E., Snow, K.K., Kosinski, M. SF-36(R) Health Survey: Manual and Interpretation Guide. Lincoln, RI: QualityMetric Incorporated, 1993, 2000.

Limitations Grid

This grid is a visual representation of four dichotomous summary limitation indicators. The indicators identify limitations patients reported in four different health categories. The limitation indicators and their criteria for activation are: Physical Limitation (PF<100), Emotional Limitation (MH<53), Role Disability (RP<100 or RE<100) and Personal Evaluation (GH<56). When an indicator is "activated," a black box appears across from the indicator name, under the appropriate date of survey administration.

Reported Change in Health

This section of the report reports how a patient rates their general health in comparison to a year ago (if the standard version of the SF-36 is used) or a week ago if the acute version is used). (See discussion of the Standard and Acute versions in the Data Quality section, below.) Response options appear on the left, and responses on initial, previous, and current administrations are indicated in a box on the right. The length of the bar corresponds to the degree to which the patient rates his or her general health compared to the past: a longer bar above the "about the same" line indicates greater improvement, while a longer bar below the line indicates greater worsening of general health. If the patient reported that their health is "about the same", an asterisk appears across from this response option.

Data Quality

This section indicates the SF-36 version administered during the current administration (standard or acute). The two versions differ in the recall period used in the items included in the RP, BP, VT, SF, RE, and MH scales. The standard version uses a 4 week recall period, whereas the acute version uses a 1 week recall period. The standard version is most frequently used. General population norms and confidence intervals are available on the standard version only.

The Data Quality section also indicates a rating of the overall quality of the data, the percent of items complete and the percent consistency of responses based on the current administration. *Item completeness* and *response consistency*, two indicators of data quality, are assessed each time a patient completes the SF-36. The closer each of these percentages is to 100 percent, the better the data quality. Item completeness is assessed by calculating the percent of items completed by the patient. Response consistency is assessed by evaluating 15 pairs of items for agreement in the pattern of responses. Taking these two indicators into account, the data quality of each SF-36 form is assigned a rating of *Excellent, Satisfactory, or Problematic*. (See next column for interpretation of problematic data.)

Missing/Double Marks and Inconsistency Report

If there are any missing data (percent items complete<100) or inconsistent responses (percent consistency<100), then a second page is printed. The top of the page notes which questions were not answered or had multiple responses (and are therefore considered missing). The bottom of the page indicates which of the 15 consistency checks were failed. The numbers listed above the inconsistency check box represent the questions involved in the consistency check. For example, if a patient responds "all of the time" to both questions 9a ("Did you feel full of pep?") and 9i ("Did you feel tired?"), then a check mark is listed under "9a vs 9i" because these responses are inconsistent.

Interpreting Problematic Data

- On a given date for a given patient, any of the following conditions result in a data quality rating of Problematic:
  1. Less than half of the items were completed for one or more of the scales, resulting in one or more missing scale scores.
  2. Inconsistent response pattern (response consistency ≤85 percent).
  3. Combination of both 1 and 2.

- A low response consistency (percent) could mean two things:
  1. The patient had difficulty understanding the questions.
  2. The patient was not paying attention to the way he/she responded to some or all of the questions (random answers).

- Items complete (percent) and response consistency (percent) can help identify patients who repeatedly have trouble completing the form and/or have trouble responding in a consistent manner.

Treat Problematic Data with Caution

Problematic data are by nature less reliable. This is especially true if there is a problem with response consistency. It is often useful to examine the individual items causing the inconsistent responses for individual patients.

References

1. Ware JE, Jr., Sherbourne C. A 36-item short-form health survey (SF-36): I. Conceptual framework and item selection. Med Care 1992, 30:6.
2. Ware JE. SF-36 Health Survey Manual and Interpretation Guide. The Health Institute, New England Medical Center, Boston MA, 1993.
3. Response Technologies, Inc. The RT 2000/SF-36 Report Formats. © 1992 Response Technologies, Inc.

Appendix D
Normative Values

NORMS FOR THE GENERAL U.S. POPULATION, TOTAL SAMPLE

Total Sample (N=2,474)

	PF	RP	BP	GH	VT	SF	RE	MH
Mean	84.15	80.96	75.15	71.95	60.86	83.28	81.26	74.74
25th Percentile	70.00	50.00	61.00	57.00	45.00	75.00	66.67	64.00
50th Percentile *(median)*	90.00	100.00	74.00	72.00	65.00	100.00	100.00	80.00
75th Percentile	100.00	100.00	100.00	85.00	75.00	700.00	100.00	88.00
Standard Deviation	23.28	34.00	23.69	20.34	20.96	22.69	33.04	18.05
Range	0-100	0-100	0-100	5-100	0-100	0-100	0-100	0-100
% Ceiling	38.79	70.85	31.85	7.40	1.50	52.32	71.01	3.91
% Floor	0.84	10.33	0.58	0.00	0.52	0.64	9.61	0.00

Ages 65 & over Males (N=293)

	PF	RP	BP	GH	VT	SF	RE	MH
Mean	65.79	59.72	68.76	58.62	57.80	79.66	76.94	77.37
25th Percentile	45.00	25.00	51.00	47.00	40.00	62.50	66.67	68.00
50th Percentile *(median)*	75.00	75.00	72.00	62.00	60.00	100.00	100.00	84.00
75th Percentile	90.00	100.00	84.00	77.00	75.00	100.00	100.00	92.00
Standard Deviation	28.31	42.51	25.37	22.05	22.55	26.00	37.48	17.42
Range	0-100	0-100	0-100	5-100	0-100	0-100	0-100	16-100
% Ceiling	6.6	45.9	22.8	1.8	1.7	50.7	68.3	7.6
% Floor	3.0	24.4	0.9	0.0	1.0	1.5	14.9	0.0

NORMS FOR COMORBID CONDITIONS: CHRONIC OBSTRUCTIVE PULMONARY DISEASE (COPD) WITH HYPERTENSION

	PF	RP	BP	GH	VT	SF	RE	MH
Mean	56.91	34.38	54.82	45.29	44.95	71.82	59.73	68.06
25th Percentile	35.00	0.00	31.00	35.00	30.00	62.50	0.00	56.00
50th Percentile *(median)*	61.11	25.00	52.00	42.00	50.00	75.00	66.67	72.00
75th Percentile	80.00	75.00	72.00	60.00	55.00	100.00	100.00	84.00
Standard Deviation	29.14	38.73	26.14	18.94	19.55	31.40	44.61	19.68
Range	0-100	0-100	10-100	5-87	0-90	0-100	0-100	13-100
% Ceiling	5.88	14.12	10.59	0.00	0.00	32.94	48.24	2.35
% Floor	2.35	42.35	0.00	0.00	1.18	2.35	27.06	0.00

Copyright(C) 1993, 2000 by John E. Ware, Jr., Ph.D.
SF-36(R) is a registered trademark of Medical Outcomes Trust
Ware, J.E., Snow, K.K., Kosinski, M. SF-36(R) Health Survey: Manual and Interpretation Guide. Lincoln, RI: QualityMetric Incorporated, 1993, 2000.

Appendix E

MOS SF-36™ HEALTH SURVEY

SITE: 1
ID: 12345986500 SEX: Male
DATE: 12-05-1996
AGE: 65-74

HEALTH SCORES

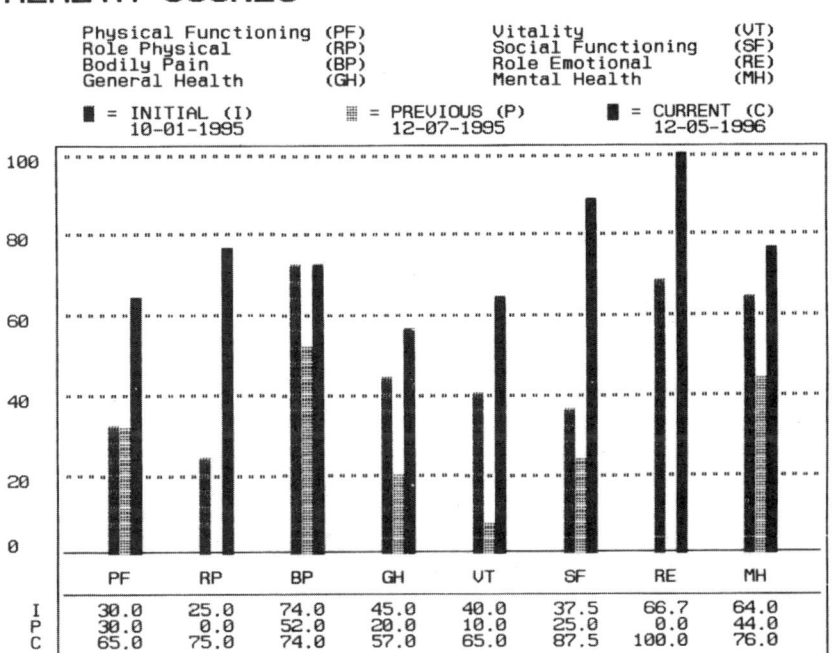

Physical Functioning (PF) Vitality (VT)
Role Physical (RP) Social Functioning (SF)
Bodily Pain (BP) Role Emotional (RE)
General Health (GH) Mental Health (MH)

■ = INITIAL (I) 10-01-1995   ▒ = PREVIOUS (P) 12-07-1995   ■ = CURRENT (C) 12-05-1996

	PF	RP	BP	GH	VT	SF	RE	MH
I	30.0	25.0	74.0	45.0	40.0	37.5	66.7	64.0
P	30.0	0.0	52.0	20.0	10.0	25.0	0.0	44.0
C	65.0	75.0	74.0	57.0	65.0	87.5	100.0	76.0

LIMITATIONS GRID

                              I P C
Physical Limitation ....
Emotional Limitation ....
Role Disability ....
Personal Evaluation ....

REPORTED CHANGE IN HEALTH

                              I P C
Much better now ....
Somewhat better now ......
About the same ....
Somewhat worse now ....
Much worse now ....

DATA QUALITY

	INITIAL 10-01-1995	PREVIOUS 12-07-1995	CURRENT 12-05-1996
VERSION USED	STANDARD	STANDARD	STANDARD
OVERALL QUALITY	EXCELLENT	SATISFACT	EXCELLENT
ITEMS COMPLETE (%)	100.0	100.0	100.0
CONSISTENCY OF RESPONSES (%)	100.0	93.3	100.0

Copyright(C) 1993, 2000 by John E. Ware, Jr., Ph.D.
SF-36(R) is a registered trademark of Medical Outcomes Trust
Ware, J.E., Snow, K.K., Kosinski, M. SF-36(R) Health Survey: Manual and Interpretation Guide. Lincoln, RI: QualityMetric Incorporated, 1993, 2000.

TYPES OF ECONOMIC AND HUMANISTIC OUTCOMES ASSESSMENTS

Answers to Self-Assessment Questions

1. Answer: B

Pharmacoeconomics is part of the larger area of research known as outcomes research. The two are not synonymous; therefore, Answer A is incorrect. Not all outcomes research is pharmacoeconomic research (Answer D). Proponents of outcomes research include clinical, economic, and humanistic variables as dependent or as the outcome variables. Outcomes research includes clinical assessments, the patient's perspective about their functioning and wellbeing, as well as the economics of the intervention; therefore, Answer C is incorrect.

2. Answer: D

The economic, clinical, and humanistic outcomes (ECHO) model represents economic, clinical, and humanistic outcomes. Each of these endpoints involves intermediate steps or intermediate outcomes. Humanistic intermediaries can include specific behaviors of an individual or a group of people. The behaviors themselves are not outcomes in this model. One example is the behavior of patients' adherence to their drug regimen. Compliance can be affected by nonbehavioral factors also, such as the cost of the drug or the patient's belief system, or attitude toward taking drugs. All of these influences can have an impact on the outcome and the patients assessment of the outcome. In a statistical model, adherence to drug regimens is considered both a dependent and an independent variable. As an independent variable, adherence can be evaluated for its effect on the dependent variable of humanistic outcomes. In this way, it is an intermediary, or an intermediate step.

3. Answer: A

Economic outcomes have been defined as the total costs of medical care associated with treatment alternatives balanced against clinical or humanistic outcomes (see Reference 13). Clinical outcomes are defined as medical events that occur as a result of a disease or treatment (Answer B). Humanistic outcomes are defined as the consequences of disease or treatment on patient functional status or quality of life (Answer C). Researchers have proposed that the evaluation of pharmaceutical products should include an assessment of each of these three outcome types.

4. Answer: D

Direct medical costs are the costs incurred for medical products and services used for the prevention, detection, and treatment of a disease, such as transportation. Examples of other direct costs include drugs, supplies, and hospitalizations. Pain (Answer A) is an example of an intangible cost. Mortality (Answer C) is an example of an indirect cost. Transportation (Answer B) is a direct nonmedical cost.

5. Answer: C

Indirect costs are those costs resulting from morbidity and mortality. They are costs valued as real money that are not directly paid for the treatment of an illness or disease, such as transportation. Morbidity costs are incurred from missing work (lost productivity), whereas mortality costs are the costs incurred due to premature death.

6. Answer: B

Economic evaluations can be conducted from single (Answer A) or multiple perspectives, as long as it is clear what the perspective(s) is and the costs and consequences are relevant to the perspective(s) chosen. Popular perspectives for conducting economic evaluations include the patient (Answer C), provider, payer, and society. In countries with nationalized medicine, society is the predominate perspective; however, it is not the only valid perspective (Answer D).

7. Answer: D

Direct costs of importance to providers are expenses paid by the provider to care for patients. The amount paid out-of-pocket by patients directly to their physicians for a clinic visit is a direct expense to patients (Answer A). Patient charges for visits to an emergency department (Answer B) and the prescription cost of insulin at the community pharmacy (Answer C) both are direct expenses to third-party payers and to patients (for the amount of their co-payment). Salaries of clinical pharmacists who monitor patients' therapies are direct expenses from the perspective of the provider.

8. Answer: B

Indirect costs are composed of costs due to work loss and decreased productivity due to illness. From the perspective of an employer, costs related to lost days of work and decreased functioning of employees are pertinent indirect costs. A drug that reduces an employee's ability to function certainly falls into this category. Loss of income (Answer C) is an indirect cost from the perspective of the patient, whereas family care-giving expenses (Answer D) are direct nonmedical costs. The patient's share of hospitalization costs (Answer A) are a direct cost from the patient perspective.

9. Answer: A

Costs from a patient's perspective are essentially the uninsured portion of what they pay, or are charged, for a product or service. The provider's perspective is represented by the true cost of providing a service (Answer B). The charges allowed for a health care product or service (Answer C) represent cost from the perspective of a payer. Cost from a societal perspective includes the cost of giving and receiving medical care, including morbidity and mortality (Answer D).

10. Answer: B

A full economic evaluation is one that encompasses two basic characteristics: 1) a comparison of two or more treatment alternatives is made; and 2) both the costs and the consequences of the alternatives are examined (see Reference 7). A partial economic evaluation encompasses only one of these characteristics. A complete evaluation should identify, measure, and compare the costs and consequences associated with competing programs or treatment alternatives.

11. Answer: D

A partial economic evaluation provides a descriptive assessment of resource use or outcome. By definition, partial evaluations do not provide both a comprehensive assessment and comparison of the costs and consequences of competing alternatives; therefore, Answer A is incorrect. A simple cost comparison without regard for outcomes, as well as comparison of only outcomes without regard for costs, are both examples of partial economic assessments. A third example of partial economic assessment is the description of costs and outcomes for a single treatment alternative.

12. Answer: C

Although partial economic evaluations may serve as a useful starting point in outlining or describing the costs or consequences of drug therapy, they are not a component of a full assessment (Answer A). A full economic assessment necessitates evaluation of both the costs and consequences of competing alternatives. In the absence of a full evaluation, a partial evaluation may provide some insight into important cost and outcome parameters for a given disease state, but should never serve as the basis for selection of an alternative.

13. Answer: D

Cost-minimization analysis should not be used if there is any doubt regarding the therapeutic equivalence of two or more treatment alternatives being compared. This methodology does not take into account differences in clinical outcomes between agents. The appropriate use of this method could be to compare agents in the same therapeutic class with documented equivalence in safety and efficacy. Although the costs of these agents would be identified, measured, and compared, the analysis should extend beyond drug acquisition costs, and include all relevant costs incurred for administering, monitoring, and preparing the agent.

14. Answer: A

The results of a cost-benefit analysis are typically expressed as either a cost-benefit ratio, or as net cost or net benefit. When comparing two or more treatment alternatives, the alternative with the greatest cost-benefit ratio, or net benefit, is considered the most efficient use of resources. However, caution must be exercised when using cost-benefit ratios. The values can be misleading; therefore, the relative magnitude of the cost-benefit ratio must be considered. The net benefit associated with a program or treatment alternative is often the preferred expression of study results.

15. Answer: A

A cost-benefit analysis is the best economic evaluation method to compare two or more programs when it is best to translate benefits into a dollar value. For example, if quantifying the value of a new pharmacy service, such as a Therapeutic Drug Monitoring Service, the cost of implementing and managing the program (the pharmacist's salary, laboratory tests), and the benefit of the program (decreased drug costs, decreased patient lengths of stay), can both be translated into dollar values.

16. Answer: A

A product or service may be considered cost-effective compared to a competing alternative when any of the following three conditions are met: 1) the alternative is less expensive and at least as effective as the comparator; 2) the alternative is more expensive and provides an additional benefit that is worth the additional cost; or 3) the alternative is less expensive and less effective and the lost benefit was not worth the extra cost of the comparator. Cost-effectiveness analysis attempts to determine the optimal alternative, which is not always the least expensive alternative, for obtaining a desired effect.

17. Answer: A

Cost-effectiveness analysis is the best economic evaluation method to apply when two or more treatment alternatives have different efficacy and safety profiles. An appropriate application of this method could be to compare treatment alternatives from different therapeutic categories that are used to treat the same disease. A complete evaluation would identify, measure, and compare all of the costs and consequences relative to the perspective(s) chosen. Relevant costs assessed in this evaluation should extend beyond drug treatment costs, and include the costs of treatment failures and adverse drug reactions.

18. Answer: C

The incremental cost-effectiveness ratio represents the incremental or additional cost required to obtain an incremental or additional benefit when comparing a treatment alternative to the next most intensive or expensive treatment option. Summary measurements of efficiency (Answer A) typically describe cost-effectiveness ratios. The cost per benefit of a new strategy independent of other alternatives (Answer B) describes the classic average cost-effectiveness ratio, where the average cost to obtain a specific therapeutic objective is spread over a large population. The cost per quality-adjusted life-year gained (Answer D) is a description of a cost-utility ratio.

19. Answer: A

Cost-utility analyses can compare cost, quality, and quantity of patient-years. Thus, when evaluating treatment alternatives that are life-extending with serious side effects, such as cancer chemotherapy, is the best economic evaluation technique. Cost-utility analysis is also an appropriate methodology to use when evaluating alternatives that produce reductions in morbidity instead of mortality, such as arthritis treatments.

20. Answer: C

The primary role of discounting in economic evaluation is to incorporate the effects of differential timing into the decision process. Whenever a cost or benefit is realized more than 1 year into the future, discounting should be performed. There is no standard discount rate to use, although 5 percent is commonly used.

21. Answer: C

There is no one standard discount rate for use in pharmacoeconomic analyses. Many investigators recommend that costs should be discounted to their present value using a rate of 3–8 percent per annum. However, a commonly used rate in recently published evaluations is 5 percent.

22. Answer: A

Sensitivity analysis is a standard approach to manage uncertainty in an economic evaluation. Due to the almost universal need to make assumptions when conducting economic evaluations, it is critical to perform sensitivity analyses. By varying sensitive variables over a range of plausible results, one can test the robustness of the study conclusions.

23. Answer: D

No one single factor can absolutely ensure that drug-use policies will have a positive effect on prescribing patterns. However, having pharmacoeconomic data to support the appropriate and cost-effective use of a pharmaceutical product typically increases its acceptance by health care providers and society. Strategic implementation of strategies using verbal, written, and on-line communication, based on sound pharmacoeconomic data, will also enhance the success of these policies in a health care organization.

24. Answer: D

For formulary management, the best uses of pharmacoeconomic data are for formulary decisions regarding the inclusion or exclusion of treatment options. Although a formulary is often viewed as a cost-containment tool, a formulary should not be a list of the cheapest alternatives. The purpose of today's formulary should be to optimize therapeutic outcomes while controlling the cost of pharmaceutical products. Contemporary formulary management decisions have begun to extend beyond an evaluation of only safety and efficacy, or only cost, and include an assessment of the pharmacoeconomic value of pharmaceutical products and services.

25. Answer: B

Health-related quality of life refers to those aspects of life dominated, or significantly influenced, by personal health and activities performed to maintain health. Health is only one aspect of quality of life. Quality of life encompasses more than a person's lifestyle (Answer A). There are 12 different domains of life proposed in the literature. Marital status, education, and religious beliefs more accurately describe quality of life, rather than health; therefore, Answer D is incorrect.

26. Answer: B

Only physical functioning is a dimension of health. Activities such as the ability to carry a bag of groceries (Answer A), playing sports (Answer C), and bathing and dressing (Answer D), are all items used to inquire about a degree or state of physical functioning. Knowing that a patient has no limitations in bathing or dressing, but has some limitations in playing sports, gives one information to describe a range of physical functions that the person can perform.

27. Answer: C

Distress and well-being describe two extreme points, or boundaries, in the range of mental health states. To be complete, it is recommended that the dimensions included within health status questionnaires go beyond the absence of the negative health state. For example, a patient who experiences relief of his psychological distress would not necessarily have achieved his ultimate health goal unless he achieved an experience of psychological well-being, or was happy, and not just not sad.

28. Answer: A

Traditional means of collecting clinical data, such as laboratory tests, radiographs, and physical examinations, are usually performed by a technician, a machine, or a clinician. Health status assessments, as described in this module, are patient self-administered questionnaires. Collection of information from patients is not a new phenomenon; what is new are the attempts to standardize the collection of this information; therefore, Answer B is incorrect. Clinicians can use the information from health status assessments in clinical decision-making; therefore, Answer C is incorrect. Although there is some controversy surrounding the application of the results of the questionnaires, the results are being used. The methods of assessing health status use the discipline of psychometrics, enabling one to assess objectively the subjective aspects of health. Thus, an argument can be made that health status measures are also "hard data;" therefore, Answer D is incorrect.

29. Answer: A

Measurement of health status across the spectrum of patient age, race, and socio-demographics is unique when using generic measures. If generic status measurements were applied to a disease population, the measurement would be too burdensome to the patient and include concepts that were not applicable to some patients in the population. The dimensions of health addressed in the measurement definitely need to be comprehensive, but cannot contain too many questions that would overburden the patient. Measurement frameworks (Answer C) should extend across the entire range of a dimension for *both* general and disease-specific assessments. In addition, measurements must be sensitive to change over time for *both* types of assessments; therefore, Answer D is incorrect.

30. Answer: B

Quality of care can be evaluated in areas of structure, process, and outcome (see Reference 5). This can be a confusing concept because one can achieve quality in the structure of a care setting, in the process of care, or in the outcome of care; however, Donnabedian proposed that to achieve true quality of care, quality must be achieved in all three areas. Although the categories are intimately related, success in one area does not imply success in another. Until the recent attention to outcomes assessment, the system had focused on achieving quality in structure and process only. Patient satisfaction with care (Answer A) is a component of quality outcomes, as is patient self-assessment of the health care system (Answer D). Although the information gained from knowing about the structure, the process, and the outcomes of a health care delivery system can give a representation of the quality of care, it is really only a starting point for changes in health policy (Answer C).

31. Answer: C

There are no national regulations for the use of patient-based assessments. The Joint Commission on Accreditation of Healthcare Organizations recommends patient satisfaction be assessed for accreditation; however, it is not a mandate; therefore, Answer A is incorrect. To date, there is no regulatory body that requires health-related quality-of-life measures for drug approval (Answer B); however, manufacturers must now provide evidence of scientifically valid conclusions to make labeling claims about quality of life. *Both* patient satisfaction and health status are measured using psychometric techniques; therefore, Answer D is incorrect.

32. Answer: A

Ware has proposed that everyday use of health status assessments could ensure that all important dimensions of functional status and well-being are considered consistently to detect, explain, and track changes over time (Answer B). Their use would make it possible to better consider the patients total functioning when choosing among therapies (Answer C). Health status assessments also could guide the efficient use of community resources and social services (Answer D), as well as more accurately predict the course of chronic disease. Although health status assessments have great potential to improve care, they are not meant to serve as a replacement for current, more detailed assessments of function, such as that used by physical therapists, or of emotional well being, such as is assessed by psychiatrists and social workers.

33. Answer: D

Existing health outcome assessments drawn from classic test theory, along with item response theory, offer exciting opportunities for appreciably expanding applications of patient based health assessments in biomedical and health services research, clinical practice, and decision-making, and policy developments. Answers A, B, and C all discuss true characteristics of the measurement and use of individual level patient self-reported health status information.

POLICY, PRACTICE, AND REGULATORY ISSUES

LISA A. BOOTHBY, PHARM.D., BCPS

COLUMBUS REGIONAL HEALTH CARE SYSTEM
COLUMBUS, GEORGIA

POLICY, PRACTICE, AND REGULATORY ISSUES

LISA A. BOOTHBY, PHARM.D., BCPS
COLUMBUS REGIONAL HEALTH CARE SYSTEM
COLUMBUS, GEORGIA

Learning Objectives:

1. Identify and describe the purpose of the following: Health Insurance Portability and Accountability Act (HIPAA), Institutional Review Board (IRB), and Informed Consent.

2. Outline the history of drug therapy legislation and regulation, and describe the current US Food and Drug Administration's process for review of drug therapies prior to prescription drug approval.

3. Describe the distributive, administrative, and regulatory functions of an investigational drug service within a department of pharmacy.

4. Discuss the purpose and function of Joint Commission on Accreditation of Healthcare Organizations (JCAHO) and the National Committee on Quality Assurance (NCQA), as well as the utility of the ORYX initiative, Standardized Core Measures, Shared Visions-New Pathways, and the Health Plan Employer Data and Information Set.

5. Interpret regulatory and practice policy issues within the context of case studies.

Self-Assessment Questions:

Answers to these questions may be found at the end of this chapter.

1. You are a member of an academic teaching hospital's Institutional Review Board. You are asked to present a new phase 1 trial evaluating the pharmacokinetics and pharmacodynamics of tiotropium in healthy volunteers before and after methacholine challenge. The sponsor wants to advertise on campus to recruit young, healthy students. Participation in this study will pay $3,000 per day. Which one of the following recommendations is the most ethical?
   A. Recommend approval with informed consent since this is a common research method.
   B. Recommend rejection due to the unnecessary risks versus perceived benefits in these volunteers.
   C. Recommend approval if ads do not disclose the amount of monetary compensation provided.
   D. Recommend rejection due to the unfair influence a large stipend creates for students with financial woes.

Questions 2 and 3 refer to the following case.
The Medication Safety pharmacist at your institution who conducts frequent medication use evaluations, as well as documents JCAHO Standard Core Measures for benchmarking and accreditation purposes, has become concerned that his job functions may violate HIPAA.

2. Which one of the following is the best answer regarding personal health information used for institutional quality improvement?
   A. This data collection violates HIPAA; personal health information must remain confidential at all times.
   B. This does not violate HIPAA if Informed Consent and IRB review are requested prior to data collection.
   C. This data collection is exempt as long as all patient identifiers are removed from the limited data set.
   D. This data collection is exempt if the research is conducted for publication and dissemination.

3. Prior to data collection for a medication use evaluation, this pharmacist recognized that once collected, this information may benefit patient care at another institution. Which of the following actions would be necessary?
   A. The pharmacist can share confidential information between hospitals as long as both sign a gag order.
   B. The pharmacist may request expedited IRB review, documenting a minimum confidentiality risk.
   C. This type of research is exempt as long as all patient identifiers are removed from the limited data set.
   D. This type of research must undergo full IRB review because patient safety and ethics are at stake.

Questions 4 through 6 refer to the following case.
A randomized, controlled, parallel clinical trial (n=100) was conducted to evaluate the efficacy of a new drug therapy for patients with hypertension. It was compared to 50 mg of atenolol once daily. The following efficacy and safety data were collected.

	Investigational drug (n=50)	Atenolol (n=50)	p-value
Blood pressure (mean)	125/75	120/70	0.08
Angioedema	2	0	0.40
Orthostatic hypotension	0	1	0.50
Rash	1	1	1.0

4. Which one of the following is the most correct response regarding the primary efficacy end point?
   A. The study did not detect a difference in blood pressure control between the groups.
   B. The study almost detected a difference; there is a decreasing trend in favor of atenolol.
   C. The study drugs are equal for the primary efficacy end point.
   D. Atenolol is more efficacious for blood pressure lowering than the investigational drug.

5. Which one of the following is the most correct response regarding the safety end point?
   A. The study did not detect a difference in adverse effects between the groups.
   B. The study almost detected a difference; angioedema may be more frequent with the study drug.
   C. The study drugs are equivalent when examining their adverse effect profiles.
   D. Angioedema occurred frequently with the investigational drug but not with atenolol.

6. What phase clinical trial is this study most likely?
   A. Phase I.
   B. Phase II.
   C. Phase III.
   D. Phase IV.

7. When would you expect the Food and Drug Administration to request a phase IV clinical trial be conducted?
   A. When more efficacy data is needed to determine which drug should be first line.
   B. When safety data is insufficient to characterize the adverse effect profile of a drug.
   C. When a preclinical signal suggests that there are no major side effects of the drug.
   D. When the drug will be used in a small population for a rare disease state.

8. During a JCAHO accreditation visit, the surveyor analyzed all of the procedures, medical tests, and drug therapies that a particular patient experienced while at the hospital. Which one of the following statements best describes this process?
   A. The shared pathway-new visions process that assesses JCAHO compliance on a continuum of care.
   B. The ORYX initiative integrates outcomes and other performance measures into the accreditation process.
   C. This describes the new HEDIS processes that allow for JCAHO and NCQA accreditation for hospitals.
   D. This is the new tracer methodology that examines health care services and how departments work together.

Questions 9 and 10 refer to the following case.
You are a member of the IRB at your institution. This investigational drug has already been shown to relieve hot flushes and preserve bone density similar to estrogen in other studies, with a positive effect on lipid profiles. The objective of the current trial is to determine if the investigational drug reduces the risk of fractures. About 4100 women over age 55 with no history of breast cancer or venous thromboembolic events and bone density T-score ≤ 1.5 were randomized to receive the investigational drug 1.25 mg or identical placebo. Mean follow-up is now about 2.5 years of a planned total of 5 years follow-up. The committee was presented with the following interim data:

	Investigational drug (n=2093)	placebo (n=2061)	p-value
Spine fracture	50	110	0.0001
Hip fracture	8	15	0.15
Other fractures	64	98	0.005
Breast cancer	25	40	0.053
Venous thromboembolic events	21	9	0.04
Coronary heart disease events	61	96	0.06

9. Which one of the following describes the appropriate action of this committee?
   A. The trial should be stopped because benefits outweigh risks and the primary end point has been reached.
   B. The trial should continue because the difference in coronary events has not yet reached significance.
   C. The trial should continue because the difference in breast cancer incidence has not reached significance.
   D. No conclusions may be made from this preliminary data at this time.

10. Based upon these data, what would be the logical next step for the sponsors of this study?
    A. Submit a New Drug Application to the Food and Drug Administration.
    B. File an Investigational New Drug Application with the Food and Drug Administration.
    C. Submit an Amended New Drug Application to the Food and Drug Administration.
    D. Begin recruitment for another clinical trial to corroborate these data.

Patient Case

You are a clinical pharmacist who practices in the area of medication safety. The Pharmacy and Therapeutics (P&T) Committee requests that you evaluate whether metformin is being used appropriately at your institution. The data collection form was presented and approved by the P&T Committee prior to data collection. After data collection, you tally the following results:

Dosage
64% (21/33) Dose between usual starting dose and maximum dose
21% (7/33) Usual starting dose (500 mg/day)
15% (5/33) 2000 mg/day

Duration
64% (21/33) Metformin prior to admission
36% (12/33) Metformin initiated in hospital

Monitoring
100% Blood glucose monitoring performed
100% Serum creatinine monitoring performed prior to dose administration [Scr values = 0.955 ± 0.237; (mean ± SD) (Max = 1.4)]
21% HgA1c monitoring performed [HgA1c = 8.1± 2.32; (mean ± SD)]

Contraindications
3% (1/33) Renal dysfunction (Scr = 1.4 mg/dL in a female)
3% (1/33) Decompensated heart failure

Outcomes
67% (22/33) Hyperglycemia with no subsequent dose titration
21% (7/33) Patient meets blood glucose goal (70–120 fasting)
9% (3/33) Hyperglycemia with dose subsequently titrated upward
3% (1/33) Hypoglycemia with no subsequent dose adjustment

1. Which one of the following statements best describes use of metformin at your institution?
    A. The use of metformin is optimal at your institution; no process changes are indicated.
    B. Process changes are indicated due to monitoring, contraindications, and outcomes data.
    C. Process changes are indicated due to inadequate dosing and duration of drug therapy.
    D. Conclusions about metformin use cannot be drawn until patients are separated by gender.

2. After presentation to the P&T Committee, these data can be used for which one of the following?
    A. Publication as a retrospective chart review in a pharmaceutical journal.
    B. Presented to a JCAHO surveyor during an accreditation site visit.
    C. Shared with other hospitals as part of a research project on diabetes outcomes.
    D. It must be shredded immediately after the committee meeting.

I. HIPAA, IRB, AND INFORMED CONSENT

A. Definitions
 1. Health Insurance Portability and Accountability Act (HIPAA) HIPAA of 1996 was designed to protect the privacy of medical information for all Americans, as well as to improve the portability and continuity of health insurance coverage.
 2. Institutional Review Board (IRB) IRB is a specially constituted review body established or designated by a health care system or agency to protect the welfare of human subjects recruited to participate in biomedical or behavioral research.
 3. Informed Consent A person's voluntary agreement, based on adequate knowledge and understanding of relevant information to participate in research, or to undergo a diagnostic, therapeutic, or preventive procedure. In giving informed consent, subjects may not waive their legal rights, or release the investigators, sponsor, or institution from liability for negligence.

B. Description of purpose and function
 1. HIPAA
    a. HIPAA is the first federal legislation to address privacy and security of health information.
    b. Each institution or health plan assigns a privacy officer and a contact person.
    c. HIPAA allows health care organizations to use and disclose personal health information for treatment, payment, and health care operations.
       i. Personal health information
          (a) Includes health information in any form: electronic, written, or spoken
          (b) Is created or received by a covered entity (e.g., health care providers, health plans)
          (c) Relates to individuals past, present, or future physical or mental health
       ii. What is not personal health information?
          (a) Does not identify an individual; all patient-specific information removed
          (b) Limited Data Set [45 CFR §164.514 (e)] of the Privacy Rules
             (1) Research
             (2) Public health
             (3) Health care operations
          (c) Copies of data use agreements for research use of Limited Data Sets must be submitted to the IRB with applications for initial review, exemption or change of protocol
       iii. When can personal health information be disclosed?
          (a) General consent (optional)
          (b) Notice and written acknowledgments
             (1) Hospitals provide one written acknowledgment at admission.
             (2) Strongly encouraged in community pharmacies, but not mandatory as of August 2002
                (A) "Notice of Privacy Practices"
                (B) Describes the types of disclosures made without consent or authorization.
                (C) State that other disclosures not listed would require a separate authorization.
                (D) State that the "covered entity" is required to maintain confidentiality.
                (E) Explain the patients' right to restrict what is disclosed.
                (F) An accounting of what has been disclosed is maintained.
                (G) All disclosures must be documented and kept for 6 years

d. HIPAA also gives patients the right to request:
   i. Copies of their health information
      (a) If records are stored off site, provider has 60 days to respond.
   ii. Corrections of personal health information in their records
   iii. Confidential communications
   iv. A list of disclosures for purposes other than treatment, payment, or operations
   v. Limitations on how their information can be used
e. Patients' health care information must be respected and must remain confidential; patient cases should not be shared with anyone not directly involved in the treatment of the patient or the collection of payment for health care services.
   i. Implications for human research
f. Consequences of noncompliance with HIPAA
   i. Fines ranging from $100 to $250,000 per person per year plus 10 years in jail

C. History of drug regulation and clinical research involving human subjects
  1. Food and Drug Law of 1906
     a. First law requiring food purity
  2. Food, Drug, and Cosmetic Act of 1938
     a. First law requiring the establishment of drug safety prior to marketing
  3. Durham-Humphrey Amendment of 1951
     a. Provides statutory basis and criteria for differentiating prescription and nonprescription drugs.
  4. Kefaufer-Harris Amendments of 1962
     a. Establish efficacy, safety, and purity of drugs.
     b. Submit results of two double-blind trials as part of a New Drug Application (NDA).
     c. Obtain informed consent from research subjects.
     d. Advertise and recruit study subjects in an accurate and ethical manner.
  5. Declaration of Helsinki in 1964
     a. Worldwide standard for medical personnel who conduct human research
  6. Belmont Report of 1979
     a. Federally funded review that resulted in increased protection for human research subjects, attention to beneficence, and justice for human research
  7. Investigational New Drug (IND) rewrite of 1987
     a. Redefined IND requirements
  8. Dietary Supplement Health and Education Act (DSHEA) of 1994
     a. Regulation of nutritional supplements and vitamins
     b. Structure/function claims are not allowed.
     c. Must be safe for human consumption under ordinary conditions of use.
  9. FDA Modernization Act of 1997
     a. Streamline clinical research on drugs.
     b. Expedite fast track drugs.
     c. Pharmacy compounding exemption and rules
     d. Pediatric clinical studies
  10. HIPAA of 1996 to present
     a. Privacy and Informed Consent

D. Institutional Review Board (IRB)
  1. Pursuant to the Food and Drug Administration's (FDA) Code of Federal Regulations [21 CFR 56], the IRB or ethics committee protects the rights, safety, and well being of all study subjects.

a. Composition
    i. At least 5 members
    ii. One member with primarily nonscientific interests
    iii. One member that is independent of the institution
    iv. Only members that are independent of the investigator and sponsor may vote
b. Considerations
    i. Qualifications of investigator
    ii. Relevant ethical concerns are addressed.
    iii. Payment of subjects is reasonable/no undue influence.
    iv. Merit and need for study
c. Purpose
    i. To assure, both in advance and by periodic review, that appropriate steps are taken to protect the rights and welfare of humans participating as subjects in research
    ii. To accomplish this purpose, IRBs use a group process to review research protocols and related materials (e.g., informed consent documents and investigator brochures) to ensure protection of the rights and welfare of human subjects of research.
d. IRB reviews clinical trials before start of research, and periodically to monitor continuing research progress.
    i. Either approves study
    ii. Requests modifications prior to approval
    iii. Disapproves study
    iv. Terminates prior approval
e. All of the following documents are reviewed by the IRB

Trial protocols	Informed Consent forms	Protocol and consent updates
Advertisements	Written information for subjects	Investigators brochure
Safety data	Compensation information (payments)	Investigators curriculum vitae
Other supportive documents requested by IRB		

f. What type of research requires IRB approval?
    i. Retrospective chart reviews
    ii. Observational studies
    iii. Experimental studies
g. What is expedited review?
    i. An expedited review procedure consists of a review of research involving human subjects by the IRB chairperson or by one or more experienced reviewers designated by the chairperson from among members of the IRB in accordance with the requirements set forth in [45 CFR 46.110]
    ii. Regulations [21 CFR 56.110] permit an IRB to review certain categories of research through an expedited procedure if the research involves no more than minimal risk.
    iii. The IRB may also use the expedited review procedure to review minor changes in previously approved research during the period covered by the original approval; under an expedited review procedure, review of research may be carried out by the IRB chairperson or by one or more experienced members of the IRB designated by the chairperson.
    iv. The reviewer(s) may exercise all of the authorities of the IRB, except disapproval. Research may only be disapproved following review by the full committee; the IRB is required to adopt a method of keeping all members advised of research studies that have been approved by expedited review.

h. Types of research that can have expedited review
   i. Research on drugs for which an IND (21 CFR Part 312) is not required
   ii. Collection of blood samples by finger stick, heel stick, ear stick, or venipuncture as follows:
      (a) From healthy, nonpregnant adults who weigh at least 110 pounds
      (b) The amount of blood drawn may not exceed 550 ml in an 8-week period, and collection may not occur more frequently than 2 times per week; or
      (c) From other adults and children: the amount drawn may not exceed the lesser of 50 ml or 3 ml per kg in an 8-week period, and collection may not occur more frequently than 2 times per week.
      (d) Prospective collection of biological specimens for research purposes by noninvasive means: hair and nail clippings, deciduous teeth at time of exfoliation or if routine patient care indicates a need for extraction, permanent teeth if routine patient care indicates a need for extraction, external secretions (including sweat), un-cannulated saliva collected either in an un-stimulated fashion or stimulated by chewing gum base or wax or by applying a dilute citric solution to the tongue, placenta removed at delivery, amniotic fluid obtained at the time of rupture of the membrane prior to or during labor, supra- and subgingival dental plaque and calculus, provided the collection procedure is not more invasive than routine prophylactic scaling of the teeth and the process is accomplished in accordance with accepted prophylactic techniques, mucosal and skin cells collected by buccal scraping or swab, skin swab, or mouth washings, sputum collected after saline mist nebulization
   iii. Research involving materials (e.g., data, documents, records, or specimens) that have been collected, or will be collected solely for nonresearch purposes (such as medical treatment or diagnosis)
   iv. Collection of data from voice, video, digital, or image recordings made for research purposes
   v. Research on individual or group characteristics, behavior, research employing survey, interview, oral history, focus group, program evaluation, human factors evaluation, or quality assurance methodologies

E. Informed consent
   1. The agreement of a person (or his or her legally authorized representative) to serve as a research subject, or to receive a certain drug therapy or procedure that documents the person's full knowledge of all anticipated benefits and risks of the treatment
   2. Persons with mental disorders that affect decision-making capacity
      a. The NIH Points to Consider document is generally consistent with the NBAC report, but is intended to provide practical guidance now for investigators and IRBs working in these fields
      b. Legally effective refers to informed consent as specified in [45 CFR Part 46] and to applicable state and local law and regulation.
      c. Human Subject Protection Regulations [45 CFR 46.109(b), 46.111(b) and 46.116]
      d. When some or all of the subjects are likely to be vulnerable to coercion or undue influence, including those with cognitive limitations, the IRB must be sure that additional safeguards have been included in the study to protect the rights and welfare of these subjects [45 CFR 46.111 (b); 21 CFR56.111 (b)].

General Template for Informed Consent with HIPAA-Approved Language

> **INSTITUTION NAME**
> **CONSENT AND AUTHORIZATION TO BE A RESEARCH SUBJECT**
>
> What PHI of yours the Researchers will look at; who will collect your PHI; who will use your PHI; with whom your PHI will be shared and why it is shared each time; the date or event, if any is set, after which we won't use or disclosure your PHI any more; and your rights under HIPAA to ask us not to use your PHI any more; you may choose to join in this research. If you do you will be agreeing to let the Researchers and any other persons, companies or agencies described below use and share your PHI for the study in the ways that are set forth in this section. So please review this section carefully.
>
> What PHI the Research Team will Use: *(Required. Specifically describe all health information that the Researchers will be using and disclosing. If you will use the entire medical file, then you must mention this fact specifically).*
>
> *Example: "The Researchers will look at your entire medical file, which contains all of your personal identifying information and health insurance information; health care providers notes; results of laboratory tests, x-rays and other medical tests; results of physical examinations, and any other information that your health care provider may have recorded about your health or health care."*
>
> Who will Collect the PHI: *(Required. Specifically name and/or describe the person or class of persons who is/ are authorized to collect the PHI and use it or disclose it, e.g., the Researchers; vendors with whom you contract to perform surveys, etc.)*
>
> *Example: "The Researchers will collect and copy the PHI described above. If any of the PHI is to be shared with other persons, as described later on in this section, then the Researchers also will be responsible for making these disclosures."*
>
> Who will Use the PHI; With Whom will it be Shared; and For What Purpose(s) Will it be Used or Shared: *(Required. Specifically name and/or describe the person or class of persons (a) who will use the PHI; or (b) with whom the PHI will be shared and describe the purpose for each use or disclosure. Persons who may use or to whom PHI may be disclosed include the Researchers, study sponsors, clinical research organization, laboratories, IRB, committees and personnel charged with oversight of clinical research, and governmental agencies charged with oversight of clinical research, including the FDA, OHRP, etc. If you have a multi-site study, you should disclose this fact in this section by including the multi-site study insert listed below. If there are only a limited number of specific persons or companies by whom/to whom the OHI will be used/disclosed, then you may specifically name them. If there are larger groups or classes of persons/companies by whom/to whom the PHI will be used/disclosed, then clearly describe the group or class.)*
>
> We have told you of our need to collect your PHI in order to conduct the study. We will share your PHI with the following persons, agencies or companies. List here.
>
> Expiration Date or Event: *(Required. You must include a date or event after which the PHI collected pursuant to the Authorization will no longer be used. For research purposes, you may state that the Authorization remains in effect until the "end of the study and any applicable records retention period," or, if the data is being collected to compile a research database, or for a similar purpose, then you may state that there is no expiration date.*
>
> *Examples: "The Researchers will continue to use your PHI until the date or event listed below, at which point your Authorization to use your PHI will end and all identifiers will be removed from your information making it impossible to link you to the study, or "At the time at which the study is closed and the period for which any records relating to the study must be retained has ended."*
>
> Your Right Under HIPAA to Revoke Your Authorization and Ask Us Not to Use Your PHI Any More: (Required.) It is your free choice to give the Researchers your OK to use and share your PHI. The term for this OK is called your "authorization." At any time you may take back your authorization for the Researchers to use and share your PHI. The term we use for taking back your authorization is "revoke." Revoking your authorization means the Researchers may no longer be able to treat you as they do now because you are in the study. But revoking your authorization will not have a bad affect on your current or future health care. Revoking your authorization also does not involve a penalty. And it does not involve the loss of any benefits that you could get otherwise.

It is a simple process to revoke your authorization for us to use your PHI. You may do this by completing and signing what we call a "revocation letter." We will give you a copy of that letter along with your copy of this Combined Informed Consent/HIPAA Authorization form. You would fill it out and sign it if you choose to revoke your authorization. Then you would give it to the researchers. The Researchers will give you another copy at any time you want one. You must make a written request to revoke your authorization to use your PHI. We will act at once if we get a letter from you revoking your authorization to use your PHI. We will not make any other use of your PHI or share it with anyone else, except as follows:

We will tell the study sponsor (if any) that you have revoked the authorization to use your PHI. We will not ask the study sponsor (if any) to return any study data we gave them. Nor will we ask any other parties to return data we gave them before you revoked your authorization. We will still give data to the study sponsor (if any) or to others to whom we promised it even after we get the letter revoking your authorization. We will do that to preserve the integrity of the research study. We will give PHI data to any governmental or University personnel, departments, or committees that may need it to comply with any laws, regulations, or policies. We will also give PHI data to any of these groups that need it to investigate the failure to comply with laws, regulations, or policies, or adverse events from the study.

Signature and Date: *(Required.)* The Researchers will ask you to sign and date this form. A copy of your signed and dated consent/authorization will be placed in your medical record(s).

Parents Signing for Children and Personal Representatives Signing for Participants who are Unable to Sign due to Incapacity: *(Required if a parent(s) is/are signing the form for a child or if person representative is signing the form for a participant who is unable to sign due to physical or mental incapacity. If a parent is signing for a minor child, attempt to get the signature of both parents if possible.)*

Parent(s): I/we certify that I/we am/are the parents/legal guardians of _____, a child who is under 18 years of age and who has been invited to participate in this study. I/we further certify that I/we have legal custody of the child and that I/we have full legal authority to make decisions concerning the child including decisions regarding health care and health care information.

Personal Representative: I certify that I _____, am over 18 years of age and that I am the personal representative of _____ ("Participant"), a person over 18 years of age, who has been invited to participate in this study but who is unable to sign this form due to physical or mental incapacity. I certify that legally I have been designated as the personal representative of the Participant because …]. I further certify that I have full legal authority to make decisions concerning the participant, including decisions regarding health care and health care information.

PHI May be Re-disclosed: (Required.) If we disclose your PHI to one of the other parties described above, that party might further disclose your PHI to another party. If your PHI is further disclosed, then the information is no longer covered by HIPAA.

Your name and other facts that might point to you will not appear when we present this study or publish its results.

Compensation: *(required when research involves more than minimal risk)*

This section should include the following: If subjects are to be paid, the anticipated amount of payment should be stated in the consent. For study-related injuries a statement should be include that immediate medical care will be provided. Make clear whether the sponsor/investigator will pay for the care. Name and phone number of someone to contact if injury occurs must be included.

Costs: *(Required when there may be costs to the subjects) If the subject is likely to incur any costs, this must be stated. The Institutional Review Board feels that, even if there will not be any costs to subjects; it is good practice to say that in the consent form. This section is often combined with the Compensation section.*

Contact Persons: *(Required in all consent forms)* If you have any questions about this study call [name of contact, can be the PI or study coordinator]. Call [name of contact]if you have been harmed from being in this study. Call the research Coordinator, _____, if you have any questions about your rights as a participant in this research study. Their telephone numbers are _____.

New Findings: *(required when appropriate)* *This section should be included whenever the possibility exists that new risks or dangers could emerge that the subject could avoid by dropping out of the study. The Institutional Review Board requires some variation of the following statement in all consent forms:* We may learn new things during the study that you may need to know. We can also learn about things that might make you want to stop participating in the study. If so, you will be notified about any new information.

Voluntary Participation and Withdrawal: *(Required in all consent forms) This section should state that the subject's participation is voluntary; an explanation of any medical consequences of study withdrawal; clear explanation of any circumstances under which participation may be discontinued by the investigator or the sponsor; additional statements in this section that are required "when appropriate." Such a statement is appropriate in any consent form, but is required in studies if there is a realistic possibility that subjects might raise serious objections to being terminated from participating in the study. An example of this situation would be if the research study involves treatment that subjects might consider beneficial, or if the study pays subjects for participation and payment would be lost if the subject is dropped.*

The following is an example of how such a statement might be worded. It should be modified as appropriate. The study doctors have the right to end your participation in this study for any of the following reasons. It would be dangerous for you to continue. You do not follow study procedures as directed by the study doctors. The sponsor decided to end the study. *Such a statement would be appropriate in studies where discontinuation of study treatment could have a deleterious effect, and where substitute treatment may be necessary. Examples would include treatment for hypertension; diabetes; psychosis; other chronic diseases; studies of contraception; implanted devices, etc. The following is acceptable wording for this statement:* Your participation is completely voluntary and you have the right to refuse to be in this study. You can stop at anytime after giving your consent. This decision will not affect in any way your current or future medical care or any other benefits to which you are otherwise entitled. The study doctor/investigator and/or sponsor may stop you from taking part in this study at any time if they decide it is in your best interest, or if you do not follow study instructions.

The following is acceptable wording for this statement: We will give you a copy of this consent form to keep.

If you're willing to volunteer for this research, please sign below.

I have read this authorization form and have been given the chance to ask questions about it. I am signing this form voluntarily and I understand that by signing I will be authorizing the Researchers to use and disclose my PHI as described in this form.

_____	_____	_____
Subject's name	Date	Time
_____	_____	_____
Subject's legally authorized representative	Date	Time
_____	_____	_____
Witness (if required)	Date	Time
_____	_____	_____
Person Obtaining Consent	Date	Time

Rev. Date __/__/____

Page __ of __

The International Conference on Harmonisation (ICH) guideline recommends that a copy of the signed and dated consent form be given to participants. As stated above, subjects are also entitled to receive an unsigned copy of the consent form whether they agree to participate or not. Leave room for IRB stamp of approval

e. The informed consent form above contains HIPAA authorization elements in addition to the traditional disclosures contained in an Informed Consent form; this obviates the need for two separate forms.
f. These documents are stored confidentially within the confines of the Investigational Drug Service, or by the principal investigator; copies may be included in the patient's medical record for inpatient clinical trials to disseminate information necessary for the patient's medical care during the person's inpatient hospital stay.

Patient Case

3. A sponsor conducts preclinical studies on an antinausea drug therapy in mice and rabbits. At supratherapeutic concentrations, decreased birth weight and some spontaneous abortions occurred. Phase I through Phase III Clinical trials were conducted in males with few adverse effects noted. The investigational antinausea agent is more effective than placebo in phase III clinical trials. The sponsor submits a New Drug Application to the FDA. Which one of the following is the best response from the FDA?
    A. Conduct preclinical toxicology studies in a mammalian model with therapeutic doses.
    B. Conduct another phase III clinical trial that includes pregnant and lactating women.
    C. Conduct a head-to-head clinical trial that compares this drug to the standard of care.
    D. Approve this drug if the sponsor agrees to start a registry for pregnancy outcomes.

II. PRESCRIPTION DRUG APPROVAL PROCESS

A. Preclinical studies
   1. Laboratory and animal studies that assess safety and biological activity in various model systems.
       a. ED50 is the amount of drug required to produce a specific effect in 50% of animals tested.
       b. LD50 is the amount of drug required to cause death in 50% of animals tested.
   2. Toxicological signals
       a. Effects on the fetus in pregnant mice, rats, rabbits, or baboons
       b. May or may not translate into human fetal adverse effects
       c. Fetal effects in humans may occur that were not observed in animal studies.
       d. Basis for pregnancy categories B, C, and some D
   3. Once complete, Investigational New Drug Application is drafted.
       a. Submit to the Food and Drug Administration.
       b. Review and approve prior to human experimentation.

B. Phase I
   1. Test a new drug or treatment.
       a. Small group of people (approximately 20–80 volunteers)
       b. Usually healthy young male adults
   2. Evaluate drug metabolism.
   3. Evaluate structure-activity relationships.
   4. Determine mechanism of action in humans.
   5. Evaluate pharmacokinetic profile to determine a safe dosage range.
       a. Initially based upon mg/kg dosing from animal studies
       b. Monitor for common side effects.
       c. Not powered to detect most adverse effects

C. Phase II
   1. Study drug or treatment in patients with disease or condition
      a. Larger group of people (approximately 80 to hundreds of patients)
      b. Number of patients included depends on many factors:
         i. Drug therapy
         ii. Disease state prevalence
         iii. Type of data (end point)
   2. Early controlled clinical studies
      a. Preliminary data on effectiveness
      b. Identify most common short-term adverse effects.

D. Phase III
   1. Study drug or treatment is given to large groups of people.
      a. Approximately many hundreds to thousands of patients.
   2. Gather additional efficacy data.
      a. Should be powered to detect differences in efficacy.
   3. Monitor side effects, and compare to commonly used treatments.
      a. Collect information on safe usage.
      b. Most are not powered to detect differences in adverse effects of moderate to rare frequency.
      c. Need enough information to weight benefits and risks.
   4. Approximately 1/3 of investigational new drugs make it to this stage.
   5. Once phase III is complete, a New Drug Application is submitted to the FDA.

E. New Drug Application (NDA)
   1. NDA is the vehicle through which drug sponsors formally propose that FDA approve a new pharmaceutical for sale and marketing in the U.S.
   2. FDA approves an NDA only after determining that the data are adequate to show the drug's safety and effectiveness for its proposed use and that its benefits outweigh the risks.

Components of the NDA

Index	Nonclinical Pharmacology and Toxicology
Summary	Human Pharmacokinetics and Bioavailability
Chemistry, Manufacturing, and Control	Microbiology (for anti-microbial drugs only)
Samples, Methods and Labeling	Clinical Data
Safety Update Report*	Case Report Forms
Statistical analysis	Patent Information
Case Report Tabulations	Patent Certification
Other pertinent information	

*The safety update report is usually submitted 120 days after the NDA submission.

F. FDA's Center for Drug Evaluation and Research classifies new drug applications with a code that reflects both the type of drug being submitted and its intended uses. The numbers 1 through 7 are used to describe the type of drug:
   1. New Molecular Entity

2. New Salt of Previously Approved Drug
3. New Formulation of Previously Approved Drug
4. New Combination of Two or More Drugs
5. Already Marketed Drug Product (i.e., new manufacturer)
6. New Indication (claim) for Already Marketed Drug (includes switch in marketing status from prescription to over-the-counter [OTC])
7. Already Marketed Drug Product: no previously approved NDA The following letter codes describe the review priority of the drug: S= Standard review for drugs similar to currently available drugs. P= Priority review for drugs that represent significant advances over existing treatments.
    a. Not all phase III drugs get approved.
    b. FDA can impose a Clinical Hold at any stage.
    c. Some drug therapies that are widely used in other countries never see the light of day in the U.S.
        i. e.g., atosiban, acamprosate, and many others

G. Phase IV
   1. After the drug or treatment has been marketed
      a. Verify effectiveness of the drug or treatment.
      b. Focus on special populations.
         i. May not have been included in clinical trials.
         ii. May mandate pharmacoepidemiology studies.
         iii. May mandate large scale prospective safety studies.
         iv. Some manufacturers are asked to start prospective registries if preclinical toxicology signals exist.
   2. Identify rare, but serious adverse effects.
      a. Determine true side effect profile.
         i. Increased external validity
         ii. Used in special populations
             (a) Thalidomide in Europe
      b. Sequelae and outcomes with long-term use

H. Fast-tracked drugs
   1. Drugs that meet unmet medical needs
   2. Patients with serious, life threatening conditions
      a. HIV drugs, certain chemotherapy agents
      b. Speeds time to market by years

I. Nutritional supplements
   1. Not regulated as drugs (DSHEA 1994)
   2. No disease-modifying, structure/function claims allowed
   3. Must be safe for human consumption
      a. Clinical trials to prove safety are not mandated
      b. Amount of active principle in preparations vary
         i. No standardization
         ii. Different manufacturers
         iii. Timing, place of harvest
         iv. Content in capsules

c. FDA may remove a dietary supplement from the market if it presents a significant or unreasonable risk of illness or injury under ordinary conditions of use.
  i. Ephedra alkaloids (Ma Huang)
    (a) Deemed not safe for human consumption
    (b) Deaths due to cardiovascular events
    (c) FDA promulgates rule that declares ephedra containing supplements "adulterated" due to unreasonable health risks (February 2004).

J. Nonprescription drugs
  1. FDA has published monographs, or rules, for a number of nonprescription drug categories.
  2. These monographs, published in the Federal Register, state requirements for categories of nonprescription drugs, such as what ingredients may be used and for what intended use.
  3. Some nonprescription drug categories covered by nonprescription drug monographs are:
    a. acne medications
    b. treatments for dandruff, seborrheic dermatitis, and psoriasis
    c. sunscreens
  4. Prescription drugs may become nonprescription if their "switch" to nonprescription drug status is approved via the NDA system.
  5. The sponsor must prove that the potential nonprescription drug is safe and effective if used per labeling instructions by persons in the lay public.

Patient Case
4. A neonate with a family history of ornithine transcarbamylase deficiency presents in the neonatal intensive case unit with hyperammonemia, tachypnea, apnea, and failure to thrive. You do a literature search to determine the appropriate therapy for this infant and find that the only effective drug therapy for this patient is an investigational drug with orphan drug status called sodium phenylacetate. Which one of the following is the best first step in the treatment of this neonate?

A. Transfer the neonate to another hospital that has experience treating this disorder.
B. Call the Investigational Drug Service to inquire about IV sodium phenylacetate compassionate use.
C. Send the neonate to hemodialysis immediately to prevent permanent cognitive dysfunction.
D. Manage the hyperammonemia with a low-protein infant formula and adequate hydration.

III. INVESTIGATIONAL DRUG SERVICE

A. Definitions
  1. Drug
    a. The Food, Drug, and Cosmetic Act defines drugs by their intended use, as "(A) articles intended for use in the diagnosis, cure, mitigation, treatment, or prevention of disease, and (B) articles (other than food) intended to affect the structure or any function of the body of man or other animals" [FD&C Act, sec. 201(g)(1)].
  2. Investigational drug
    a. A drug is not generally recognized as "safe and effective" unless it is used per its official labeling as approved by the FDA; FDA regulations specify when an Investigational New Drug Application is required.

3. New drugs
    a. A "new drug" may have been in use for many years; if a product is intended for use as a drug, no matter how ancient or "traditional" its use may be, once the FDA has made a final determination on the status of a nonprescription drug product, it must have an approved New Drug Application or comply with the appropriate nonprescription monograph to be marketed legally in interstate commerce.
    b. Certain OTC drugs may remain on the market without New Drug Application approval pending final regulations covering the appropriate class of drugs.
    c. An investigational drug shall be considered as any new drug that is not approved by the Food and Drug Administration (FDA) for use in humans; this definition specifically includes any newly invented or discovered substance undergoing phase I, II, or III investigation.

B. Purpose
    1. Investigational Drug Service
        a. To ensure that the use of investigational drugs is conducted ethically, and
        b. In full conformity with all applicable laws and regulations
    2. Investigational Drug Service serves as the coordinator and control center for investigational drugs.
        a. Assume responsibility for maintaining records of the drugs delivered to the Service.
        b. Maintain drug inventory.
    3. Dispensing of drugs to research subjects
        a. Return to the sponsor or alternative disposition of unused product.
        b. Responsibilities include maintaining records of an investigational drug delivery to the site.
        c. Inventory at the site
        d. Use of the drug by each research subject
        e. Return of unused product to the sponsor
        f. Maintaining appropriate storage conditions
        g. Investigators will maintain records that document dosing mandated in the protocol.
        h. The Investigational Drug Service will store and dispense the investigational drug as specified by the sponsor and in accordance with applicable regulatory requirements.
    4. Both inpatient and outpatient services are provided.
    5. IRB participation
        a. Representative(s) from the Investigational Drug Service
        b. Voting member of the IRB
            i. Responsibilities include
                (a) Reviewing incoming and existing research protocols within the institution
                (b) Reviewing potential and continuing research in the community
                (c) Goal is to insure ethical, humane treatment.
    6. New Uses for already approved drugs
        a. Commercially available drugs used in new ways or on new patient populations in connection with a research study are also considered investigational drugs.
        b. Studies with commercially available substances are usually considered to be undergoing phase IV clinical trials.
        c. Other studies with commercially available substances may be undergoing various phase trials based on a new patient population.

Patient Case

5. You start a new job with the University of the Tropical Islands College of Pharmacy. New employees are offered the choice of a PPO or an HMO health plan. Here are the data you are provided to aid in your decision-making.

HEDIS PERFORMANCE MEASURES	HMO	PPO
Optimal practitioner contact	20%	19%
Acute treatment phase	58%	61%
Continuation treatment phase	44%	46%
Comprehensive Diabetes Care		
HbA1c testing	82%	85%
Eye exam	55%	64%
Low density lipoprotein C	82%	80%
Prenatal and Postpartum Care		
Timeliness	86%	92%
Postpartum care	77%	81%
Beta Blocker Treatment	93%	95%
Breast Cancer Screening	76%	83%
Cervical Cancer Screening	80%	87%
Cholesterol Management After Cardiac Events	76%	84%
Childhood Immunization Status		
Diphtheria, tetanus, pertussis	82%	81%
Oral polio virus	86%	85%
Measles, Mumps, and Rubella	90%	87%
H Influenza type B	84%	79%
Hepatitis B	80%	78%
Chicken pox vaccine (varicella zoster)	76%	64%

How do the HEDIS measures help you to decide on a health plan?
A. If key health interventions are similar, decisions can be based on cost and convenience.
B. Statistical comparisons between the health care plans help ensure the right choice.
C. These data are the same data JCAHO surveyors are looking for during site visits.
D. These data are not helpful in the decision process because no outcomes data are provided.

IV. JCAHO, ORYX, NCQA, AND HEDIS

A. Definitions
1. Joint Commission on Accreditation of Healthcare Organizations (JCAHO)
   a. JCAHO is an independent, not-for-profit organization that sets the standards for accreditation in health care.
2. Tracer methodology
   a. This method of evaluation conducted during an on-site survey traces the health care experiences that a patient had while at the hospital.
3. ORYX
   a. A JCAHO strategic initiative that integrates outcomes and other performance measurement data into the accreditation process; a component of the ORYX initiative is the Standardized Core Measures.

4. Shared Visions-New Pathways
   a. A new JCAHO initiative that began in January 2004 represents a paradigm shift away from intermittent survey preparation and toward continuous operational improvement.
5. National Committee on Quality Assurance (NCQA)
   a. NCQA is an independent organization, 501(c)(3) non-profit organization whose mission is to improve health care quality everywhere.
6. Health Plan Employer Data and Information Set (HEDIS)
   a. HEDIS are performance measures drafted and sponsored by the NCQA to benchmark health care plans in the U.S.

B. Purpose and function
   1. JCAHO
      a. Evaluates and accredits more than 16,000 health care organizations and programs in the United States.
         i. JCAHO is the nation's predominant standards-setting and accrediting body.
         ii. JCAHO develops clinical and administrative health care standards.
         iii. Institutional compliance is compared with these benchmarks.
      b. Accreditation surveys generally occur once every 3 years.
         i. Unannounced surveys are scheduled to start in 2006.
   2. Tracer methodology (new)
      a. A JCAHO method of evaluation conducted during an on-site survey
      b. Designed specifically to "TRACE" the health care experiences that a patient had while at the hospital
         i. A 3-day survey will have about 11 tracer activities.
         ii. Focus on priority focus areas
         iii. Focus on past deficiencies (type 1 recommendations)
         iv. Purpose is to assess compliance with JCAHO standards.
      c. Surveyor follows specific patients through the hospital process.
         i. Looks at care, treatment, and services for patients.
         ii. Looks at how departments work together.
   3. ORYX
      a. This initiative integrates outcomes and other performance measures into the accreditation process.
      b. A component of the ORYX initiative is the Standardized Core Measures.
         i. Core Measures
            (a) Data on standardized performance measures
            (b) Collected by JCAHO accredited institutions
            (c) Evidence-based outcomes designed to permit more rigorous comparisons
            (d) The first four initial core measures for hospitals include:
               (1) Acute myocardial infarction
               (2) Heart failure
               (3) Community-acquired pneumonia
               (4) Pregnancy and related conditions
            (e) Acute myocardial infarction core measures document the proportion of AMI patients that:
               (1) Expire during hospital stay.
               (2) Receive aspirin at arrival.
               (3) Have aspirin prescribed at discharge.

(4) Receive adult smoking cessation counseling.
(5) Are on β-blocker therapy at admission.
(6) Have β-blocker therapy prescribed at discharge.
(7) Receive thrombolytic agent within 30 minutes of hospital arrival.
(8) Percutaneous coronary intervention within 120 minutes of hospital arrival
(f) Congestive heart failure core measures document the proportion of patients that receive:
(1) Discharge instructions for appropriate activity level, diet, discharge medications, follow-up appointment, weight monitoring, and what to do if symptoms worsen
(2) Left ventricular function (LVF) assessment before arrival, during hospitalization, or planned for after discharge
(3) An ACE Inhibitor prescription for left ventricular systolic dysfunction
(4) Adult smoking cessation advice/counseling
(g) Community-acquired pneumonia core measures document the proportion of patients that:
(1) Receive an oxygen assessment within 24 hours of arrival.
(2) Pneumococcal screening and or vaccination
(3) Blood cultures prior to antibiotics or within 24 hours
(4) Antibiotic treatment consistent with IDSA guidelines within 4 hours of arrival
(5) Smoking cessation advice and counseling for adults and pediatrics
(6) Influenza screening and vaccination
(h) Pregnancy core measures document the proportion of patients that:
(1) Have prenatal care and treatment selection, especially in those with a history of cesarian section.
(2) Have live born neonates that expire within 28 days after birth.
(3) Have vaginal deliveries with third-degree or fourth-degree perineal laceration.
ii. JCAHO is currently developing new measure sets
(a) Surgical infection prevention
(b) ICU care
(c) Pain management
(d) Children's asthma care
iii. More core measures will be identified in the future.
(a) Beginning this year, core measure data will be used by JCAHO.
(b) Assist in focusing on-site survey evaluation activities
(c) Institutional compliance with core measures will be reported on the JCAHO Web site.
2. Shared Visions-New Pathways (2004)
a. Focus on continuous operational improvement.
i. 15 months after last survey, JCAHO sends Periodic Performance Review (PPR) access.
ii. Instructions on how to proceed accompany this PPR information
iii. Hospital has 3 months to complete the PPR.
b. Hospital must devise plan of action with measures for success for any areas that are deemed "noncompliant," using elements of performance standards.
i. Three months later, this plan is submitted electronically via a secure extranet link.

ii. One month later, the plan is reviewed, and feedback is given via teleconference.
iii. Six months before next site visit, hospital completes electronic application for accreditation.
iv. Three months prior, the survey dates are scheduled.
v. Two weeks prior to the survey, the hospital receives the Priority Focus Process component as do the surveyors.
c. Survey occurs, using tracer methodology.
i. 48 hours later, survey report is available on the extranet site
ii. Hospital has 90 days to submit Evidence of Standards Compliance if requirements for improvements were found to maintain Full Accreditation Status vs. Provisional Accreditation.
iii. Quality Report is then made available to the public on JCAHO's Quality Check Internet site.
3. NCQA
a. NCQA evaluates health care in three different ways:
i. Rigorous on-site review of key clinical and administrative processes
ii. Health Plan Employer Data and Information Set
iii. Comprehensive member satisfaction survey
b. Accreditation and certification programs are voluntary.
i. More than half of the U.S. HMOs currently participate.
c. Almost 90 percent of all health plans measure their performance using HEDIS.
i. JCAHO and NCQA have partnered.
ii. Goal is to standardize research accreditation.
(a) Review and accredit research programs.
(1) Public and not-for-profit hospitals
(2) Academic medical centers
(3) Other research facilities
4. HEDIS
a. Health Plan Employer Data and Information Set
i. Used in more than 90 percent of the nation's managed care organizations
ii. A set of standardized measures
iii. Measures performance in key areas
(a) Immunization rates
(b) Mammography screening
(c) Cholesterol management
(d) Customer satisfaction
(e) Others
b. Patients, employers, and others use HEDIS data to compare health care plan performance.

REFERENCES

HIPAA, IRB, and Informed Consent

1. UTHSCSA Investigator's Handbook - Table of Contents. Available at *http://www.uthscsa.edu/irb/forms.asp*. Accessed February 28, 2006.
2. Giacalone RP, Cacciatore GG. HIPAA and its impact on pharmacy practice. Am J Health-Syst Pharm 2003;60:433-45.
3. OCR HIPAA Privacy. December 3, 2002. Revised April 3, 2003. Research. [45 CFR 164.501, 164.508, 164.512 (i)]. Cited 19 March 2004. Available at *http://www.hhs.gov/ocr/hipaa/guidelines/research.pdf*. Accessed February 28, 2006.
4. Title 21–Food and Drugs. Chapter I–Food and Drug Administration, Department of Health and Human Services. Part 50–Protection of Human Subjects, Code of Federal Regulations, Title 21, Volume 1, revised as of April 1, 2003. From the U.S. Government Printing Office via GPO Access [CITE: 21CFR50] [Page 284-295] Available at *http://www.access.gpo.gov/ nara/cfr/waisidx_00/21cfr50_00.html*. Accessed March 1, 2006.

Food and Drug Administration's Prescription Drug Approval Process

1. Guidance for Industry: Good Clinical Practice Consolidated Guideline. Available at *http://www.fda.gov/cder/guidance/959fnl.pdf*. Accessed February 28, 2006.
2. Clinical Studies (Overview). Available at *http://www.fda.gov/cder/handbook/clinstud.htm*. Accessed February 28, 2006.

Functions of an Investigational Drug Service

1. Rockwell K, Bockheim-McGee C, Jones E, Kwon IG. Clinical research: national survey of US pharmacybased investigational drug services-1997. Am J Health- Syst Pharm 1999;56:337-46.
2. U.S. Food and Drug Administration, Center for Drug Evaluation and Research Clinical Investigators Federal Regulations for Clinical Investigators. Available at *http://www.fda.gov/cder/about/smallbiz/CFR.htm*. Accessed February 28, 2006.

JCAHO, NCQA, ORYX, HEDIS

1. Joint Commission. Comprehensive Accreditation Manual for Hospitals: The Official Handbook. Joint Commission on Accreditation of Healthcare Organization:2004.
2. Goodwin A. Quality Improvement Initiatives in Managed Care, in Managed Care Pharmacy Practice. Navarro, RP, eds. Gaithersburg, MD: Aspen; 1999.

ANSWERS AND EXPLANATIONS TO PATIENT CASES

1. Answer: B
A careful analysis of the MUE data demonstrated that only 21% of the patients document HgA1c monitoring. This is not acceptable since Healthy People 2010 objectives include at least yearly HgA1c measurements for 80% of patients with diabetes. In addition, one patient had renal dysfunction and another had congestive heart failure, both of which are contraindicated with metformin drug therapy. Equally problematic are the 22 patients that had hyperglycemia without dose titration or additional drug therapies added to reach normoglycemic goals. Clearly process changes are indicated. Because these patients are in the hospital versus an ambulatory care setting, duration of therapy is less meaningful.

2. Answer: B
The HIPAA privacy act mandates IRB review of personal health information prior to publication and dissemination. Because these data were collected for institutional quality assurance, it cannot be published or shared with other institutions. It can be kept with other Pharmacy and Therapeutics Committee materials (e.g., packet, minutes) for JCAHO accreditation purposes. All patient health information with patient identifiers must be shredded.

3. Answer: A
It is unethical to conduct clinical trials in pregnant women, especially if fetal adverse effects are suspected. The preclinical data provided some toxicological signals that there may be human fetal adverse effects with this drug; however, the preclinical trials were not conducted in a mammalian system. Thalidomide, for example, was not teratogenic in rats and rabbits, but was in baboons. This will help assess the true fetal risk. Then, if deemed so by the FDA, if the drug is approved and there is a signal that the drug may have fetal adverse effects in humans, a prospective registry should be created.

4. Answer: B
The Investigational Drug Service may already be registered with the sponsors of the IV sodium phenylacetate investigation drug study and compassionate use program. This is the most desirable option for the family and for the neonate. However, if the drug cannot be obtained at your facility, the neonate must be transferred to a level III NICU that does have access to the investigational drug study. Rarely are neonates hemodialyzed for hyperammonemia as adults are often treated. Although a low-protein diet is a good plan after the immediate crisis, it will do little in the acute phase to control the hyperammonemia.

5. Answer: A
HEDIS performance measures for both plans look similar. Ultimately, the patient will pick the program that is most convenient at a reasonable cost. None of the performance measures directly measure outcomes, only preventative measures. Outcome data would be more definitive if it were provided. JCAHO surveyors are looking for some of these measures, but few of the Standardized Core measures are included in this data set.

ANSWERS AND EXPLANATIONS TO SELF-ASSESSMENT QUESTIONS

1. Answer: C
Large stipends were one of several examples provided in the IRB Code of Ethics that could present undue influence or coercion on the volunteer if economically challenged. Although the methacholine challenge study design is widely used and has been published, it is not without risk. Advertising that there is a stipend for participation, but not disclosing the amount, seems more ethical.

2. Answer: C
Personal health information that is used solely for quality assurance purposes within an institution is exempt from the need for Informed Consent, according to HIPAA. All patient identifiers must be removed to ensure that patients cannot be identified. These data may not be published or shared with other institutions without informed consent or a wavier of the need for informed consent from Expedited IRB review and approval.

3. Answer: B
If the pharmacist recognizes prior to data collection that there may be a need to use this information for research purposes or dissemination outside the hospital, an IRB review is necessary. Either full or expedited IRB review is necessary to determine whether Informed Consent is necessary to protect the patients' rights.

4. Answer: A
The p-value, or test statistic for the efficacy comparison was 0.08, which is greater than 0.05; therefore, unless the study was powered to detect a difference in blood pressure control and stated so a priori, then the appropriate interpretation is that the study did not detect a difference in blood pressure control between the two antihypertensives. We can't conclude that one is more effective than the other. This is a potential type 2 error.

5. Answer: A
All p-values for the safety end points were greater than 0.05; thus, the study did not detect a difference in these adverse effects between the groups. If it were powered to detect a difference, then we could say that there is no difference in adverse effect profiles. It is inappropriate to discuss trends. This is a potential type 2 error.

6. Answer: B
Phase II clinical trial because it has a relatively small sample (n=100). It was conducted in patients with hypertension, and the primary end point was efficacy of blood pressure lowering. As demonstrated in questions 4 and 5, phase II clinical trials are rarely powered to detect differences in adverse effects, but sometimes are powered to detect differences in continuous end points such as blood pressure.

7. Answer: B
Phase IV clinical trials are usually conducted at the request of the FDA when there are questions about the safety or adverse effects associated with a drug therapy, or when long-term outcomes data are needed for evidence-based decision-making. They may also be conducted if preclinical data suggest that a certain adverse effect may occur that was not corroborated in clinical trials, because the clinical trials may not have had a large enough sample size to detect these adverse effects.

8. Answer: D
The new tracer methodology allows JCAHO surveyors to trace the path of several patients throughout the health care system. Surveyors are looking for Core measure compliance as well as how departments work together for the total care of the patient. This differs from the new Shared pathway-new visions process that requires continual compliance with JCAHO standards, or the ORYX initiative of which the Standard Core measures is a part. JCAHO and NCQA have combined efforts for accreditation for clinical research only up to the time of this writing.

9. Answer: A
This large, well-designed, phase III study met its primary end point and found a statistically significant difference in spine and other fractures with the investigational drug versus placebo. It also detected a difference in venous thromboembolic adverse effects. To continue this study would deny the women with a high risk of fractures receiving the placebo the chance to take effective therapy if they so chose. Yes, it is true that if the study was continued, we may see a statistically significant difference in coronary heart disease events between the groups, but this was not the primary end point. Patients could be followed up after unblinding to monitor coronary heart disease events prospectively. This would have the level of evidence of an observational study, but at least the patients on placebo would have the choice to take the active drug therapy or not. 2-332

10. Answer: A

The sponsor should compile all required data and submit a New Drug Application to the FDA. An Investigational New Drug Application is submitted after preclinical studies and before clinical trials to obtain permission to begin human testing, and an Amended New Drug Application is submitted for generic drugs that wish to demonstrate bioequivalence to a branded proprietary drug. A third phase III trial is not necessary prior to submitting the New Drug Application.

2010 CANDIDATE'S GUIDE

APPLY ONLINE AT WWW.BPSWEB.ORG

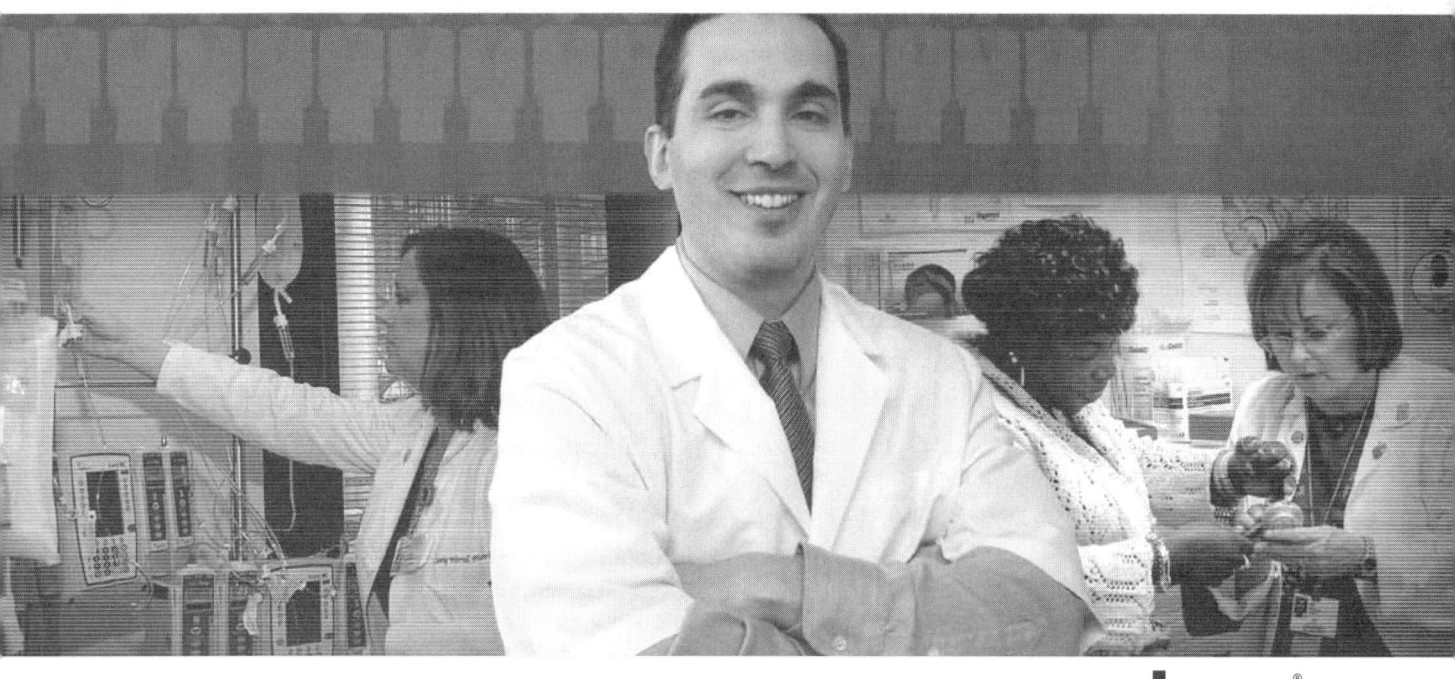

Board of Pharmacy Specialties bps

2010 Candidate's Guide

Specialty Certification in:
Nuclear Pharmacy
Nutrition Support Pharmacy
Oncology Pharmacy
Pharmacotherapy
Psychiatric Pharmacy

Test Date: October 2, 2010
Application Deadline: August 1, 2010

bps® Board of Pharmacy Specialties

Thank you for your interest in becoming certified in your chosen field of specialty practice. As the delivery of health care becomes more sophisticated and more complex, there is a concomitant need for pharmacy to identify practitioners who are qualified to meet these challenges. The recognition of areas of specialized practice and the certification of pharmacist specialists go a long way towards assuring society that its pharmaceutical care needs are being properly addressed.

For nearly 35 years, the Board of Pharmacy Specialties has provided specialty-level certification programs for pharmacists – both nationally and internationally. The founding of BPS by APhA in 1976 resulted from a five-year effort during which the entire profession studied and deliberated the issue of specialization in pharmacy. Nuclear pharmacy, nutrition support pharmacy, oncology pharmacy, pharmacotherapy and psychiatric pharmacy exist today as bona fide specialties due to ongoing collaborative efforts by all segments of the profession. A sixth BPS specialty, Ambulatory Care Pharmacy is currently under development and is scheduled to be available in 2011. BPS will continue to develop new specialties to meet the needs of the public and the profession..

The Board, with assistance from several professional organizations and their members, has continued to provide vital leadership and support for the recognition of specialties and the certification of pharmacist specialists. As a result, BPS and its Specialty Councils are now the principal entities through which these activities are carried out for the pharmacy profession. Each of the Specialty Councils works diligently with test development consultants to ensure that the entire certification process is psychometrically sound and legally defensible. BPS is also working with its strategic partner organizations to promote the value of specialty recognition and certification to the profession, other health care professionals, employers, and the public.

Quality pharmacist care requires a cadre of well-trained, experienced, and motivated pharmacists. Your interest in specialty certification illustrates your commitment to advancing our profession. BPS salutes your interest and commitment to quality patient care. The American public requires nothing less of our profession.

Richard J. Bertin

Richard J Bertin, PhD, RPh
Executive Director

Board of Pharmacy Specialties • 2215 Constitution Ave., NW • Washington, DC 20037-2985
(202) 429-7591 • FAX: (202) 429-6304 • www.bpsweb.org • www.bpsweb.org

The Board of Pharmacy Specialties (BPS) is an autonomous division of the American Pharmacists Association (APhA), founded in January 1976 to recognize specialties and certify pharmacists in specialized areas of pharmacy practice.

GENERAL INFORMATION

Board of Pharmacy Specialties

The Board of Pharmacy Specialties (BPS) is an independent non-governmental certification body that provides recognition of persons involved in the advanced practice of pharmacy specialties. BPS was created on January 5, 1976 by the American Pharmaceutical Association (now the American Pharmacists Association, APhA), and exists today as an autonomous division of APhA.

The Board is composed of eight pharmacists, five of whom represent BPS specialty practices, two health care professionals other than pharmacists and one public member. The Executive Director and one member of the APhA Board of Trustees are non-voting Board members, *ex officio*.

BPS establishes a Specialty Council for each recognized specialty. Specialty Councils work with the Board to develop and administer psychometrically sound and legally defensible certification processes, consistent with public policy regarding the credentialing of health care professionals. A Specialty Council is composed of six pharmacists practicing in the specialty area and three other pharmacists.

The Five Point Purpose of the Board of Pharmacy Specialties Certification Program:

1. To grant recognition of appropriate pharmacy practice specialties based on criteria established by the Board of Pharmacy Specialties
2. To establish standards for certification and recertification of pharmacists in recognized pharmacy practice specialties
3. To grant qualified pharmacists certification and recertification in recognized pharmacy practice specialties
4. To serve as a coordinating agency and informational clearing house for organizations and pharmacists in recognized pharmacy specialties
5. To enhance public/consumer protection by developing effective certification programs for specialty practices in pharmacy

Importance of Certification

The primary purpose of specialization in any health care profession is to improve the quality of care individual patients receive, to promote positive treatment outcomes, and ultimately, to improve the patient's quality of life. Specialties evolve in response to the development of new knowledge or technology that can affect patient care. The rapid, dramatic advancement in drug therapy in recent decades has created a clear need for pharmacy practitioners who specialize in specific kinds of treatment and aspects of care. Specialty certification is a responsible, progressive initiative from the profession to try to ensure the best possible patient care.

Board certification has allowed more pharmacists to participate in collaborative drug therapy management which is a significant value to patients. Pharmacists certified in a specialty are frequently sought for professional consultations. As the contributions of pharmacists become more recognized we anticipate greater recognition from Medicare and Medicaid along with private payers. Employers and patients can feel secure in knowing that the Board certified pharmacist has taken the initiative to seek advanced specialized training that sets them apart.

Certification can also provide a personal reward for pharmacist specialists. Preparing for the certification exam offers an opportunity to increase advanced, specialized knowledge in the practice area. Specialty certification is a means of informing other professionals of the individual's educational and practice accomplishments, setting the specialist apart from colleagues. It is one way to demonstrate advanced knowledge and skills independent of, and in addition to, a degree program or license. Many certificants have reported enhanced respect from colleagues in other health care professions. Others tell of a "competitive edge" in applying for jobs. Many pharmacist specialists certified by BPS have also reported increased salaries or one-time bonuses. Still others have received payment from third party payers because their skills and knowledge are validated through certification.

Health care organizations have documented many cases in which the services of certified pharmacist specialists may have contributed in large measure to tangible results, including:

- Optimal use of drugs;
- Substantial reduction in adverse drug reactions;
- Fewer complications related to drug treatment;
- Shorter hospital stays (resulting in lower hospital costs);
- Reduced morbidity and mortality;
- Reduced unnecessary medication use (resulting in lower drug costs);
- Improved laboratory monitoring of drug therapy; and
- Improved patient satisfaction.

Recognition of BPS Certification

BPS-certified pharmacist specialists are recognized for their advanced level of knowledge, skills, and achievement by many government agencies and educational organizations. Following are examples of specific benefits that may be realized by BPS-certified pharmacist specialists:

- U.S. Nuclear Regulatory Commission: specialists may be recognized as Authorized Nuclear Pharmacists
- U.S. Department of Defense: specialists may receive bonus pay
- U.S. Department of Veterans Affairs: specialists may serve at a higher pay step
- U.S. Public Health Service: specialists may receive bonus pay
- New Mexico and North Carolina State Boards of Pharmacy: specialists may apply for specified prescribing privileges
- Many schools/colleges of pharmacy award advanced placement in non-traditional PharmD programs on an individual basis and may recognize BPS certification in this process
- Increasing numbers of employers are recognizing BPS-certified specialists with monetary reward or promotion/hiring preference.

bps® 2010

BOARD OF PHARMACY SPECIALTIES
Sharon M. Durfee
Sandra Edwardson
Rebecca S. Finley (Chair)
Susan Goodin
Dick R. Gourley
George H. Hinkle (Chair Elect)
Melinda Joyce
Beth Mertz
Maria Llana Posey
Marsha A. Raebel
Terry L Schwinghammer (Past Chair)
Suzanne R. White

SPECIALITY COUNCIL ON NUCLEAR PHARMACY
Carmen Aceves Blumenthal
Carolyn C. Brackett
Allegra DePietro Bruce
Wendy Galbraith (Chair)
Fred P. Gattas, III (Vice Chair)
Scott P. Knisha
Walter Miller
John J. Sterzinger
Norman Tomaka

SPECIALTY COUNCIL ON NUTRITION SUPPORT PHARMACY
Phil Ayers
Jacqueline R. Barber (Chair)
Joseph Boulatta
Todd W. Canada (Vice Chair)
Catherine Crill
Jane M. Gervasio
Jay E. Mouser
Michael D. Reed
Lawrence A. Robinson

SPECIALTY COUNCIL ON ONCOLOGY PHARMACY
Lisa Davis
David W. Henry (Chair)
Thomas E. Hughes
Becky A. Nagle
Margaret E. McGuiness
Joseph J. Saseen
Rowena Schwartz
J. Andrew Skirvin (Vice Chair)
Timothy Mark Woods

SPECIALTY COUNCIL ON PHARMACOTHERAPY
Laura M. Borgelt (Chair)
Mary E. Burkhardt
Elizabeth Ann Chester
Brian Erstad
Karen M. Gunning
Curtis E. Haas
Eric J. MacLaughlin (Vice Chair)
Todd Sorenson
Scott K. Stolte

SPECIALTY COUNCIL ON PSYCHIATRIC PHARMACY
Nancy C Brahm
Steven Brughart
Louise Cohen
Carla B. Frye
Jessica L. Gören (Vice Chair)
Julie M. Koehler
Jerry McKee (Chair)
Ruth E. Nemire
Jose A. Rey

TABLE OF CONTENTS

GENERAL INFORMATION
Importance of Certification 3
Recognition of BPS Certification 3
Important Dates 5

OVERVIEW
Non Discrimination Policy 5

APPLICATION INFORMATION
General Information 5
Name and/or Address Changes 5
Test Dates 5
Alternate Test Date 6
Test Sites 6
DANTES Program 6
Alternate Test Sites 6
Transferring Test Sites 6
Exception to Eligibility Requirements 6
Processing Applications 7
Withdrawals 7
Retaking the Examination 7
Americans with Disabilities Act 7

FEES AND PAYMENT METHODS
Fee Payments 7
Application Fee 7
Declined Credit Cards, Returned Checks and Handling Fees.. 7
Withdrawals 7

INFORMATION FOR FOREIGN TRAINED/ FOREIGN LICENSED CANDIDATES 8

PREPARING FOR THE EXAMINATION
Information Sources 8

ON THE DAY OF YOUR EXAMINATION
Inclement Weather and Cancellations 9
Examination Format and Content 9
Administration of the Examination 9
Security 10
Confidentiality Statement 10
Use of Calculators 10

FOLLOWING THE EXAMINATION
Score Reporting 10
Confidential Score Reports 11
If You Pass the Examination 11
If You Do Not Pass the Examination 11

REVOCATION OF CERTIFICATION
Appeal Process 11

RECERTIFICATION 11

ANNUAL REGISTRATION 11

BPS SPECIALTIES
Nuclear Pharmacy 11
Nutrition Support Pharmacy 12
Oncology Pharmacy 13
Pharmacotherapy 13
Psychiatric Pharmacy 14

SAMPLE EXAMINATION QUESTIONS 14

OVERVIEW

This Candidate's Guide is intended for use by pharmacists who are interested in being certified as specialists by the Board of Pharmacy Specialties (BPS) in any of the BPS-recognized specialty practice areas. This Guide provides information on BPS certification processes: eligibility requirements, application procedures, examination administration, annual registration, and recertification.

This document is ONLY A GUIDE. The information, procedures, and fees detailed in this publication may be amended, revised, or otherwise altered at any time and without advance notice by the Board of Pharmacy Specialties. The provision of this Guide does not confer any rights upon an applicant. The information contained in this Guide supersedes information contained in all previous editions of the BPS Candidate's Guide.

All correspondence and requests for information concerning the administration of BPS specialty certification examinations should be directed to:

Board of Pharmacy Specialties
2215 Constitution Avenue, NW
Washington, DC 20037
TEL 202-429-7591 • FAX 202-429-6304
bps@aphanet.org • www.bpsweb.org

It is the candidate's responsibility to submit a fully completed application by the postmark deadline of August 1. Incomplete applications or those submitted after the indicated deadline may be returned to candidates without being processed.

Non Discrimination Policy
BPS endorses the principles of equal opportunity and nondiscrimination. BPS does not discriminate with regard to age, gender, ethnic origin, race, religion, disability, marital status, veteran status, sexual orientation, or any other category protected by federal or state law.

APPLICATION INFORMATION

General Information
All questions pertaining to BPS certification should be directed to the Board as noted above. BPS office hours are Monday through Friday, 8:30am-5:00pm (Eastern Time). The Board offices are closed on all federal holidays.

All applicants are encouraged to submit their applications online from the BPS web site (www.bpsweb.org). A valid credit card account number is required for all online applications. The online application process uses a secure server.

Applications on paper must be accompanied by a check, cashier's check, money order, or credit card account number. Purchase orders will NOT be accepted.

Applications may be submitted by facsimile (FAX) with payment charged to a valid credit card account (American Express, MasterCard, VISA). A faxed copy of a check is NOT acceptable.

IMPORTANT DATES

Deadline for requesting an alternate site * or alternate date **
July 1, 2010   July 1, 2011

Postmark deadline for applications
August 1, 2010   August 1, 2011

Last day to withdraw or change test site
September 1, 2010   September 1, 2011

EXAMINATION DATE
October 2, 2010 (All BPS Specialties)
October 3, 2011

* Established test sites are listed on page 6. A group of ten (10) or more applicants may request that an examination be administered at an alternate site. Requests for alternate sites in Alaska, Hawaii, and foreign countries will be reviewed on a case by case basis, if the requirement of 10 candidates cannot be met. Complete details on requesting an alternate examination site, including appropriate forms, are available online at www.bpsweb.org/resources. Requests for alternate sites, along with all application forms, must be submitted, no later than July 1.

**Candidate's who because of religious reasons cannot sit for an examination on Saturday, may request an alternate test date. See page 6 for details.

Do not mail a hard copy of an application transmitted by facsimile or submitted online..

It is the candidate's responsibility to submit an application that is completely and accurately filled out by the postmark deadline of August 1. Incomplete applications will not be processed. All applications are processed within 20 working days of receipt. Applications submitted after the August 1 deadline may be returned unprocessed.

Name and/or Address Changes
All applicants are responsible for immediately notifying BPS of any address change or legal name change.
Notification for admission to the examination, mailing of test results, maintenance of certified status and renewal of certification depend on the Board having current information. An applicant or certificant who legally changes his/her name should immediately notify BPS by mail and enclose a copy of a government issued document reflecting the legal name change. The documentation (such as a marriage certificate) must be issued by a federal, state, or local government.

Test Dates
The dates of upcoming BPS Specialty Certification Examinations are **Saturday, October 2, 2010** and **Saturday, October 3, 2011.** All BPS specialty certification examinations are administered once a year, on the same date, at the same sites. While BPS examinations are normally administered on Saturdays,

BPS policy does provide for an alternate test date (normally the following Sunday) for religious reasons (see below).

Alternate Test Date

BPS will provide an alternate date for administration of certification examinations in order to accommodate candidates whose religious affiliations prevent them from participating in an examination on a Saturday. The alternate date is usually the Sunday immediately following the administration of the examination (Sunday, October 3, 2010 and October 4, 2011). The fee to secure and staff a test site on an alternate date is $750, payable by the requestor. This fee is in addition to the certification application fee which is $250 if the group cannot provide an approved test center.

Requests for an alternate date administration must be submitted, in writing, to BPS, along with the completed application and appropriate fees. This request is due on or before July 1. The request must be accompanied by an original letter, on letterhead, from a leader of the applicant's religious community indicating specific reasons for the request. All candidates requesting an alternate test date will be advised of their eligibility to sit for the examination, as well as their test date and site by August 1.

Test Sites

BPS will establish test sites in 35 cities for the administration of its specialty certification examinations in 2010. Notification of the exact location of testing room is provided with the candidate's Admission Permit and posted on the BPS web site. Applicants must indicate their preferred test site in the space provided on the application form.

The Board reserves the right to cancel a site if there is an insufficient number of applicants for the site. BPS also reserves the right to close a test site to those who wish to change test sites after the application deadline (August 1), if the number of original applicants fills a site to capacity.

US Test Sites
Atlanta, GA
Baltimore, MD
Boston, MA
Chapel Hill, NC
Charleston, SC
Chicago, IL
Cincinnati, OH
Dallas, TX
Denver, CO
Detroit, MI
Houston, TX
Indianapolis, IN
Jacksonville, FL
Kansas City, MO
Los Angeles, CA
Memphis, TN
Miami, FL
Minneapolis, MN
Omaha, NE
Philadelphia, PA
Phoenix, AZ
Pittsburgh, PA
Portland, OR
Rochester, NY
St. Louis, MO
Salt Lake City, UT
San Francisco, CA
San Antonio, TX
Seattle, WA
Tampa, FL

Foreign Test Sites
Al Ain, United Arab Emirates
Jeddah, Saudi Arabia
Madrid, Spain
Riyadh, Saudi Arabia
Seoul, Korea

The Board does not provide hotel or travel recommendations. Candidates are encouraged to use their own travel agent or one of the search engines on the world wide web to locate hotel accommodations near a test site, maps, and driving instructions for a particular test site.

DANTES Program

Overseas military pharmacists may sit for BPS certification using the DANTES program through the Military Education Centers. For additional information, contact BPS directly or visit *www.dantes.doded.mil*

Alternate Test Sites

Any group of ten or more interested individuals may request an alternate test site. The applicant group may represent any combination of BPS-recognized specialties (Nuclear Pharmacy, Nutrition Support Pharmacy, Oncology Pharmacy, Pharmacotherapy, and Psychiatric Pharmacy). The applicant group may contain candidates for both certification and recertification examinations.

Within the contiguous 48 states: Applicant groups must have at least 10 individuals committed to sitting for a BPS exam. No additional fee will be charged for establishing an alternate test site in the contiguous 48 states. Alternate exam sites must be at least 200 miles from any of the BPS-designated test sites listed above, or be preapproved by BPS.

Alaska, Hawaii, Puerto Rico and foreign countries: Groups with fewer than 10 applicants in Alaska, Hawaii, Puerto Rico and foreign countries that request an alternate site will be required to pay a fee of $750. If the group cannot identify a test center that meets BPS specifications, BPS' testing consultant will provide a site for an additional fee of $250. Payments must accompany the request for establishing an alternate site.

All requestors: Request forms and complete details on requesting an alternate test site are available from BPS and can also be accessed on the BPS web site (www.bpsweb.org). Requests for alternate sites must be submitted, in writing, to BPS by **July 1,** and must be accompanied by ALL applications and fees from those requesting the alternate site. All applicants requesting an alternate site will be advised of their eligibility to sit for the examination, as well as the designation of the alternate site, by August 1. BPS will not be responsible for notifying other candidates or the profession-at-large of these designated alternate sites.

Examination dates for BPS specialty certification examinations are set by the Board and remain the same regardless of site.

Transferring Test Sites

Candidates wishing to transfer test sites must do so IN WRITING and the request must be received by BPS by **September 1** for the October test date. Requests should be sent to: BPS, 2215 Constitution Avenue, Washington, DC 20037; Fax: 202-429-6304; E-mail: *bps@aphanet.org*.

Exception to Eligibility Requirements

Candidates for certification, who are within six (6) months of fulfilling the eligibility requirement for time in practice or completion of a residency, will be permitted to sit for the certification examination. If a passing score is achieved, certification will be granted following receipt of documentation that the individual has fulfilled this eligibility requirement.

Processing Applications

All applicants will be notified by postal mail or email of their eligibility to sit for the examination within 20 working days of BPS' receipt of their application and fee. If for any reason an application is rejected, the entire fee is refunded and the original application and all documentation are returned to the applicant along with an explanation of why the application was not accepted. Incomplete applications may be returned to candidates by mail without being processed. Applicants who submit applications electronically will be notified if their application is incomplete or rejected.

For identification purposes, a unique Candidate Number is assigned to each eligible applicant by BPS when an application is processed. Candidates should keep a record of this number and use it in all correspondence with BPS.

An Admission Permit will be electronically mailed to each candidate at least two weeks prior to the examination date. This permit notes the candidate's name and address as they appear in the official BPS files, Candidate Number, testing site and room name, and starting time for the examination. This admission permit, along with valid picture identification with a signature, MUST be presented at the examination site to gain admission to the testing room. If an applicant has not received this permit at least 5 days before the examination, BPS should be notified immediately by phone (202-429-7591) or *email:bps@aphanet.org*

Withdrawals

Candidates may withdraw from the certification process up to the withdrawal deadline of **September 1.** Candidates must inform the Board of their withdrawal in writing. This request may be sent by fax, regular mail, or e-mail. The request must be received by the Board on or before the deadline of **September 1.**

Requests for medical and personal emergency withdrawals after the September 1 deadline are reviewed by the BPS Executive Director and decisions are made on a case-by-case basis. The request, with supporting documentation (e.g., physician's letter, police report), must be in writing and must be received at the BPS office no later than **SEVEN** days after the examination date.

Candidates who withdraw from the certification process will be refunded the fee paid, less an administrative charge of $100. Refunds will be processed within three to five weeks after the examination date.

Retaking the Examination

If a candidate fails to achieve a passing score on the examination, retaking the examination is permitted. BPS will contact applicants who have failed an examination in the previous year with an application authorization. The fee for retaking the examination is $300. If the candidate does not retake the examination within a two-year period, submission of the complete application will be required, along with payment of the full fee in effect at that time. **An individual who fails one specialty examination may NOT apply for another specialty examination as a retake candidate.**

Retake candidates who then withdraw from taking the examination are processed as described in the section "Withdrawals" above. If the candidate does not retake the examination within a two-year period, a new application must be submitted with required documentation of a current license and payment of the full fee in effect at that time.

Americans with Disabilities Act

The Board of Pharmaceutical Specialties complies with the relevant provisions of the American with Disabilities Act (ADA). If you have a disability and require accommodations under this Act during the certification examination, please complete and submit the "Accommodation Request Form," along with the application form. All application forms and requests for accommodations must be submitted no later than **August 1.**

It is the individual's responsibility to complete all applicable parts of this form if an accommodation is being requested. Supporting documentation must be supplied regardless of the method of submitting the application (electronic, fax, mail). Professionals submitting documentation in support of a candidate's request for accommodation may be contacted by BPS for clarification of any information provided concerning the requested accommodations. Failure to notify the Board of needed accommodations by August 1 may result in the accommodations not being available at the time of the examination.

FEES AND PAYMENT METHODS

Fee Payments

Payments are made in US dollars by **credit card** (VISA, MasterCard, American Express), **check, cashier's check, or money order** made payable to Board of Pharmacy Specialties. Purchase orders can *NOT* be accepted.

Application Fee

The application fee payment must accompany each completed application. The fee for first-time applicants for specialty certification is six hundred ($600 dollars). Candidates who failed an examination within the past two years will be permitted to retake the examination during this period at the cost of $300.

Declined Credit Cards and Returned Checks

When a credit card transaction is declined, or a check is returned for non-sufficient funds payment must be sent by a certified check or money order for the amount due.

Forfeiture of Fees

Candidates who fail to arrive at the Testing Centers on the date and time they are scheduled for examination and who have failed to get an approved withdrawal will forfeit their examination fees and must re-register by contacting BPS. Examination fees may NOT be transferred to another date.

Candidates arriving more than 15 minutes late for an examination will not be admitted, and will forfeit their examination fee.

All fees are subject to change at the sole discretion of the Board.

INFORMATION FOR FOREIGN TRAINED/ FOREIGN LICENSED CANDIDATES

BPS certification is oriented primarily toward pharmacists licensed and practicing in the USA. Foreign applicants are encouraged to apply online, and all required documentation should be submitted as attachments with the application. Applicants who received their pharmacy education and training outside the USA but who are licensed to practice in the USA need only provide a copy of their current, active state pharmacy registration certificate/license, along with their application form.

Applicants who received their pharmacy education outside the USA and who are not licensed to practice pharmacy in the USA must provide the Board with the following:

- copy of certificate, diploma or other official document indicating that the individual has completed an educational program preparing him/her for basic pharmacy practice; and
- documentation of current active legal authorization to practice pharmacy in their country of origin or residence.

Note eligibility restrictions for the nuclear pharmacy specialty on page 12.

If these documents are not in English, notarized English translations must be provided by the candidate, at the candidate's expense.

Throughout BPS specialty certification examinations, all measurements from laboratory test results are expressed in traditional units. For those candidates whose pharmacy practice site is outside the United States, a conversion chart from traditional units to standard international units will be provided.

The Board is aware that examination questions dealing with procedures or regulatory issues in the USA are not necessarily pertinent to candidates who practice in foreign countries. However, all candidates are given the same examination and are held to the same standard of achievement, regardless of the country in which they practice and the regulations under which they practice.

Please note BPS certification does not confer the privilege to practice pharmacy in the USA or in any other country.

PREPARING FOR THE EXAMINATION

The Board publishes the content outline specific to each examination and strongly encourages candidates to become thoroughly familiar with this document. Content outlines are occasionally modified to reflect changes in practice. Candidates should ensure that they are using the current outline for their specialty. Current content outlines are posted on the BPS web site or are available upon request from BPS.

Suggested preparation for the examination might include:

- residency or other formal training
- the study of journal articles, textbooks or other publications related to the content outline;
- continuing education programs and courses in specialized pharmacy practice;
- study groups and examination preparation courses;
- reviewing sample test questions printed in this Guide or on the BPS website.

Potential applicants may contact the organizations noted below which offer review/preparatory courses and materials for the specialty or specialties listed to determine program content, relevance to the BPS examinations and availability. BPS and its Specialty Councils neither sponsor nor endorse training or educational opportunities in specialized practice areas, or review/preparatory courses for any of the BPS examinations.

Contact the organization for more information. This is not intended to be a comprehensive list of sources.

For Oncology Pharmacy and Pharmacotherapy:
American College of Clinical Pharmacy
(913) 492-3311 • FAX (913) 492-0088
www.accp.com

For Nuclear Pharmacy:
University of New Mexico College of Pharmacy
Office of Continuing Pharmacy Education
(505) 272-3125 • FAX (505) 272-6749
hsc.unm.edu/pharmacy/radiopharmacyCE

For Nutrition Support Pharmacy:
American Society for Parenteral and Enteral Nutrition
(301) 587-6315 • FAX (301) 587-2365
www.clinnutr.org

For Oncology Pharmacy and Psychiatric Pharmacy:
American Society of Health-System Pharmacists
(301) 657-4383 • FAX (301) 652-8278
www.ashp.org

For Oncology Pharmacy
Hematology Oncology Pharmacy Association
(877) 467-2791
www.hoparx.org

For Psychiatric Pharmacy:
College of Psychiatric and Neurologic Pharmacists
(402) 476-1677
www.cpnp.org

ON THE DAY OF YOUR EXAMINATION

Inclement Weather and Cancellations

The safety of all candidates is of the utmost concern to BPS. Reasons for canceling an examination administration may include, but not be limited to, adverse weather conditions and natural disasters. BPS will consult with its testing agency and on-site Chief Examiners to determine the status of affected test sites. If the examination administration is canceled, BPS will work with its testing agency and the on-site Chief Examiner to place notices with local news services indicating the examination's cancellation. Notice will also be posted on the BPS web site (www.bpsweb.org). No alternate date will be scheduled.

Candidates are urged to contact the Board (202-429-7591 or bps@aphanet.org) or visit the BPS web site (www.bpsweb.org) on the day prior to the examination, if weather conditions are such that the cancellation of other civic activities and/or the closing of airports appear to be imminent.

If an examination administration is canceled for weather-related and/or safety concerns, candidates will be offered a refund of their full fee paid. BPS, however, is not responsible for any personal costs or expenses incurred by candidates in the event that an examination administration is canceled.

Examination Format and Content

There are 200 questions on each BPS specialty certification examination. The multiple-choice format is used exclusively. Four possible answers are provided for each question, with only ONE designated as the correct or best choice. It is to the candidate's advantage to answer every question on the examination, since the final score is based on the total number of questions answered correctly. There is no penalty for selecting an incorrect choice. Each question is carefully written, referenced, and validated to determine its accuracy and applicability.

A specialty certification examination does not attempt to test all of a candidate's knowledge in the specialized practice area. The examination samples the knowledge and skills required to perform the tasks in each of the major areas of responsibility of the specialty as defined through a role delineation study. Mastery of the knowledge and skills involved in this defined scope of specialized practice is necessary for board certification, regardless of the particular activities in which an applicant is currently involved.

BPS specialty certification examinations are constructed according to test specifications derived from task analyses. Technical support in conducting task analyses, establishing test specifications and constructing examinations is provided by an independent testing company that specializes in the assessment of the knowledge, skills and abilities of professionals.

A Content Outline, listing the domains, tasks, and knowledge statements specific to each specialty practice, is provided for the information of prospective candidates on the BPS website or upon request. The Content Outline also notes the percentage of items per domain. Examination content outlines are developed through a nationwide study of the work pharmacy specialists perform in a variety of practice settings.

Examinations are not structured domain by domain. Items testing each domain are distributed randomly throughout the total examination. While BPS examinations test the stated domains of each specialty, candidates are advised that the examinations will probably NOT address all of the knowledge statements listed under the domains in the content outline of the examination.

New regulations, drugs and therapies are incorporated annually into the examinations. All BPS specialty certification examinations reflect current, best practice at the time they are constructed – approximately six months prior to test administration. Official United States Adopted Name (USAN) generic names are used on all BPS examinations for all drug products, when possible.

Administration of the Examination

The examination day schedule is provided below. Candidates may complete and return the examination materials to proctors before the scheduled end of either test session.

Activity	Time
Admit Candidates to Room	8:00 am
Test Instructions	8:30 am
First Session (100 items)	9:00 am
Lunch Break	11:30 am
Admit Candidates to Room	12:45 pm
Test Instructions	1:15 pm
Second Session (100 items)	1:30 pm
End of Examination	4:00 pm

On the day of the examination, all candidates MUST present their Admission Permits AND valid photo identifications with signature (e.g., driver's license, hospital identification, passport) in order to be admitted to the testing room. Candidates who arrive after the examination has begun and candidates without valid photo identification and an admission permit may not be admitted to the examination. If that occurs, their fees will be forfeited.

Candidates will not be permitted to enter the exam room unless proper identification as described above is presented.

Candidates must provide their own sharpened #2 (or 2B) pencils, good eraser and hand-held, silent, non-printing, battery or solar powered calculator for use during the examination. Candidates will **NOT** be permitted to have reference books, study notes, or certain personal items in the examination room, including:

Cell phones
Cameras
PDAs (personal digital assistants)
Pagers
Radio or headset devices
Recorders
Purses
Briefcases

Food or drink
Hats (other then ceremonial or religious headwear)
Jackets
Personal papers
All non-test materials listed above must be stored in areas designated for that purpose.

Test instructions will be provided to candidates on the use of the answer sheet. Only answers properly marked on the answer sheet will be scored. Answers written in the test book will not be scored. The test booklet and the answer sheet are the property of BPS. **BOTH must be returned to the proctors at the end of EACH session of the examination.**

Security

BPS and its testing agency maintain examination administration and security standards that are designed to assure that all candidates are provided the same opportunity to demonstrate their abilities. The testing sites are monitored by proctors for security purposes. Candidates will be allowed to leave the room during the test administration to use the rest room facilities. Only one person will be excused from the room at a time and a proctor will accompany the individual to and from the rest room. Candidates are encouraged to place their answer sheet inside the examination booklet whenever they leave their seats.

Before beginning the examination, candidates will be asked to read and sign the *Statement of Confidentiality*. This statement restricts candidates from sharing any information about the examination with other individuals, including discussions with fellow test takers following the examination, and the sharing of information with colleagues who might be planning to take the examination in the near future.

Chief Examiners are authorized by BPS and its testing consultant to maintain a secure and proper test administration environment. This may include the relocation of candidates prior to or during the examination and/or the dismissal of candidates from the examination. Candidates will be inspected for devices such as hand-held scanners, cameras, tape recorders, or other electronic equipment. Areas around the testing room (e.g. hallways, restrooms, telephone stalls) are monitored throughout the examination for security purposes.

Candidates may not communicate with other candidates during the examination. Anyone who provides or receives assistance during the test administration will be dismissed from the testing room. Candidates may not photograph, record, or memorize any examination material. Other causes for dismissal include, but are not limited to: using notes, references, or any test aids; using unauthorized calculators; causing a disruption to the test environment; and removing any examination material from the testing site. Candidates who are dismissed from the testing room forfeit all fees.

Candidates' calculators and wristwatches will be checked prior to admission to the testing room for word processing capabilities. If either is found to be a word processor, it will be confiscated by a proctor and returned at the end of the test day.

Personnel from the Board of Pharmacy Specialties, its Specialty Councils, the BPS testing agency, and/or their delegates will proctor the examination. No one is permitted in the testing room during the examination except for the candidates and persons authorized by BPS and/or by the testing agency.

Statement of Confidentiality for BPS Examinations:

1. This examination and the test questions contained herein are the exclusive
2. property of BPS.
3. This examination and the test questions contained herein are protected by
4. copyright law. No part of this exam may be copied or reproduced in part or whole by any means whatsoever, including memorization.
5. The theft or attempted theft of an examination booklet is punishable as a felony.
6. My participation in any irregularity occurring during this examination, such as
7. giving or obtaining unauthorized information or aid, as evidenced by observation or subsequent analysis, may result in termination of my participation, invalidation of the results of my examination or other appropriate action.
8. Further discussion or disclosure of the contents of the examination orally, in writing or by any other means is prohibited

My signature indicates that I have read, understood and agree to be bound by the statement of confidentiality. Failure to comply can result in termination of my participation, invalidation of the results of my examination or other appropriate action.

Use of Calculators

In order to provide a realistic environment for performing calculations in the solution of practice problems, hand-held, silent, non-printing, battery or solar powered calculators may be used. Hand-held calculators that contain addition, subtraction, multiplication, division, and log functions are appropriate for the examination. Candidates may NOT use calculators or any other devices that have either word processing or word storage capabilities (complete A-Z keypad). All calculators will be examined by a proctor before a candidate is admitted to the examination area. Candidates are responsible for providing their own calculators.

FOLLOWING THE EXAMINATION

Score Reporting

Specialty certification examinations are prepared by BPS Specialty Councils to assess practice-based knowledge and skills. Candidates' scores are determined by the total number of items answered correctly. Criterion-referenced standard-setting procedures are used to establish the passing score for all BPS examinations. A detailed description of this process is posted at the BPS web site (*www.bpsweb.org*).

Answer sheets are scored electronically. Candidates who do not achieve a passing score on the examination may request a hand scoring of their answer sheets. Requests for hand scoring of the answer sheets must be submitted to BPS, in writing, within 90 days of the candidate's receipt of his/her score report. A check or money order for fifty dollars ($50) must accompany the request for hand scoring.

Confidential Score Reports

Confidential score reports are sent directly to each candidate by mail. Each score report contains the following information: passing score, candidate's score, maximum score, average score, standard deviation and range of scores. Total scores are reported, as well as scores by domains.

The standard turn-around time required to score, analyze, report scores and grant certification is approximately sixty days. A certificate suitable for framing and a BPS lapel pin are sent to newly certified specialists approximately sixty days after notification of certification.

Application to take the certification examination constitutes written authorization for the testing agency to release that candidate's score to BPS and to the examinee ONLY. Group performance data will be utilized by the testing agency, the Specialty Council, or others designated by BPS, for purposes of research and development and for reporting to the profession. Access to a candidate's score report is limited to those staff at BPS and the Board's testing agency who are involved in the processing and mailing of these reports. BPS will not release personal exam information (other than name/address of certified individuals under established policy) without written authorization.

In order to protect the security and integrity of the specialty certification examinations, neither BPS nor its testing agency release examination questions, answer sheets, or the answer key to any individual or organization. While all efforts are made by BPS, its Specialty Councils, and its testing agency to produce completely accurate examinations, occasional errors do occur. If a candidate believes there is an error in an examination question, the on-site proctor should be advised at once and/or the candidate should contact BPS immediately after the examination.

If You Pass the Examination

Once scores have been validated, BPS sends official notices to candidates who have achieved passing scores on the examinations. BPS will NOT report individual scores by telephone, fax, or email. Candidates who do not receive score reports within 75 days after the test date should contact BPS in writing and a duplicate report will be issued at no cost.

If You Do Not Pass the Examination

If you do not achieve a passing score on the examination, you may re-apply to take the examination. The fee for retaking the examination is $300. If the candidate does not retake the examination within a two-year period, submission of the complete application will be required, along with payment of the full fee in effect at that time. **An individual who fails one specialty examination may NOT apply for another specialty examination as a retake candidate.**

REVOCATION OF CERTIFICATION

The certification of an individual may be revoked by BPS for any of the following reasons:

- Failure to complete or fulfill the requirements for certification or recertification;
- Failure to maintain professional licensure;
- Determination that certification or recertification was improperly granted;
- Misrepresentation or misstatement of facts submitted upon application for certification or recertification;
- Violation of Conflict of Interest and/or confidentiality/ non-disclosure attestations to BPS

Appeal Process

A reconsideration and appeal process is available to individuals seeking a redress of an action by BPS. All requests must be made in writing. The process and procedures for appeal are available at *www.bpsweb.org*, or upon request from the BPS office.

RECERTIFICATION

To maintain "Active" BPS status, recertification is required every 7 years. Recertification requirements are listed in the BPS Specialties section (pages 11 to 14). Certificants are expected to keep their certification current. If requirements are not completed at the end of the seven year cycle, certification lapses. Once certification has lapsed, an individual will need to meet all current requirements to take and pass the certification exam.

ANNUAL REGISTRATION

All BPS-certified pharmacists are required to register annually with the Board and pay an annual fee, currently $100. An invoice notice for the annual fee is sent to each certificant generally in the spring. Pharmacists holding more than one BPS certification are assessed only one annual fee.

Failure to pay the annual fee results in removal of the individual's name from BPS' official list of certified pharmacists for that year. This list of BPS-certified specialists "in good standing" is published on the Board's web site and elsewhere. Upon applying for recertification, all outstanding annual fees and a 5% penalty must be paid.

BPS SPECIALTIES

NUCLEAR PHARMACY

Nuclear Pharmacy seeks to improve and promote the public health through the safe and effective use of radioactive drugs for diagnosis and therapy. A nuclear pharmacist, as a member of the nuclear medicine team, specializes in the procurement, compounding, quality control testing, dispensing, distribution, and monitoring of radiopharmaceuticals. In addition, the nuclear pharmacist provides consultation regarding health and safety issues, as well as the use of non-radioactive drugs and patient care. Those who are granted certification in this specialty may use the designation Board Certified Nuclear Pharmacist and the initials BCNP, as long as certification is valid.

Eligibility Requirements:

The minimum requirements for certification in nuclear pharmacy are:

- Graduation from a pharmacy program accredited by the Accreditation Council for Pharmacy Education (ACPE) or program outside the U.S. that qualifies the individual to practice in the jurisdiction. Foreign trained pharmacists must pass the Foreign Pharmacy Graduate Examination Committee (FPGEC) examination.
- Current, active license to practice pharmacy in the U.S. or another jurisdiction
- 4,000 hours of training/experience in nuclear pharmacy practice
- Achieving a passing score on the Nuclear Pharmacy Specialty Certification Examination

The required 4,000 hours of experience may be earned in a variety of settings.

Academic-up to 2,000 hours:

- Undergraduate courses in nuclear pharmacy: up to 100 hours experience for every quarter credit hour or 150 hours experience for every semester credit hour, to a maximum of 1,500 hours
- Postgraduate courses in nuclear pharmacy: up to 100 hours experience for every quarter credit hour or 150 hours experience for every semester credit hour, to a maximum of 1,500 hours
- MS or PhD degree in nuclear pharmacy: 2,000 hours
- Successful completion of the Nuclear Pharmacy Certificate Program offered by Purdue University (217 hours) or The Ohio State University (214 hours), or the Nuclear Education Online (NEO) Program offered by the Universities of New Mexico and Arkansas (250 hours). Credit for other courses will be assessed on a case-by-case basis.

Training/Practice-up to 4,000 hours:

- Residency* in nuclear pharmacy: hour-for-hour credit to a maximum of 2,000 hours
- Internship to satisfy requirements of state boards of pharmacy: hour-for-hour credit in a licensed nuclear pharmacy or facility authorized to handle radioactive materials, to a maximum of 2,000 hours
- Nuclear pharmacy practice: hour-for-hour credit in a licensed nuclear pharmacy or health care facility approved by state or federal agencies to handle radioactive materials, to a maximum of 4,000 hours.

Effective January 1, 2013, only residencies accredited by the American Society of Health-System Pharmacists or other BPS recognized bodies are creditable for this purpose.

Examination Content (Refer to the Nuclear Pharmacy Content Outline for details.)

Domain 1: Drug Order Provision (66% of the examination)

- Subdomain A: Procurement (8% of the examination)
- Subdomain B: Compounding (26% of the examination)
- Subdomain C: Quality Assurance (9% of the examination)
- Subdomain D: Dispensing (23% of the examination)

Domain 2: Health and Safety (24% of the examination)
Domain 3: Drug Information Provision (10% of the examination)

Recertification

Recertification for Board Certified Nuclear Pharmacists (BCNP) is a three-step process:

- Self-evaluation: Review of the nuclear pharmacy practice activities/functions that have changed since initial certification or last recertification
- Peer review: Documentation of nuclear pharmacy practice activities over the seven year certification period, which are then reviewed by the Specialty Council on Nuclear Pharmacy
- Formal Assessment: This assessment of a practitioner's knowledge and skills will be accomplished through one of two methods: 1) achieving a passing score on the 100-item, multiple-choice objective recertification examination based on the content outline of the certification examination; OR 2) earning 70 hours of continuing education credit provided by a professional development program approved by BPS.

A current, active license to practice pharmacy is required for recertification.

As part of the recertification process, every BCNP is asked to complete an annual practice report form provided by BPS. The information is compiled by BPS at the beginning of the recertification process and sent to the BCNP for verification and updating. At the time of recertification, the BCNP is also required to certify that (s)he is not currently under suspension by either the U.S. Nuclear Regulatory Commission or a state Radiation Control Organization.

NUTRITION SUPPORT PHARMACY

Nutrition support pharmacy addresses the care of patients who receive specialized nutrition support, including parenteral and enteral nutrition. The nutrition support pharmacist has responsibility for promoting maintenance and/or restoration of optimal nutritional status, designing and modifying treatment according to the needs of the patient. The nutrition support pharmacist has responsibility for direct patient care and often functions as a member of a multidisciplinary nutrition support team. Those who are granted certification in this specialty may use the designation Board Certified Nutrition Support Pharmacist and the initials BCNSP, as long as certification is valid.

Eligibility Requirements

The minimum requirements for this specialty certification are:

- Graduation from a pharmacy program accredited by the Accreditation Council for Pharmacy Education (ACPE) or program outside the U.S. that qualifies the individual to practice in the jurisdiction.
- Current, active license to practice pharmacy in the U.S. or another jurisdiction.

Completion of three (3) years practice experience with at least 50% of time spent in nutrition support pharmacy activities (as defined by the BPS Nutrition Support Content Outline)
OR Completion of a specialty (PGY2) residency* in nutrition support pharmacy.
Achieving a passing score on the Nutrition Support Pharmacy Specialty Certification Examination.

Effective January 1, 2013, only residencies accredited by the American Society of Health-System Pharmacists or other recognized bodies are creditable for this purpose.

Examination Content (refer to the Nutrition Support Pharmacy Content Outline for details)

Domain 1: Clinical Practice/Provision of Individualized Nutrition Support to Patients (68% of the examination)

    Subdomain A: Assessment (21% of the examination)
    Subdomain B: Develop and Implement a Therapeutic Plan of Care (21% of the examination)
    Subdomain C: Monitoring and Clinical Management (26% of the examination)

Domain 2: Management of Nutrition Support Operations (20% of the examination)

    Subdomain A: Patient Care Management (12% of the examination)
    Subdomain B: Compounding Operations (8% of the examination)

Domain 3: Advancement of Nutrition Support Practice (12% of the examination)

Recertification

Recertification for Board Certified Nutrition Support Pharmacists (BCNSP) is based on the following activities:

Earning a minimum of 3.0 continuing education units (CEU) in nutrition support with no less than 1.0 CEU earned every two years. These CEU must be from providers approved by the Accreditation Council for Pharmacy Education (ACPE). NOTE: 1.0 CEU equals 10 hours of approved continuing education.
Achieving a passing score on the 100-item, multiple-choice recertification examination, which is based on the content outline of the certification examination

A current, active license to practice pharmacy is required for recertification.

ONCOLOGY PHARMACY

Oncology pharmacy specialists recommend, design, implement, monitor and modify pharmacotherapeutic plans to optimize outcomes in patients with malignant diseases. Those who are granted certification in this specialty may use the designation Board Certified Oncology Pharmacist and the initials BCOP, as long as certification is valid.

Eligibility Requirements

The minimum requirements for this specialty certification are:

Graduation from a pharmacy program accredited by the Accreditation Council for Pharmacy Education (ACPE) or a program outside the U.S. that qualifies the individual to practice in the jurisdiction.

- Current, active license to practice pharmacy in the U.S. or another jurisdiction.
- Completion of four (4) years of practice experience with at least 50% of time spent in oncology pharmacy activities (as defined by the BPS oncology pharmacy content outline)
OR
- Completion of a specialty (PGY2) residency* in oncology pharmacy plus one (1) additional year of practice with at least 50% of time spent in oncology pharmacy activities (as defined by the BPS oncology pharmacy content outline)
- Achieving a passing score on the Oncology Pharmacy Specialty Certification Examination

* Effective January 1, 2013, only residencies accredited by the American Society of Health-System Pharmacists or other BPS recognized bodies are creditable for this purpose.

Examination Content (Refer to the Oncology Pharmacy Content Outline for details)

Domain 1: Clinical Skills and Therapeutic Management. (60% of the examination)
Domain 2: Generation, Interpretation, and Dissemination of Information. (20% of the examination)
Domain 3: Guidelines, Policies, and Standards. (15% of the examination)
Domain 4: Public Health and Advocacy. (5% of the examination)

Recertification

Recertification for Board Certified Oncology Pharmacists (BCOP) requires assessment of a practitioner's knowledge and skills through one of two methods:

- Achieving a passing score on the 100-item, multiple-choice objective recertification examination, based on the content outline of the certification examination;
OR
- Earning 100 hours of continuing education credit provided by a professional development program approved by BPS.

A current, active license to practice pharmacy is required for recertification.

PHARMACOTHERAPY

Pharmacotherapy is that area of pharmacy practice that is responsible for ensuring the safe, appropriate, and economical use of drugs in patient care. The pharmacotherapy specialist has responsibility for direct patient care, often functions as a member of a multidisciplinary team and is frequently the primary source of drug information for other healthcare professionals. Those who are granted certification in this specialty may use the designation Board Certified Pharmacotherapy Specialist and the initials BCPS, as long as certification is valid.

Eligibility Requirements

The minimum requirements for this specialty certification are:

- Graduation from a pharmacy program accredited by the Accreditation Council for Pharmacy Education (ACPE) or a program outside the U.S. that qualifies the individual to practice in the jurisdiction.

- Current, active license to practice pharmacy in the U.S. or another jurisdiction.
- Completion of three (3) years of practice experience with at least 50% of time spent in pharmacotherapy activities (as defined by the BPS Pharmacotherapy Content Outline) OR completion of a PGY1 residency*
- Achieving a passing score on the Pharmacotherapy Specialty Certification Examination

*Effective January 1, 2013, only residencies accredited by the American Society of Health-System Pharmacists or other BPS recognized bodies are creditable for this purpose

Examination Content (Refer to the Pharmacotherapy Content Outline for details.)

Domain 1: Patient-specific Pharmacotherapy
(55% of the examination)

Domain 2: Retrieval, generation, interpretation and dissemination of knowledge in pharmacotherapy
(30% of the examination)

Domain 3: Health System-related Pharmacotherapy
(15% of the examination)

Note: This is subject to change in early 2010 as the result of job task analysis update. Obtain the most current content outline at www.bpsweb.org

Recertification

Recertification for Board Certified Pharmacotherapy Specialists (BCPS) is an assessment of a practitioner's knowledge and skills through one of two methods:

- Achieving a passing score on the 100-item, multiple-choice objective recertification examination, based on the content outline of the certification examination;
  OR
- Earning 120 hours of continuing education credit provided by a professional development program approved by BPS.

A current, active license to practice pharmacy is required for recertification.

PSYCHIATRIC PHARMACY

Psychiatric pharmacy addresses the pharmaceutical care of patients with psychiatric-related illnesses. As a member of a multidisciplinary treatment team, the psychiatric pharmacy specialist is often responsible for optimizing drug treatment and patient care by conducting such activities as monitoring patient response, patient assessment, recognizing drug-induced problems, and recommending appropriate treatment plans. Those who are granted certification in this specialty may use the designation Board Certified Psychiatric Pharmacist and the initials BCPP, as long as certification is valid.

Eligibility Requirements

The minimum requirements for this specialty certification are:

- Graduation from a pharmacy program accredited by the Accreditation Council for Pharmacy Education (ACPE) or a program outside the U.S. that qualifies the individual to practice in the jurisdiction.
- Current, active license to practice pharmacy in the U.S. or another jurisdiction.
- Completion of four (4) years of practice with at least 50% of time spent in psychiatric pharmacy activities (as defined by the BPS Psychiatric Pharmacy Content Outline)
  OR
- Completion of a specialty (PGY2) residency* in psychiatric pharmacy plus one (1) additional year of practice with at least 50% of time spent in psychiatric pharmacy activities (as defined by the BPS Psychiatric Pharmacy Content Outline)
- Achieving a passing score on the Psychiatric Pharmacy Specialty Certification Examination

*Effective January 1, 2013, only residencies accredited by the American Society of Health-System Pharmacists or other BPS recognized bodies are creditable for this purpose

Examination Content (Refer to the Psychiatric Pharmacy Content Outline for details.)

Domain 1: Clinical Skills and Therapeutic Management
(65% of the examination)

Domain 2: Education and Dissemination of Information
(25% of the examination)

Domain 3: Clinical Administration
(10% of the examination)

Recertification

Recertification of Board Certified Psychiatric Pharmacists (BCPP) requires an assessment of a practitioner's knowledge and skills through one of two methods:

- Achieving a passing score on the 100-item multiple choice recertification examination, based on the content outline of the certification examination;
  OR
- Earning 100 hours of continuing education credit provided by a professional development program approved by BPS.

A current, active license to practice pharmacy is required for recertification.

SAMPLE EXAMINATION QUESTIONS

The following sample questions provide candidates with an opportunity to review the FORMAT of questions used on BPS specialty certification examinations. Four possible answers are provided for each question, with only ONE designated as the correct or best choice. This multiple-choice format is used exclusively on BPS examinations.

Practice tests for each specialty are also available on the BPS website at www.bpsweb.org. Consult them for additional specialty-specific examples of questions.

SAMPLE:
A 35-year-old, 70 kg patient was examined by his family physician for a complaint of right-sided abdominal pain for 6 weeks, and nausea. A CT scan of the abdomen revealed a solid bulky mass within the retroperitoneum. The patient underwent an exploratory laparotomy and the mass (8.0 x 7.0 cm) was removed. The patient was diagnosed with advanced testicular cancer and underwent a right orchiectomy. He has now been admitted for his first cycle of cisplatin, vinblastine,

and bleomycin (PVB). In addition to corticosteroids, which of the following is the best choice for an antiemetic to provide for prevention of acute emesis?

*1. Ondansetron
2. Metoclopramide
3. Prochlorperazine
4. Haloperidol

SAMPLE:

The GUSTO-1 trial evaluated four thrombolytic strategies for acute myocardial infarction. The investigators studied 41,021 patients with evolving myocardial infarction. A total of 1,081 hospitals in 15 countries participated in the trial, which was conducted from December 1990 to February 1993. The authors found a 14% reduction in the mortality for accelerated tissue plasminogen activator (t-PA) as compared with two streptokinase-only strategies (p=.001). The mortality rates for the four treatment groups are reported below:

Regimen #	Thrombolytic Strategy	30-day mortality rates
1	Streptokinase and i.v. heparin	7.4%
2	Accelerated t-PA and i.v. heparin	6.3%
3	Streptokinase and s.c. heparin	7.2%
4	t-PA and streptokinase and i.v. heparin	7.0%

Considering these results, for every 100 patients treated, how many more patients would benefit (i.e., demonstrate reduced 30-day mortality) after receiving accelerated t-PA (Regimen #2) rather than streptokinase and i.v. heparin (Regimen #1)?

(1) 0.1   *(2) 1   (3) 7   (4) 11

SAMPLE:

For a state of equilibrium to occur in a radionuclide generator:

*1. The parent/daughter half-life ratio must be greater than 1.
2. The daughter radionuclide must be a stable isotope.
3. Elution must occur daily.
4. The daughter radionuclide should exhibit branched decay.

SAMPLE:

An 80-year-old ambulatory female patient with hypertension receiving captopril 50mg twice daily requires a second antihypertensive agent for optimum blood pressure control. History includes diet-controlled diabetes mellitus, chronic obstructive pulmonary disease, mild left ventricular hypertrophy (LVH) and mild dementia. Serum creatinine = 2.5 mg/dL; BUN = 30 mg/dL. Which of the following antihypertensive agents should be added to the regimen?

1. Prazosin
2. Verapamil
*3. Metoprolol
4. Hydrochlorothiazide

SAMPLE:

A patient with Type 2 diabetes reports vomiting, somnolence, epigastric pain, anorexia, hyperventilation, diarrhea, and thirst. Medications include enalapril 20 mg daily; hydrochlorothiazide 25 mg daily; metformin 1000 mg twice daily; and digoxin 0.25 mg daily. Serum creatinine = 2 mg/dL, blood glucose = 365 mg/dL, pH = 7.2, anion gap = 20. Which adverse drug effect is the patient most likely experiencing?

1. Renal tubular acidosis secondary to enalapril
2. Lactic acidosis secondary to metformin
3. Respiratory acidosis secondary to compensation for metabolic alkalosis from hydrochlorothiazide
4. Metabolic acidosis secondary to hydrochlorothiazide/digoxin

SAMPLE:

A 67-year-old patient with Parkinson's disease presents with mildly erythematous scaly plaques distributed in a butterfly-like pattern across the face and extending into the nasolabial folds. Scaling and flaking are also present in the patient's beard, eyebrows, scalp and behind his ears. His medications include: phenytoin, 300 mg h.s., for seizures following a stroke that occurred last year; amantadine, 100 mg b.i.d., for mild bradykinesia and rigidity; and augmentin, 850 mg b.i.d. x 10 days, for a recent upper-respiratory infection. The patient has no fever and claims that the lesions, which itch "a little bit," have been present for several years but have become more noticeable over the past month. Which of the following best describes how this problem should be managed?

*1. Explain that the condition is seborrheic dermatitis, common in patients with Parkinson's disease and is not caused by drug therapy; treat with hydrocortisone cream 1% to affected areas b.i.d.
2. Call the patient's neurologist for evaluation and monitoring of the lesions for possible progression to Stevens-Johnson syndrome; discontinue phenytoin and substitute valproic acid.
3. Recommend that the patient stop using the augmentin, because of drug allergy, and call the patient's prescriber.
4. Explain that the condition is livedo reticularis, a harmless reaction to amantadine that requires no treatment.

SAMPLE:

A well-nourished 36 year-old male was transferred to the surgical ICU following an exploratory laparotomy for a gun shot wound to the abdomen. Transfer orders included continuous nasogastric suction, IV morphine for pain, cefoxitin, 2 g IVPB q8 hr, and D5-Normal Saline, 85 ml/hr. On admission to the SICU, his serum electrolytes were normal. The patient remained NPO due to continued intestinal ileus, the nasogastric suction volume averaged 2000 ml daily, and the patient's weight was unchanged.

Laboratory values on the 3rd post-op day were:

Sodium	137 mEq/L	(normal = 135-147 mEq/L)
Potassium	3.8 mEq/L	(normal = 3.5-5.0 mEq/L)
Chloride	89 mEq/L	(normal = 95-105 mEq/L)
CO3	37 mEq/L	(normal = 22-28 mEq/L)
Glucose	111 mg/dL	(normal = 70-110 mg/dL)
BUN	22 mg/dL	(normal = 8-18 mg/dL)
Creatinine	1.2 mg/dL	(normal = 0.6-1.2 mg/dL)

Which of the following therapeutic recommendations is appropriate at this time?

1. initiate TPN due to prolonged period of NPO status
*2. initiate parenteral pantoprazole to reduce gastric acidity
3. increase IV infusion rate to match nasogastric output volume
4. change IV infusion to D5-Lactated Ringers at same infusion rate

* Correct choice

VISION STATEMENT

The Board of Pharmacy Specialties will be the premier post-licensure certification agency serving the needs of the pharmacy profession and the public.

MISSION STATEMENT

The Mission of the Board of Pharmacy Specialties is to improve patient care through recognition and promotion of specialized training, knowledge, and skills in pharmacy and specialty board certification of pharmacists.

We will accomplish this mission by:

- *Providing leadership for the profession of pharmacy in the discussion, evolution, direction and recognition of specialty board certification of pharmacists;*
- *Establishing and promoting, in collaboration with stakeholders, the value of pharmacy specialization and board certification;*
- *Establishing the standards for identification and recognition of pharmacy specialties;*
- *Establishing standards of eligibility, knowledge, and skills as the basis for board certification;*
- *Developing and administering a valid process to evaluate the knowledge and skills of pharmacists.*

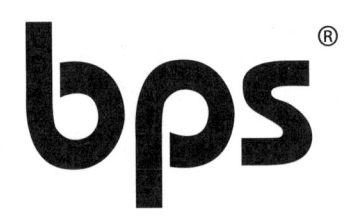

bps®

Board of Pharmacy Specialties
2215 Constitution Avenue, NW
Washington, DC 20037
202-429-7591 • FAX 202-429-6304
bps@aphanet.org
www.bpsweb.org

©Copyright 2010, Board of Pharmacy Specialities. All Rights Reserved.